TERMINOLOGY CHANGES NEW IN THIS EDITION — cont'd

Chapter 9 Bony Thorax

body	(gladiolus)
jugular notch	(manubrial notch)
xiphoid process	(ensiform cartilage)

Chapter 10 Thoracic Viscera

cardiac impression	(cardiac fossa)
costodiaphragmatic recess	(costophrenic, or phrenicostal sinus)
hilum	(hilus)
impression	(fossa)
jugular notch	(manubrial notch)
pulmonary pleura	(visceral)
superior thoracic aperture	(thoracic inlet)

Chapter 11 Long Bone Measurement

limb	(extremity)

Chapter 12 Contrast Arthrography

limb	(extremity)

Chapter 13 Foreign Body Localization and Trauma Radiography Guidelines

limb	(extremity)

Chapter 14 Mouth and Salivary Glands

MOUTH

frenulum tongue	(frenulum linguae)
soft palate	(velum)
sublingual fold	(plica sublingualis)

SALIVARY GLANDS

parotid duct	(Stensen's duct)
sublingual caruncle	[new]
sublingual ducts	(ducts of Rivinus, or Bartholin's duct)
submandibular duct	(submaxillary, or Wharton's duct)
submandibular gland	(submaxillary gland)

Chapter 15 Anterior Part of Neck

auditory tubes	(eustachian tubes)
choanae	[new]
cricothyroid ligament	(cricothyroid interval)
inferior constrictor muscle	(cricopharyngeus muscle)
laryngeal inlet	(laryngeal orifice)
laryngeal pharynx	(hypopharynx)
lymphoid	(lymphadenoid)
piriformis recess	(piriformis sinus)
rima vestibuli	(vestibular slit)
valleculae epiglottica	(epiglottic valleculae)
vestibula folds	(false vocal cords)

Chapter 16 Digestive System: Abdomen, Liver, Spleen, Biliary Tract

LIVER

hepatopancreatic ampulla	(ampulla of Vater)
hilum	(hilus)
porta	(porta hepatis)
sphincter choledochus	(sphincter of Oddi)
visceral surface of liver	(posterior surface of liver)

PANCREAS AND SPLEEN

accessory pancreatic duct	(duct of Santorine)
pancreatic duct	(duct of Wirsung)
pancreatic islets	(islets of Langerhans)

Chapter 17 Digestive System: Alimentary Tract

STOMACH

angular notch	(incisura angularis)
cardia	[new]
cardiac notch	(cardiac incisura)
esophagogastric junction	(esophageal orifice, or cardiac sphincter)
gastric folds	(rugae)
pyloric antrum	(pyloric vestibule)
pyloric canal	[new]
pyloric orifice	[new]

SMALL INTESTINE

first portion	(superior portion)
second portion	(descending portion)
third portion	(horizontal portion)
fourth portion	(ascending portion)
common hepatic duct	(hepatic duct)
duodenojejunal flexure	(angle of Treitz)

LARGE INTESTINE

left colic flexure	(splenic flexure)
right colic flexure	(hepatic flexure)

Chapter 18 Urinary System

glomerular capsule	(capsule of Bowman)
hilum	(hilus)
major calyces	(infundibula)
renal papilla	(apex)
spongy portion [of male urethra]	(cavernous portion)
straight tubule	(descending and ascending limbs of the loop of Henle)
suprarenal glands	(adrenal glands)

Chapter 19 Male Reproductive System

ductus deferens	(vas deferens)
spongy portion [of male urethra]	(cavernous portion)

Chapter 20 Female Reproductive System

cervix	(neck)
intestinal surface	(posterior surface [of uterus])
isthmus	(superior cervix)
isthmus	(internal os)
lateral angles	(cornua)
ovarian vesicular follicles	(ovisac)
perineal body	[new]
uterine ostium	(external os, or external orifice of cervix)
uterine tube	(fallopian tube) [oviduct deleted]
vesical surface	(anterior surface)

Chapter 21 Skull

FRONTAL BONE

frontal tuberosity	(frontal eminence)
nasal spine	(frontal spine)
superciliary ridges	(superciliary arches)
supraorbital notch	(supraorbital foramen)

ETHMOID BONE

ethmoidal air cells	(ethmoid cells)
lateral labyrinths	(lateral masses)
nasal conchae	(turbinates)

PARIETAL BONES

parietal tubercle	(parietal tuberosity or eminence)

SPHENOID BONE

chiasmatic groove	(optic groove, or sulcus)
hypophysis	(pituitary body)
optic canal	(optic foramen)
sphenoidal sinuses	(sphenoid sinuses)
sphenoidal air cells	(sphenoid air cells)

Continued on inside back cover.

MERRILL'S ATLAS OF

RADIOGRAPHIC POSITIONS and RADIOLOGIC PROCEDURES

VOLUME THREE

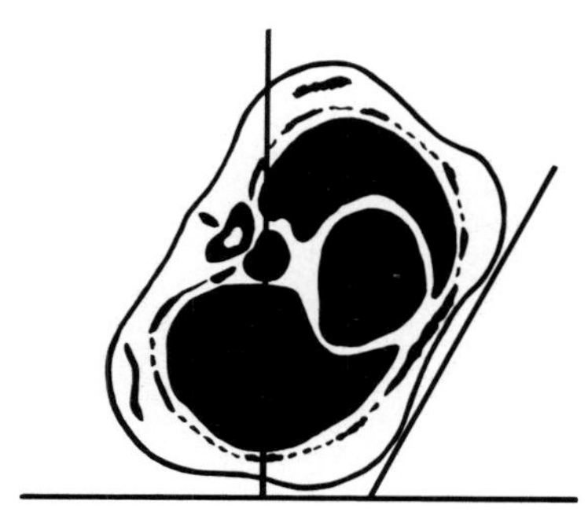

VOLUME THREE

MERRILL'S ATLAS OF

RADIOGRAPHIC POSITIONS and RADIOLOGIC PROCEDURES

PHILIP W. BALLINGER, M.S., R.T.(R)

Director and Assistant Professor, Radiologic Technology Division
School of Allied Medical Professions
The Ohio State University
Columbus, Ohio

Seventh Edition

with **2987** illustrations, including **9** in full color

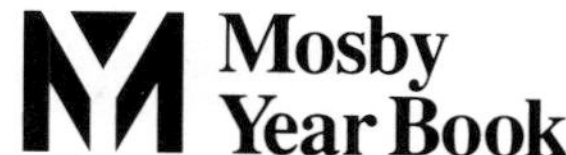

St. Louis Baltimore Boston Chicago London Philadelphia Sydney Toronto

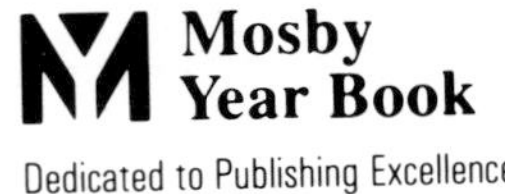

Dedicated to Publishing Excellence

Editor: David Culverwell
Developmental Editor: Elaine Steinborn
Assistant Editor: Ellen Baker Geisel
Production Editing Manager: Mark Spann
Production Editor: Mary Stueck
Design: Gail Morey Hudson
Illustrations prepared by Graphic Works, Inc.

SEVENTH EDITION

A Mosby imprint of
Mosby–Year Book, Inc.

Printed in the United States of America

Mosby–Year Book, Inc.
11830 Westline Industrial Drive, St. Louis, Missouri 63146

Library of Congress Cataloging in Publication Data

Ballinger, Philip W.
Merrill's atlas of radiographic positions and radiologic procedures—7th ed./Philip W. Ballinger.
p. cm.
Includes bibliographical references.
Includes index.
IBSN 0-8016-0195-9
IBSN 0-8016-0170-3 (set)
1. Radiography, Medical—Positioning—Atlases. I. Title.
II. Title: Atlas of radiographic positions and radiologic procedures
[DNLM: 1. Technology, Radiologic—atlases. WN 17 B192m]
RC78.4.B35 1990
616.07'572—dc20

C/MV/MV 9 8 7 6 5 4 3

CONTRIBUTORS

THOMAS J. BECK, Sc.D.
Assistant Professor
Department of Radiology
The Johns Hopkins Hospital
Baltimore, Maryland

JANINE BLOME, R.N.
Manager of Product Surveillance and Epidemiology
Department of Medical Affairs
Berlex Laboratories, Inc.
Wayne, New Jersey

JEFFREY A. BOOKS, R.T.(R)
Chief Technologist
Department of Radiology
Cabarrus Memorial Hospital
Concord, North Carolina

MICHAEL G. BRUCKNER, B.S., R.T.(R)
Division of Cardiovascular and Interventional Radiology
Department of Radiology
The Ohio State University Hospitals
Columbus, Ohio

TERRI BRUCKNER, M.A., R.T.
Columbus, Ohio

JOHN P. DORST, M.D.
Director Emeritus
Division of Pediatric Radiology
The Johns Hopkins Hospital
Baltimore, Maryland

PAUL J. EARLY, B.S., DABSNM
Director, Medical Physics Services
NMA Medical Physics Consultation
Mallinckrodt Medical, Inc.
Cleveland, Ohio

JAMES H. ELLIS, M.D.
Associate Professor
Director, Abdominal Division
Department of Radiology
University of Michigan Medical Center
Ann Arbor VA Medical Center
Ann Arbor, Michigan

WILLIAM F. FINNEY, III, M.A., R.T.(R)
Assistant Professor
Radiologic Technology Division
School of Allied Medical Professions
The Ohio State University
Columbus, Ohio

JOSEPH FODOR, III, M.S., R.T.(R), F.A.S.R.T.
Assistant Director
Barrett Center for Cancer Prevention, Treatment, and Research
University Hospital
Cincinnati, Ohio

SANDRA L. HAGEN-ANSERT, B.A., R.D.M.S.
Program Director, Ultrasound
Department of Radiology
Division of Ultrasound
Clinical Research Sonographer
Division of Pediatric Cardiology
UCSD Medical Center
University of California
San Diego, California

MARCUS W. HEDGCOCK, Jr., M.D.
Chief of Computed Imaging
DVA Medical Center;
Assistant Professor of Radiology
University of California
San Francisco, California

RICHARD D. HICHWA, Ph.D.
Associate Professor
Director PET Imaging Center
Department of Radiology
University of Iowa
Iowa City, Iowa

KENNETH C. JOHNSON, M.S.
President, Kenneth Johnson and Associates, Inc.
Columbus, Ohio

NINA KOWALCZYK, M.S., R.T.(R)
Assistant Director
Department of Radiology
Riverside Methodist Hospital
Columbus, Ohio

JACK C. MALOTT, A.S., R.T.(R), F.A.S.R.T., F.A.H.R.A.
Director, Radiologic Administration
Associate Professor
University of Cincinnati Hospital
University of Cincinnati College of Medicine
Cincinnati, Ohio

CHARLES H. MARSCHKE, B.A., R.T.(R)(T)
Director, Radiation Therapy Program
University of Vermont
Burlington, Vermont

JOHN O. OLSEN, M.D.
Associate Professor
Department of Radiology
The Ohio State University
Columbus, Ohio

RICHARD C. PASKIET, Jr., B.A., R.T.(R)

Regional Sales Manager
Fuji Medical Systems, Inc., U.S.A.
Stanford, Connecticut

WALTER W. PEPPLER, Ph.D.

Clinical Associate Professor
Department of Medical Physics
University of Wisconsin—Madison
Madison, Wisconsin

ALAN H. ROWBERG, M.D.

Assistant Professor
Department of Radiology
University of Washington
Seattle, Washington

ANN HRICA SEGLINSKI, R.T.(R)

Chief Technologist, Pediatric Section
Department of Radiology
The Johns Hopkins Hospital
Baltimore, Maryland

JANE A. VAN VALKENBURG, Ph.D., R.T.(R)(N)

Director, Radiological Sciences Program
Weber State University
Ogden, Utah

RONALD D. WEINSTEIN, Ph.D., R.T.(R)

Director, School of Cardiovascular Technology
St. Luke's Episcopal Hospital
Texas Children's Hospital
Texas Heart Institute
Houston, Texas

JOAN A. WODARSKI, R.N., B.S.N.

Senior Clinical Nurse
Department of Pediatric Radiology
The Johns Hopkins Hospital
Baltimore, Maryland

PREFACE

Hardly is the ink dry on one edition when new knowledge, different procedures, and technological advancements dictate that the revision process begin. Such was the case with this edition of *Merrill's Atlas of Radiographic Positions and Radiologic Procedures*.

One of the more noticeable changes can be attributed to the Twelfth International Congress of Anatomists, which met in London in 1985. Substantial alterations of nomenclature were adopted; these results were published in the 1989 sixth edition of *Nomina Anatomica,* the third edition of *Nomina Histologica,* and the third edition of *Nomina Embryologica*. Because the terminology authorized by the International Congress is the standard terminology for anatomy, this seventh edition of *Merrill's Atlas* reflects these nomenclature changes.

To make the transition to the new anatomic terminology easier, the decision was made to list the new term first and the older term parenthetically. An example of the change is that of the carpal navicular; the accepted name is the scaphoid, so it is printed in the text as *scaphoid (navicular)*. Some reviewers of the early manuscript did not like all of the terminology changes, but we as health care professionals must adopt the terminology used in anatomy textbooks and taught to radiography students, medical students, and residents in radiology. I personally prefer *odontoid process* to the term *dens,* and *extremity* to *limb,* but in the new edition these examples are printed as *dens (odontoid process),* and *limb (extremity)*. To assist the reader of *Merrill's Atlas* in identifying which anatomic terms have changed since the sixth edition, a summary listing the new and old terms is printed on the inside cover.

Other changes were designed to make using the text easier. The phase of patient respiration has been consistently placed in this edition. *Respiration* instructions have been included just before the central ray for those procedures involving the head and torso. For all chapters involving radiography of the head, *italics* were added to the primary positioning landmarks to help the user to quickly identify the positioning lines and points needed to accurately position the patient. The terms *position* and *projection* have been changed to reflect the terminology adopted by The American Registry of Radiologic Technologists. Descriptions of all positioning terms are included in Chapter 3 on p. 43 to 50, including summary Table 3-2 on p. 45. The entrance and exit points for the central ray were expanded and clarified to more precisely identify the centering points when positioning the patient. Similarly, some centering points were slightly changed to reflect the anatomical centering points of the body part, which are required when using positive beam limitation equipment. Other changes include placing the running heads on the edges of the pages. This makes locating a chapter or a specific position much easier.

The organization of the book remains essentially unchanged; Volumes 1 and 2 contain the radiologic procedural examinations, and Volume 3 contains descriptions of the radiology specialties. This organization was planned so, as an option, a student radiographer might purchase Volume 1 for the first term in the educational program, Volume 2 for the second educational term, and Volume 3 during the second year of professional radiography education.

Two entirely new chapters were added to Volume 3: Digital Subtraction Angiography and Computed Radiography. In addition, all chapters received substantive revisions with the addition of new illustrations and text.

Before, during, and after revising the textbook, many reviewers made significant contributions by offering suggestions for clarifying the information for the reader. Grateful appreciation is extended to three radiologists, Javier Beltran, M.D., Jerome J. Cunningham, M.D., and James Jerele, D.O., who reviewed selected chapters and offered suggestions for improvement. Several technologists devoted extensive time and effort in reviewing new chapters and new material and, in general, offering suggestions for improvement. Thanks and my true appreciation are extended to Michael W. Drafke, M.S., R.T. (R), from the College of DuPage in Glen Ellyn, Illinois; Eugene D. Frank, B.S., R.T. (R), FASRT, from the Mayo Clinic and Foundation in Rochester, Minnesota; Michael L. Fugate, M.Ed., R.T. (R) from Southwest Virginia Community College in Richlands, Virginia; Bruce W. Long, M.S., R.T.(R) from the Indiana University School of Medicine in Indianapolis, Indiana; Kenneth Roszel, B.S., R.T., from Geisinger Medical Center in Danville, Pennsylvania; Jeffrey L. Rowe, M.S., R.T.(R), from Muskingum Area Technical College in Zanesville, Ohio; Dennis Spragg, M.S.Ed., R.T.(R), from Lima Technical College in Lima, Ohio; and Anton R. Zembrod, M.Ed., R.T.(R) of Wichita Falls, Texas. I also want to thank Professor Spragg for his evaluation of the material from *Merrill's Atlas* that was published in the first edition of the *Pocket Guide to Radiography* published by Mosby-Year Book, Inc. in 1989. Mark Smith, R.T. and Debra Saunders, R.T., colleagues and graduate students at The Ohio State University, assisted me by critiquing manuscript, reviewing new material, assisting in obtaining new radiographs, proofreading manuscript, and responding to multiple requests for assistance. Your work was appreciated, and I gained a great deal of respect for each of you. I'm sure your futures will be bright.

Literally thousands of journal articles must be searched for and reviewed in revising each edition. Terry Kempton, R.T. devoted extensive time and effort to search for, locate, and review thousands of journal articles. As a result, over 1300 articles written by over 2800 authors were reviewed and added to this edition in the bibliographic sections of all three volumes. The task was extremely demanding and would not have been possible without Ms. Kempton's help.

Two anatomists at The Ohio State University assisted greatly in revising this edition. Margaret Hines, Ph.D reviewed the anatomy sections following the publication of the 1989 editon of *Nomina Anatomica*. Dr. Hines' comments were extremely valuable and timely in making the changes in terminology possible. Her continual support and assistance are truly appreciated. Professor John Chidley also reviewed the anatomy sections and offered suggestions for changes.

Eva James, R.T., reviewed the comments of the anatomists and those received from users, synthesized them, compared them with *Nomina Anatomica,* and organized the anatomy sections of the chapters for consistency and clarity. In addition, Ms. James reviewed the final manuscript and prepared a summary of the anatomic terms that have changed from the previous edition.

Sincere thanks are extended to Julie Gilhousen, R.T.(R)(N) from Picker International, Inc. for her cooperation in arranging for the use of the radiographic equipment needed to produce new photographic illustrations. Picker International, Inc. has demonstrated strong support for this *Atlas* through all seven editions and that support is truly appreciated.

Although every effort has been made to ensure accuracy and consistency of information, an occasional mistake escapes. When such occurs, you can assist me by marking the error on a photocopy of the page and mailing it directly to me. Suggestions for improvement are also welcome, for it is only with the assistance of concerned professionals that the text is strengthened.

This *Atlas* requires extensive visual support and without the professional staff of the medical illustrators, medical photographers, and the concerned staff of the Biomedical Communications Division in the School of Allied Medical Professions and The Ohio State University, the illustrations printed in this textbook would not be of such high quality. Particular thanks are extended to chief photographer Robert Jones for his patience and cooperation in shooting, printing, and reprinting the illustrations to show just what is desired. Thanks also to Mr. Harry Condry and Mr. Matthew Eppley for their responding to my many, sometimes impossible, requests.

Sincere thanks are extended to scores of individuals (R.T.s, students, and physicians) who assisted by locating radiographs for this edition. As is the custom, whenever a radiograph is printed in the *Atlas,* the name of the individual supplying the original radiograph is printed adjacent to the image. Unfortunately there were a few radiographs I was not able to print because they were duplicates. Thanks again to all who assisted by supplying illustrations of excellent quality for this edition.

Sincere thanks are extended to Eileen Buckholz who has served as secretary to the Radiologic Technology Division at The Ohio State University (and manager of my schedule) for several years. Her ability to assist the faculty and students, get me to classes with students, attend university meetings, respond to phone calls, and many other tasks while keeping track of me is truly appreciated. Thanks again, Eileen, for all your help.

To David Culverwell, Peggy Fagen, Christi Mangold, Cecilia Reilly, Elaine Steinborn, Mary Stueck, and the entire professional staff of Mosby-Year Book, Inc., I enjoyed working with you in our mutual quest to produce a quality textbook. Although some of the deadlines were a little tight, we generally made them.

Without the total support of my family this project would not have been possible. To my father-in-law, L. Neil Hathaway, thanks for your understanding and encouragement. I also thank my parents, D.W. and Mildred Ballinger, for their love and encouragement demonstrated throughout my career and their continuing support and assistance. They are always there when they are needed and I apologize for taking that for granted. To my wife, Nancy, loving appreciation is extended for her understanding and assistance. In addition to being an understanding wife (well, most of the time), my multiple requests for her help have generally been answered. Many times the family schedule has been revised or something rescheduled because I was out of town or "just had to work." Thanks for your love and support over the years. My son, Eric, and daughter, Monica, are relatively understanding of the neverending revision process. I apologize for the many times I should have been doing things to assist and support them, but was instead working on the book or attending a professional meeting. Over the years Eric and Monica have learned to stop asking, "Is the book done yet?" because they know that as soon as it is complete, it and other projects will compete for my attention. Eric and Monica, I love you and appreciate your patience. I only wish that sometimes when you see my travel schedule posted on the refrigerator door, instead of asking, "Now where are you going?" you'd ask, "When will you be back?"

Philip W. Ballinger

Columbus, Ohio

CONTENTS

VOLUME ONE

VOLUME TWO

VOLUME THREE

Contents

MERRILL'S ATLAS OF

RADIOGRAPHIC POSITIONS and RADIOLOGIC PROCEDURES

VOLUME THREE

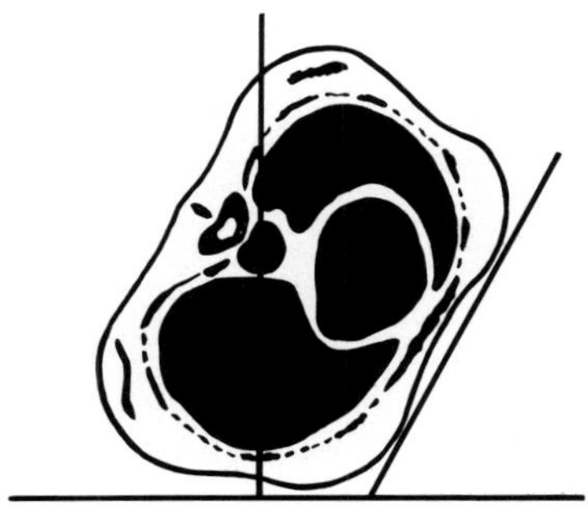

Chapter 25

PEDIATRIC RADIOGRAPHY

JOHN P. DORST
ANN HRICA SEGLINSKI
MARY J. BLOME
THOMAS J. BECK
JOAN A. WODARSKI

Radiographic examinations are fundamentally the same whether the patient is an adult or a child. Consequently, when judiciously modified, most of the techniques described in the first two volumes are applicable to children and infants. There are some important differences of course. Protection from unnecessary radiation is especially important. There are some fundamental differences in imaging requirements, such as that high kVp chest radiographs are of limited usefulness. For the technologist, however, the most obvious difference is that many of the patients are either too young or too frightened to cooperate with the examination.

If physicians and nurses are to provide quality care for infants and children, they must perform unpleasant or painful procedures on these patients at many of their medical visits during their early, impressionable years. For example, they must give hypodermic injections for the routine immunizations and perform throat cultures, which make most children gag and some vomit. Therefore many young children begin to cry whenever they are approached by anyone in a white uniform. Indeed, in many pediatric centers the nurses and technologists no longer wear uniforms for just this reason.

Fortunately, most of the radiologic procedures necessary for children are not painful. Yet, small children often vigorously resist such examinations because they have learned to anticipate that medical procedures are likely to hurt. Their fear increases if they are taken from the security of their parents and increases again when they see the large size of the x-ray machine.

Does taking a radiograph have to be so unpleasant for a small child? Usually not. Most children are reasonably adaptable patients when approached on their terms. This takes time, but usually less time than is needed to perform a good examination on a child who is frightened and uncooperative.

Approach to the Child

One who wishes to have a successful relationship with children must like children—and not only happy, well children but also sick children, who are often tired, cranky, and frightened.

The next prerequisites are understanding, patience, and honesty. One must understand as well as possible the fears, needs, and desires of children. One must recognize that a child's immature concept of the world and of illness frequently leads to frightening misconceptions of what may happen in a hospital or a physician's office. Indeed, what is a small child to think of the "very large camera that takes pictures of what is inside him"? Also, certain words may frighten children. If one technologist calls "shoot" to another to indicate the moment to make the exposure, the child is likely to be startled and cry, because the word *shoot* often connotes a hypodermic injection or a gunshot. Other words that may upset children, depending on their ages, include needle (same connotation as shoot), hurt, pain, remove, cut out, cut off, dye (misinterpreted as die), surgery, operation, cancer, leukemia, and many others. Medical personnel who deal with children should try to develop a sensitivity to how children may react to or misinterpret what is said to them.

Patience is required to greet each child in the waiting room, to learn what name or nickname is preferred, to learn the child's interests, and then to explain in simple terms what the child will experience. It is most effective if one communicates at the child's eye level, which means that one might kneel for small children. Frequently the child will ask for a description of the procedure a number of times, and such repetitions may indeed test one's patience.

Understanding and patience will be of little value, however, if one is not honest when the procedure is likely to be disagreeable or painful, such as drinking a barium suspension, having an enema, or receiving an injection for an intravenous urogram. *Never tell a child that a painful procedure will not hurt.* Children old enough to understand should have advance explanation.

To help parents, physicians, and nurses prepare children, some hospitals have illustrated pamphlets that describe, in age-appropriate language, intravenous urography and the common fluoroscopic procedures (Fig. 25-1). It is perhaps best left to the parents to decide when to tell a child about a forthcoming examination. If told too early, many children will fret and lose sleep worrying about an only moderately or briefly unpleasant examination. Yet, most children do better if they are told what is in store for them before they leave home or their hospital bed.

Technologists need to learn to observe and quickly evaluate each child's level of maturity and ability to communicate. The following vignettes of children of various ages may help to determine a child's maturity. To find a much more detailed discussion see Whaley and Wong.[1]

YOUNG INFANTS

Infants to about 6 months of age do not make a sharp distinction among persons who care for them. They often are playful or sleepy when warm and well fed. Reaction to pain stimulates total body movement and loud crying that may cease upon distraction. When there is time, prolonged crying can be quieted by taking the child from the room so that others may be examined. Ask the parent or an aide to hold the child, speak softly and soothingly, and offer a bottle of water or formula if not contraindicated.

[1]Whaley LF and Wong DL: Nursing care of infants and children, ed 4, St Louis, 1990, Mosby–Year Book Inc.

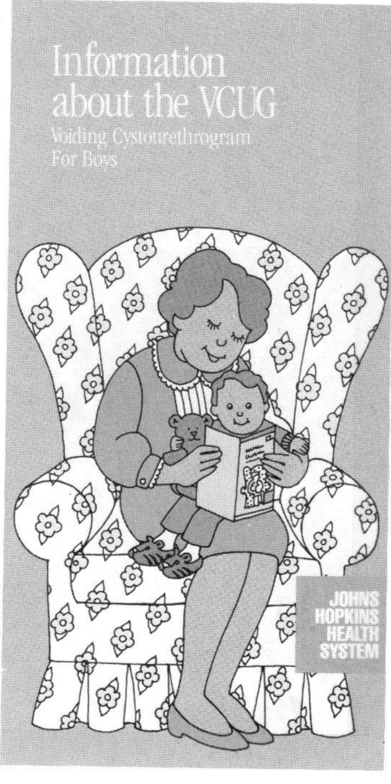

Your doctor needs you to have an X-ray test called a VCUG—an abbreviation for voiding cystourethrogram.

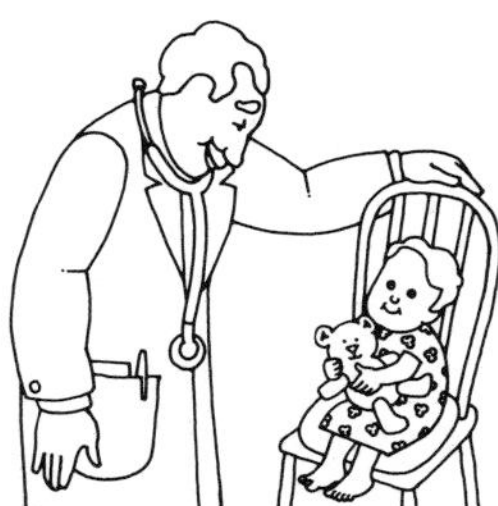

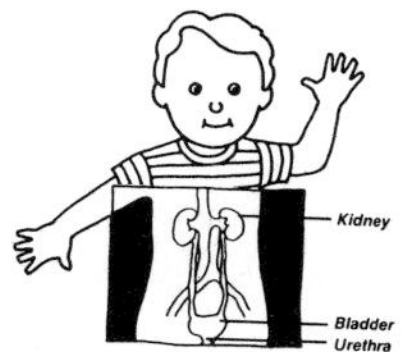

What is a VCUG?

The VCUG is a special X-ray test that shows the doctor what the inside of your bladder and urethra look like. (See picture.) The bladder stores your urine, often called "pee." When you go to the bathroom, your urine comes out through your urethra, which is inside your penis.

Can my parents come with me to the X-ray room?

Yes. When it is your turn to have the VCUG, your X-ray technologist (the person who will take your X-ray pictures) will meet you in the waiting area and accompany you to the X-ray room. Your parents may go into the room with you. You may also bring your favorite stuffed animal or blanket.

Is there a place for me to change clothes in private?

Yes. There is a private dressing room by the X-ray room where you may change into a patient gown.

What is the X-ray room like?

The room has two large machines with special cameras that take X-ray pictures of the inside of your body. There is also a television set where you will be able to see special moving X-ray pictures of yourself.

The X-ray room may seem chilly at first because the machines work better when the room is kept cooler than normal. And the special X-ray table may feel hard. The people taking care of you will try to make you as comfortable as possible, with plenty of sheets and blankets.

Do the machines hurt?

No, they won't hurt you. During the test, one of the machines will come close to you, but it won't touch you. During much of the exam, the lights in the room will be turned down so that it is easier for you and the doctor to see the moving X-ray pictures on the TV.

What happens during the test?

Your X-ray technologist will ask you to lie on your back and will take an X-ray picture of you. Then your X-ray nurse or doctor will come into the room and talk to you to help you get ready for the test. She or he will ask you to lie down on your back with your legs slightly spread. The nurse or doctor will wash your penis with special liquid soap, which may feel cool. (In a hospital or doctor's office, it is O.K. for doctors or nurses to touch the "private parts" of your body when it is necessary to find out if there is a problem.) Then they will gently slide a small, soft tube into your bladder through your urethra. This will feel strange, but it will hurt very little or not at all *if* you relax by breathing in and out through your mouth slowly and deeply.

Your doctor will let some liquid from a bottle run through the tube into your bladder. You and your doctor can watch your bladder fill on the TV. When you feel you have to go to the bathroom, the doctor will take an X-ray picture of your full bladder, and then take more X-ray pictures as you urinate (another word meaning "pee") into a bedpan while lying on the X-ray table. Every child having this test needs to do this, and the tube will come out as you urinate. Someone will help to make you comfortable once again after the test.

(continued on back page)

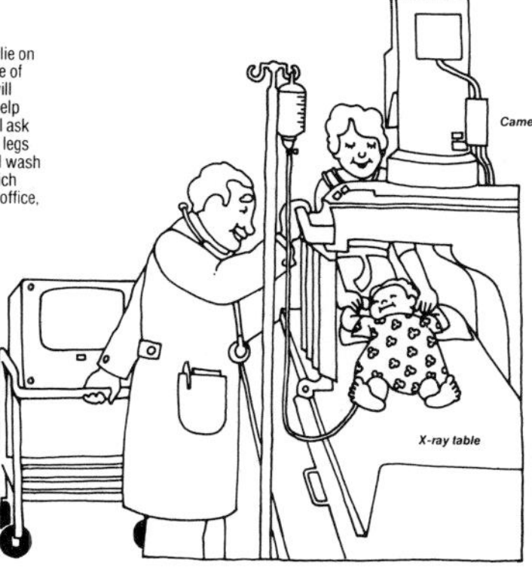

How long will the test take?

The test usually takes about one hour. It may be shorter or longer depending on the number of X-ray pictures that the doctor needs. When all of the X-ray pictures have been taken, the X-ray technologist will show you to the dressing room so you may change into your own clothes.

How can I prepare for the test?

No special preparations are needed. You may eat and drink as you normally do.

Where should I go for the test?

The test will be done in the Division of Pediatric Radiology of The Johns Hopkins Hospital, on level B-1 of the Nelson/Tower Building. It is easiest to take the Nelson/Tower elevators by the Hospital's main entrance on Wolfe Street to the B-1 level and follow the radiology signs until you reach Children's X-ray. If you need further directions, feel free to ask along the way. Information receptionists are located by the Wolfe Street entrance. Patient parking is conveniently located by the Hospital in the first building of the garage on Broadway.

If you have questions . . .

Your doctor, nurse, X-ray technologist and others involved in your care will be happy to answer any other questions you have when you are here. You may also call us. From 9 a.m. to 4:30 p.m., Monday through Friday, you may contact the nurse by calling (301) 955-6454. In an emergency, contact the pediatric X-ray doctor (radiologist) on call by calling (301) 955-6070.

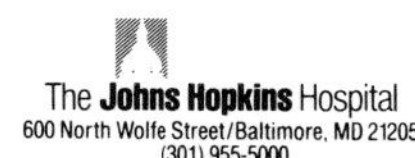

The **Johns Hopkins** Hospital
600 North Wolfe Street/Baltimore, MD 21205
(301) 955-5000

This brochure was prepared by the Division of Pediatric Radiology and the Children's Center Child Life Department of The Johns Hopkins Hospital and The Johns Hopkins School of Medicine.

Fig. 25-1. Pamphlet to help parents prepare their sons for a voiding cystourethrogram. (A sample of each of the 6 pamphlets in the series is available without charge from J Dorst, MD, Department of Radiology, The Johns Hopkins Hospital, 600 N Wolfe St, Baltimore, MD 21205.)

INFANTS TO 3 YEARS OF AGE

The principal stress factors for children 6 months to 3 years are (1) pain, (2) separation from parents, (3) limitation of by now impressive motor skills, and (4) loss of routines and rituals involving eating, sleeping, bathing, and play. A pacifier or baby bottle may often calm the infant. The technologist should approach the toddler with a smiling, friendly manner and talk with a gentle voice, possibly offering a simple toy. Immobilization is almost always necessary, and it is less disturbing to a child than having a number of adults try to hold him or her in the correct position. Once properly immobilized, most children become calm, and a technically good diagnostic examination can be completed. *Precaution: an immobilized child must never be left alone in a room except for the moment the x-ray exposure is made.*

THREE TO FIVE YEARS OF AGE

Preschoolers can understand instructions and explanations if they are offered with an understanding of the child's likely perceptions; for example, "Does your mommy or daddy take pictures of you with a camera? . . . She does? . . . Good! We are going to take pictures of you too. We have a big and special camera—bigger than your mommy's. There it is. Isn't it big? But it won't hurt. It takes a special kind of picture that will help your doctor make you well. They have to be really good pictures. So you have to lie very still on this table so that we can make a really good picture that will help your doctor. I will bring the camera over you while you lie on the table, but it will not touch or hurt you."

Preschoolers are eager to please, and a gamelike atmosphere can facilitate your work. Often the child can be "talked through" a procedure. Praise must be given when the child tries to cooperate. It will serve to reduce the child's anxiety, and it is a highly valued reward. Even with the most cooperative preschoolers, immobilization often is required, because they do not understand the need to hold still in a fixed position.

Immature concepts of illness and treatment, including the fear of invasion of their bodies (e.g., by a needle or an enema) or loss of any part of their bodies (even blood), are universal at this age. Thus Band-Aids are very important to preschoolers, since they fear that any intrusion of the body will result in their "insides leaking out"; make liberal use of Band-Aids.

SCHOOL-AGED CHILDREN

The suggestions in the preceding section also apply for school-aged children. To gain their confidence, technologists should offer full explanations of the expected experience to these older, more sophisticated children. Naturally, the explanations should be modified as the children get older; for example, "We are going to take your picture with an x-ray machine. It is like your mother and father's camera but much bigger. It doesn't hurt when your father takes your picture, does it? Well, it won't hurt when we take your picture with this special camera. It's called an x-ray machine."

Children in this age group are better able to cope with hospitalization because as they socialize in school and form attachments to their peers they are loosening their bonds with home and parents. Indeed, attaining independence is important to them, and they should be allowed freedom of choice whenever possible—for example, a choice of which projection of the chest to do first. They will have less time to worry about their strange surroundings and feelings of helplessness if the technologist talks to them throughout the procedures. The trick is to keep up one's chatter and yet be careful not to say something that demeans the child or violates the child's "personhood." *Many grade-school children are surprisingly modest, and ignoring their modesty can cause intense embarrassment.*

Restraints are often necessary if good radiographic examinations of infants and young children are to be obtained. However, any child older than 7 or 8 years should not be forced to have an examination, except during an emergency. When older children are recalcitrant, they should be taken from the radiographic room, a now-threatening atmosphere, and the parents should be enlisted for calm reassurance. Speak to the parents to make certain that they understand the procedure so that they may explain it and allay fear. Sometimes the radiologist may offer support for the technologist and share the conversation with the parents and child. The presence of a nurse or physician trusted by the child eases the trial of the moment and enables many examinations to be performed without force.

ADOLESCENTS

Adolescent patients have often developed successful mechanisms of coping with the stress of hospitalization. Yet, because many of them have a great deal of misinformation about illness and medical care, their responses to a particular examination may seem quite inappropriate. Occasionally an adolescent child will refuse an examination. Parents, older siblings, nurses, or physicians may, in that event, be of some help and should be invited to join in the discussion. *Only in life-threatening emergencies and when all explanations and arguments have failed should an adolescent patient be forced to have an imaging examination.*

The rapidly changing body image during pubertal development causes adolescents to be quite concerned about privacy and modesty, and technologists should respect these feelings.

MENTALLY RETARDED CHILDREN

Some mentally retarded children can be examined without problem if they are treated in accordance with their mental age rather than their chronologic age. Others can be examined with the help of their parents, teachers, or hospital attendants. Although a few can be examined only when sedated, sedation may often compound the problem, as discussed in the next section, and should be the last resort. Meperidine hydrochloride and promethazine hydrochloride are the drugs usually employed, since chlorpromazine hydrochloride occasionally is epileptogenic in children who have seizures, and some mentally retarded children require unusually large doses of chloral hydrate for sedation.

PARENTS IN RADIOGRAPHIC ROOM

In the past, parents frequently were not allowed to accompany their children into radiographic rooms. Today many pediatric radiologists and technologists believe that parents who wish to accompany their child should be permitted to do so. Indeed, since most parents can give their child important support, parents probably should be encouraged to accompany any child who is unduly apprehensive. When parents are overly concerned about the examination, we find that it usually works best to tell them immediately that they may be present. The technologist then explains the procedure and what the child will experience. When appropriate, the technologist may then *very gently* suggest that, since the child seems to be less concerned than the parent, the child might do better if the parent remained in the waiting room.

Unless the mother is certain that she is not pregnant, she should be in the control booth or out of the radiographic room when the exposure is made. If the parent becomes upset by any feature of the examination and is not reassured by the technologist's explanation, the examination should be discontinued until the radiologist, a trusted nurse or attendant, or the referring physician has allayed the fears.

Sedation

SEDATION FOR COMPUTED TOMOGRAPHY (CT), MAGNETIC RESONANCE IMAGING (MRI), AND NUCLEAR MEDICINE SCANS

Because patients must remain still for many minutes while CT and MRI examinations are performed, children 6 months to 4 years of age usually require sedation. Properly done, such sedation is almost always uneventful. However, complications can occur, such as respiratory arrest and vomiting with aspiration of the vomitus. Therefore the sedation should be done by a qualified nurse or physician and the child watched or monitored by qualified individuals until the sedation has worn off. When the child is brought to the radiology department sedated and returned to the nursing unit shortly after the imaging examination, it is especially important for trained personnel to accompany the child on the trips.

SEDATION FOR FLUOROSCOPY AND PLAIN FILM RADIOGRAPHY

Unlike CT and MRI, patients cannot lie still throughout most fluoroscopic and radiographic examinations. Instead they must assume specific positions for films or turn during fluoroscopy—activities that awaken most sedated children. At that point it is usually more difficult to obtain a satisfactory examination because the medication has decreased their abilities to cooperate, to understand explanations, to follow instructions, and to control their fears. For such examinations, sedation usually should be reserved for unusually fearful children, including some who are mentally retarded. It also can be useful during attempts to reduce intussusceptions.

Patient Care

GENERAL PRINCIPLES

Technologists should know how to provide basic patient care for the infants and children entrusted to them. When a child arrives in the department, the competent technologist notes a number of things: Are there specific instructions for the child's care while in the department? Does the child have physical problems that will interfere with the examination, possibly requiring use of unusual positions? Is the intravenous solution flowing at the proper rate and on time? Does the child's condition suggest the possibility of emergency treatment or other special care?

Many sick infants and children have conditions that require *special diets* or *the collection of all urine or stool*. Before giving a child anything to eat or drink or discarding a specimen, check with the nursing unit or, if the child is an outpatient, with the parents.

When a child arrives in the radiology department with an *intravenous infusion* running, it is important to check that the infusion is on time and has not infiltrated the soft tissues and that there is enough fluid in the bottle to last until the child returns to the nursing unit. When restraining the child for a radiographic examination, care is required to ensure that the tubing does not become blocked or the needle dislodged. The radiologist or the nurse should be notified as soon as any such problem develops.

Technologists must know how to care for a child with a *colostomy* or *ileostomy*—how to remove and replace the bag and how to protect the stoma. Some bags should be removed before taking any radiograph of the abdomen because the rim that attaches the bag to skin is radiopaque and can hide calculi or other abnormalities. Other bags have radiolucent rings and therefore do not require removal unless the bag is filled with feces, or with urine that contains contrast material.

Children are especially likely to have *contagious illnesses*. The radiology department should not be the place where children "catch" each other's infections. Most of the measures to avoid the spread of infection are simple and effective and should be scrupulously observed in the department and during bedside (portable) examinations: wash hands before and after examining each child, clean the radiographic table and restraining devices with a mild disinfectant solution immediately after use, and keep the department clean and neat. *The most important precaution is hand washing, but unfortunately it is the most neglected.*

When children have been placed in *respiratory or enteric isolation* or on *wound or blood precautions* and they cannot be radiographed in bed, they should be brought to the department when few or no other patients are present. They must be kept separate from other patients, examined quickly, and returned to their nursing unit promptly. Depending on the type of illness, technologists and physicians may be required to wear protective gowns, gloves, or face masks, as specified by hospital protocol. After the examination the radiographic room, table, and equipment used must be disinfected as specified by protocol.

Severely burned children and children who have immunologic deficiencies, either innate, such as dysgammaglobulinemia, or associated with chemotherapy for cancer or organ transplant, are likely to get serious and sometimes fatal infections. They require *protective isolation,* which should be provided as specified by the hospital protocol. In general, this consists of precautions taken to protect the patient from contracting an infection. These children should be examined, whenever possible, when no other patients are in the department—particularly no patients with infectious diseases. The radiographic room and equipment must be carefully cleaned *before* the patient is admitted. Technologists and physicians must wear face masks when with the patient.

Smith et al[1] have published a practical guide to handling children in the radiology department who are known to have specific infections.

Respiratory distress may develop rapidly in children. *Children restrained for an examination must never be left alone. If distress develops while the child is restrained, release him or her immediately.* Generally this remedies the situation. Sometimes it helps to raise the child into a semierect position and extend the head slightly. Periodic classes should be held to educate and reeducate all personnel who deal with pediatric patients in the recommended methods of cardiopulmonary resuscitation.

CARE OF PREMATURE INFANTS

In the radiology department, *hypothermia* is the greatest hazard to premature infants and to some full-term infants. Hypothermia is likely to intensify their illnesses and may prove fatal.[2] Since small infants may rapidly become hypothermic even in rooms most people consider uncomfortably warm, they should be examined whenever possible in the nursery with the infant in an incubator or infant warmer. When the examination must be done in the radiology department, the infant should be transported in a warm incubator by a health professional. The infant may be prepared for the examination while still in the incubator; for example, an enema tube or a nasogastric tube may be inserted or simple restraints may be applied. Removal from the incubator should be for as short a period as possible, and the infant should be returned during pauses in the examination if there is any evidence of hypothermia. *Immobilization is rarely needed for these infants; when it is, a gentle, simple method that can be applied quickly should be chosen.*

[1]Smith WL et al: Minimizing the risk of infectious diseases in the radiology department, Appl Radiol 10(4):70-73, 1981.

[2]Avery ME, Fletcher BD, and Williams RY: The lung and its disorders in the newborn infant, ed 4, Philadelphia, 1981, WB Saunders Co, pp 251, 306, 339.

No completely satisfactory method of keeping an infant warm during fluoroscopy appears to have been developed. One method is to place the infant on a relatively radiolucent warming pad and under a portable infrared heat lamp or similar warmer. The lamp must be kept a suitable distance from the infant, usually at least 3 feet. Most heat lamps become inefficient during fluoroscopy because the fluoroscope shields them from the infant. The warmers designed by Newman and Poznanski,[1] however, remain effective since they are placed on each side of the infant.

When an infant arrives in the radiology department in an incubator or radiant warmer, body temperature should be monitored while the infant is removed from that warm, monitored environment. This can be done by measuring axillary or rectal temperature with a mercury or electronic thermometer. The most accurate method is to use a remote reading thermometer (telethermomotor) with a skin probe (thermistor)—the type that comes with most incubators and warmers. The skin probe is placed over the liver, where the skin temperature should be about 36.5° C. If the skin temperature drops below 35° C, the examination should be interrupted and the infant returned to the incubator.[2]

[1]Newman DE and Poznanski AK: A simple device for infant warming during radiography, Radiology 97:439, 1970.

[2]Poznanski AK: Practical approaches to pediatric radiology, Chicago, 1976, Year Book Medical Publishers, Inc, pp 14-16.

SPECIAL PATIENT CARE PROBLEMS

Several pediatric conditions may present problems to radiologic technologists.

Myelomeningocele

Myelomeningocele is a birth defect characterized by a cystic protrusion of meninges and nerve roots or spinal cord from the back that causes varying degrees of permanent paralysis and is often associated with hydrocephalus. Most infants with myelomeningoceles should be examined prone until the defect has been surgically repaired and the wound healed.

Omphalocele

An *omphalocele* is a birth defect that resembles an enormous umbilical hernia. It has a thin, translucent wall and contains bowel and liver. It must be carefully supported so that the sac is not broken, and it must be kept moist and warm. In *gastroschisis,* a similar congenital anomaly, a portion of bowel protrudes through a defect near the navel. It is even more important that this bowel be kept moist and warm, since it is not contained in a sac. Whenever possible, the referring physician or a specially trained nurse should remain with such infants in the radiology department since they may rapidly become hypothermic.

Osteogenesis imperfecta

Osteogenesis imperfecta is an inherited condition characterized by bones that are likely to break. There is great variation in severity, from individuals who suffer only a few fractures during their lives and often do not realize that they are different from anyone else to infants who are born with multiple fractures. All infants and children with osteogenesis imperfecta must be handled with extreme care; otherwise, a fracture may be caused. The technologist should explain to the parent, nurse, or physician who accompanied the child to the radiology department the correct position for each required radiograph. The attendant, rather than the technologist, should help the child assume that position. If the attendant believes the child cannot safely assume this position, an alternative approach must be used. It is often possible to obtain a properly positioned radiograph by angling the x-ray tube, the film, or both. The technologist who does not believe it is possible to obtain a satisfactory radiograph or who has any question about handling the child should consult the radiologist before proceeding.

Arthrogryposis

Arthrogryposis, also known as *arthrogryposis multiplex congenita* and *amyoplasia congenita,* is an inherited disorder characterized by severe limitation of motion in more than one joint. The muscles in the affected limb or limbs are extremely thin, and the bones are thin, are osteoporotic, and may fracture easily. The suggestions in the preceding paragraph about handling patients with osteogenesis imperfecta also apply to handling patients with arthrogryposis.

Child abuse

When preparing a child for an examination or when viewing the radiographs, the technologist may be the first person to suspect that the child has been abused. Many states require all health professionals to report suspected cases of abuse. The technologist should speak with the radiologist, if available, or the attending physician. Following the discussion, the decision of whether or not to report the suspicion is made.

Identification of an abused child will be aided by familiarity with the list of typical types and sites of abuse given in the box that follows on p. 8. The technologist should not be reassured if the child appears clean and well dressed since the parents of an abused child may feel remorse and guilt following the incident and may therefore bathe and dress the child in clean clothes to make a good impression.[1] Helfer and Kempe[2] have published two helpful lists of features that should sensitize health professionals to the possibility of child abuse.

Technologists should approach examining an abused child in the same way as they approach examining any other injured or ill child. The child *and the parents* must be accorded the same kindness and care. A critical attitude or remark toward the parents may seriously jeopardize the child's opportunity to grow up to be a socially productive and reasonably normal adult.

Although children of all ages may be abused, physical abuse is most likely to result in fractures when the victim is an infant. These fractures frequently are multiple and involve the growing ends of the bone in a fairly characteristic manner. A normal radiographic examination never excludes abuse since the majority of physically abused children do not have fractures or dislocations.[3] Sexually abused children rarely have radiographic abnormalities.

[1]Weston JT: The pathology of child abuse. In Helfer RE and Kempe CH, editors: The battered child, ed 2, Chicago, 1974, University of Chicago Press, pp 69-70.

[2]Helfer RE and Kempe CH: The child's need for early recognition, immediate care and protection. In Kempe CH and Helfer RE, editors: Helping the battered child and his family, Philadelphia, 1972, JB Lippincott Co, p 73.

[3]Rodriquez A: Handbook of child abuse and neglect, Flushing, NY, 1977, Medical Examination Publishing Co, Inc, p 22.

The usual radiographic examination of an infant or young child for possible fractures caused by abuse includes radiographs of the skull (frontal, Towne, and lateral images), chest (frontal projection with good rib detail), spine (lateral positions of the cervical, thoracic, lumbar, and sacral spine), and upper and lower limbs (frontal images that include the hands, pelvis, and feet).

Abused children may suffer from many injuries other than fractures. They include subdural hematomas and hygromas, cerebral contusions, intraventricular hematomas, pulmonary contusions, pleural effusions, pericardial effusions, hematomas of the bowel (usually of the duodenum), pancreatitis, pancreatic pseudocysts, and lacerations of the bowel, liver, kidney, and/or spleen.

VISUAL DIAGNOSIS OF NONACCIDENTAL TRAUMA[1]

I. Typical sites
- A. Buttocks and lower back (paddling)
- B. Genitals and inner thighs (sexual abuse)
- C. Cheeks (slap marks)
- D. Earlobes (pinch marks)
- E. Upper lip and frenulum (forced feeding)
- F. Neck (choke marks)

II. Inflicted bruises
- A. Human hand marks (pressure bruises), oval grab marks (fingertips), trunk encirclement bruises, linear marks (fingers), handprints, pinch marks
- B. Human bite marks
- C. Strap marks, linear bruises (belt or whip), loop mark bruises (doubled-over cord)
- D. Bizarre marks, bruises from blunt instruments, tattoos and fork mark punctures, circumferential tie marks (ankle, wrist), gag marks
- E. Bruises at different ages of healing:

Age	Color
0 to 2 days	Swollen, tender
0 to 5 days	Red, blue
5 to 7 days	Green
7 to 10 days	Yellow
10 to 14 days	Brown
2 to 4 weeks	Clear

III. Normal bruises
- A. Facial scratches on babies with long fingernails
- B. Knee and skin bruises
- C. Forehead bruises
- D. Bruises over bony prominences

IV. Other types of abuse
- A. Inflicted burns
  1. Cigarette burns
  2. Match tip or incense burns
  3. Dry contact burns (from forced contact with heating devices, e.g., electric hot plate)
  4. Branding burns (from heated metals)
  5. Scalds (from forced immersion)
- B. Head injuries
  1. From direct blows
     a. Skull fractures
     b. Scalp swelling and bruises
     c. Retinal hemorrhages
  2. From violent shaking
     a. No skull fractures
     b. No scalp swelling or bruises
     c. Retinal hemorrhages
- C. Abdominal injuries (from being kicked or hit)
  1. Ruptured liver or spleen
  2. Ruptured blood vessel
  3. Intestinal perforation
  4. Kidney injury
  5. Pancreatic injury
  6. Intramural hematoma of duodenum or proximal jejunum
- D. Bone injuries
  1. Usual fractures
  2. Fractures at different stages of healing
  3. Repeated fractures at same site
  4. Unusual fractures (ribs, scapula, sternum)

[1]Prepared by Barton D. Schmitt, M.D., Department of Pediatrics, University of Colorado Medical Center, Denver, 1978.

Protection of the Child

PROTECTION FROM INJURY

It is the responsibility of the radiology department to see that a child neither injures himself or herself nor is injured while in the department. To avoid injury the department must provide supervision of all children while in the department and frequently during their passage to and from the department. Infants and young children must be watched with particular care. Even the best available methods of immobilizing infants and young children are slightly hazardous. Immobilization should be done only by experienced technologists, and the immobilized child must be watched at all times.

PROTECTION FROM UNNECESSARY RADIATION

Children are more sensitive than adults to both the latent somatic effects and the genetic effects of radiation.

The *latent somatic effects* of radiation are those that may occur months or years later in the person who is irradiated. They include nonspecific life shortening and the induction of malignancies. Immature growing tissues in many of the child's organs are considerably more sensitive to radiation damage than the mature tissues of an adult. Moreover, a child is more likely than an adult to live long enough to develop a malignancy or other change induced by radiation administered possibly 30 years earlier.

The malignancies most likely to be induced by irradiating a child are lung and thyroid cancer and leukemia.[1] Consequently, the tissues at greatest risk are the thyroid gland, the lungs, and the hematopoietically active bone marrow, which in the child younger than 7 years is present throughout most of the skeleton. In postpubescent girls, the breasts are also at risk for developing cancer.

Although *genetic effects* are caused by irradiation of a person's testicles or ovaries, they cause no recognizable damage in the irradiated person. The potential damage takes the form of mutations in that person's sperm or ova that increase the likelihood that his or her descendants will have a serious disease. Because their entire reproductive periods lie ahead, children as a population are particularly susceptible to the genetic effects of radiation.

[1]The effects on populations of exposure to low levels of ionizing radiation. Report of the Advisory Committee on the Biological Effect of Ionizing Radiation, National Academy of Science, 1980.

Provided that reasonable precautions are taken, the likelihood that a diagnostic x-ray examination will cause a harmful somatic or genetic abnormality is quite small. For example, if 1 million small children are each given 1 rad to their hematopoietic bone marrow, 32 to 68 more cases of leukemia are likely to result during the next 25 years than if they had received no radiation.[1] To put this into perspective, if 10 million 1-year-old children each have one AP abdominal radiograph, one of them is likely to develop radiation-induced leukemia within 25 years.[1,2]

[1]The effects on populations of exposure to low levels of ionizing radiation. Report of the Advisory Committee on the Biological Effect of Ionizing Radiation, National Academy of Science, 1980.

[2]Technique: 10 mAs, 65 kVp, single phase, 8:1 grid, Kodak Lanex regular screens with Ortho G film; estimated marrow dose 0.002 rads. Dose computed from Rosenstein M, Beck TJ, and Warren GG: Handbook of selected organ doses for projections common in pediatric radiology, HEW Publication (FDA) 79-8079, May 1979.

When the gonads lie within the x-ray field, they should be shielded unless shielding will interfere with the procedure. The testicles are much more easily shielded than the ovaries. When obtaining radiographs of the abdomen or pelvis, a lead rubber shield (0.5 mm lead equivalent or greater) can usually be positioned so that it covers the testicles and does not obscure pertinent anatomy (Fig. 25-2). Alternatively, a shadow shield may be used. The shadow shield is attached by a moveable arm to the x-ray collimator housing. With the collimator light turned on, the arm is adjusted so the shadow of the shield covers the testicles.

An ovarian shield, however, can be used only occasionally because it almost always obscures important portions of the body. Fortunately, the unshielded ovaries lie near the midplane of the body and consequently receive significantly less radiation in similar examinations than the superficial testicles. Intravenous urograms should be tailored so that the ovaries are outside the x-ray beam on as many of the radiographs as possible. Similar planning is occasionally possible with other abdominal examinations.

A

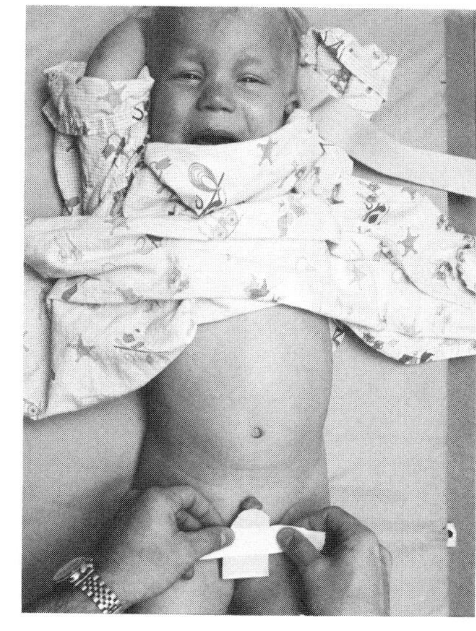

B

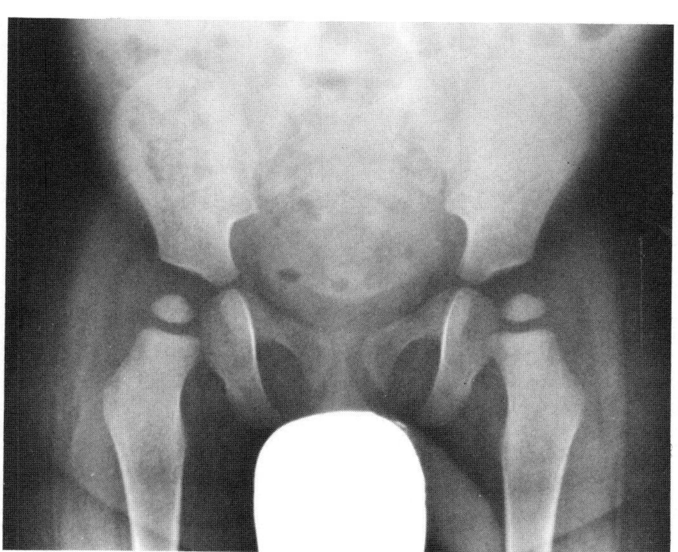

Fig. 25-2. A, The male gonadal shield is positioned so that the convex upper margin lies just beneath the concave lower margin of the pubic and ischial bones. **B,** Radiograph showing correctly positioned male gonadal shield that covers the testicles but does not obscure any of the bones.

The practice of gonadal shielding is important to protect the population as a whole. In diagnostic radiography of children, however, a greater concern is the risk (quite small) of inducing a latent cancer. This cancer risk is minimized by reducing both the quantity of radiation used and the amount of sensitive tissue irradiated. One of the most important tissues at risk is the active bone marrow. This risk is largely influenced by the amount of bone marrow exposed by the x-ray beam. Since the active marrow is distributed throughout the skeleton in a small child, the larger the x-ray field the greater the bone marrow dose. Therefore careful *collimation to expose only the area of interest is extremely important.* Whenever possible, care should be taken to shield or exclude from the x-ray field those tissues at risk for somatic effects. When practical, the breasts of a postpubescent girl should be excluded from the beam. This can be accomplished when examining for scoliosis by careful collimation and/or having the girl wear a special vest that provides lead shielding of the breasts. Moreover, use of PA projections of the thorax rather than AP projections results in a significant reduction in the amount of radiation received by the breasts. The same considerations apply to the thyroid gland when making radiographs that include the neck—many chest radiographs include the neck.

Whenever possible, the highest kilovoltage consistent with the desired level of contrast and fast film-screen systems should be used in pediatric radiography to minimize the amount of radiation received during the examination. At the same time it must be recalled that the smaller size of pediatric organs places a conflicting demand on the resolution of the imaging system. Small body parts require higher resolution systems to be satisfactorily visualized. Ideally, the pediatric film-screen system should have higher resolution than that used in adult radiography, and it should also be faster! Fortunately, recent film-screen technology has resulted in systems that combine excellent resolution with reasonably fast speed. For most general pediatric radiography, the best combination appears to be a reduced crossover (antiprint-through) film combined with moderately fast rare earth screens that provide a system speed of about 400. The same film combined with medium speed rare earth screens to yield a speed of about 200 is a good compromise for radiography of the forearms, hands, and feet. Brodeur and his associates[1] carry this more than a step further and use three different film-screen combinations. Additional suggestions for minimizing radiation exposure are given in the following section on patient motion.

Computed tomography (CT) poses an unnecessary radiation hazard to children unless one fundamental difference between CT and conventional radiography is kept in mind. In CT, use of more radiation than is necessary does not result in an overexposed image as it does in conventional radiography. It is possible to use the identical technical factors for a specific CT examination of a small child and of a large adult and get a good study of each! A technologist would never consider doing this in radiography, in part because it would result in a seriously overexposed radiograph of the child. CT, however, corrects for the overexposure of the child and the images look fine. Yet most modern CT systems can provide excellent images of small patients at reduced mAs values. This is done in second- and fourth-generation systems by selecting either a low mA value or a shorter scan time; in pulsed third-generation systems, a lower mAs value is selected. The use of a lower kVp value will result not only in a reduction in dose (for the same mAs) but also in improved image contrast.

If care is not exercised, computed radiography (CR) systems (see Chapter 35) that employ photostimulatable phosphor plate technology also can deliver unnecessary radiation to children. In such systems the film and screens used in conventional radiography are replaced by a special radiation-sensitive phosphor plate. The plate is put in a cassette and exposed in exactly the same way a conventional x-ray film is exposed, but the image is stored on the phosphor plate rather than on an x-ray film. After the exposure the plate is removed from the cassette and the image "developed" in a special laser reader. Because the phosphor plate is difficult to overexpose or underexpose, one can use the same technique on almost every patient. Therefore it is easy to give a child much more radiation than is necessary. Fortunately, these CR systems can also decrease the radiation dose to children. Exposure factors must be chosen carefully, however, since too little exposure results in an image in which subtle tissue contrasts cannot be recognized. As this is written, a number of radiology departments are evaluating which factors give the best images with the least radiation dose using this type of CR.

It should be emphasized that this concern for radiation protection of the child should *never* compromise the quality or efficacy of a clinically indicated radiologic examination. A poorly performed or incomplete examination gives the child unnecessary radiation!

Once girls begin to menstruate they can become pregnant, and the immature tissues of the embryo and fetus are even more sensitive to radiation damage than the tissues of the child. To avoid unnecessary irradiation of an unborn child, *elective radiographic examinations of the abdomen, pelvis, and upper thighs should only be done during the first 10 days of the menstrual period.* All girls older than 11 years (or their parents) should be questioned about their menstrual history, and if indicated the girls should be spoken to privately to learn if they are sexually active and use effective birth control. Because of the adolescent's concern for modesty, gentle questioning by a sympathetic, mature woman is most likely to elicit honest responses.

Suggestions for minimizing radiation to parents are given in an earlier section about parents in the radiographic room.

[1]Brodeur AE, Silberstein MJ, Graviss ER, et al: Three-tier rare-earth imaging system, AJR 136:755, 1981.

The Principal Problem: Patient Motion

Infants and young children are charming wigglers at best, screaming fighters at worst. The secrets of obtaining good radiographs are (1) establishing a good rapport, which was previously discussed in the section "Approach to the Child," (2) equipment that permits fast exposures with appropriate factors, and (3) proper positioning aids, with immobilization when necessary.

APPROPRIATE X-RAY EQUIPMENT

Appropriate, fast exposures are largely dependent on suitable radiographic equipment and technical factors. Generators used for pediatric examinations should permit exposure times as brief as 1 or 2 milliseconds. Kilovoltages up to 140 are useful, but 125 kV is adequate for all studies. Such generators offer optimum exposure flexibility when used with fast film-screen systems.

Field size and patient thickness are frequently smaller in pediatric than in adult radiology. When they are, less scattered radiation is produced. Consequently, grid ratios greater than 8:1 are rarely necessary. Depending on the kilovoltage, the replacement of a 12:1 grid with an 8:1 grid approximately halves the patient dose.[1] Abdominal radiographs of hypersthenic or obese adolescents may require a higher grid ratio. A 10:1 grid is a good compromise. Fine-line stationary grids or high-speed Potter-Bucky mechanisms are necessary for the short exposures that are used in many examinations.

[1]Nickoloff EL, Beck TJ, and Leo FP: Variations in patient entrance exposures for selected x-ray procedures. Proceedings of Medicine VIII Meeting of Society of Photo Optical Engineers, April 20-22, 1980, Las Vegas, Nevada.

Radiographic machines sold in the United States must have collimators that automatically adjust the x-ray beam to the same size as the film. Although selection of the proper film size with collimation to the margins of that film is usually adequate for adults, this practice almost always results in excessively large fields for infants and children because small errors in collimation give unnecessary radiation to a proportionately much greater amount of their small bodies. Therefore in pediatric radiography the collimator almost always needs to be adjusted further so that the radiograph includes only the pertinent anatomy.

The highest kilovoltage consistent with the desired level of contrast and fast film-screen systems should be used to minimize exposure times, thereby reducing the chance that patient motion will reduce the usefulness of the radiograph and possibly require a repeat examination. Since these measures also reduce the radiation the patient receives, they are discussed at more length in the preceding section "Protection of the Child."

A rigorous quality control program is required to ensure optimum performance from radiographic machines, cassettes, film, and film processors over the years.

IMMOBILIZATION

Even the best available methods of immobilizing infants and young children have a slight potential for harm. Therefore immobilization should only be performed by experienced technologists. Before starting, the procedure should be explained to the parents and to any child old enough to understand. *The immobilized child must not be left unattended at any time,* except for the instant when the exposure is made, and even then a technologist or another trained medical person must always watch the child.

Immobilization is used to ensure correct patient position and to minimize, but *not* completely stop, voluntary motion; other motion is minimized by fast exposures. *An infant or child must never be immobilized so tightly that small movements are impossible.*

The following items are useful for positioning and immobilizing children, and most of them should be available: bed sheets, diapers, adhesive tape, stretch gauze bandages, elastic bandages, orthopedic stockinettes, sponges, sandbags, compression bands, plastic compression panels, and head clamps or sponges. If many infants and young children are studied in a department, there are a number of commercial immobilizing devices that are well worth their cost.[1]

Adhesive tape is used in many ways for immobilization. One way is to attach one end of the tape to the edge of the x-ray table, pass the tape over the child, and attach the other end of the tape to the other side of the table (see Fig. 25-4 in the next section). It is best not to let the adhesive surface of cloth adhesive tape touch a child's skin or hair. Either the skin or hair is covered by a cloth or a paper napkin, or else the tape is turned as it crosses the child so the smooth side is next to the skin or hair. When necessary to *attach* adhesive tape to a child's skin, first attach a piece of paper tape or special plastic tape that causes minimal irritation to the skin and then attach the cloth adhesive tape to the paper or plastic tape already on the skin. *The skin of premature infants is easily injured by adhesive tape. Most premature nurseries use a special type of adhesive tape* that is unlikely to injure the skin, and the same tape should be used when premature infants are examined in radiology.

Sandbags should be available in many sizes: small, firm sandbags weighing 3 to 7 pounds; long, firm sandbags weighing 10 to 30 pounds; and many, long, floppy sandbags of the same weights. All should have covers that can be cleaned or changed after each use. The long, firm sandbags are placed on each side of an infant or young child to help ensure that he or she does not roll off the table.

[1]A list of the devices found useful is available from J. Dorst, M.D., Department of Radiology, The Johns Hopkins Hospital, Baltimore, Maryland 21205.

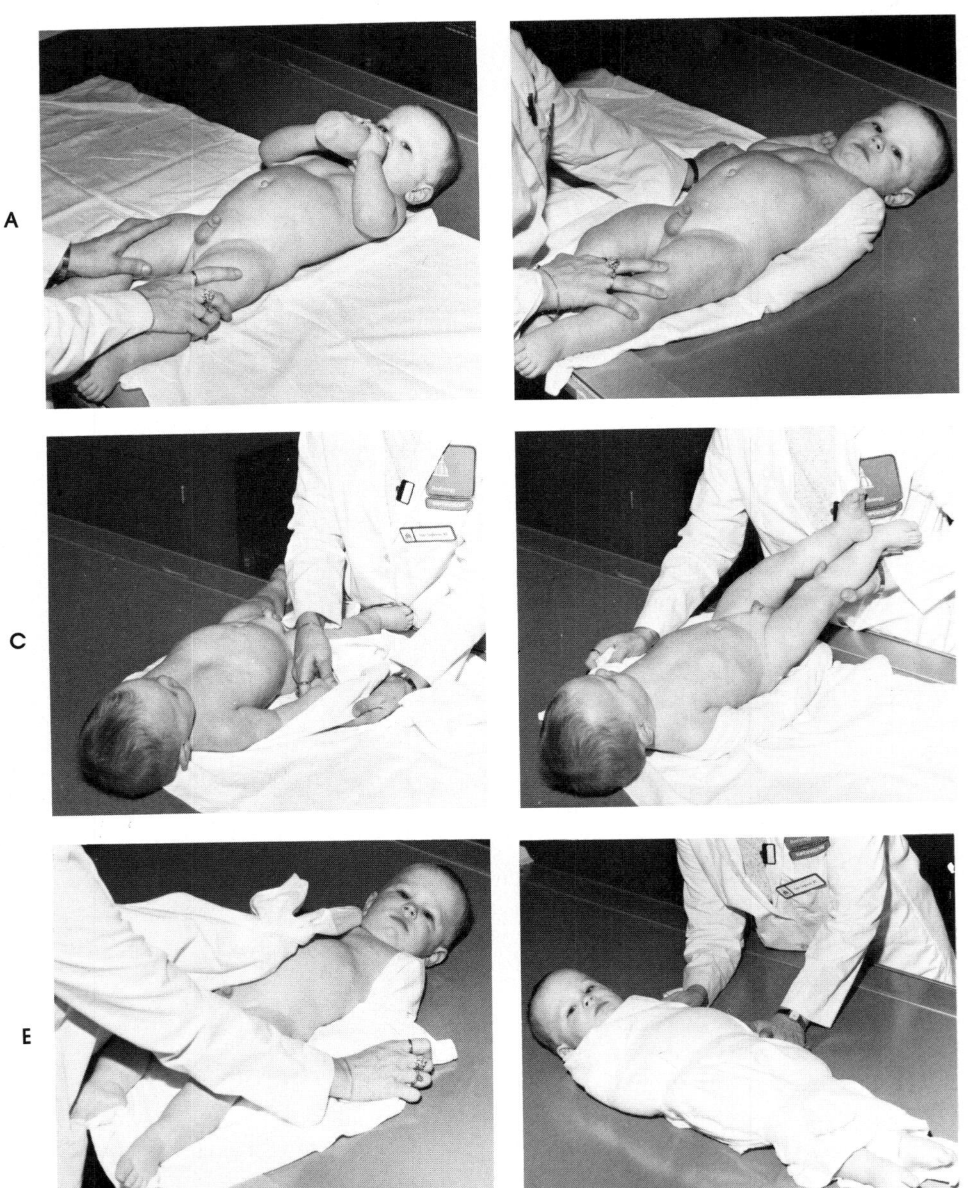

Fig. 25-3. Swaddling or "mummifying" an infant or young child. **A,** The child is placed in the center of a sheet folded lengthwise so that it extends from axillae to between the knees and ankles. **B,** One end of the sheet is brought over the child's left arm, under the body and pulled comfortably tight. **C,** The same end of the sheet is then brought over the child's right arm. **D,** It is brought back under the body and pulled comfortably tight. **E,** The other end of the sheet is now brought over the child, then under the child, and over again. **F,** Finally it is secured with three or four pieces of adhesive tape.

They can also be used to anchor the ends of a diaper or towel that is stretched over the child to hold him or her in the correct position. The long, floppy sandbags can take the place of a diaper or towel; the sand is run into the ends of the bag, which are placed on each side of the child, and the empty portion of the bag is stretched over the child.

Swaddling the body and limbs of an infant or young child is a gentle method of immobilization that is invaluable in certain situations. This method is demonstrated in Fig. 25-3. Since the result slightly resembles the wrapped mummy found when an Egyptian mummy case is opened, the technique is often referred to as *mummifying*. To immobilize a child for radiographs of an upper limb, that limb is left out of the swaddle. Similarly, for radiographs of the lower limbs only the body and upper limbs are swaddled.

Involuntary movement (for example, respiration) and small body movements are best minimized by *short exposures*. Even with equipment that permits exposures of 1 to 2 milliseconds (0.001 to 0.002 second), the technologist must make the exposure at the right instant, as explained in the following section.

Common Pediatric Examinations

CHEST RADIOGRAPHY

Infants and children younger than 4 years old are best examined supine (Fig. 25-4) unless a special device is used to hold them erect.[1] The arms are held next to the ears within a sleeve formed by a diaper, pillowcase, or orthopedic stockinette that passes behind the head. The legs and pelvis should be encased in a similar sleeve; this one may conveniently be made of stretch gauze bandage or elastic bandage *not* wrapped too tightly. For the frontal projection (Fig. 25-4, *A*), the patient is placed supine on the x-ray film cassette, a compression band is placed over the pelvis, and a second band or adhesive tape is used to immobilize the legs. The head and arms are cradled between two sandbags. The head must not be turned even slightly to the side because often this will oblique the chest. The head can be held straight by a head holder or by a length of cloth adhesive tape attached to paper adhesive tape on the child's forehead and to the sides of the x-ray table. For the lateral position, the supine child is elevated on a firm sponge or a low nonmetallic platform to minimize fogging the film by radiation scattered by the metallic edge of the x-ray table (Fig. 25-4, *B*). Lateral radiographs can also be obtained by turning the child onto his or her side and immobilizing the child in a manner similar to the positioning for the AP (Fig. 25-4, *C*).

[1]Poznanski AK: Practical approaches to pediatric radiology, Chicago, 1976, Year Book Medical Publishers, Inc, pp 30-34.

A

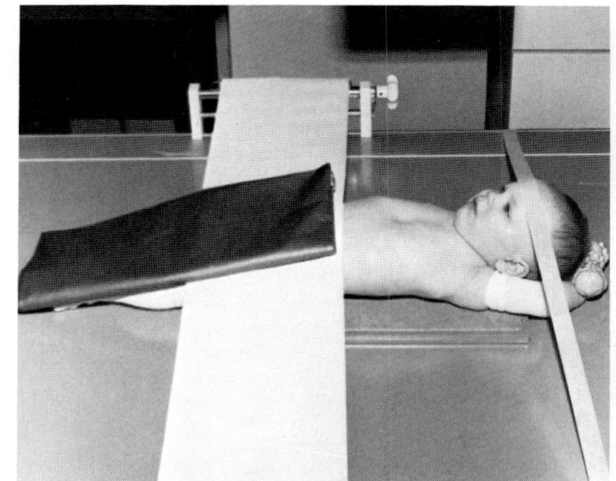

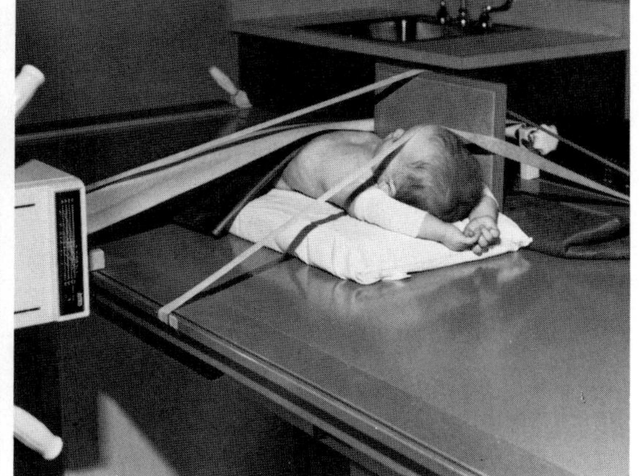

B

C

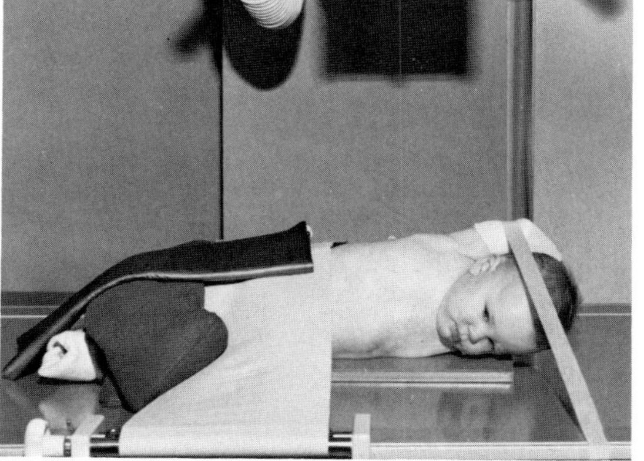

Fig. 25-4. Positioning for chest radiography. A sleeve, made in this instance from two layers of surgical stockinette, is passed over both arms and behind the head. A second sleeve of stockinette is pulled over the lower limbs and pelvis. A length of paper adhesive tape, which does not stick to the hair, is attached to the forehead and the edges of the x-ray table to hold the head straight. For added strength, a piece of cloth tape may be placed over the paper tape. A compression band is positioned to hold the child so that the attendant may leave the room. It is covered with a sheet of lead rubber for gonadal protection. If the child struggles, a sandbag may be placed tightly against each arm or a head clamp used. **A,** Position for AP radiograph. **B,** Position for lateral radiograph, using a horizontal x-ray beam. Note that the child is raised above the x-ray table to avoid scattered radiation from the metal edge of the table. In this instance the patient was placed on a decubitus sponge placed in a clean pillowcase. **C,** Alternative position for lateral radiograph. The positioning for a lateral decubitus chest radiograph is similar to that used for the abdomen (see Fig. 25-5).

Children who are old enough to stand straight for the examination, without turning to the side or twisting their bodies, and to take a deep breath when requested, yet young enough to be apprehensive, are best examined in the AP body position with their arms held over their heads. This is done so the patient may watch the technologist. Older children and adolescents may be examined in the PA or AP body position; the AP position delivers less radiation to the bone marrow but more to the thyroid and breasts.[1] It seems to work best if children and adolescents hold their arms over their heads or drape their arms over the x-ray cassette holder, since they often have trouble holding the usual adult position (hands on hips with elbows and shoulders rotated forward) as they take a deep breath.

Precise timing is especially important in chest radiography. *To obtain a radiograph showing deep inspiration of an infant or child too young to follow directions* the technologist should start the exposure at the beginning of expiration. This sounds paradoxical, yet it works because expiration is considerably longer than inspiration. The technologist watches the child breathe a number of times, moving his hand in time with the respirations. When the technologist sees the child take a deep breath, he makes the exposure at the instant that expiration starts. *If the child is on a respirator,* the technologist should watch the needle of the respirator and make the exposure the instant expiration begins.

[1]Archer BR et al: Bone marrow dose in chest radiography: the postero-anterior vs. anteroposterior projection, Radiology 133:211-216, 1979.

ABDOMINAL RADIOGRAPHY

Frontal radiographs of the abdomen should be made with the feet inverted about 20 degrees, which places the hips in a true AP position. Otherwise, positioning for a supine abdominal radiograph is much the same as for a supine chest radiograph (Fig. 25-5, *A*). There are a number of advantages to taking the frontal radiograph with the child prone (PA) (Fig. 25-5, *B*) rather than supine: (1) the air is redistributed in the colon so that (a) it is less likely to obscure the kidneys and adrenal glands and (b) it often becomes possible to exclude a bowel obstruction; (2) a small pneumoperitoneum may be recognized; and (3) duodenal obstruction may be disclosed.[1] The disadvantages are that young children may be frightened when placed prone and it is difficult to place the lead testicular shield correctly.

Abdominal radiographs of young children and infants standing or held erect are difficult to obtain. The left lateral decubitus position, made with the child's left side down and the x-ray beam horizontal (Fig. 25-5, *C*), is easily made and gives more information, since small amounts of free intraperitoneal air are more likely to be shown on the decubitus projection. When the child should not be turned on the side for some reason, an abdominal radiograph can be made using a horizontal x-ray beam while the child lies supine (Fig. 25-5, *D*). This radiograph will usually also show free intraperitoneal air when present, but it is frequently more difficult to interpret correctly than the left lateral decubitus projection. We have found it to be the most sensitive radiograph, however, when looking for free intraperitoneal air in a premature infant who has been lying supine.

[1]Berdon WE, Baker DH, and Leonidas J: Advantages of prone positioning in gastrointestinal and genitourinary radiographic studies in infants and children, Am J Roentgenol Radium Ther Nucl Med 103:444, 1968.

Except when examining premature infants, *all abdominal radiographs should be made with a stationary grid or a Potter-Bucky diaphragm.* Technologists inexperienced in pediatric radiology frequently think that an infant's or child's abdomen is so small that a grid is unnecessary, but radiation fog often obscures important detail on such radiographs.

When a newborn infant has an *anorectal malformation* (imperforate anus), it is important to determine whether the colon ends above or below the levator ani muscles. In the past this assessment was usually made on a lateral radiograph of the abdomen obtained with the infant held inverted and a lead marker placed on the anal dimple. This examination is seldom done today since most pediatric surgeons believe that physical examination provides a more accurate assessment of where the colon ends.[1]

[1]Berdon WE et al: A radiographic evaluation of imperforate anus: an approach correlated with current surgical concepts, Radiology 90:466-471, 1968.

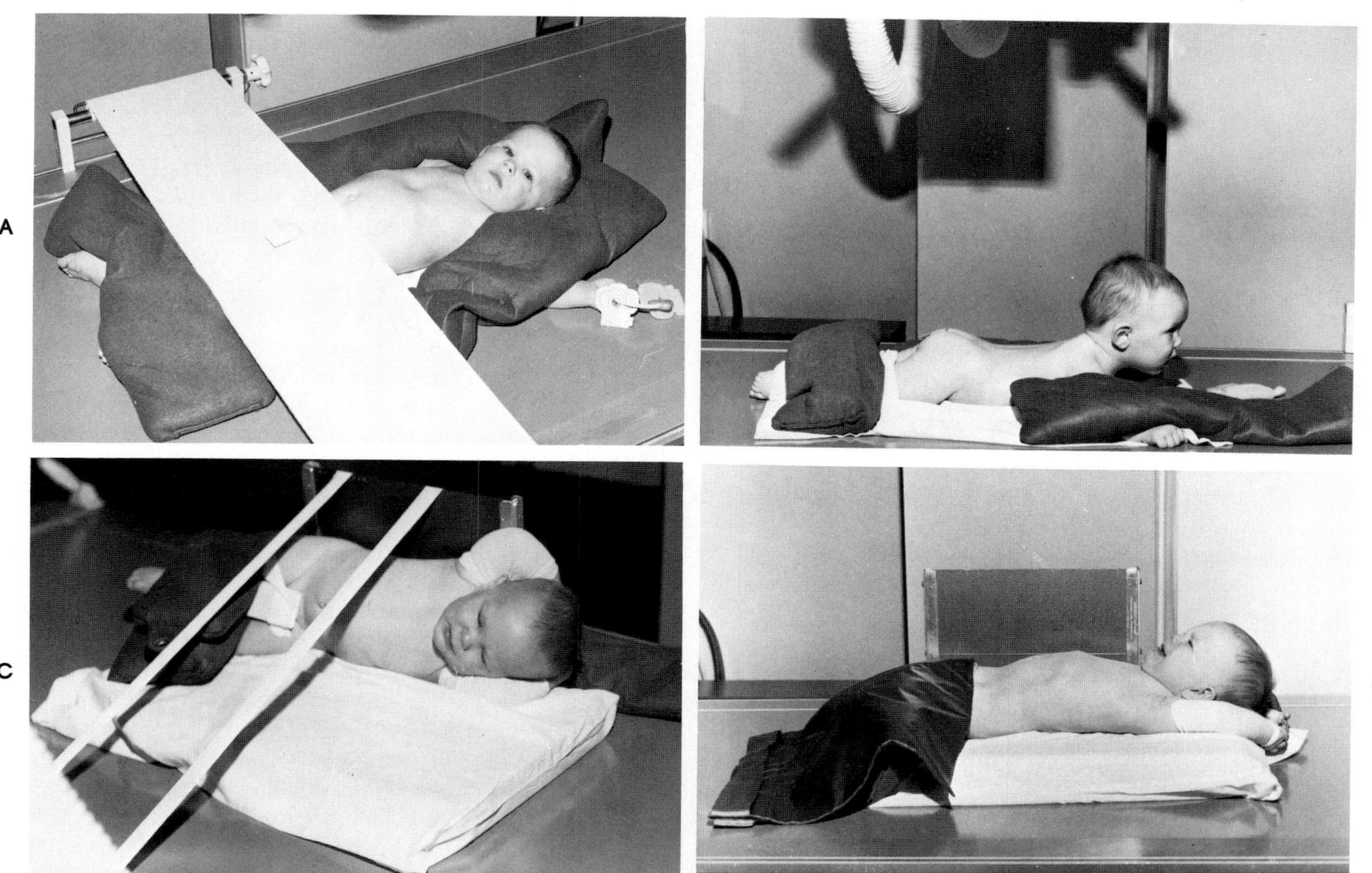

Fig. 25-5. Positioning for abdominal radiograph using long, floppy sandbags. Position for **A,** supine AP radiograph, **B,** prone PA radiograph, **C,** left lateral decubitus radiograph, and **D,** lateral abdomen radiograph using a horizontal x-ray beam. For two positions **(C** and **D),** the arms are immobilized beside the head using a sleeve formed of surgical stockinette, a diaper, or a towel. Note placement of gonadal shield on all illustrations.

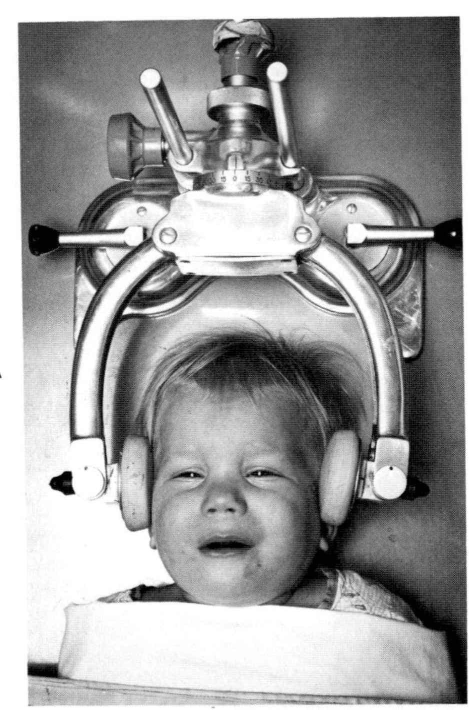

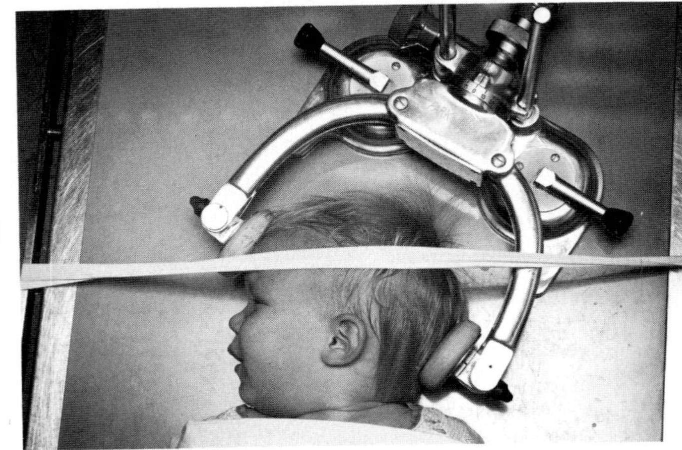

Fig. 25-6. Use of head clamps for frontal and lateral skull radiographs. The child has been swaddled and is held by a restraining band. On the lateral position, a length of adhesive tape secured to the edges of the x-ray table supplements the head clamp. The center of the tape has been twisted so that the adhesive does not touch the child and will not stick to his hair. **A,** AP, and **B,** lateral.

SKULL RADIOGRAPHY

Until a child is old enough to cooperate, skull radiography is best performed with the child supine on the radiographic table. If the infant or young child is swaddled as seen in Fig. 25-3 and secured between two long, firm sandbags with a compression band, it is relatively simple to position the head correctly and hold it with a head clamp (Fig. 25-6) or between two large, firm, clean sponges. A U-shaped sponge can also be employed (Fig. 25-7). A series of such sponges of various sizes can be fashioned, and they are also available commercially. Using such a sponge, the lateral skull radiograph is made using a horizontal x-ray beam (Fig. 25-7, *C*). Most technologists find it easier to obtain a perfect lateral radiograph using this technique than with a vertical x-ray beam (Fig. 25-6, *B*).

Compared to the size of the trunk, the skull of an infant or young child is relatively large. Lying supine, the neck is somewhat flexed. Consequently the x-ray tube needs to be angled less than the usual 30 degrees for the Towne radiograph. It should be angled so the plane of the central ray passes through the anterior hairline and the external auditory meatuses. For a true AP projection, the tube is angled somewhat cranially so the central ray is directed along the canthomeatal line. When the skull is deformed and asymmetric, best results usually are obtained if the skull is positioned with the line through the external auditory meatuses parallel to the tabletop for all frontal projections and perpendicular to the tabletop for all lateral images.

A

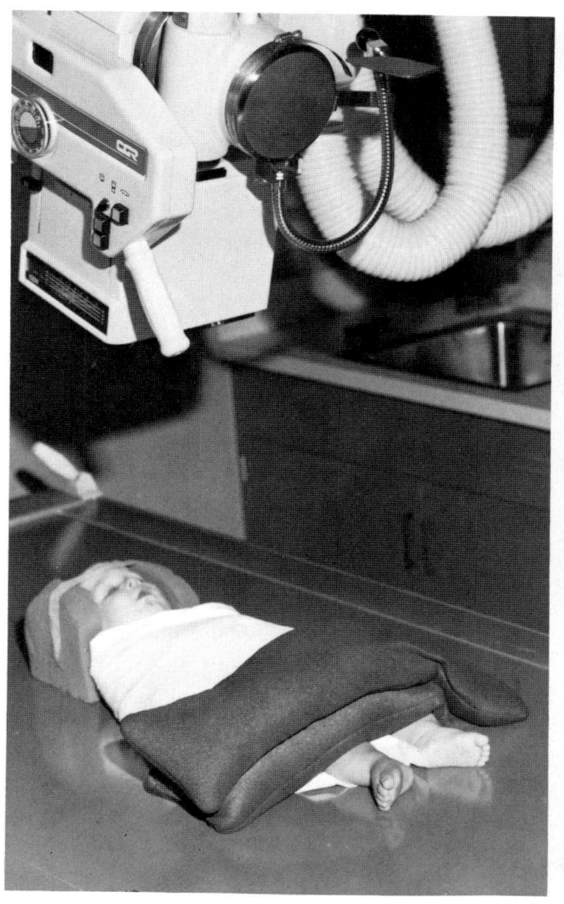

B

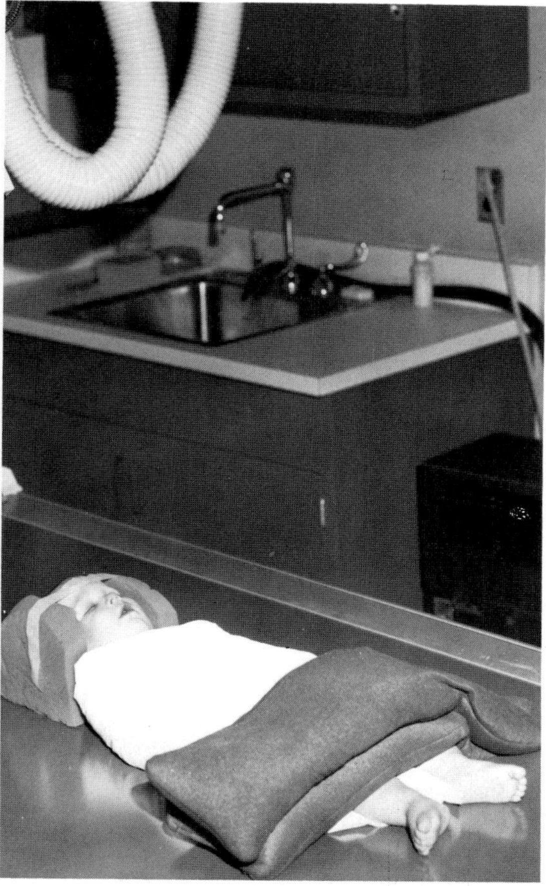

C

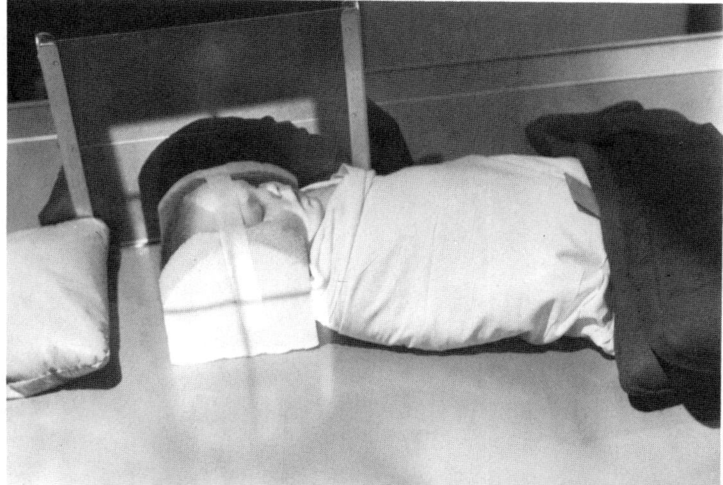

Fig. 25-7. Skull radiography using a U-shaped sponge, which has been pulled against the sides of the head by a length of paper adhesive tape. For additional immobilization a sandbag may be placed on each side of the sponge or a piece of adhesive tape used as seen in Fig. 25-6, *B*. The child has been swaddled and his lower limbs have been immobilized by two floppy sandbags. Positioning for, **A,** AP projection, **B,** AP axial (Towne) position, and **C,** lateral skull with horizontal central ray.

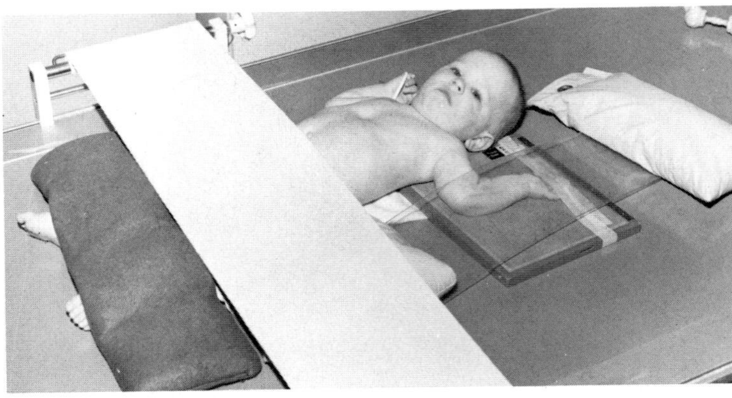

Fig. 25-8. Convenient position for making a single radiograph of the upper limb of an infant or young child. This position is useful when a single image of the limb is desired, even though it provides a *lateral* image of the humerus, elbow, and ulna but a *frontal* projection of the radius and hand. The limb is immobilized by a slightly flexible plastic panel weighted at each end by a sandbag. The rest of the infant may be immobilized in a variety of ways. Floppy sandbags and a compression band were used above. It is often necessary to hold the other upper limb under a floppy sandbag.

A

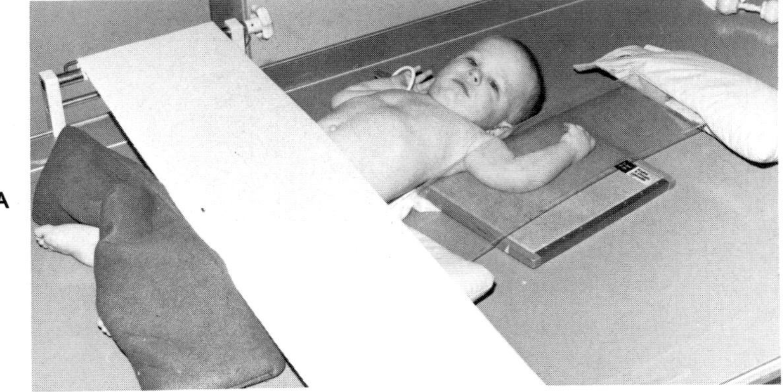

B

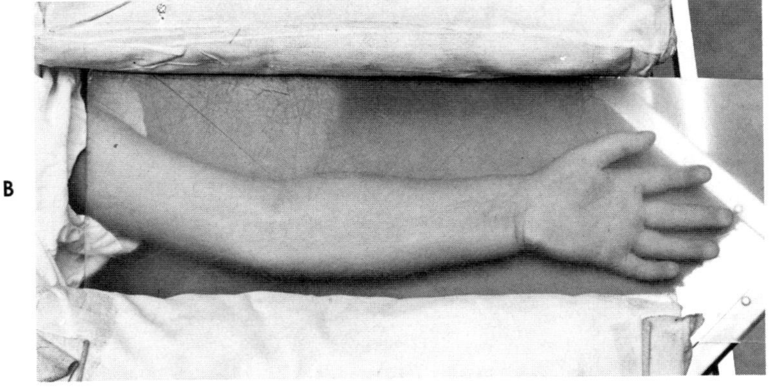

Fig. 25-9. Positioning for conventional projections of the upper limb. **A,** A lateral radiograph is obtained by abducting the shoulder 90 degrees, flexing the elbow 90 degrees, and placing the hand lateral. Sponges may be needed to hold the hand in position. The limb is immobilized beneath a slightly flexible plastic panel held at each end by a sandbag. **B,** A frontal (AP) radiograph is obtained by abducting the shoulder 90 degrees and keeping the elbow straight and the hand flat. The plastic panel is held in position by a long sandbag along each edge and a small sandbag distal to the hand (not shown on photograph). For both radiographs, the body and other limbs are immobilized as demonstrated.

LIMB RADIOGRAPHY

When the child is too young to cooperate, limbs can be held in position with a plastic panel held by sandbags (Figs. 25-8 to 25-10). A true lateral radiograph of the elbow or forearm may be obtained with a child supine if the arm is abducted 90 degrees, the elbow is flexed 90 degrees, and the lateral aspects of the forearm and hand are placed against the radiographic table as seen in Fig. 25-9, *A*.

An *examination for a possible fracture* requires special care. Rough handling can increase the displacement of the bone fragments, causing further damage to blood vessels and other soft tissues and possibly causing a portion of the bone to break the skin. While positioning the limb, the technologist must be sensitive to the child's responses and never *force* the limb into the desired position. If there is any question, only one exposure should be made. By using a horizontal x-ray beam or by putting the cassette in the Bucky tray, it is often possible to make this exposure without moving the limb. Otherwise, the technologists will have to lift the limb gently and slip the cassette underneath. If the radiologist or attending physician does not find a gross fracture on this first radiograph, additional exposures can be made with the limb properly positioned under the physician's supervision. The limb should be moved extremely slowly and gently into the desired positions, stopping if the child has more than mild pain.

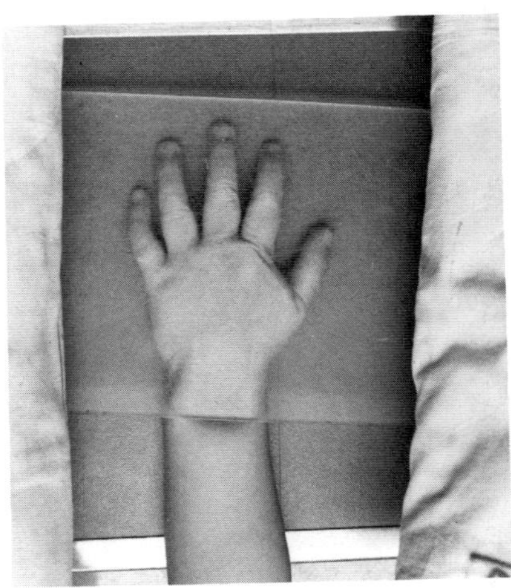

Fig. 25-10. Positioning for PA projection of hand and wrist. The hand is held by a plastic panel weighted at the ends by sandbags.

Table 25-1. Intravenous urography—dose of Conray 60, Hypaque 50, Renografin 60, and similar contrast agents

Weight of child (lb)	Dose of contrast agent
0-4	Use ultrasound if possible
5-15*	1 ml/lb*
16-50	1 ml/lb
51-100	50 ml
Over 100	0.5 ml/lb

*When small infants have heart disease, serious congenital abnormalities, chromosomal anomalies, or other serious illnesses, use another method to evaluate their urinary tracts when possible.
Data from Berdon WE: Pulmonary edema in infants who receive contrast media, Radiology 139:507, 1981.

INTRAVENOUS UROGRAPHY

Although infants and children should have an empty stomach at the start of an intravenous urogram, *they must not be permitted to become dehydrated*. Infants should be scheduled so the study is started at the time they would normally be fed. They may be fed after the contrast material has been injected and certainly should be fed if the examination lasts longer than 1 hour. Most young children tolerate going without fluids for 6 to 8 hours. The amount of contrast material injected is determined by the child's weight. Examples of dosage are listed in Table 25-1.

Positioning for the AP projection is the same as for the abdomen (Fig. 25-5, *A*). Oblique images are frequently useful. To minimize radiation to the gonads many of the radiographs made during intravenous urography can often be limited to the kidneys. Unless the history or radiographic findings indicate a reason to obtain more radiographs of the pelvis and urinary bladder, they are included on only two radiographs—the preliminary radiograph and one late radiograph.

FLUOROSCOPY

During fluoroscopic examinations of small children it is good practice to cover most of the radiographic tabletop with lead rubber (0.5 mm lead equivalent). Properly positioned, the lead will shield from radiation exposure the parts of the child one does not wish to examine and the people holding and feeding the child. For example, during a barium enema only the abdomen and pelvis are not protected by lead. Once the rectum and low sigmoid colon of a boy have been examined, he can be moved down slightly so that his testicles are shielded during the rest of fluoroscopy.

Special Pediatric Examinations

BONE AGE

Most children are evaluated using the Greulich and Pyle method[1] or the Tanner-Whitehouse 2 method.[2] Both methods require a single frontal radiograph of the left hand and wrist. The hand is placed palm down with the fingers slightly separated so that they do not touch and the thumb making an angle of about 30 degrees with the second metacarpal. The SID is 30 inches, and the x-ray tube is centered to the head of the third metacarpal.[2]

For children younger than 3 years of age, the Sontag, Snell, and Anderson method, modified to minimize gonadal radiation, can be used.[3] The following radiographs are needed: (1) an AP projection of the left humerus that includes the distal one half of the clavicle, the shoulder, and the elbow, (2) a PA projection of the left hand and wrist, (3) AP and lateral images of the left knee, and (4) AP and lateral images of the left foot and ankle. If the radiologist is available to check the radiographs before the child leaves the department, (3) and (4) are modified. A single lateral position of the knee and a single oblique image of the foot and ankle are made and checked by the radiologist to determine whether an AP projection of the knee or an additional projection of the foot and ankle is needed.

[1]Greulich WW and Pyle SI: Radiographic atlas of skeletal development of the hand and wrist, ed 2, Stanford, Calif, 1959, Stanford University Press.
[2]Tanner JM et al: Assessment of skeletal maturation and prediction of adult height (TW2 method), New York, 1975, Academic Press, Inc.
[3]Schuberth KC, and Zitelli J, editors: The Harriet Lane handbook, ed 8, Chicago, 1978, Year Book Medical Publishers, Inc, pp 261-262.

CLUBFOOT RADIOGRAPHY

For a description of positioning to demonstrate clubfoot deformity, see Volume 1, Chapter 6, Figs. 6-67 to 6-75 of this atlas.

TRACHEA AND LARYNX

Radiographic studies of the trachea and larynx are obtained to evaluate acute and chronic upper respiratory problems in infants and children. Examples of acute problems include croup and acute epiglottitis; the most common chronic problems are complications of previous endotracheal intubation. Children with either type of problem can suddenly develop severe respiratory distress during the examination. They must be watched carefully at all times. Restraints should be used only if necessary and removed immediately if there is any evidence of increased respiratory difficulty. If a child is examined for possible *acute epiglottitis* a single soft tissue lateral image is made of the neck centering on the larynx with the *child sitting erect and the physician in attendance*. Only if evaluation of this radiograph shows no evidence of epiglottitis is it safe to proceed with the usual study (below), and the child must be watched particularly carefully for any evidence of increasing distress.

AP projections

A special Thoraeus filter of 0.40 mm tin, 0.50 mm copper, and 0.75 mm or 1.0 mm aluminum is placed in front of the x-ray collimator for the frontal, but not for the lateral, radiographs. The *tin side of the filter must face the x-ray tube,* and the aluminum side must face the patient. Exposures are made using as high kilovoltage as is available—140 kVp probably is optimum.[1]

[1]Joseph PM et al: Upper airway obstruction in infants and small children: improved radiographic diagnosis by combining filtration, high kilovoltage and magnification, Radiology 121:143, 1976.

Correct positioning is critical. The child is placed supine with the shoulders supported by a folded sheet or a sandbag to extend the neck so that a line joining the inferior aspect of the body of the mandible and the most inferior portion of the occipital bone (which can be identified fairly well by palpation) is perpendicular to the x-ray film. The central ray is centered just below the larynx if the examination is limited to the cervical airway; it is centered to the suprasternal notch if the examination includes the larynx, all of the trachea, and the central bronchi.

Two radiographs are taken, one with the patient phonating (crying or saying a word such as "see" for as long as possible) and the second during inspiration.

Lateral position

The patient is not moved. The Thoraeus filter is removed, and the x-ray tube is positioned for a horizontal beam lateral exposure of the neck. The cassette is positioned vertically beside the neck. A soft tissue technique is used for this position, which is best made during phonation. It should *not* be made as the child swallows.

DEFECOGRAPHY

Defecography is used principally to evaluate the rectum and anal canal of children who are incontinent of feces, especially children who previously had surgical repair of an anorectal malformation (imperforate anus) or Hirschsprung's disease. The child is examined while sitting on a radiolucent potty or toilet seat. Barium paste is smeared on the anal verge, and the enema tube is inserted. The tube is not secured to the patient but held in place by means of a long sponge forceps. Barium is run in, and, when the child indicates a desire to defecate, the enema tube is removed. The child is told to start defecating, stop, and start again as a recording is made on videotape. The examination sometimes is repeated, with one fluoroscopic spot radiograph made as the child defecates and another after he or she stops.[1] An excellent modification of this technique using a semisolid contrast material has been described by Poznanski.[2]

[1]Kelly JH: Cine radiography in anorectal malformations, J Pediatr Surg 4:538-546, 1969.
[2]Poznanski AK: The use of a semisolid contrast medium in defecography, Radiology 97:82, 1970.

Final Thought

This chapter has a number of hints and suggestions about ways to make friends with children at the same time as one makes radiographs of them. The best teachers, however, are the children themselves. If we carefully observe how their faces and bodies respond to what we do and say, they will teach us the best ways to do our work.

Technologists who make the effort to learn from children will find working with them a richly rewarding experience.

SELECTED BIBLIOGRAPHY

Gyll C, Blake NS, and Thornton A: Paediatric diagnostic imaging, New York, 1986, John Wiley & Sons.

Wilmot DM and Sharko GA: Pediatric imaging for the technologist, New York, 1987, Springer-Verlag.

Chapter 26

TOMOGRAPHY

JEFFREY A. BOOKS

Since its inception in the 1890s, radiography has presented the problem of trying to record accurately three-dimensional body structures on two-dimensional films. This unavoidably results in the superimposition of structures, which often obscures important diagnostic information. One familiar method used to attempt to overcome this problem is the technique of right-angle images. Over the years many other techniques have been developed that partially circumvent the problem of superimposition, such as multiple radiographs, stereoscopic images, and subtraction techniques in angiography.

The partial or complete elimination of obscuring shadows by the effect of motion on shadow formation is a common technique used in radiography. This effect is frequently used with conventional projections. For example, in conjunction with a long exposure time, breathing motion is used to reduce rib and pulmonary shadows to a background blur on frontal images of the sternum and on lateral radiographs of the thoracic spine.

Body-section radiography, or more appropriately tomography, is a term used to designate the radiographic technique with which most of the problems of superimposed images are overcome.

*Tomography** is the term used to designate the technique whereby a predetermined plane of the body is demonstrated in focus on the radiograph. Other body structures above or below the plane of interest are eliminated from the image or are rendered as a low-density blur caused by motion.

The origin of tomography cannot be attributed to any one person; in fact, tomography was developed by several different gifted individuals experimenting in different countries at about the same time without any knowledge of each other's work.

*All italicized words are defined at the end of this chapter.

In 1921 one of the early pioneers in tomography, a French dermatologist, Dr. André-Edmund-Marie Bocage, described in an application for a patent many of the principles used in modern tomographic equipment. Many other early investigators made significant contributions to the field of tomography. Each of these pioneers applied a different name to his particular device or process of body-section radiography. Bocage (1922) termed the result of his process moving film roentgenograms; the Italian Vallebona (1930) chose the term *stratigraphy;* the Dutch physician Ziedses des Plantes (1932) who made several significant contributions called his process *planigraphy*. The term *tomography* came from the German investigator Grossman as does the *Grossman principle,* which will be discussed later in this section. Tomography was invented in the United States in 1928 by Jean Kieffer, a radiologic technologist, who developed the special radiographic technique to demonstrate a form of tuberculosis that he had. His process was termed *laminagraphy* by another American, J. Robert Andrews, who assisted Kieffer in the construction of his first tomographic device, the laminagraph.[1]

A great deal of confusion arose over the many different names given to the general process of body-section radiography. To eliminate this confusion the International Commission of Radiological Units and Standards appointed a committee in 1962 to select a single term to represent all of the processes. *Tomography* is the term that the committee chose, and it is this term that is now recognized throughout the medical community as the single appropriate term for all forms of body-section radiography.[2]

[1]Littleton JT: Tomography: physical principles and clinical application, Baltimore, 1976, The Williams & Wilkins Co, pp 1-13.

[2]Vallebona A and Bistolfi F: Modern thin-section tomography, Springfield, Ill, 1973, Charles C Thomas, Publisher.

In tomography, as in conventional radiography, there are three basic requirements: an x-ray source, an object, and a recording medium (film). However, in tomography, to create an image of a single plane of tissue a fourth requirement must be met—synchronous movement of two of the three essential elements during the x-ray exposure. This is achieved by moving the x-ray source and film in opposing directions about the stationary patient. The basic tomographic blurring principle is demonstrated in Fig. 26-1. At the beginning of the exposure the tube and film are at positions T_1 and F_1, respectively. During the exposure the tube and film travel in opposite directions, and their movements are terminated at the end of the exposure at positions T_2 and F_2. The *focal plane* is at the level of the axis of rotation or the *fulcrum* and is considered parallel with the tabletop. Structures at the same level of the focal plane remain in focus, whereas structures in other planes above and below this level are blurred from view. Tomography may be thought of as a process of controlled blurring. Note that the object located at point B is projected at the right side of the film at the beginning of the exposure. Next observe that at the end of the exposure the relative position of the projected object has now moved to the left of the film. Since this is not a static image but a dynamic one, this structure is now nothing more than a blurred density on the film. An object at point A located at the level of the focal plane, however, is projected at the same place on the film throughout the entire exposure and therefore is not blurred but remains in focus. It is important to realize that the sharpness of detail of the structures demonstrated in the focal plane is not enhanced in tomography. Tomography is a process of controlled blurring. Therefore the focal plane structures are merely less blurred than the focal plane structures.

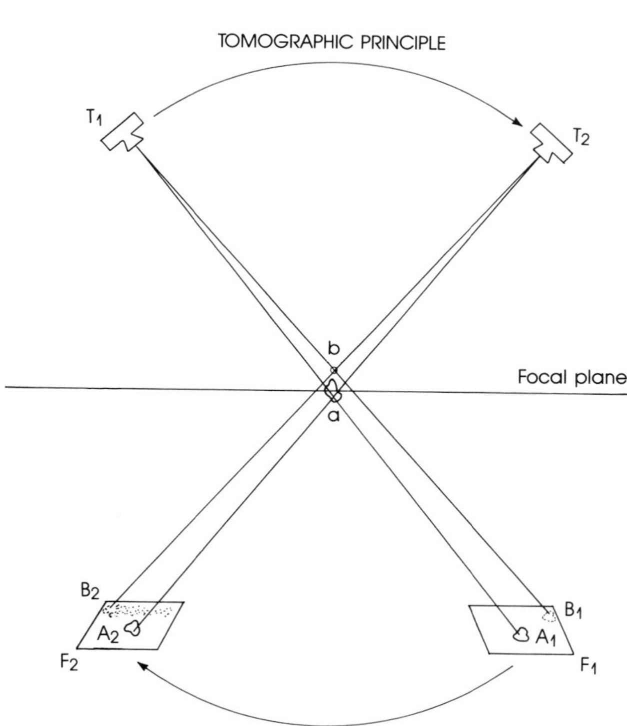

Fig. 26-1. X-ray tube *(T)*, focal plane (patient), and x-ray film *(F)*.

Tomographic sections at different fulcrum heights may be obtained by altering the level of the focal plane. This may be accomplished by one of two methods, depending on the principle utilized in the design of the tomographic device. These two principles, the *planigraphic principle* and the *Grossman principle,* are the basis of all modern tomographic equipment (Fig. 26-2). The Grossman principle utilizes a fixed fulcrum system in which the axis of rotation, or the fulcrum, remains at a fixed height. The focal plane level is changed by raising and lowering the tabletop and patient through this fixed point to the desired height. In contrast, the planigraphic principle utilizes an adjustable fulcrum system (Fig. 26-3). The actual fulcrum or pivot point is raised or lowered to the height of the desired focal plane level, whereas the tabletop and patient remain stationary at a fixed height.

The *exposure angle* (Fig. 26-4) is that angle of arc that is described by the movement of the tube and film during the tomographic exposure. The width of the focal plane or the plane of tissue that is in maximum focus is called the *section thickness* (Fig. 26-5). The thickness of the tomographic section may be changed by altering the exposure angle. Tomograms using wide exposure angles will demonstrate thin sections; conversely, smaller exposure angles will demonstrate comparatively thicker sections.

The range of section thickness produced by wide-angle tomography is approximately from 1 to 5 mm, and that with narrow-angle tomography, or zonography, is from slightly less than 1 cm to about 2.5 cm. *Zonography,* or the tomographic technique used to demonstrate relatively thick sections or zones of tissue, was first described by Zeidses des

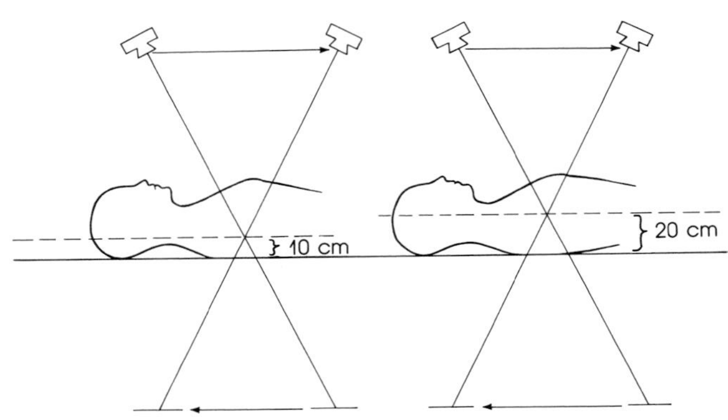

Fig. 26-2. Planigraphic principle (adjustable fulcrum). Pivot point height is changed to alter fulcrum level.

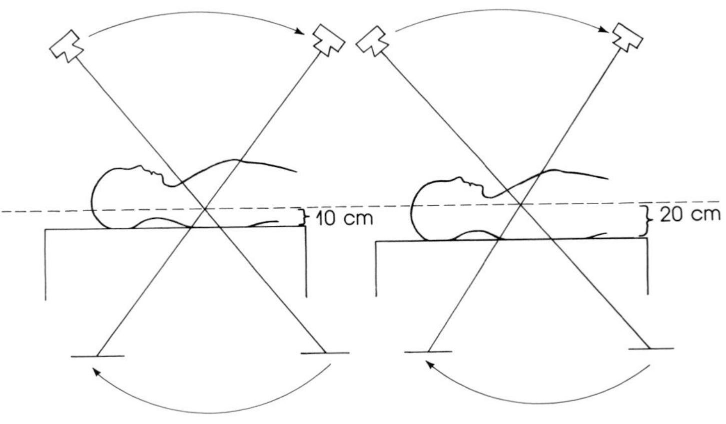

Fig. 26-3. Grossman principle (fixed fulcrum). Tabletop height is changed to alter fulcrum level.

Plantes, who recommended it for examining sections of the cranium and the spinal column. Zonography is now used for a number of other regions and is particularly useful in tomographic examinations of the abdominal structures.

The degree to which definition decreases with distance from the focal plane is dependent on the width of the angle described by the tube motion. This depends on the width of the angle described by the tube. Wide angles of the tube movement provide excellent blurring of structures close to the focal plane, as well as of those remote from it. Narrow angles of tube movement provide excellent blurring of structures remote from the focal plane but only moderate to slight blurring of structures close to the focal zone.

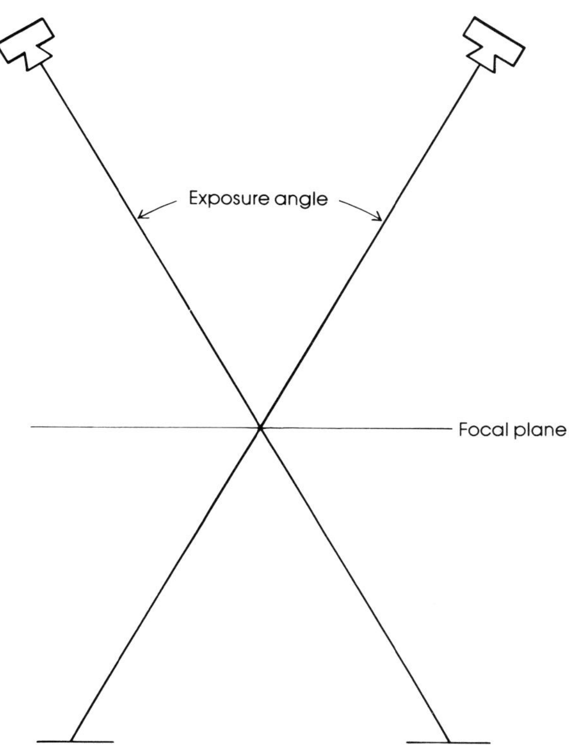

Fig. 26-4. Exposure angle.

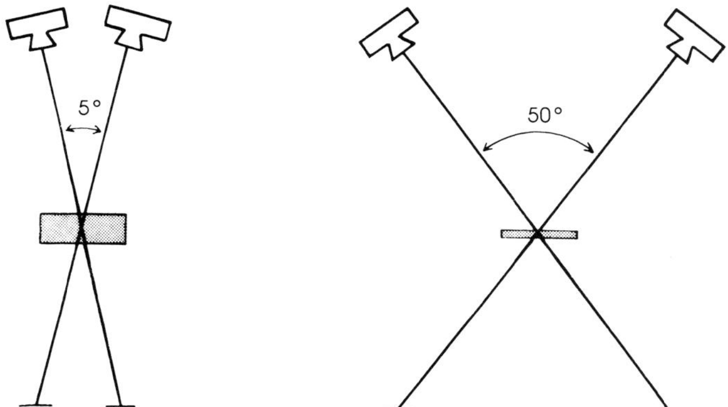

Fig. 26-5. Narrow exposure angles yield thick tomographic sections; wide exposure angles yield thin tomographic sections.

Although visibility of the objective area is greatly enhanced by the partial or complete elimination of obscuring shadows, the appearance of the tomogram is quite different from that of a conventional radiograph. The customary sharp definition and clear contrast are diminished, and the contours of all but the thinnest structures are absent. The contrast is reduced because of the blurring action diffusing elements in other planes over the focal plane image. This creates an overall increase in the density on the tomogram that results in an overall decrease in contrast in the structures demonstrated. The formation of the tomographic image is a cumulative process. The shadows of structures in the plane of focus accumulate on the film as the area traversed by the beam of radiation swings over the arc. The images are not sharp, since the radiation traverses structures from many angles, outlining clearly only those boundaries to which it is momentarily tangential in its passage.

Zonograms are comparable in appearance to conventional radiographs, because (1) the cuts are thick enough to show structural contours; (2) the narrow arc described by the tube directs the radiation at only slightly oblique angles, so that it projects structural contours more nearly true to shape; and (3) because of less blurring, contrast and detail are superior to those of the tomograms. However, this is not to say that there is more diagnostic information in a zonogram than in a wide-angle tomogram; each has its place in tomography. The choice between using a wide or narrow exposure angle primarily depends on the thickness of the structure or structures to be in the tomogram and their proximity to other structures outside the focal plane.

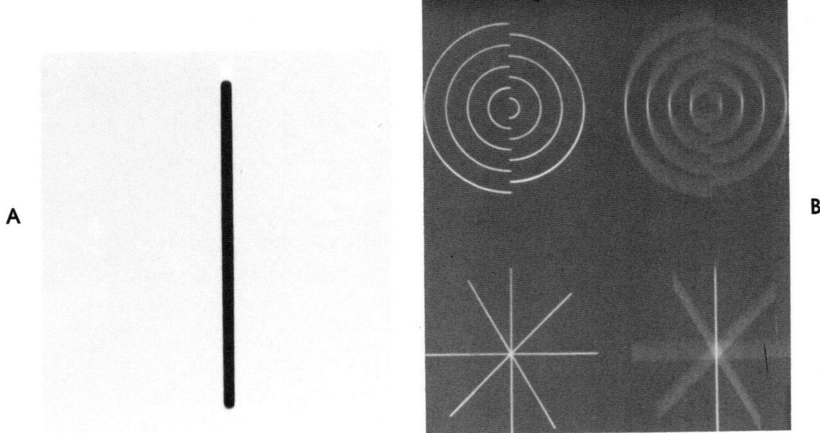

Fig. 26-6. A, Pinhole tracing of 45-degree longitudinal linear motion. B, Tomogram of test object at 45-degree longitudinal linear motion. Left pattern is at level of focal plane. Right pattern is 5 mm above level of focal plane. With linear motion the best blurring occurs to elements of test object oriented perpendicular to movement of tube and the least blurring to elements oriented parallel.

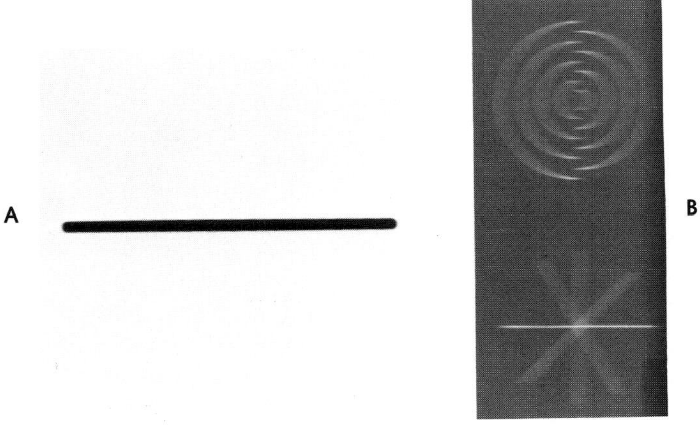

Fig. 26-7. A, Pinhole tracing of 45-degree transverse linear motion. B, Tomogram of test object at 45-degree transverse linear motion.

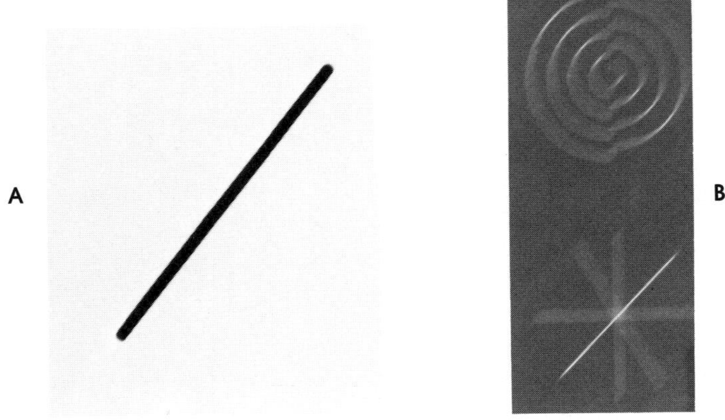

Fig. 26-8. A, Pinhole tracing of 45-degree oblique linear motion. B, Tomogram of test object at 45-degree oblique linear motion.

Blurring Motions

Modern tomographic equipment offers a variety of different blurring patterns. These blurring motions fall under two separate categories: *unidirectional,* or *linear,* and *pluridirectional,* or *complex, motions,* which include circular, elliptical, hypocycloidal, and spiral motions. A basic understanding of the characteristics of these blurring patterns is necessary for understanding their advantages as well as their limitations.

LINEAR MOTION

The basic tomographic blurring pattern is the undirectional, or linear, motion. The blurring action of linear motion is provided by elongation of structures outside of the focal plane so that they become indistinguishable linear streaks or blurs over the focal plane image. Maximum blurring occurs to those elements of structures outside the focal plane that are oriented perpendicular to the relative motion of the tube (Figs. 26-6 to 26-8). In linear tomography, therefore, elements of structures oriented parallel to the motion of the tube are incompletely blurred and can form false shadows over the focal plane image. This results in an inaccurate representation of the focal plane because of the summation of the focal plane image and images of some structures outside the plane of focus. This characteristic is demonstrated in the following tomogram of a test object.

The test object consists of two wire patterns: pattern 1 is located at the level of the focal plane (left-hand image in Fig. 26-6, *B*); pattern 2 (right-hand image) is 5 mm away from the level of the focal plane and therefore exhibits the effects of the blurring motion used.

The best blurring occurs to those elements of the patterns that are perpendicular to the tube movement, and the least occurs to those parallel. In linear tomography it is important to orient those structures to be blurred at right angles to the tube movement. For example, in tomography of the chest the tube movement is oriented perpendicularly to the ribs for maximum blurring of those structures.

A more efficient blurring motion would be one in which all of the elements of an object would be perpendicular to the movement of the tube at some time during the exposure. This is the principle of the second type of blurring motion, the multidirectional, or pluridirectional, motion.

CIRCULAR MOTION

The basic pluridirectional motion is the circular pattern (Fig. 26-9). The circular motion does not blur by mere elongation as in linear motion but by evenly diffusing the densities of those structures outside the focal plane over the focal plane image. Tomograms using a circular or any other complex motion therefore exhibit more even but less contrast than do linear tomograms with their characteristic linear streaking. Note that all elements of the test pattern are equally blurred regardless of their orientation. The circular motion maintains a constant radius and angle throughout the exposure, which results in a sharp cutoff margin of the blurred structures. This in turn may result in the formation of phantom images superimposed over the focal plane image.

The phenomenon of phantom images occurs more often in circular tomography using small angles as in circular zonography. The phantom images are created by the fusion of the margins of the blurred shadows of structures slightly outside the focal plane or by annular shadows of dense structures again slightly outside the focal plane.

These phantom images are usually less dense and distinct than the actual focal plane images. They can be identified as such on successive tomograms as the real structure or structures come into focus.

The characteristics of wide-angle circular tomography are identical to small-angle circular tomography, with one exception. The wider angle results in greater displacement of the blurred shadows, reducing the possibility of phantom image formation.

ELLIPTICAL MOTION

The elliptical motion, having both linear and circular aspects to the pattern, exhibits blurring characteristics of both (Fig. 26-10). It requires the same perpendicular orientation as the linear motion and exhibits similar phantom shadow characteristics to both the linear and circular motions. Although it is a more efficient blurring motion than the simple linear motion, the quality of blur is much less than the circular motion or the more complex motions, *hypocycloidal* and *spiral motion*.

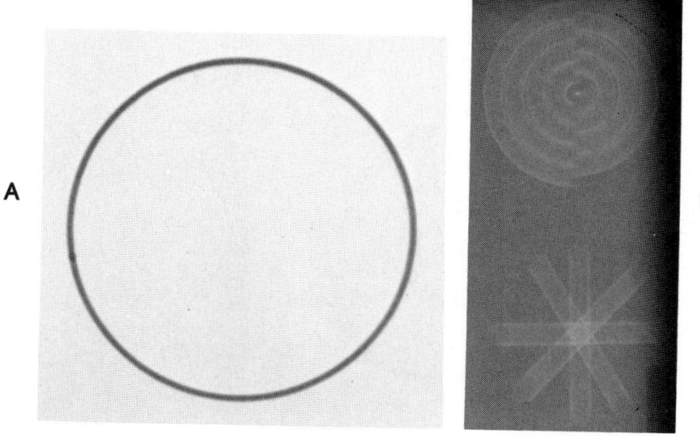

Fig. 26-9. Circular motion of 45 degrees. **A,** Pinhole tracing. **B,** Tomogram of test object demonstrating annular shadow formation and fusion of marginal blur pattern—characteristics of circular motion.

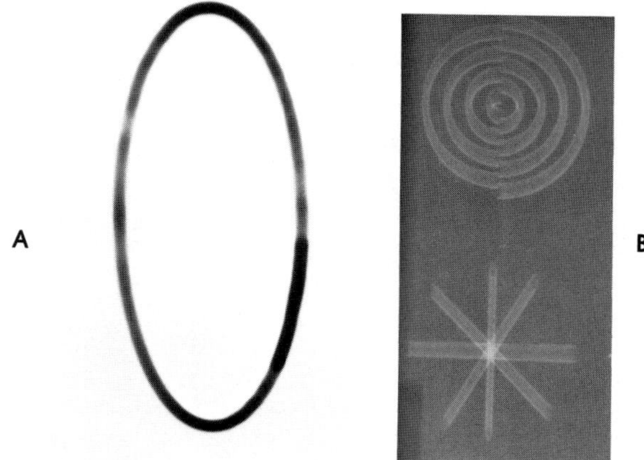

Fig. 26-10. Elliptical motion. **A,** Pinhole tracing. **B,** Tomogram of test object demonstrating characteristics of both linear and circular motions.

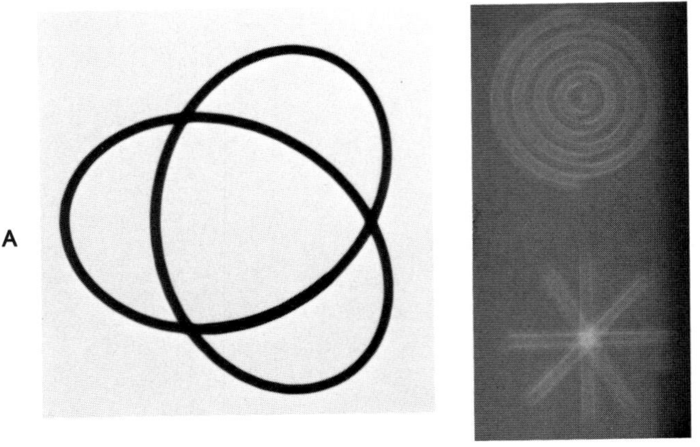

Fig. 26-11. Hypocycloidal motion. **A,** Pinhole tracing. **B,** Tomogram of test object demonstrating excellent blurring characteristics.

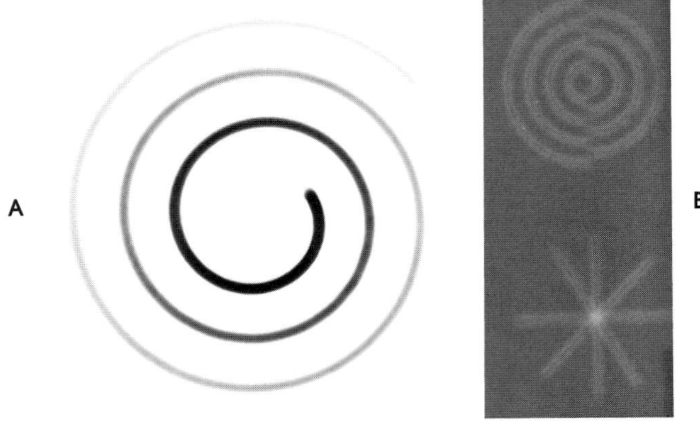

Fig. 26-12. Trispiral motion. **A,** Pinhole tracing. **B,** Tomogram of test object demonstrating excellent blurring characteristics.

HYPOCYCLOIDAL MOTION

The hypocycloidal motion offers excellent displacement of the marginal blur pattern, nearly eliminating the possibility of phantom image formation (Fig. 26-11). It provides excellent blurring of structures both close to and remote from the focal plane and has a focal plane thickness of slightly less than 1 mm.

SPIRAL MOTION

Tomographic equipment capable of producing a spiral motion is usually designed for a three-spired motion or a five-spired motion (Fig. 26-12). The spiral motion, although different in pattern from the hypocycloidal motion, also offers excellent displacement of the marginal blur pattern, exceptional resolving power, and an extremely thin section thickness of less than 1 mm.

These excellent blurring characteristics make both the hypocycloidal and spiral motion useful in examinations of any area of the body, and they are especially useful in tomographic examinations of the skull, where structures are very small and compact and require greater separation of tissue planes (Fig. 26-13).

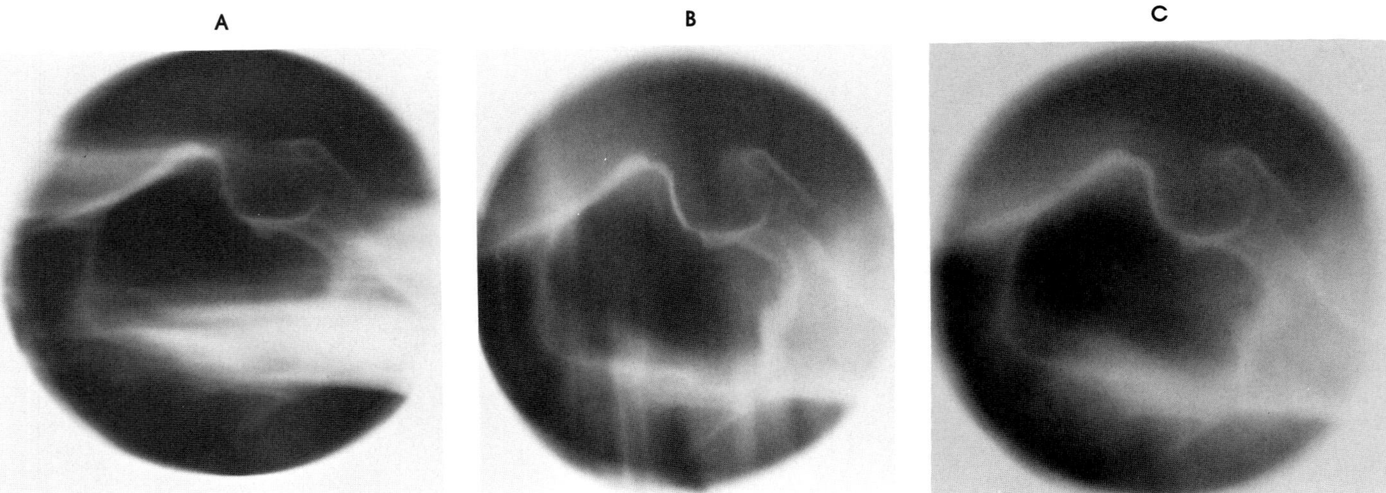

Fig. 26-13. Tomograms of sella turcica in lateral position through midplane. **A,** Transverse linear motion. **B,** Longitudinal transverse motion. **C,** Trispiral motion demonstrating the sella turcica much more clearly and without parasitic linear streaking that is found in **A** or **B.**

Factors Affecting Tomographic Image

"The difference between a high quality tomogram and a poor one is very slight; hence, it is extremely important that attention be given to all the parameters which contribute to the focal plane image."[1] The factors that affect the tomographic image can be divided into two categories: (1) patient variables and (2) equipment variables.

PATIENT VARIABLES

As in conventional radiography, proper positioning of the patient and centering of the central ray are of critical importance. Another and equally important factor that must be considered in tomography is the selection of the proper focal plane level. The part must be adequately immobilized because any motion will add unwanted blur to the focal plane image. Object size and the relative density of structures will affect density and contrast of the image.

EQUIPMENT VARIABLES

The tomographic principle utilized will affect several different properties of the image, with magnification being affected the most. Tomographic machines utilizing the *fixed fulcrum,* or Grossman, principle will maintain a constant magnification factor at any focal plane level because the distance between the focal plane and the film remains the same at any level. Conversely, with the *adjustable fulcrum,* or planigraphic, system, the focal plane–film distance changes as the fulcrum height is varied, resulting in different magnification of the focal plane image at different fulcrum heights. This magnification is, however, at most working levels, less than the fixed rate of magnification of the fixed fulcrum machines.

The degree to which structures outside the focal plane are blurred is a function of the geometry of the blurring pattern and the angle of the tomographic arc. The more complex the blurring pattern is, the greater the effacement will be of those structures outside the focal plane. Wide exposure angles provide greater blurring of structures close to the focal plane as well as those that are remote. The exposure angle also determines the thickness of the focal plane image. As previously mentioned, the wider the exposure angle, the thinner the section thickness will be, and, conversely, the narrower the exposure angle, the thicker the section thickness.

Each blurring pattern requires a specific amount of time to complete its motion. Therefore the exposure time must be of sufficient length to allow completion of the motion before terminating the exposure. Linear motions generally take less time to complete than do the more complex pluridirectional movements. Exposure time is one half of the mAs formula, but, since there are restrictions for certain exposure times for each different pattern, the mA and kV must be altered to change the density. Since contrast levels are inherently low in tomography, high mAs and relatively low kV techniques are used in most examinations to enhance the contrast between structures.

Collimating to the smallest possible field size also improves the contrast of the image.

The focal spot size will affect the detail of the focal plane image. In areas in which great detail is required, such as the skull, cervical spine, and extremities, the smallest available focal spot should be used. In other areas, fine detail may not be required; therefore, to prolong the life of the x-ray tube, the large focal spot should be used when possible. Extreme care must be taken not to exceed the recommended tube limits or cooling rate.

Tomographic machines must provide synchronous, vibration-free movement of the tube and film because any mechanical instability may transmit unwanted motion and create additional blur to the focal plane image. For this reason, most manufacturers have designed tomographic equipment to begin the exposure after the motion has begun, allowing enough time for any unwanted motion and vibration to be stabilized that may have been caused by the rapid acceleration of the tube and film. The exposure is then terminated just before the end of the movement to avoid any motion that may occur during the rapid deceleration of the tube and film.

Since the thicknesses of cassettes vary with each manufacturer, one type of cassette should be used throughout the entire examination. Otherwise, the focal plane images will not be successively consistent from level to level because the height of the film and therefore the focal plane image will vary with each different cassette used.

The film-screen combination will greatly affect the tomographic image. Very low speed film-screen combinations will produce images with very good detail, but they require a prohibitive amount of radiation. A faster combination produces images with good detail and contrast with much less radiation. Other combinations using rare earth screens are available that produce films with excellent detail but slightly lower contrast.

Equipment

Tomography machines may be varied in appearance and function, but all have three basic requirements in common. Aside from the usual features of any radiographic machine, such as an x-ray source, timer, and mA and kVp selector, any x-ray machine capable of producing a tomographic image must have the following additional features: (1) the machine must have some type of linkage connecting the x-ray source and film carriage that will provide synchronous, vibration-free movement of the tube and film in opposite directions during the tomographic exposure; (2) there must be a means of imparting motion to the tube and film carriage for each different tomographic movement; and (3) there must be a means of adjusting the fulcrum height for tomograms at different levels.

As the x-ray tube moves in one direction, the film carriage will always move in the opposite direction. The film will move synchronously with the movement of the tube, maintaining a constant relationship with each other as they move. This mechanical type of linkage is the basic type of linkage that most tomographic machines utilize, from the simplest machines to the highly sophisticated pluridirectional units. The major difference between the two is that in the multidirectional machines the simple metal rod is replaced by a heavier metal beam or a parallelogram of thick rods that attach at either end to the x-ray tube and film carriage. The heavier material used for the linkage is required to withstand the great centrifugal force created by the tube and film carriage as it swings rapidly through the complex motions.

[1]Littleton JT: Tomography: physical principles and clinical application, Baltimore, 1976, The Williams & Wilkins Co, p 33.

There is another type of linkage that has been made possible by advances in computer technology. One manufacturer has developed a radiographic machine capable of linear tomography with no direct mechanical linkage between the tube and film carriage. The x-ray tube is mounted on the ceiling and is electronically linked to the film carriage through a microcomputer. The microcomputer controls separate drive motors that maintain the tube and film in alignment throughout the linear motion. This revolutionary design allows for greater mobility of the x-ray tube for radiographic examinations since it is free floating when not in the tomographic mode, which makes it much more versatile than the standard radiographic/tomographic unit.

The second requirement is that there must be a means of imparting motion to the tube and film carriage for each tomographic motion. Modern machines employ motors that drive the tube and film for the blurring movement. The motor drive and the linkage mechanism must provide stable, vibration-free movement of the tube and film. Any unwanted motion may cause additional blurring of the focal plane image.

All tomographic machines must also have some means of adjusting the height of the fulcrum. In machines utilizing the adjustable or planigraphic principle, the motor drive alters the actual pivot point of the tube-film carriage assembly by raising and lowering the axis of rotation. Tomographic machines utilizing the fixed fulcrum, or Grossman, principle have a tabletop that is raised or lowered by a motor to the desired height.

Tomographic equipment has changed considerably since the early days of Vallebona and des Plantes. Their first machines were crude although ingeniously designed contrivances operated with ropes, pulleys, and hand cranks. Present-day equipment is motor driven and ranges from simple radiographic tables that can change over to linear tomography to highly sophisticated machines designed primarily for pluridirectional tomography. The more elaborate tomographic machines offer several automatic functions, such as automatic fulcrum height adjustment and motorized cassette shift for multiple exposures on one film. The pluridirectional machines are capable of several different complex motions as well as the simple linear movement.

TESTING OF TOMOGRAPHIC EQUIPMENT

Tomographic equipment is carefully checked and calibrated by the manufacturer's service representative when it is installed. The tube-film movement must be stable and exactly balanced, and there must be synchronization of the travel time and exposure time at each of the exposure angles and tomographic movements. These are checked with a pinhole test device. The pinhole test device is a lead plate with a very small beveled hole in the middle, which is positioned on the tabletop directly in line with the central ray. Pinholes must be placed either above or below the focal plane. The tomographic exposure is made, tracing on film the actual pattern of the tomographic motion used. Any mechanical instability or aberration in the correct exposure time can be noted on the pinhole tracing. Examples of pinhole tracings can be found in the section on blurring motions.

Another test device called a tomographic test phantom is used to determine the accuracy of the fulcrum height indicator and the section thickness of the different exposure angles and blurring motions. The blurring characteristics of the different motions may be determined with the phantom also (see Figs. 26-6 and 26-13). Different phantoms are available, but most manufacturers of tomographic equipment recommend the test phantom developed by Dr. J.T. Littleton. This is the type of device used in Figs. 26-6 to 26-12.

Clinical Applications

Tomography is a proven diagnostic tool that can be of significant value when a definitive diagnosis cannot be made from conventional radiographs, since confusing shadows can be removed from the point of interest. Tomography may be used in any part of the body but is most effective in areas of high contrast, such as in bone and lung. Body-section radiography is used to demonstrate and evaluate a number of different pathologic processes, traumatic injuries, and congenital abnormalities. A basic familiarization with the clinical applications of tomography will help the tomographer to be more effective in the performance of his or her job. Some of the major areas of clinical applications are described below, although the versatility of tomography lends itself to other applications.

PATHOLOGIC PROCESSES IN SOFT TISSUES

One of the most frequent uses of tomography is to demonstrate and evaluate benign processes and malignant neoplasms in the lungs. Differentiation between benign lesions and malignancies cannot always be made with conventional chest radiography. With tomography it is possible to define the location, size, shape, and marginal contours of the lesion. Differentiation between benign and malignant tumors depends on the characteristics of the lesion itself. Benign lesions characteristically have smooth, well-marginated contours and frequently contain bits of calcium. The presence of calcium in a chest lesion usually confirms it as being benign. The benign lesions most commonly found in the lungs are granulomas, which form as a tissue reaction to a chronic infectious process that has healed.

Conversely, carcinogenic neoplasms characteristically have ill-defined margins that feather or streak into the surrounding tissue and rarely contain calcium (Figs. 26-14 and 26-15). Lung cancers may originate in the lung, in which case the neoplasm would be termed a primary malignancy. Bronchogenic carcinoma is an example of a primary malignancy that may develop in the chest. Lung cancers may develop as the result of the spread of cancer from another area of the body to the lungs. These malignancies are termed secondary or metastatic tumors. Breast cancer and testicular cancer, as well as others, may metastasize to the lungs.

When there is an apparent solitary nodule noted on a conventional chest radiography, the presence or exclusion of other lesions may be determined with general tomographic surveys of both lungs. These "whole lung" or "full lung" tomograms are used to exclude the possibility of metastatic disease from other organs. Frequently these lesions cannot be visualized by conventional radiographic methods, and tomography is the only means to identify these occult nodules. The demonstration of the number of tumors, their location, size, and relation to other pulmonary structures is crucial to the physician's plan of treatment and the prognosis for the patient. Reexamination by tomography may be performed at a later date to check on the progress of the disease and the effectiveness of the therapy.

A

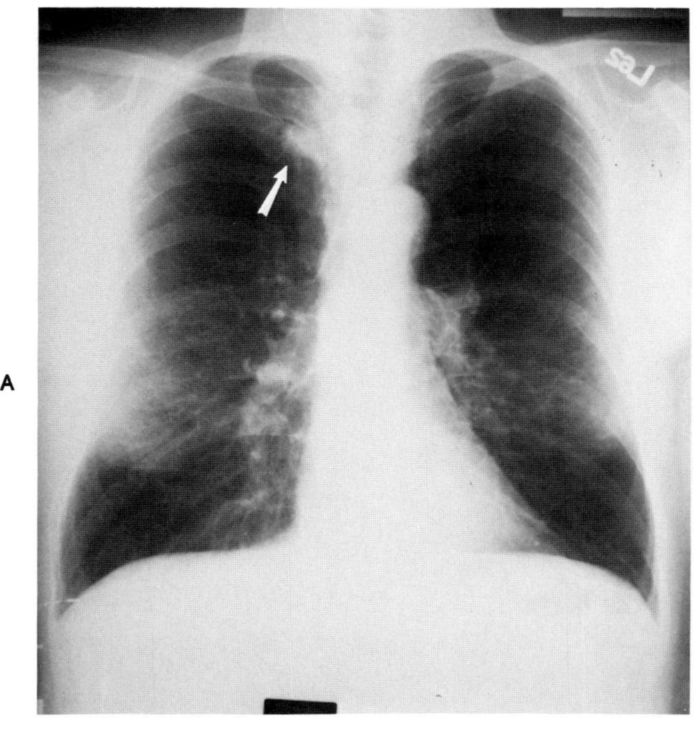

Fig. 26-14. **A,** PA chest radiograph demonstrating ill-defined density *(arrow)* in right upper chest. **B** and **C,** Collimated AP tomograms of patient in **A** demonstrating lesion in posterior chest plane with ill-defined margins that feather or streak into surrounding lung tissue, characteristic of malignant chest

B

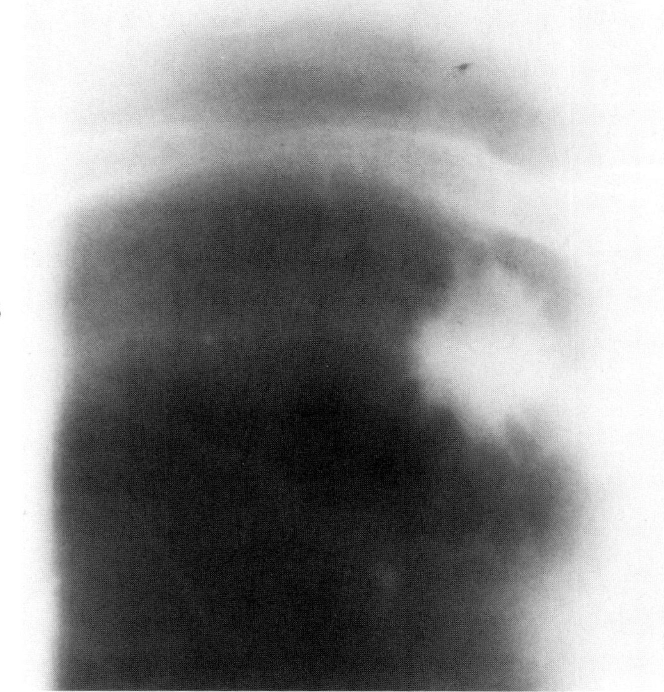

C

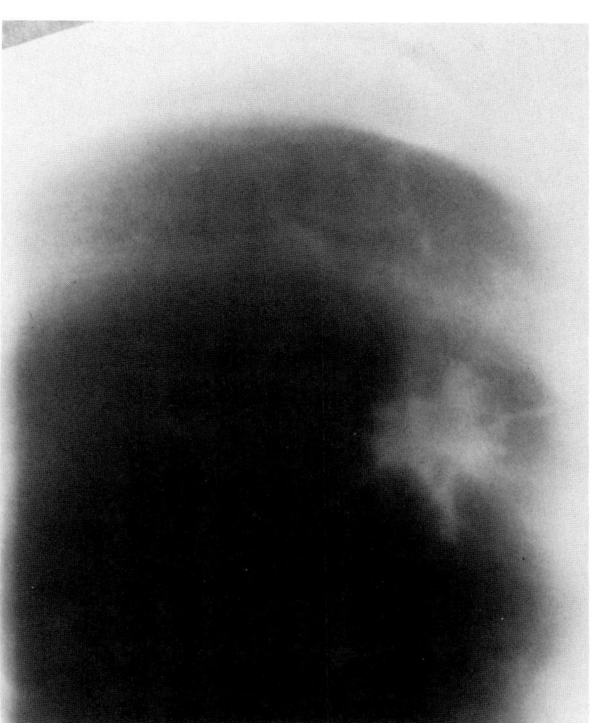

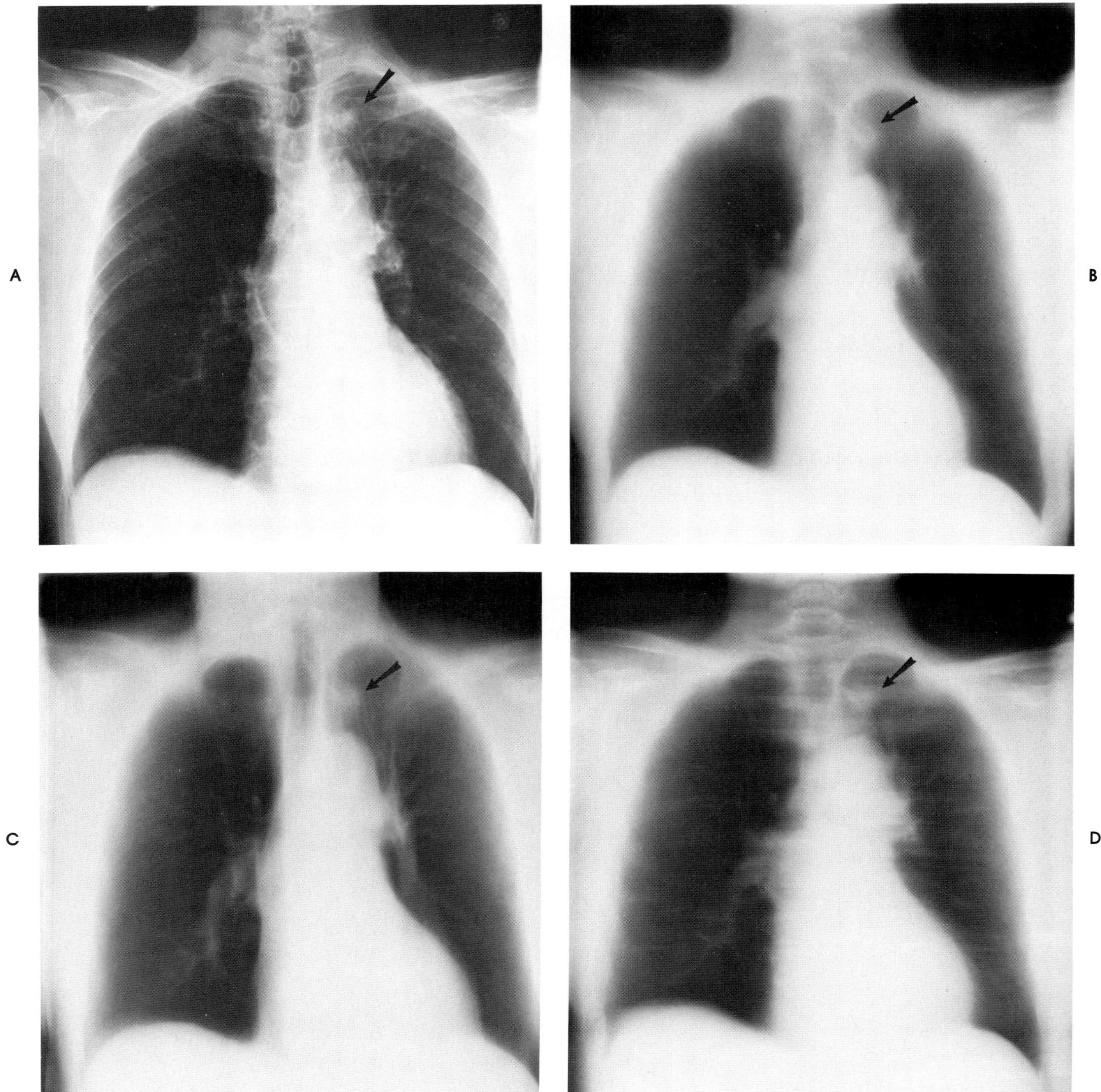

Fig. 26-15. A, AP chest radiograph with vague density *(arrow)* over medial end of left clavicle. **B** to **D,** AP full lung tomograms of patient in **A** taken to exclude possibility of other occult lesions. **B,** Trispiral tomogram 1 cm anterior to hilar plane at level of tumor. Radiographic appearance of lesion *(arrow)* is consistent with malignant chest neoplasm. **C,** Longitudinal linear tomogram of 40 degrees at same fulcrum level as **B.** Visualization of lesion *(arrow)* is decreased because of linear streaking and incomplete blurring of other structures outside focal plane. **D,** 40-degree transverse linear tomogram at same level as **B** and **C,** again demonstrating poor visualization of lesion *(arrow)* because of linear blurring characteristics. Blurring of anterior ribs is incomplete.

PULMONARY HILA

Neoplasms involving the pulmonary hila are very effectively evaluated by tomography. It is possible with tomography to determine if and to what degree the individual bronchi are patent or obstructed. This partial or complete obstruction may occur when a neoplasm develops within the bronchus and bulges into the bronchial airspace or if a tumor grows adjacent to the bronchus. As the lesion grows, it may press against the bronchus, causing a reduction in the size of the lumen and thus restricting or obstructing the airflow to that part of the lung. Pneumonia, atelectasis, and other inflammatory or reactive changes that may occur with the obstruction may further hinder conventional imaging of this area. Demonstration of bronchial patency through a density is strong evidence that the lesion is inflammatory and not malignant (Fig. 26-16).

SOFT TISSUE LESIONS AFFECTING BONY STRUCTURES

Another major application of tomography is to demonstrate and evaluate soft tissue neoplasms in the presence of bony structures. Because of the high density of bone and the relatively low density of the soft tissue neoplasms, it is usually not possible to demonstrate the actual lesion, but it is possible to demonstrate with great clarity the bony destruction caused by the presence of the tumor.

For example, neoplasms involving the pituitary gland usually cause bony changes or destruction of the floor of the sella turcica, which would indicate the presence of a pituitary adenoma. In addition to demonstrating destruction caused by the tumor, it is possible with tomography to demonstrate the bony septations in the sphenoidal sinus, which aids the surgeon removing the tumor (Fig. 26-17).

A

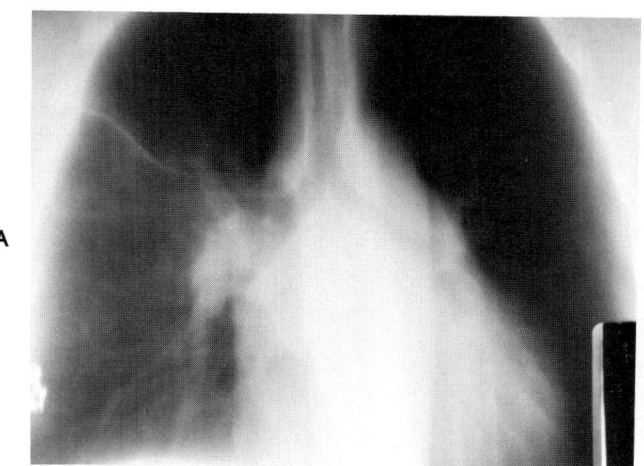

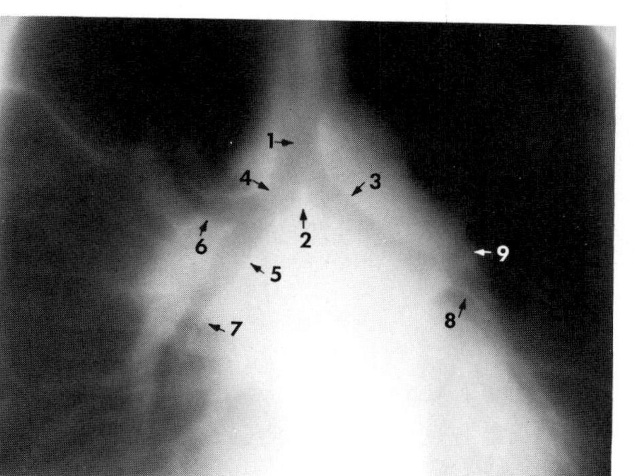

B

Fig. 26-16. Normal bronchotomogram through midplane of hilum. **A,** Linear tomogram. **B,** Trispiral tomogram demonstrating more clearly the hilar structures: *1,* trachea; *2,* carina; *3,* left main-stem bronchus; *4,* right main-stem bronchus; *5,* intermediate bronchus; *6,* right upper lobe bronchus; *7,* right lower lobe bronchus; *8,* left lower lobe bronchus; *9,* left upper lobe bronchus.

A

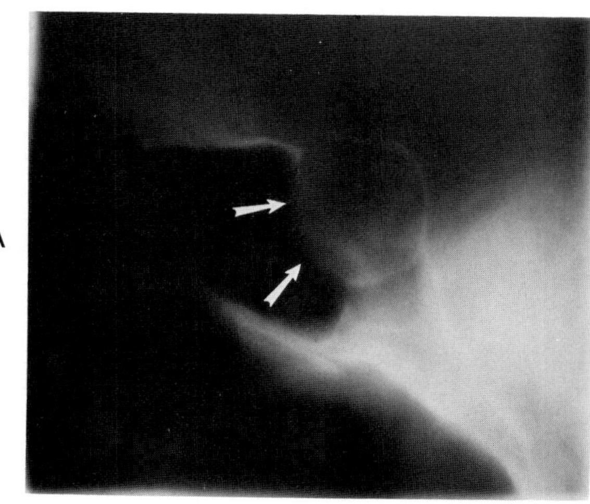

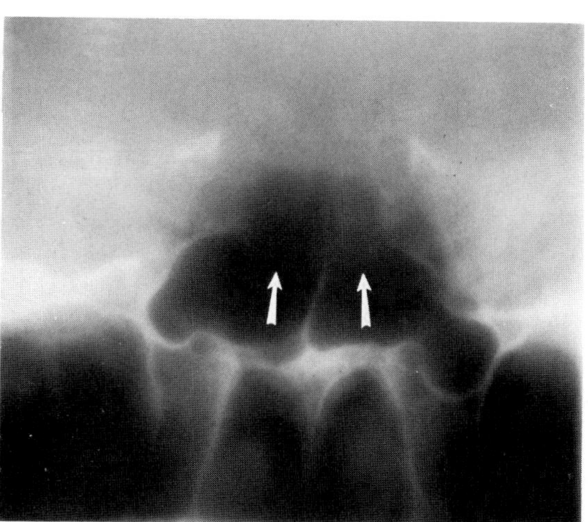

B

Fig. 26-17. Tomograms through midplane of sella turcica demonstrating destruction of floor *(arrows)* caused by presence of pituitary adenoma. **A,** Lateral tomogram. **B,** AP tomogram.

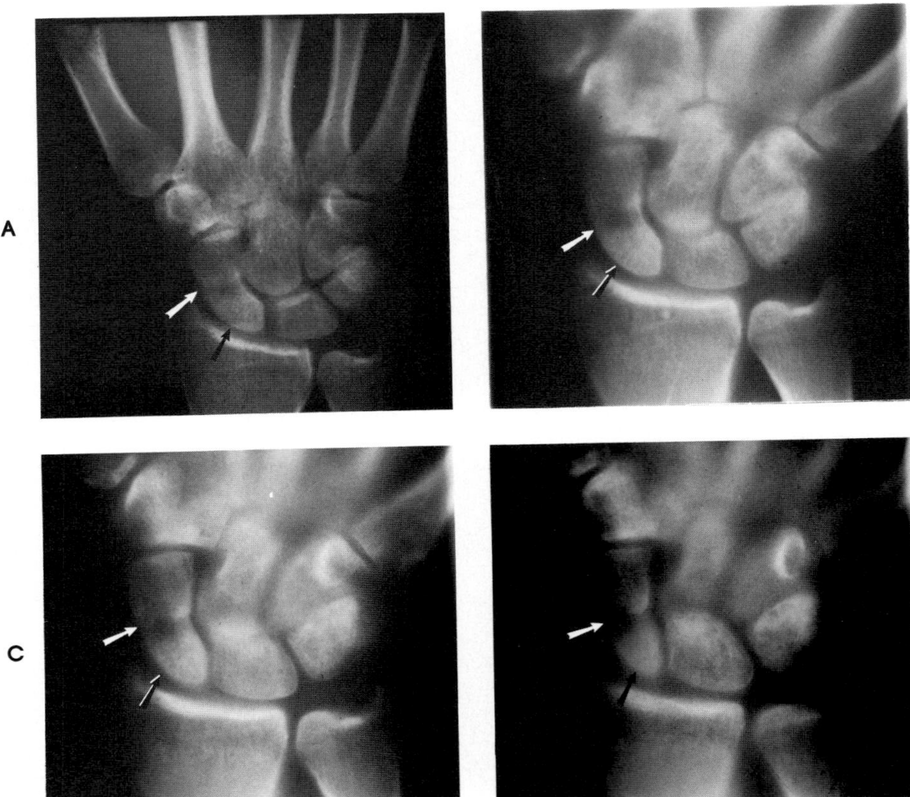

Fig. 26-18. **A,** PA radiograph demonstrating healing fracture *(white arrow)* of scaphoid bone and increased density *(black arrow)* of proximal end. **B, C,** and **D,** Tomograms at 3 mm intervals demonstrating fracture site *(white arrows)* with dense area *(black arrows)* of sclerotic bone at proximal end of scaphoid bone, consistent with aseptic necrosis.

LESIONS IN BONE

Subtle changes that may occur as a result of a pathologic process in bone tissue may be noted on conventional radiographs, but in many instances only with the aid of tomography can the true nature and extent of the involvement be determined (Fig. 26-18). Pathologic processes involving bony structures are normally characterized by bone destruction and/or changes in the bone tissue or the surface margins. More specifically, in tomography the attempt is made to identify the extent of bone destruction, the status of the cortex of the bone (i.e., whether destruction extends through the cortical bone), the presence of any periosteal reaction to the lesion, changes in the bone matrix, new bone formation, and the status of the zone of the bone between the diseased and normal bone.

Destruction of bone or other alterations in the bone may be the result of a multitude of different benign or malignant processes that manifest themselves in different ways. Some benign processes such as osteomyelitis are presented as areas of bone destruction, whereas others such as osteomas are presented as abnormal growths of bone from bone tissue. Some processes may exhibit a combination of bone destruction and new growth, as occurs in Paget's disease and rheumatoid arthritis.

Malignant neoplasms in bone tissue may occur in the form of primary lesions or secondary lesions resulting from the metastatic spread of cancer from another area of the body.

Some forms of cancer occurring in bone will exhibit areas of both destruction and new growth, whereas others exhibit only areas of extensive destruction.

FRACTURES

The three major clinical applications for tomography when dealing with known and suspected fractures are (1) identification and evaluation of occult fractures, (2) better evaluation of known fractures, and (3) evaluation of the healing process of fractures.

If a fracture is suspected clinically but cannot be ruled out or identified by conventional imaging methods, tomography may be indicated. Tomography is often used when fractures are suspected in areas of complex bone structures such as the cervical spine. The cervical spine projects a myriad of confusing shadows, often hiding fracture lines, making an accurate diagnosis impossible. With tomography it is possible to identify and evaluate these occult fractures (Fig. 26-19). Knowledge of these fractures can be crucial to the patient's plan of treatment and prognosis. Another area that frequently requires tomographic evaluation for occult fractures is the skull. The skull has many complicated bone structures that often make identification and evaluation of fractures in some areas extremely difficult without the use of tomography. The facial nerve canal that courses through the temporal bone is just one of many areas in the skull that is difficult to evaluate for fractures without tomography. Blowout fractures of the orbital floor also frequently require tomographic evaluation because of the difficulty in identifying and evaluating fractures and fragments of the thin bone of which the floor and medial wall of the orbit are composed (Fig. 26-20).

Tomography may also be used to evaluate known fractures with greater efficiency than is possible with conventional radiography. In some instances a fracture may be visualized on a conventional radiograph, but, because of the complex nature of the fracture or superimposition of shadows from adjacent structures, the fracture site cannot be adequately evaluated without the use of tomography. This often is the case in fractures of the hip involving the acetabulum. In acetabular fractures, portions of the acetabulum are often broken into many fragments. These fragments may be difficult to identify, but with tomography the fragments and any possible femoral fracture can be evaluated before any attempt is made to reduce the fracture.

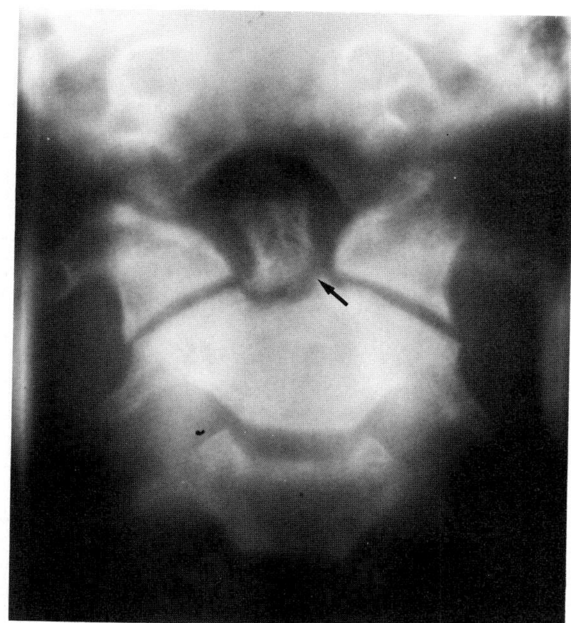

Fig. 26-19. AP tomogram of C1-3 demonstrating complete fracture at base of dens *(arrow)*.

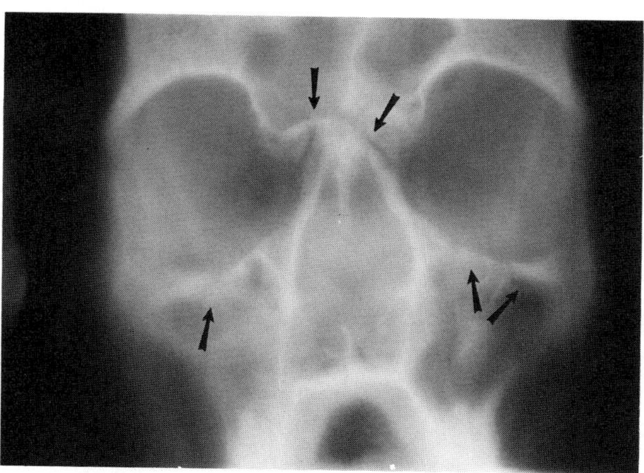

Fig. 26-20. Frontal tomogram in reverse Caldwell method demonstrating multiple facial fractures *(arrows)*.

HEALING FRACTURES

Tomography may also be used to evaluate the healing process of fractures when, because of overlying shadows of fixation devices, adjacent structures, or the bone callus, conventional imaging methods may prove inadequate. In these cases it may be impossible to tell if the bone is healing properly throughout the fracture site without the use of tomography. With tomography it is possible to identify the areas of the fracture when incomplete healing exists (Fig. 26-21).

ABDOMINAL STRUCTURES

Because of the relatively homogeneous densities of abdominal structures both radiographic imaging and tomographic imaging of this area are most effectively performed in conjunction with the use of contrast materials. Zonography is usually preferred for tomographic evaluation of these organs. As previously stated, zonography produces focal plane images of greater contrast than is possible with thin-section tomography. This increased level of contrast aids in the visualization of the relatively low-density organs of the abdomen. The extensive blurring of remote structures that occurs with wide-angle tomography is not necessary in the abdomen since there are relatively few high-density structures in this area that would compromise the zonographic imaging of the abdominal structures. Thick sections of organs are depicted with each zonogram, and entire organs can be demonstrated in a small number of tomographic sections.

A circular motion with an exposure angle of 8 or 10 degrees is recommended for use in the abdomen. Occasionally, an angle of 15 degrees may be necessary to eliminate bowel gas shadows if the smaller angle does not provide adequate effacement (blurring) of the bowel.

Zonography using a linear movement is not recommended because it does not provide adequate blurring of structures outside the focal plane. If a linear movement is used, an exposure angle of 15 degrees should be used to provide adequate blurring. It should be remembered that linear tomography does not produce accurate focal plane images because of the incomplete blurring effect of structures oriented parallel to the tube movement. Although the possibility of false image formation does exist with circular tomography, the image of the focal plane is far more accurate than with linear tomography. Linear tomograms are higher in contrast than circular tomograms, but this is actually because of the linear streaking caused by the incomplete blurring characteristics of the linear motion. The circular motion, on the other hand, will produce an accurate focal plane image with slightly less but even contrast.

The most common tomographic examinations of the abdomen are of the kidneys and biliary tract. These examinations are normally performed with contrast material.

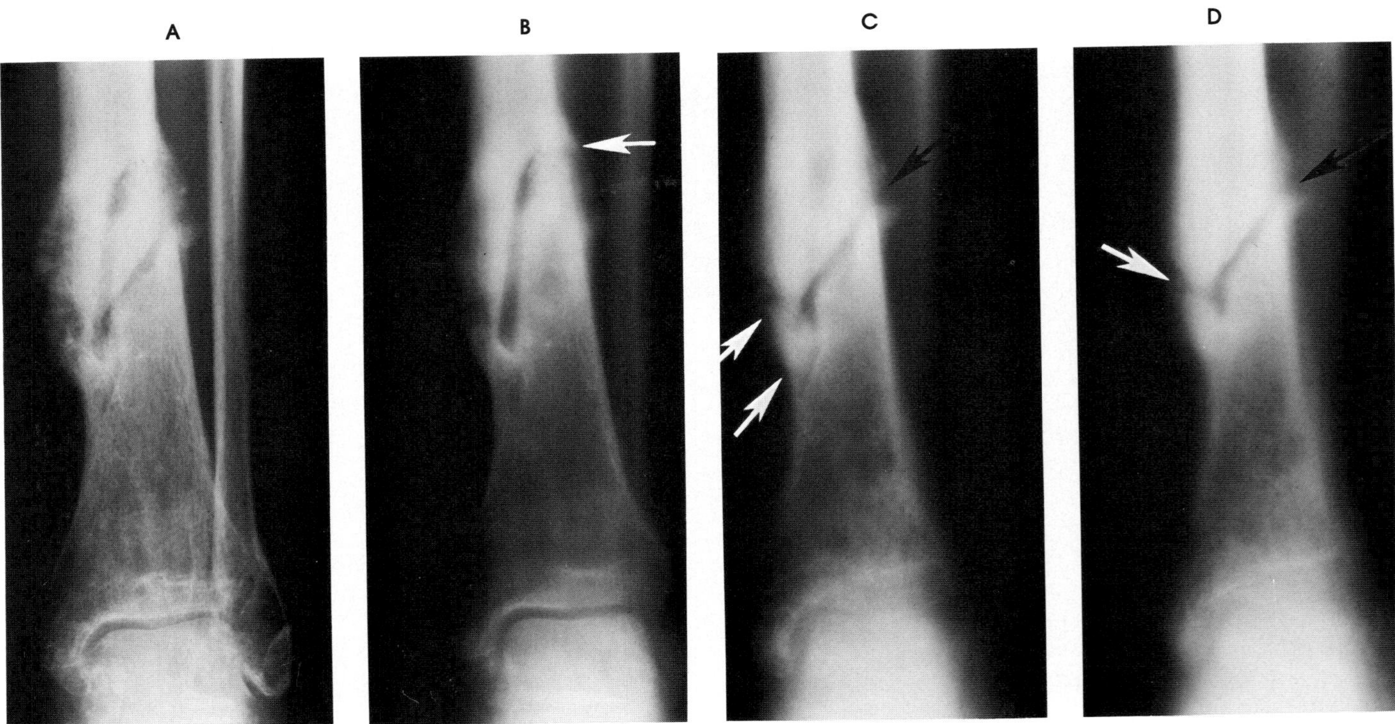

Fig. 26-21. A, AP radiograph of distal tibia demonstrating questionable complete union of fractures. **B,** AP tomogram of same patient as in **A,** demonstrating incomplete union of longitudinal fracture *(arrow).* **C** and **D,** Tomograms demonstrating incomplete union of oblique fractures *(arrows)* through shaft of tibia of same patient as in **A** and **B.** **C,** 0.5 cm and, **D,** 1 cm posterior to **B.**

RENAL TOMOGRAPHY

Many institutions routinely include tomography of the kidneys as part of the intravenous urography (IVU) procedure (Fig. 26-22). The tomograms are usually taken immediately following the bolus injection of the contrast material. At this time the kidney is entering the nephrogram phase of the IVU in which the nephrons of the kidney begin to absorb the contrast material, causing the parenchyma of the kidney to become fairly radiopaque. It is then possible to demonstrate with zonography lesions in the kidney that may have been overlooked with conventional radiography alone.

Another typical renal tomographic examination is the nephrotomogram. The major difference between this and the IVU is the method of introduction of the contrast material. In nephrotomography the contrast material is drip-infused throughout the examination instead of introduced in a single bolus injection. This method allows for a considerably longer nephrographic effect, since the nephrons continuously absorb and excrete the contrast material as it is being infused and opacify the kidney.

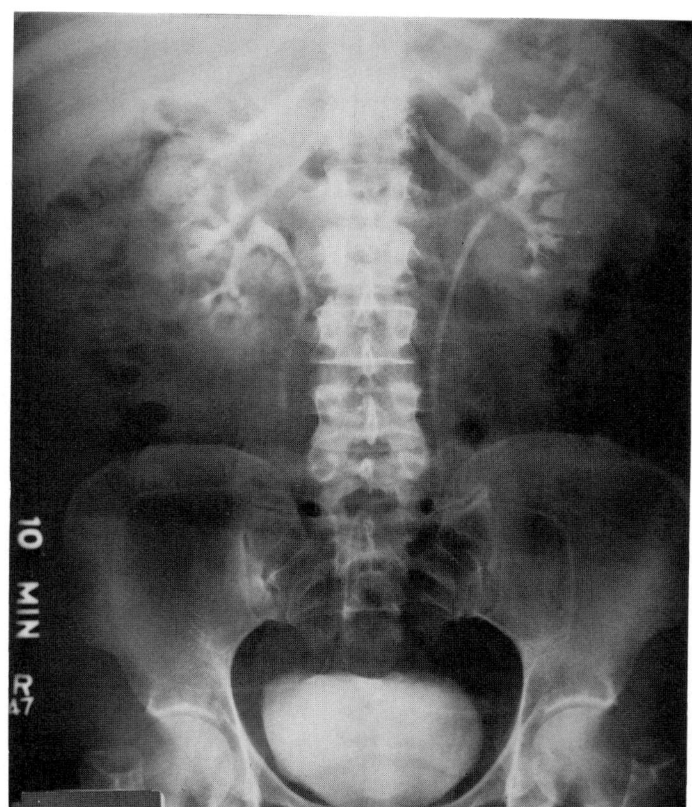

A

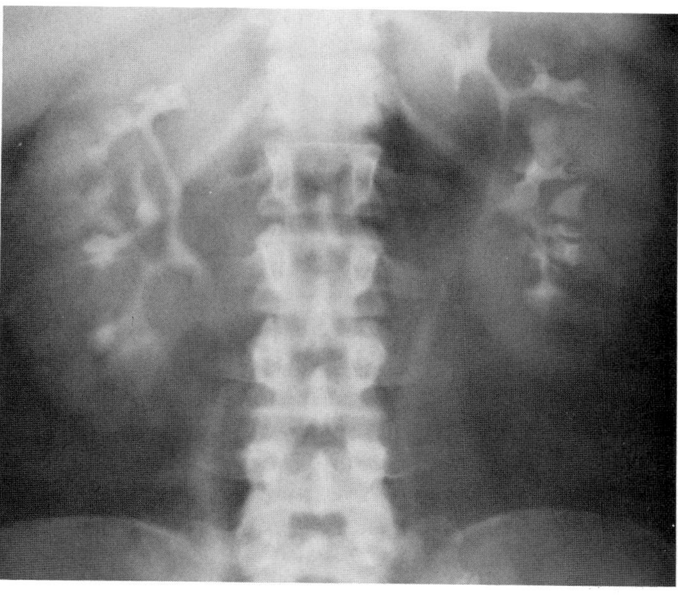

B

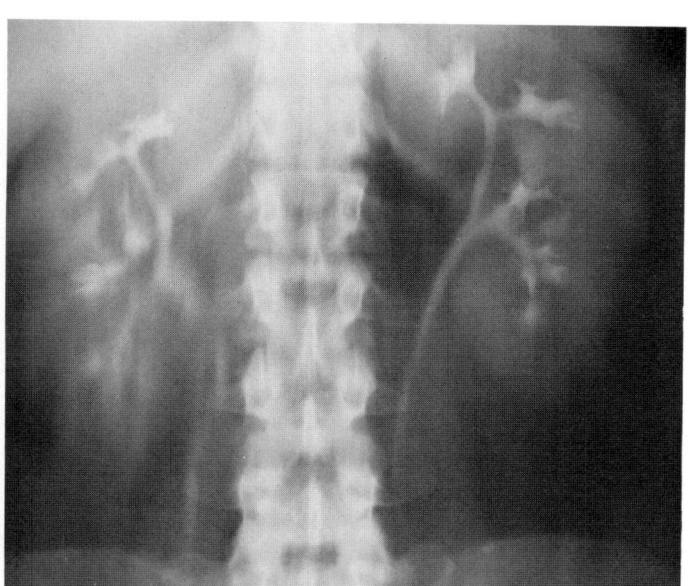

C

Fig. 26-22. A, AP radiograph of intravenous urogram. Bowel shadows obscure kidneys. **B,** AP tomogram of same patient as in **A** through midplane of kidneys using 8-degree circular motion. Bowel shadows are absent, and visualization of kidneys is improved over **C. C,** AP tomogram of same patient as in **A** and **B** and at same levels as in **B,** but employing 20-degree linear motion. Note linear streaking and loss of detail of collecting systems and kidney borders.

INTRAVENOUS CHOLANGIOGRAMS

The biliary tract is another organ system that may require tomography for adequate evaluation. If an oral cholecystogram does not yield sufficient information for a diagnosis or if biliary ductal disease is suspected in a cholecystectomized patient, then an intravenous cholangiogram (IVC) may be indicated. The IVC is performed by infusing a solution of the contrast material Cholegrafin into the bloodstream, where it is first absorbed into and then excreted by the liver into the biliary ducts. The drip infusion should be administered slowly over approximately 20 to 30 minutes to reduce the possibility of anaphylactic shock. Opacification of the ducts is generally not dense enough for adequate evaluation with conventional radiography alone. The ducts may also be partially or completely obscured by the superimposition of shadows or other structures in the abdomen. Even though the ducts may be well opacified on conventional radiographs, tomography should be performed to provide additional information not available with conventional radiography (Fig. 26-23). Zonography is normally used for IVCs; however, there may be instances in which more blurring or a thinner tomographic section is desired. For those instances, a trispiral or hypocycloidal motion may be preferred. If a linear motion is to be employed, an exposure angle of 15 to 20 degrees should be used.

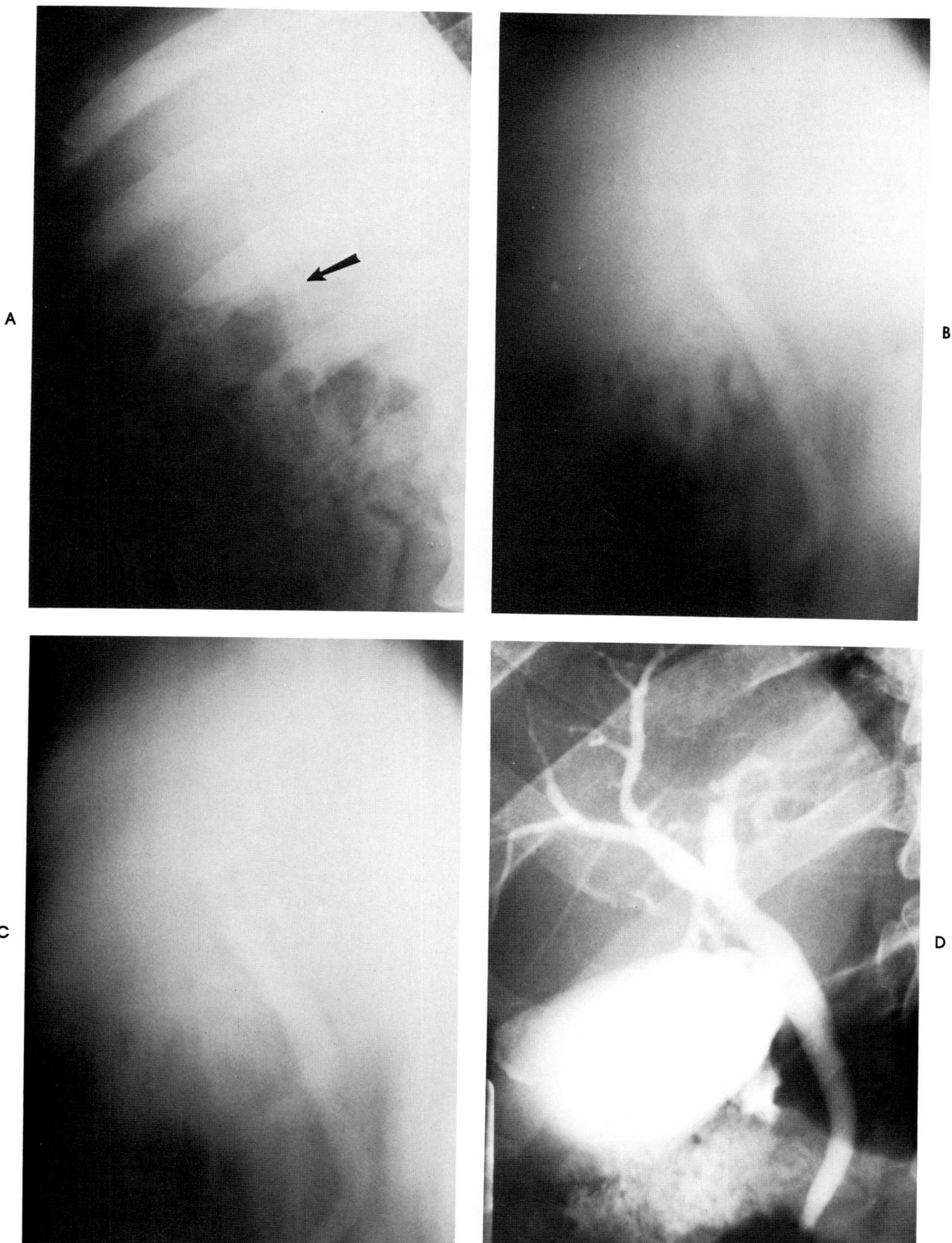

Fig. 26-23. A, RPO position radiograph of intravenous cholangiogram. Faintly opacified common bile duct *(arrow)* is obscured by bowel gas and liver. **B** and **C,** RPO position tomograms of same patient as in **A** through level of common bile duct. Visualization of duct is improved over plain film study **(A). D,** Transhepatic cholangiogram of same patient as in **A** to **C.**

Basic Principles of Positioning

In conventional radiography rarely does one single radiographic image contain all the diagnostic information necessary to make an accurate diagnosis. This is also true in tomography; one series of tomograms in a single image usually does not contain enough information to make an accurate diagnosis. As in radiography, two or more images are usually required for most tomographic examinations. In the case of bilateral structures, such as the internal auditory canals, only one radiograph may be used. In such cases, tomograms of the contralateral side are made for comparison.

Many standard radiographic positions are used in tomography. The AP and lateral images are basic to most tomographic examinations. Occasionally, a special oblique position may be necessary to optimally visualize the part under investigation. Basically, in tomography the structures should be oriented either parallel or perpendicular to the tomographic plane. For example, when evaluating structures in the base of the skull the patient's head should be positioned in a basal projection so that the base of the skull will be oriented parallel to the section plane. This parallel position not only will produce images that are more anatomically correct but also will reduce the total number of tomograms necessary to cover the area of interest. If the base of the skull is not parallel but is slightly obliqued, more tomograms are required to adequately evaluate the area of interest. This also pertains to other areas of the body in which large, relatively flat surfaces occur, such as in long bones. When making tomograms of long bones such as the femur the long axis of the bone should be adjusted to be parallel to the tomographic plane. Some structures, such as the sella turcica, are better suited to a perpendicular orientation for tomography. Since the presence of a pituitary adenoma usually affects the floor of the sella, it should be oriented perpendicular to the section plane. The AP and lateral radiographs are routinely used for this examination, and in both images the floor will remain perpendicular to the tomographic plane.

There are very few areas in radiology in which the demand placed on the knowledge and ability of the technologist are as great as in the field of tomography. The tomographer must possess a better than average knowledge of anatomy and of the spatial relationships of the structures of the body. Tomographic technologists must know where certain structures of the general body parts are located, how to best position those structures for tomographic examination, at what depth the particular structures are located, and how the tomographic image should look. There are many occasions when even the experienced tomographer must rely heavily on the knowledge and instruction of the radiologist monitoring the examination. A close working relationship between the technologist and the radiologist should exist since no two tomographic examinations are exactly alike and each case must be considered individually.

It is necessary to provide the radiologist with an adequate clinical history of the patient. This information may be obtained from the patient's medical records if it is not provided on the examination requisition or by interviewing the patient. This clinical information and any pertinent radiographs should be reviewed and discussed with the radiologist before beginning the examination. After reviewing this information the radiologist and technologist can then decide on the area of interest, the optimum position, the size of the field of exposure, the type of blurring motion and exposure angle to be used, the separation intervals between tomographic sections, and the parameters for the fulcrum height. It is recommended that the most complex motion available be used whenever possible.

All equipment preparation should be accomplished before positioning the patient. This will reduce the amount of time that the patient is required to maintain an often uncomfortable position. The technologist should briefly and simply explain the procedure to the patient and offer a rough estimate of the expected length of the examination. Many patients are under the mistaken impression that the procedure consists of just a few x-rays that can be taken in a matter of a few minutes and that they will then be permitted to leave. They are not aware that they will be required to maintain a certain position throughout the procedure. The patient who knows beforehand what to expect will be in a better frame of mind to cooperate throughout the lengthy examination.

The use of a suitable table pad is recommended for tomographic examinations. A table pad that is 4 cm thick will add an insignificant amount of distance to the overall patient thickness and will greatly increase the patient's comfort. Patient comfort is extremely important, and all attempts should be made to ensure this. If the patient is not comfortable, even the most cooperative patient will not be able to hold still for the examination. Angle sponges and foam blocks should be used to assist the patient in maintaining the correct position wherever applicable. However, foam sponges are not recommended for use in tomographic examinations of the head. Section intervals of 1 or 2 mm are often employed in this area, and foam sponges do not give firm enough support of the head. With little change in pressure the head may move, drastically altering the desired focal plane levels. Folded towels may be used to support the head; they offer greater resistance to any downward pressure of the head.

Immobilization Techniques

The most effective immobilization technique is the technologist's instructions to the patient. No amount of physical restraint will keep a patient from moving if he does not fully understand the importance of holding still from the first preliminary film to the end of the tomographic series.

Although suspension of respiration is not necessary in many tomographic examinations, it is mandatory in examinations of the chest and abdomen. Explicit breathing instructions must be given to the patient for examinations of these areas. In chest tomography the patient should be instructed to take the *same* deep breath for each tomogram. The patient should be cautioned not to strain and take in the maximum breath since the patient may have difficulty in holding the breath during the exposure. The patient should be told to take in a moderately deep breath that can be comfortably held for the duration of the tomographic exposure. This not only allows for optimum inflation of the lungs but also provides consistency between the focal plane levels throughout the tomographic series. This consistency in inspirations is vitally important if the area of interest is located near the diaphragm. Slight variations in the amount of air taken in may result in obscuring the area of interest by the elevated diaphragm. Suspension of respiration is also necessary to prevent blurring of structures by the breathing motion.

Respiration should be suspended in the expiratory phase in examinations of the abdomen to elevate the diaphragm and visualize more of the abdomen. As in chest tomography, the suspension of respiration will assist in maintaining consistency in tissue planes and reduce motion artifacts.

Occasionally, suspended respiration techniques may be necessary in tomographic examinations of the head. Unwanted motion of the head may occur when obese people or women with large breasts are positioned in the RAO position for lateral skull tomography. This problem may be resolved by having the patient suspend respiration during the exposure or by turning the patient over into an RPO position.

It is helpful to mark the entrance point of the central ray on the patient's skin. If the patient does happen to move, he or she can easily be repositioned using this mark as a reference point. This will eliminate the need to take another scout film to recheck the position. If the mark is made with a grease pencil, it can easily be removed at the completion of the examination. When performing tomographic examination of the skull in the lateral position it is helpful to place a small midline mark on the patient's nasion to facilitate measuring for the midline tomogram and to recheck the position between the scout films and the actual tomographic series. By ensuring that this mark is still at the same level from the tabletop, that the interpupillary line is still perpendicular to the tabletop, and that the central ray is still entering at the reference mark, the correct position can be maintained throughout the entire examination.

Scout Tomograms

Three preliminary tomograms are usually taken to locate the correct levels for the tomographic series. One tomogram is taken at the level presumed to be at the middle of the structure or area to be examined. The other two scout tomograms are taken at levels higher and lower than this midline tomogram. The separation interval between these tomograms depends on the thickness of the structure. Tomograms of small structures, such as those found in the skull, may be made at 5 mm or 1 cm intervals for the preliminary films. Once the correct planes have been determined, the tomographic series will be taken at smaller intervals. When the total depth of the area of interest is several centimeters thick, the separation interval for these scout tomograms is increased to 2 cm or more. Table 26-1 includes separation intervals for the preliminary tomograms and the tomographic series.

External landmarks are often used as reference points to assist in the determination of the proper fulcrum level for the scout tomograms. In some cases, such as chest lesions that can be identified on a PA and lateral chest radiograph, measurements can be taken from these radiographs to aid in the selection of the scout tomogram levels.

For example, to determine the proper level to a chest lesion for AP tomography, the distance is measured on the conventional lateral chest radiograph from the posterior chest wall to the middle of the lesion. This distance is then added to the thickness of the table pad. A scout tomogram taken at this fulcrum height should be in the middle of the lesion. A similar process can be used for tomography in the lateral position taking the measurements from the AP chest radiograph.

If the area of interest is not localized on the scout films, it may be necessary to take a plain film centered exactly as the preliminary tomograms were. This is done to confirm that the area of interest is actually in the collimated field of view and recentering is not required.

Table 26-1. Positions for tomography

Examination part	Position	Central ray position	Preliminary tomographic levels	Separation intervals	Comments
Sella turcica	AP	Glabella	1.5, 2.5, and 3.5 cm anterior to tragus	2 mm	Shield eyes.
	Lateral	2.5 cm anterior and superior to tragus	−1, 0, and +1 cm to midline of skull	2 mm	Place water bag under patient's chin for support.
Middle ear (internal acoustic canal, facial nerve canal, etc.)	AP	Midpoint between inner and outer canthi	−0.5, 0, and +0.5 mm to tip of tragus	1 or 2 mm	Shield eyes.
	Lateral	5 mm posterior and superior to external acoustic canal	At level of outer canthus and 1 and 2 cm medial	1 or 2 mm	Place water bag under patient's chin for support.
Paranasal sinuses (general survey) and orbital floors	Reverse Caldwell	Intersection of midsagittal plane and infraorbital rims	−2, 0, and +2 cm to level of outer canthus	3 or 5 mm	Infraorbitomeatal line should be perpendicular to the tabletop.
	Lateral	2 cm posterior to outer canthus	−3 and +3 cm to midline of skull	3 or 5 mm	Place water bag under patient's chin for support.
Base of skull	Submentovertex	Midpoint between angles of mandible	+1, 0, and −1 cm	2 or 3 mm	Orbitomeatal line should be parallel to tabletop.
Cervical spine	AP	To vertebral body(ies) of interest	0, −2, and −4 cm to external auditory meatus	3 or 5 mm	
	Lateral	To vertebral body(ies) of interest	−2, 0, and +2 cm from midline of back	3 or 5 mm	Place water bag under patient's chin for support and two or more on neck to equalize density for entire cervical spine.

Table 26-1. Positions for tomography—cont'd

Examination part	Position	Central ray position	Preliminary tomographic levels	Separation intervals	Comments
Thoracic spine	AP	To vertebral body(ies) of interest	3, 5, and 7 cm from tabletop	5 mm	Flex knees slightly to straighten spine.
	Lateral	To vertebral body(ies) of interest	−2 and +2 cm from midline of back	5 mm	Flex knees and place sponge against patient's back for support.
Lumbar spine	AP	To vertebral body(ies) of interest	4, 7, and 10 cm from tabletop	5 mm	Flex knees slightly to straighten spine.
	Lateral	To vertebral body(ies) of interest	−2, 0, and +2 cm from midline of back	5 mm	Flex knees and place sponge against patient's back for support.
Hip	AP	Head of femur	−2, 0, and +2 cm from greater trochanter	5 mm	Place water bag over area of greater trochanter to equalize density in hip.
	Lateral (frog leg)	Head of femur	5, 7, and 9 cm from tabletop	5 mm	Place water bag over area of femoral neck to equalize density.
Extremities	AP and lateral	At area of interest	5 mm to 1.5 cm depending on size of extremity	2-5 mm	Adjust extremity to be parallel to tabletop.
Chest (whole lung and hila)	AP	9-12 cm below sternal notch	10, 11, and 12 cm above tabletop	1 cm	Use trough filter (80-90 kVp).
	Lateral	Midchest at level of pulmonary hila	−5, 0, and +5 cm from midline of back	1 cm	Place sponge against patient's back for support.
Chest (localized lesion)	AP and lateral	Measure distance to lesion from chest wall on plain radiographs and center at this point on patient	Measure distance to lesion on lateral chest x-ray and add thickness of table pad; −2, 0, and +2 cm from measurement	2, 3, or 5 cm	Use low kVp (50-65) for high contrast.
Nephrotomogram	AP	Midpoint between xiphoid process and top of iliac crests	7 cm for small patient; 9 cm for average patient; 11 cm for large patient	1 cm	Use 8-10° of circular movement or 15-20° of linear movement.
Intravenous cholangiogram	20 degrees from RPO	10 cm lateral to lumbar spine	10, 12, and 14 cm for small patient; 12, 14, and 16 cm for average patient; 13, 16, and 19 cm for large patient	5 mm to 1 cm	Use 8-10° of circular movement or 15-20° of linear movement.

General Rules for Tomography

1. Know the anatomy involved.
2. Position the patient as precisely as possible.
3. Utilize proper immobilization techniques.
4. Use a small focal spot for tomography of the head and neck and extremities.
5. Use a large focal spot for other areas of the body where fine detail is not critical.
6. Use low kVp when high contrast is desired.
7. Use high kVp when it is necessary to reduce contrast differences between structures; for example, whole lung tomography requires high kVp (80-90) in conjunction with a trough filter.
8. Use water or flour bags in other areas when necessary to absorb primary or secondary radiation; for example, in lateral cervical spine tomography place the filter bags on the upper cervical spine area to reduce the density difference between the spine and dense shoulders.
9. Collimate the beam as tightly as possible to reduce patient exposure and improve contrast.
10. Shield the patient, especially the eyes, in examinations of the skull and upper cervical spine.
11. Use the proper blurring motion. In general, use the most complex blurring motion available. Where zonography is required, a circular motion should be used. If linear motion is the only one available, care must be taken to orient the part correctly to the direction of the tube.
12. Mark each tomogram with the correct layer height. This may be done by directly exposing lead numbers on each tomogram or by marking each tomogram after it is processed. Another method is to vertically shift the right or left marker used on each successive film. By knowing the level of the first film the technologist can determine the correct level for each successive film. If multiple tomograms are taken on one film, the same shift sequence must be followed to avoid confusion in marking the layer heights.

TOMOGRAPHY OF SKULL

Strict immobilization techniques must be utilized for any tomographic examination of the skull. Reference points should be marked on the patient for rechecking the position.

The basic skull positions are outlined in the following sections and are to be used in conjunction with Table 26-1.

AP projection

The patient's head should be adjusted to align the orbitomeatal line and the midsagittal plane perpendicular to the tabletop. The distances from the tabletop to each tragus (the tonguelike projection of the ear just in front of the external auditory meatus) should be equal if the head is positioned perfectly straight.

Reverse Caldwell position

The infraorbitomeatal line should be perpendicular to the tabletop as well as to the midsagittal plane. The tragi should be equidistant from the tabletop.

Lateral position

The midsagittal plane should be parallel to the tabletop. The interpupillary line should be perpendicular to the tabletop. The orbitomeatal line should be approximately parallel to the lower border of the film.

TOMOGRAPHY OF OTHER BODY PARTS

Standard radiographic positions (AP, lateral, and oblique) are utilized for most areas of the body. The same general rules of tomography apply to all areas. In general, the position that best shows the area of interest in a conventional radiograph is usually the best position for tomography. Selected tomograms are shown in Figs. 26-24 to 26-29.

For information on *panoramic tomography,* which is used to radiographically demonstrate the entire mandible and temporomandibular joint on one film, see Volume 2, Chapter 22 of this atlas.

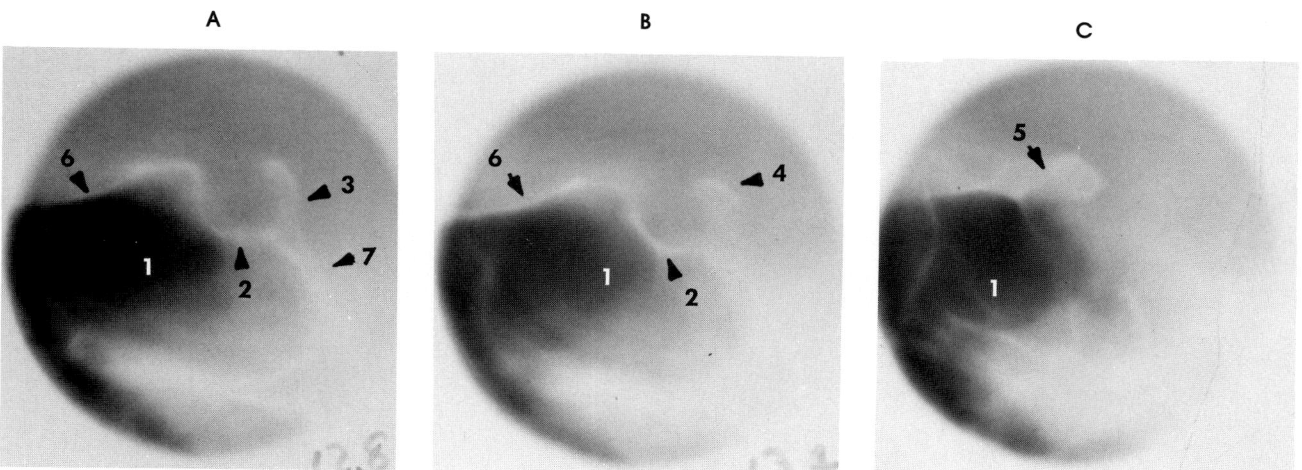

Fig. 26-24. Tomograms of sella turcica in lateral position. **A,** Through midplane of sella. **B,** 5 mm lateral to **A. C,** 1 cm lateral to **A.** *1,* Sphenoidal sinus; *2,* floor of sella; *3,* dorsum sellae; *4,* posterior clinoid process; *5,* anterior clinoid process; *6,* planum sphenoidale; *7,* clivus.

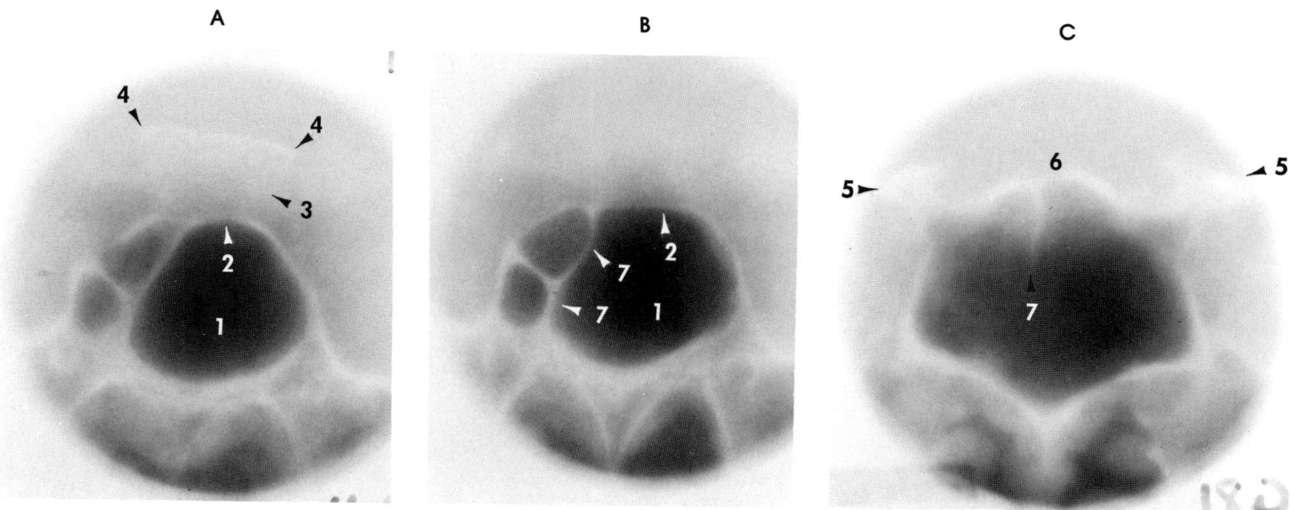

Fig. 26-25. Tomograms of sella turcica in frontal projection. **A,** Posterior plane of sella turcica in frontal projection. **B,** 1 cm anterior to **A** demonstrating floor of sella. **C,** 2 cm anterior to **A** demonstrating anterior clinoid processes. *1,* Sphenoidal sinus; *2,* floor of sella; *3,* dorsum sellae; *4,* posterior clinoid processes; *5,* anterior clinoid processes; *6,* planum sphenoidale; *7,* septations of sphenoidal sinus.

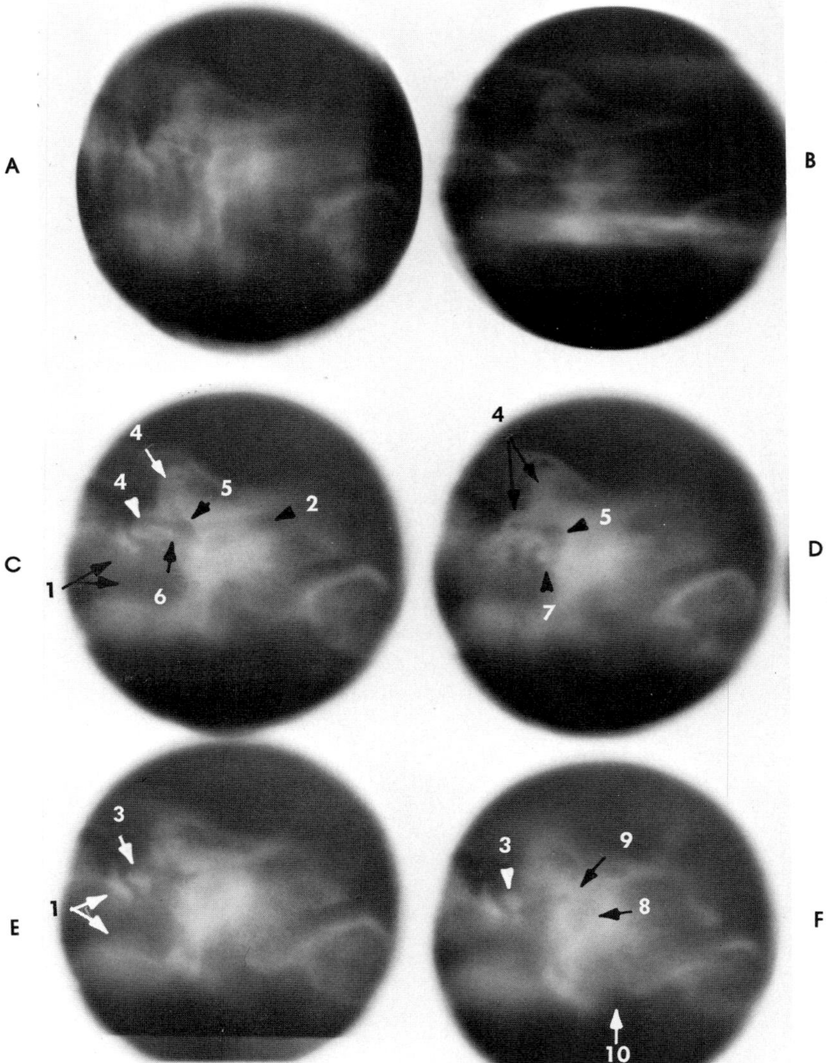

Fig. 26-26. Tomograms of middle ear in AP projection. **A,** Longitudinal linear; **B,** transverse linear; and **C,** trispiral motion are at same posterior level of middle ear. Note improved visualization of structures with trispiral motion **(C)**. **D** to **F,** Anterior to level of **C** by 2, 4, and 6 mm, respectively. *1,* External acoustic canal; *2,* internal acoustic canal; *3,* ossicular mass including malleus, incus, and lateral and superior semicircular canals; *4,* acoustic ossicles; *5,* vestibule; *6,* fenestra vestibuli; *7,* fenestra cochlea; *8,* cochlea; *9,* cochlear portion of facial nerve canal; *10,* carotid canal.

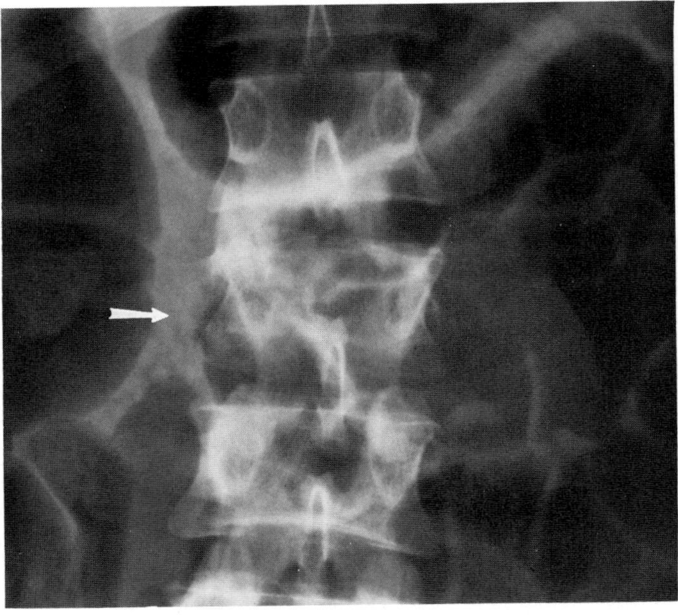

Fig. 26-27. AP radiograph of suspected fracture *(arrow)* of L2 (see Fig. 26-28).

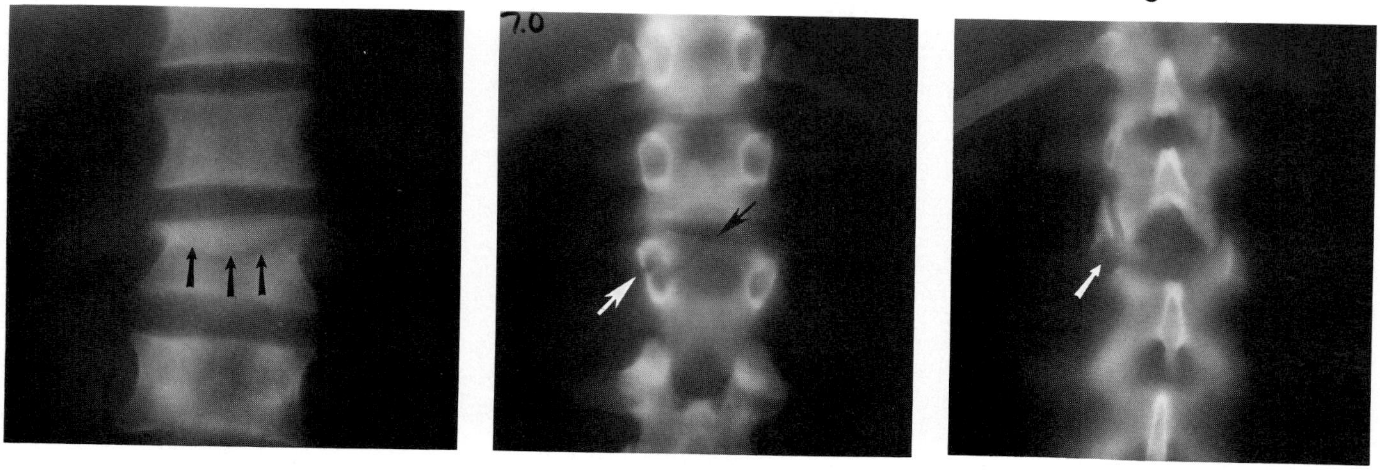

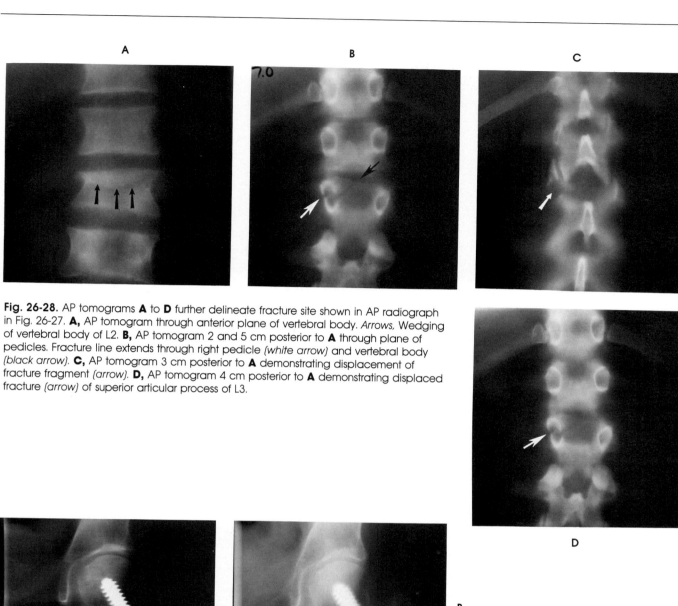

Fig. 26-28. AP tomograms **A** to **D** further delineate fracture site shown in AP radiograph in Fig. 26-27. **A,** AP tomogram through anterior plane of vertebral body. *Arrows,* Wedging of vertebral body of L2. **B,** AP tomogram 2 and 5 cm posterior to **A** through plane of pedicles. Fracture line extends through right pedicle *(white arrow)* and vertebral body *(black arrow).* **C,** AP tomogram 3 cm posterior to **A** demonstrating displacement of fracture fragment *(arrow).* **D,** AP tomogram 4 cm posterior to **A** demonstrating displaced fracture *(arrow)* of superior articular process of L3.

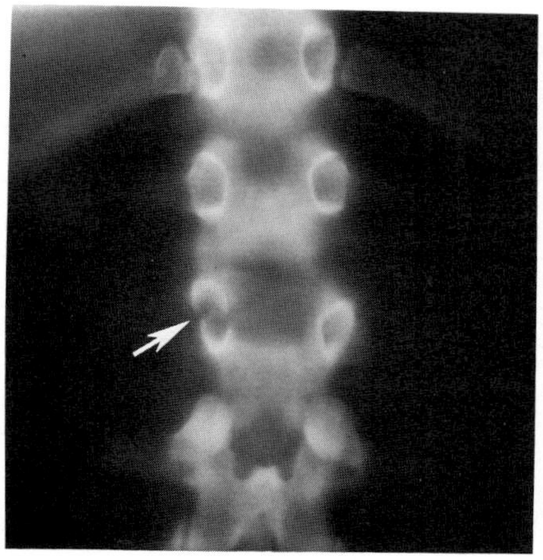

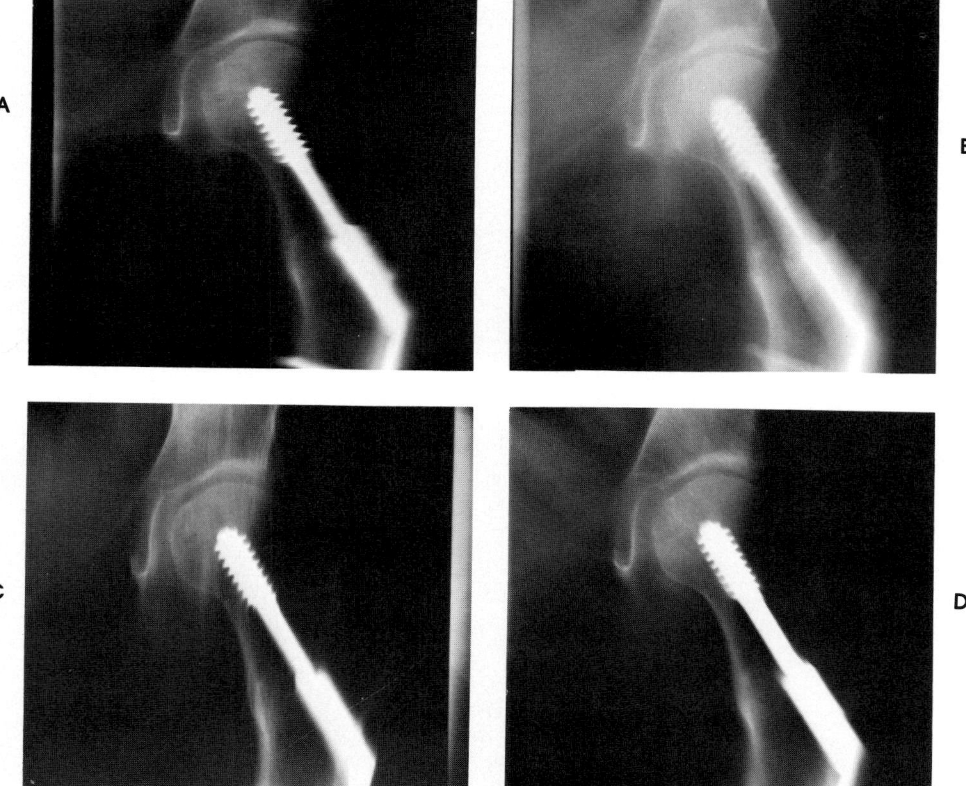

Fig. 26-29. AP tomograms of hip with fixation device at same level comparing different blurring motions; **A,** trispiral; **B,** circular; **C,** longitudinal linear; **D,** oblique linear.

Summary

Tomography has changed dramatically since the early days of Bocage and des Plantes. Their crude devices bear little resemblance to today's modern tomographic machines. Tomography has been widely accepted as an extremely useful diagnostic tool. Linear tomographic machines can now usually be found in even the smallest hospitals, and most large hospitals have one or more pluridirectional machines in addition to several linear tomographic/radiographic units in daily use.

Computed tomography (CT) and magnetic resonance imaging (MRI) have certainly proven themselves as extremely valuable diagnostic tools, and in some cases their images are far superior to those of conventional tomography. There are, however, many instances where tomography is the examination of choice over CT and MRI. Also, the extremely high cost of CT and MRI units in comparison to tomography machines is prohibitive to many hospitals. The cost to the patient per examination is also much higher than for conventional tomographic examination. Most MRI and CT scanners are extremely busy, and many cannot handle the high workload. Conventional tomography can often answer the question satisfactorily or at least screen the patient for further evaluation by the other, more sophisticated imaging modalities.

Had CT and MRI never been developed, tomography would certainly have enjoyed the tremendous technologic growth that has allowed these more recent imaging modalities to come about. With the help of digital fluoroscopy, however, tomography is slowly catching up. There are special tomography machines now under development and in limited use that, through a process called digital tomosynthesis, are in some instances equal to and even surpassing the imaging capabilities of CT and MRI. Coupled to a computer and a digital fluoroscopy unit, these tomography units are able to synthesize any tomographic plane from one single tomographic pass. In addition, the digital tomosynthesis system (DTS) enables manipulation of the image by changing the window level settings, allowing tissue characterization similar to that of CT and MRI.

Since only one tomographic slice is required, patient radiation dose is reduced drastically. Patient throughput can also be greatly increased since the patient need not even remain in the department because the images can be synthesized and manipulated at a later time.

In addition to routine tomographic studies, DTS shows great promise in the areas of angiotomography and digital subtraction angiography.

It is plain to see that tomography will remain for many years to come as a valuable diagnostic imaging tool for large hospitals as well as small. Technologic advances under development will only increase its value.

Definition of Terms

adjustable fulcrum Tomographic fulcrum that is either raised or lowered to achieve the desired fulcrum height. (See planigraphic principle.)

complex tomographic motion (See pluridirectional tomographic motion.)

exposure angle The angle of arc described by the movement of the x-ray tube and film during a tomographic motion.

fixed fulcrum Tomographic fulcrum remains at a fixed height. (See Grossman principle.)

focal plane That plane of tissue that is in "focus" on a tomogram.

fulcrum The point of axis of rotation for a tomographic motion.

Grossman principle Tomographic principle in which the fulcrum or axis of rotation remains at a fixed height. The focal plane level is changed by raising or lowering the tabletop through this fixed point to the desired height.

laminagraphy (See tomography.)

linear tomographic motion Basic tomographic movement that occurs when x-ray tube and film movement occurs with the longitudinal axis of the tomographic table.

phantom images False tomographic images that appear but do not represent an actual object or structure within the focal plane. These images are created by the incomplete blurring or the fusion of the blurred margins of some structures characteristic to the type of tomographic motion used.

planigraphic principle Tomographic principle in which the fulcrum or axis of rotation is raised or lowered to alter the level of the focal plane; the tabletop height remains constant.

planigraphy Synonymous with tomography.

pluridirectional tomographic motion Tomographic motion that moves in many different directions.

section thickness The tomographic plane that is in maximum focus.

stratigraphy Synonym for tomography.

tomographic angle (See exposure angle.)

tomography Internationally accepted term used to describe body section radiography as discussed in this chapter.

unidirectional tomographic motion Tomographic motion that moves in only a linear direction.

zonography Tomography that uses exposure angles of 10 or less depicting thick sections or zones of tissue.

SELECTED BIBLIOGRAPHY

Andrews JR: Planigraphy. I. Introduction and history, AJR 36:575, 587, 1936.

Berrett A: Modern thin-section tomography, Springfield, Ill, 1973, Charles C Thomas, Publisher.

Bocage AEM: French patent no. 536464, 1922.

Bosniak MA: Nephrotomography: a relatively unappreciated but extremely valuable diagnostic tool, Radiology 113:313-321, 1974.

Chasen MH et al: Tomography of the pulmonary hila: anatomical reassessment of the conventional 55 posterior oblique view, Radiology 149:365, 1983.

Durizch ML: Technical aspects of tomography, Baltimore, 1978, Williams & Wilkins.

Holder JC et al: Metrizamide myelography with complex motion tomography, Radiology 145:201, 1982.

Kieffer J: United States patent, 1934.

Littleton JT: Tomography: physical principles and clinical applications, Baltimore, 1976, Williams & Wilkins.

Littleton JT et al: Adjustable versus fixed-fulcrum tomographic systems, AJR 117:910-929, 1973.

Littleton JT et al: Linear vs. pluridirectional tomography of the chest: correlative radiographic anatomic study, AJR 134:241-248, 1980.

Maravilla KR et al: Digital tomosynthesis: technique for electronic reconstructive tomography, AJR 141:497, 1983.

Older RA et al: Importance of routine vascular nephrotomography in excretory urography, Radiology 136:282, 1980.

Potter GD et al: Tomography of the optic canal, AJR 106:530-535, 1969.

Stanson AW et al: Routine tomography of the temporomandibular joint, Radiol Clin North Am 14:105-127, 1976.

Valvasori GE: Laminagraphy of the ear: normal roentgenographic anatomy, AJR 89:1155-1167, 1963.

Chapter 27

MAMMOGRAPHY

JOHN O. OLSEN

Introduction and Historical Development

Mammography is the single most important innovation in breast cancer control since the introduction of the *radical mastectomy** in 1898. Mammography has done more to influence the detection and management of breast cancer than any other development since that time, and the importance of mammography is directly related to its value in the detection and management of breast cancer. If breast cancer did not exist, there would be few indications for mammography. Until 1984, breast cancer was the leading cause of death from cancer of American women, and 1 of every 11 American women will develop breast cancer in her lifetime. (In 1984 lung cancer became the leading cancer killer of women.) Although breast cancer is more common in older than in middle-aged women, the most common cause of death of women between the ages of 39 and 45 is breast cancer.

*All italicized terms are defined at the end of this chapter.

Before the development of the radical mastectomy operation by William Stewart Halstead, breast cancer was considered a hopeless and invariably fatal disease. Less than 5% of patients survived 4 years after the diagnosis, and the local recurrence rate of surgically treated breast cancer was over 80%. The 1898 Halstead procedure raised the 4-year survival rate to 40% and reduced the rate of local recurrence to approximately 10%. This was certainly a great step forward; however, over the next 60 years there was no additional improvement in breast cancer survival. Some principles of breast cancer management became clear, and those principles remain valid today. The patients who responded well to extensive surgery were those who had an early stage of the disease. Patients with advanced disease did poorly. The earlier the diagnosis of breast cancer is made, the better the chances of survival. The concept of removing all palpable breast masses in hopes of finding earlier cancers was developed, and it was recognized that careful physical examination of the breast could lead to the detection of some early breast cancers. However, most patients with breast cancer were not being diagnosed until their disease was advanced. This fact and the still dismal breast cancer survival statistics illustrated the need for a tool that would aid in the early detection of breast cancer. That need is filled by mammography (Fig. 27-1).

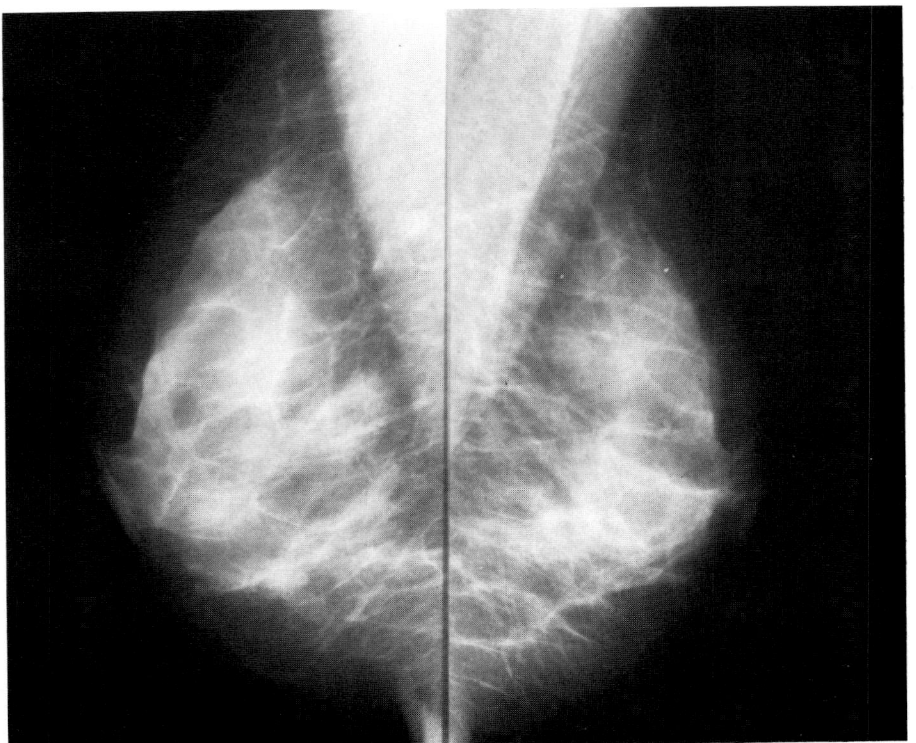

Fig. 27-1. Normal breast. Right and left mediolateral projections of the normal breast demonstrating water density, parenchymal tissue interspersed with fatty tissue, and supporting structures. Note the basic symmetry of the distribution of parenchyma in the two breasts. The fine lines *(top arrow)* extending to the skin are Cooper's ligaments. The thicker curving line *(arrowhead)* are veins.

Courtesy Karen M. Bridges, R.T.)

In 1913 a German physician named Soloman reported the radiographic appearance of breast cancers and described the mechanism of how breast cancer spread, based on x-ray studies of cancerous breasts removed at surgery. The first published radiograph of a living person's breast was made by Kleinschmidt, and it appeared in a 1927 German medical textbook on malignant tumors. During the 1930s there were publications on mammography from South America, the United States, and Europe, but there was little clinical interest in mammography for breast cancer diagnosis. A few pioneers, including LeBorgne in Uruguay, Gershon-Cohen in the United States, and Gros in Germany, published excellent comparisons of mammographic and pathologic anatomy and developed some of the clinical techniques of mammography. The significance of breast *microcalcifications* was well understood by that time. By the mid-1950s mammography was refined to the point of being a reliable clinical tool. Refinements included low kilovoltage x-ray tubes with molybdenum targets and high-detail, industrial-grade x-ray film. In the mid-1950s Egan in the United States and Gros in Germany popularized the application of mammography for the diagnosis and evaluation of breast cancer. Breast xerography was introduced in the 1960s and popularized by Wolfe and Ruzicka. Xerography substantially lowered the radiation dose received by the patient, as compared with industrial grade x-ray film. Many practitioners found the xerographic images easier to understand and evaluate, and xeromammography was widely applied to the evaluation of breast disease. The first attempts at widespread population screening began at this time.

Higher-resolution, faster-speed x-ray film used in combination with an intensifying screen was first introduced by the Du Pont Company in 1970, again substantially reducing radiation exposure to the patient. Improved film screen combinations were developed by both Kodak and Du Pont in 1975, and by this time extremely high-quality mammography images could be produced with very low patient radiation exposures. Even faster lower-dose films, magnification techniques, and grids for scatter rejection have since been introduced. It is now widely recognized that high-quality mammography coupled with careful physical examination can lead to detection of breast cancer at an early stage when it is most curable (Fig. 27-2).

In 1973 the Breast Cancer Detection Demonstration Project (BCDDP) was implemented. In this project 280,000 women underwent annual screening for breast cancer at 29 locations throughout the United States for 5 years. This project, organized by the American Cancer Society and the National Cancer Institute, demonstrated unequivocally that a program of screening, physical examination, mammography, and breast self-examination leads to the earlier diagnosis of breast cancer. In the project over 41% of all the cancers were found only with mammography, and an even greater proportion of *early* breast cancers were found only with mammography. This study was not designed to demonstrate that early detection of breast cancer would lead to increased survival rates, but there is now definite evidence from carefully controlled studies in other countries, including the Netherlands, Sweden, and Germany, that the early diagnosis of breast cancer leads to an increase in its curability. In the United States, the HIP (Health Insurance Plan) study in New York City showed the same mortality reduction from breast cancer through mammography screening in women over age 50.

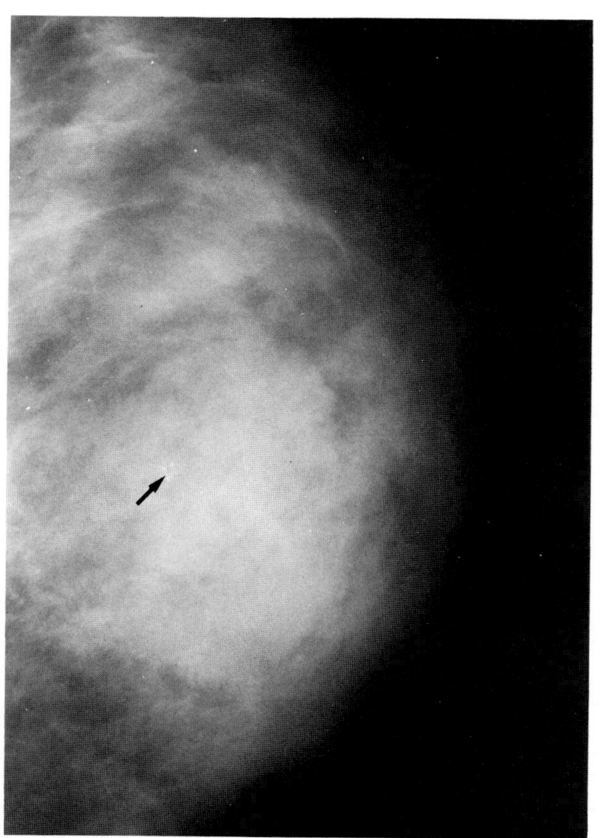

Fig. 27-2. Early breast cancer in a 36-year-old woman. A 5 mm carcinoma (*arrow*) contains microcalcifications. The physical examination was normal. The cancer was confined to the ducts (in situ) and was not yet invasive.

Risk Versus Benefit

In the mid-1970s a major controversy over mammography arose in which many members of the public developed the perception that the radiation exposure from diagnostic x-rays would cause breast cancer and would actually induce more breast cancers than would be detected. This is not the case, but fear of radiation exposure still causes some women to refuse mammography, and many women who undergo the examination are rightfully concerned about exposure levels and the resultant risk of carcinogenesis. For this reason it is necessary to understand the relationship between breast irradiation and breast cancer and to understand the relative risks of mammography in light of the natural incidence of breast cancer and the potential benefit of the examination. There is no direct evidence to suggest that the small doses of diagnostic x-rays used in mammography can induce the development of breast cancer. It has been demonstrated, however, that large doses of radiation can lead to an increased incidence of breast cancer and that the risk is dose dependent. The evidence that breast irradiation can increase the risk of breast cancer comes from three studies of groups of women who developed increased incidences of breast cancer after being exposed to large doses of radiation: (1) the population exposed to the atom bomb at Hiroshima and Nagasaki; (2) a group of women with tuberculosis who received multiple fluoroscopic examinations of the chest; and (3) a group of women who were treated with radiation for *postpartum mastitis*. In each case, the radiation received by the women was many times higher than that from mammography. Based on experience with large doses of radiation and using a linear dose response relationship, estimates of possible risks at lower levels of radiation can be made (Fig. 27-3). It can be estimated that 1 rad of radiation to the breast tissue will cause a 1% increase in the incidence of breast cancer over the natural incidence. The natural incidence of breast cancer is 8%, or 8 breast cancers for every 100 women, over their lifetime. An increase of 1% over the natural incidence would lead to a total incidence of 8.08% or almost 8.1 cancers in 100 women over their lifetime. This is the worst-case estimate because it assumes a direct linear relationship. The actual risk from 1 rad of radiation to the breast might be much lower, and it is definitely not higher. When scientists argue over whether the risk is low or very low, the uncertainty can confuse the public into thinking that the risk is unknown and therefore might be very high.

Today, the average radiation dose to the breast parenchyma in a high-quality xerographic or mammographic examination is actually much lower than 1 rad. The average mid-breast dose for a typical xerogram exposure in the BCDDP was 0.37 rad, and the average mid-breast dose for a typical film screen mammogram exposure in the BCDDP was 0.04 rad. In comparison with other risks of living, the risk of having an x-ray film screen mammogram is equivalent to the risk of smoking several cigarettes, driving 60 miles in an automobile, or being a 60-year-old man for 10 minutes.

Based on the success of the national BCDDP project in finding early breast cancer, it is possible to conservatively calculate that the *risk versus benefit* ratio of mammography is well over 25 to 1 for women who begin breast *screening* at age 50. That means that at least 25 cancers can be found and successfully treated for every cancer induced. In women 35 years of age who enroll in lifetime annual screening mammography, at least 10 cancers can be found and successfully treated for every cancer induced.

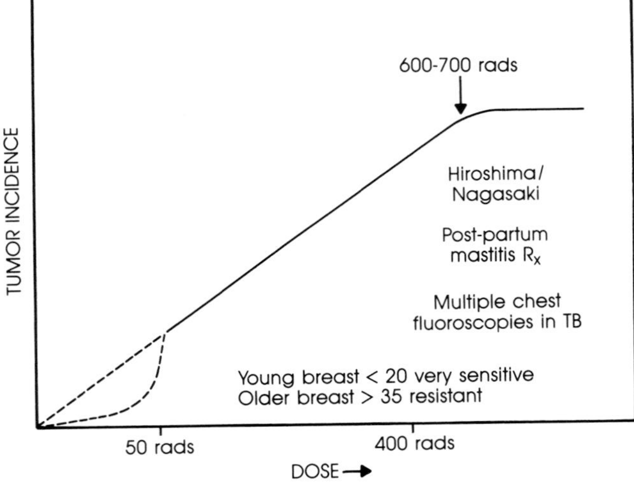

Fig. 27-3. Dose response curve for radiation-induced breast cancers. The *solid line* represents a summary of known data from three different populations exposed to large doses of radiation. Since there is no population data available that shows an increased incidence of breast cancer at doses under 50 rads, the *dotted lines* indicate estimated incidence at lower doses. The *upper straight-line* estimate is a direct extrapolation from the known data. This model is the one used in all calculations of radiation risk. The *lower curved line* is the pattern actually observed in all experimental animal studies of radiation-induced tumors. Although the curved model would predict a lower level of risk at lower levels of radiation, this model is not used in any patient risk calculations.

The current recommendations from the American Cancer Society and the American College of Radiology concerning screening mammography are that all women over the age of 50 should have an annual mammogram. Women between the ages of 40 and 50 should have an annual or biannual mammogram, and women between the ages of 35 and 40 should have a baseline mammogram. A baseline examination made sometime before the onset of menopause is useful for subsequent evaluation of the breast.

An important observation in the previously mentioned population studies illustrating the potential sensitivity of breast tissue to radiation is that the breast tissue of women in their teens to early twenties seems to be much more sensitive to radiation than the breast tissue of women over the age of 30. We must be concerned with breast irradiation, and we need to conduct our examinations with as little radiation exposure as possible consistent with accurate detection.

Let us distinguish between the words *diagnosis* and *detection*. The mammogram is an excellent tool for the detection of breast cancer, but it does not diagnose breast cancer. Some lesions seen on the mammogram may appear consistent with malignant disease, but turn out to be completely benign conditions. Breast cancer can therefore be diagnosed only by a pathologist evaluating a tissue sample from the lesion. Mammography can detect lesions that may be cancerous. Once a lesion is detected, a more specific diagnostic evaluation of the patient, which might include aspiration, breast biopsy, or an ultrasound examination, is indicated.

The preceding discussion addresses the screening of patients who do not have significant breast symptoms. All patients with clinical evidence of significant or potentially significant breast disease should undergo mammography, and all patients who are going to have a breast biopsy should have a mammogram (Fig. 27-4).

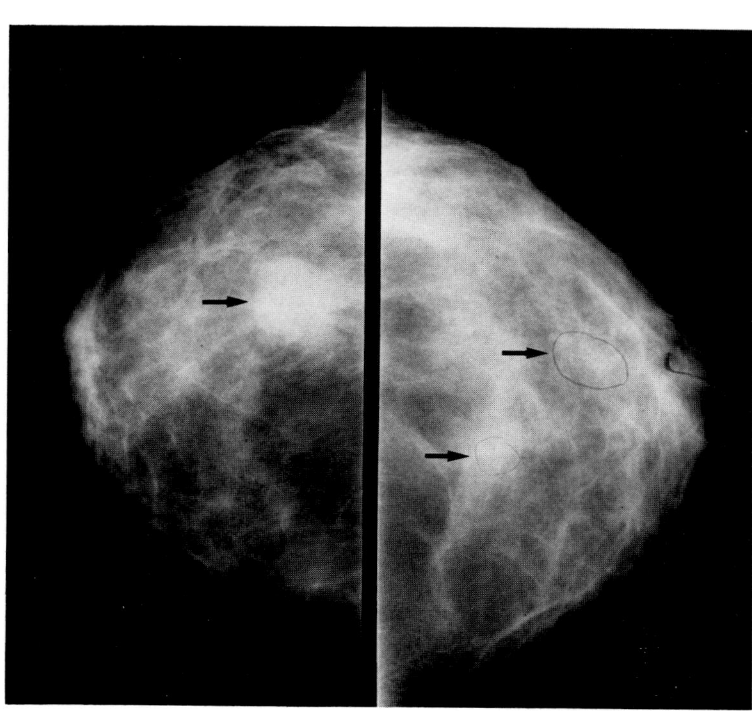

Fig. 27-4. Craniocaudal projections of the right and left breasts in a 28-year-old woman 4 months postpartum and not breast feeding. The right breast contains a large firm mass (*arrow*) palpable on physical examination. The left breast contains two smaller nonpalpable masses (*arrows*) with microcalcifications. All three lesions were breast cancers.

Anatomy and Physiology of the Breast

The terms *breast* and *mammary gland* are often used as synonyms. Anatomy textbooks tend to use the term *mammary gland,* whereas radiography texts tend to favor the term *breast*. The breasts (mammary glands) are lobulated glandular structures located within the superficial fascia of the anterolateral surface of the thorax of both males and females. The mammary glands divide the superficial fascia into anterior and posterior components, so that the mammary tissue is completely surrounded by fascia and is enveloped between the anterior and posterior layers of superficial fascia. In the female, the breasts represent one of the secondary sex characteristics and function as accessory glands to the reproductive system by producing and secreting milk during lactation. In the male, the breasts are rudimentary and without function. Rarely, they are subject to abnormalities, such as neoplasm, which require radiologic evaluation.

The female breast varies considerably in size and shape, depending on the amount of fat and glandular tissue and the condition of the suspensory ligaments. Each breast is usually cone shaped, with the base or posterior surface of the breast overlying the pectoralis major and serratus anterior muscles. These muscles extend from the second or third rib inferiorly to the sixth or seventh rib and from near the lateral margin of the sternum laterally toward the anterior axillary plane. An additional projection of breast tissue called the axillary prolongation or axillary "tail" of the breast extends from the upper lateral base of the breasts into the axillary fossa (Fig. 27-5).

The breast tapers anteriorly from the base, ending in the nipple, which is surrounded by a circular area of pigmented skin called the areola. The breasts are supported by suspensory ligaments extending from the posterior layers of the superficial fascia through the anterior fascia into the subcutaneous tissue and skin. These ligaments are called Cooper's ligaments. It is the condition of these ligaments and not relative fat content that gives the breasts firmness or lack of firmness.

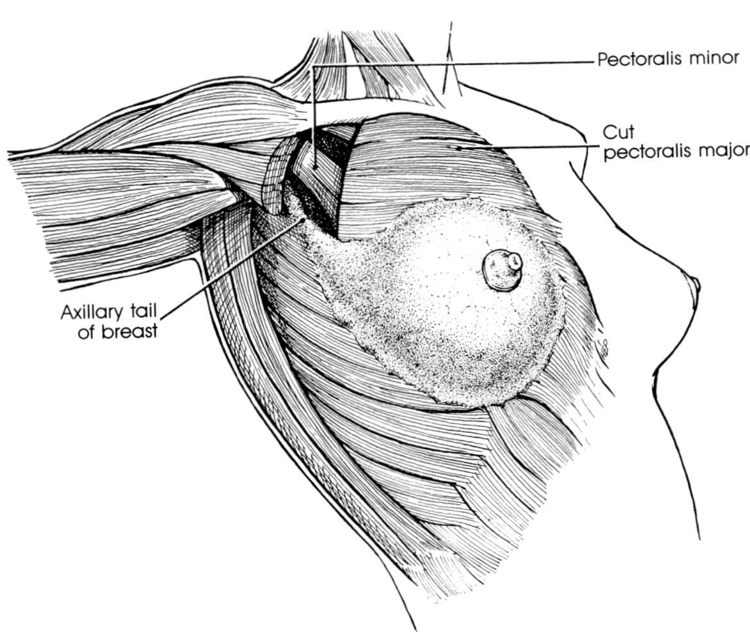

Fig. 27-5. Relationship of the breast to the chest wall is demonstrated. Note the extension of breast tissue posteriorly into the axilla.

The adult female breast consists of 15 to 20 lobes. The lobes are distributed so that there are more lobes superiorly and laterally than inferiorly and medially. Each lobe is divided into many lobules, which are the basic structural units of the breast. The lobules contain the glandular elements, or acini. Each lobule consists of several acini, draining ducts, and interlobular stroma or connective tissue. All these elements are part of the breast parenchyma and participate in hormonal changes. During the late teens to early twenties, each breast contains several hundred lobules. The lobules tend to decrease in size and number with increasing age and particularly after pregnancy. This normal process is called *involution*.

The openings of each acinus join to form lactiferous ductules that drain the lobules, which in turn join to form 15 to 20 lactiferous ducts, one for each lobe. Several lactiferous ducts may combine before emptying directly into the nipple, so that there are usually fewer duct openings on the nipple than there are breast ducts and lobes. The individual lobes are incompletely separated from each other by the Cooper's ligaments. The space between the lobes also contains fatty tissue and additional connective tissue. A layer of fatty tissue surrounds the gland, except in the area immediately under the areola and nipple (Fig. 27-6).

The lymphatic vessels of the breast drain laterally into the axillary lymph nodes and medially into the internal mammary chain of lymph nodes. Approximately 75% of the lymph drainage is toward the axilla, and 25% of the drainage is toward the internal mammary chain. The axillary nodes vary in number from 12 to 30 or more. The axilla is occasionally radiographed during breast examinations to evaluate these nodes. The internal mammary nodes are situated behind the sternum and manubrium and, if enlarged, are occasionally visible on a lateral chest radiograph.

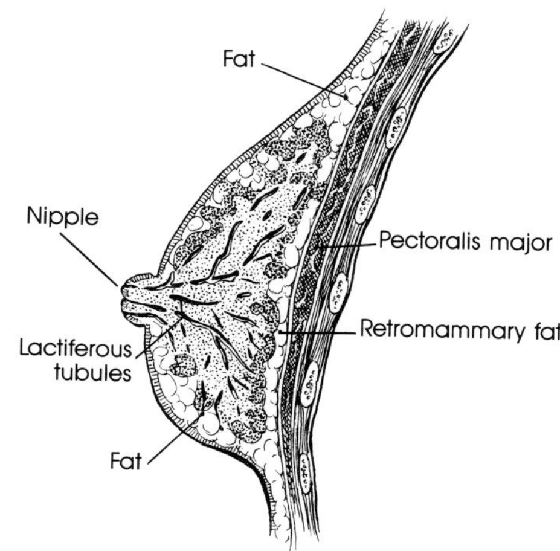

Fig. 27-6. Sagittal section through the female breast illustrating structural anatomy.

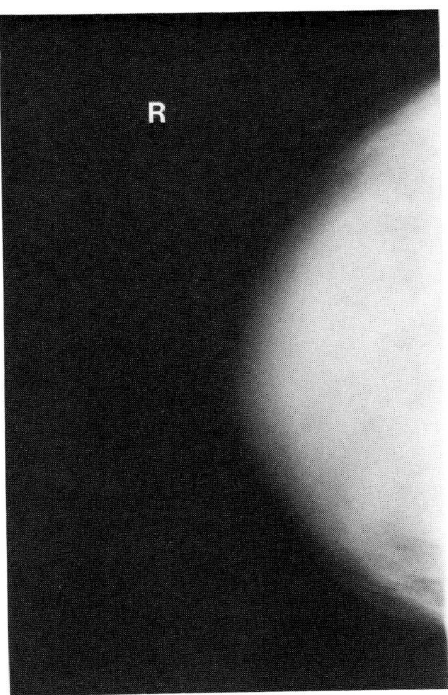

Fig. 27-7. Craniocaudal projection of normal breast of 19-year-old woman who has never been pregnant. Note dense glandular tissues with small amounts of fat. For women who do not become pregnant, breasts may remain dense for many years.

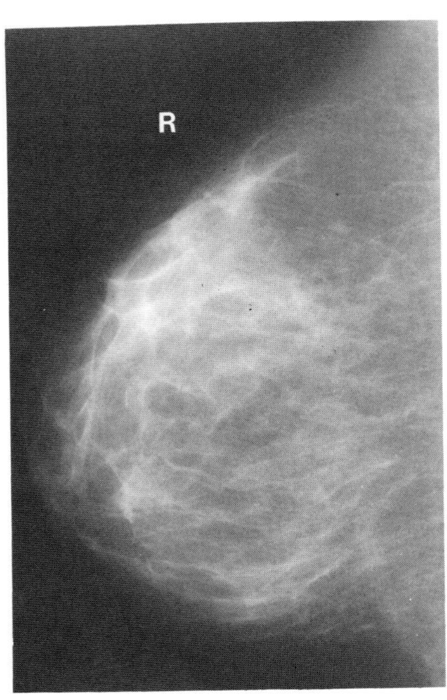

Fig. 27-8. Mediolateral projection of normal breast of 24-year-old woman who has had two pregnancies. Note decreased volume of glandular tissue and increased amount of fat.

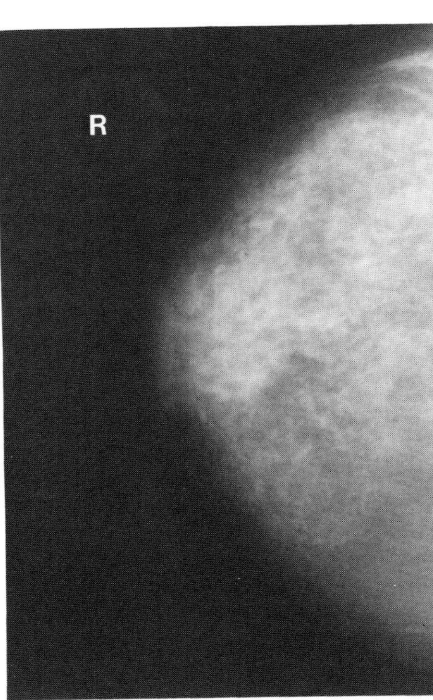

Fig. 27-9. Craniocaudal projection of breast of 42-year-old woman with fibrocystic disease illustrating prominent dilated ducts.

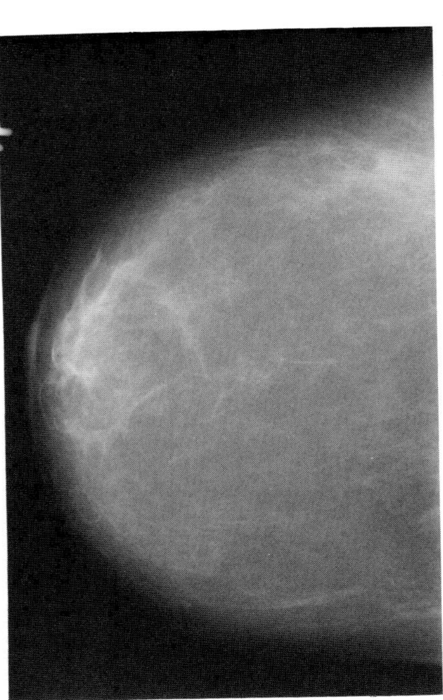

Fig. 27-10. Craniocaudal projection of normal breast of a 68-year-old woman. Most of the glandular tissue is atrophic. Some glandular tissue remains in the lateral breast posteriorly and in the retroareolar area.

TISSUE VARIATIONS

The glandular and connective tissues of the breasts are water-density structures. The ability to demonstrate radiographic detail within the breast depends on the fat within and between the breast lobules and the fat surrounding the breasts. The postpubertal adolescent breast contains primarily dense connective tissue and casts a relatively homogeneous radiographic shadow with little tissue differentiation (Fig. 27-7). Increasing development of water-density glandular tissue does not increase radiographic contrast except to the extent that the increased fat is also accumulated by the breasts. Fat accumulation varies markedly among individuals. During pregnancy, significant hypertrophy of glands and ducts within the breasts occurs. This change causes the breasts to become extremely dense and opaque. Following the end of lactation, there usually is considerable involution of glandular and parenchymal tissues, which are replaced with increased amounts of fat. This normal fat accumulation significantly increases the natural radiographic contrast within the breasts (Fig. 27-8). Patients with some forms of fibrocystic parenchymal disease may not show this involution (Fig. 27-9).

The glandular and connective tissue elements of the breast can regenerate as needed for subsequent pregnancies. After menopause, the glandular and stromal elements undergo gradual atrophy (Fig. 27-10). Major external factors such as surgical menopause and ingestion of hormones may retard this normal process. From puberty through menopause, the breast is influenced by mammotrophic hormones that induce cyclic changes. Thus the glandular and connective tissues are in a state of constant change (Figs. 27-11 to 27-15).

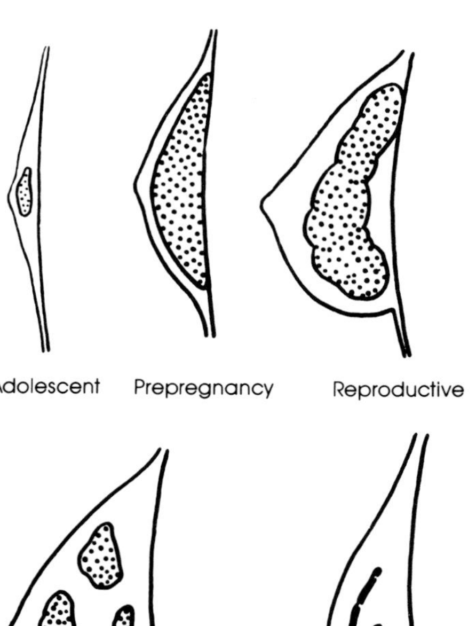

Fig. 27-11. Diagramatic profile drawings of breast illustrating the most likely variation and distribution of radiographic density (*shaded areas*) related to the normal life cycle from adolescence to senescence. This normal sequence may be altered by external factors such as pregnancy, hormone medications, surgical menopause, and fibrocystic breast disease.

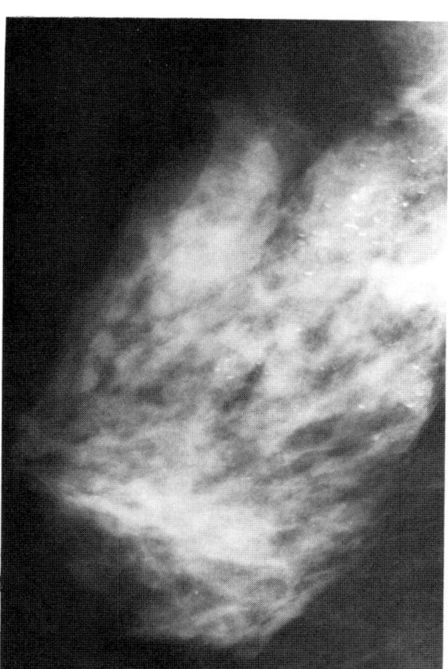

Fig. 27-12. Mediolateral projection of the breast of a 34-year-old woman with extensive fibrocystic disease.

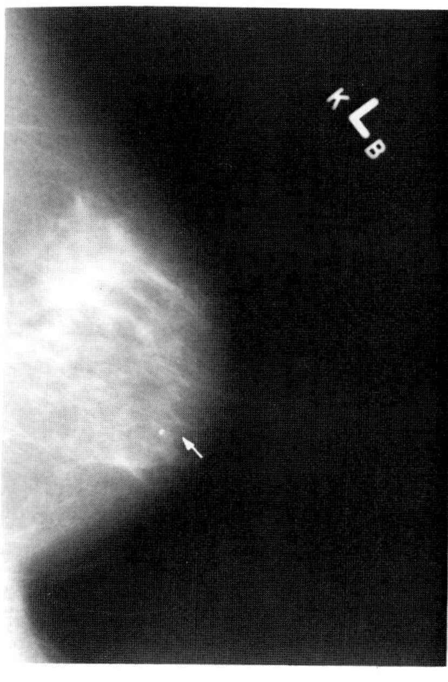

Fig. 27-13. Mediolateral projection of normal breast in a 34-year-old woman who has had three pregnancies. Some dense glandular tissue is in the upper part of the breasts. The upper and outer portions of the breast usually show the least involution. The small dense round ring-like calcification is a benign calcification in a breast duct.

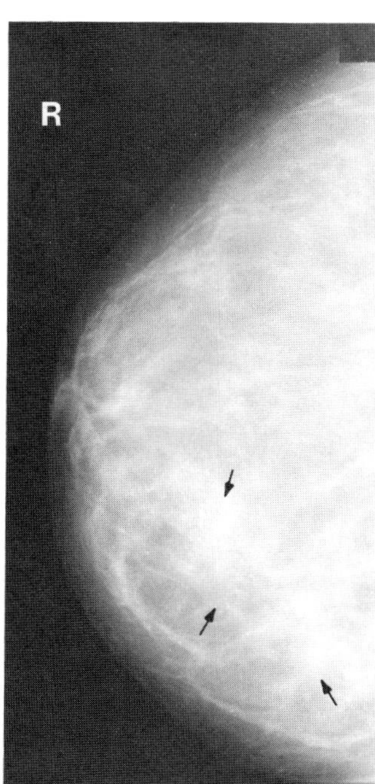

Fig. 27-14. Craniocaudal projection of breast of 37-year-old woman demonstrating extensive irregular small calcifications in carcinoma (*arrows*).

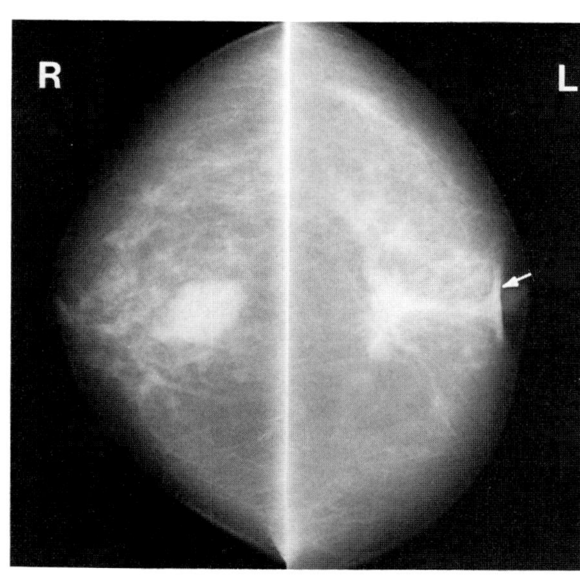

Fig. 27-15. Craniocaudal projections of bilateral breast masses. *L,* Left breast contains irregular carcinoma producing considerable spiculation and skin retraction; *arrow,* skin thickening. *R,* Right breast contains fibroadenoma.

Breast Imaging

There are two basic recording systems available for displaying x-ray images of the breast. One system uses a dry electrophotographic process called xerography and is referred to as *xeromammography*. The other system employs x-ray film and is referred to as *film screen mammography*. There is no major difference in the clinical efficacy of the two systems, but there are major differences in technical requirements. Equipment designed to work well with one image recording system is entirely inappropriate for the other.

XEROMAMMOGRAPHY

Xeromammography is a specialized radiography processing system employing a dry, electrophotographic technique. The system uses a charged aluminum plate coated with selenium powder instead of traditional x-ray film. A thin layer of the selenium powder is carefully deposited on an electrically conductive plate. The powder is then charged by applying an electrical voltage; the charge remains uniformly distributed over the plate. When exposed to x rays, the plate discharges in proportion to the quantity of radiation deposited. The remaining charge on the plate contains the latent x-ray image. This electrostatic image is made visible by dusting the selenium layer with a fine layer of charged powder, which brings out a fine-grain image. For a permanent image, the powder image is electrostatically transferred to paper. The entire developing and recharging process is performed automatically in a special Xerox processor.

There are several major differences between xeromammography and film mammography. The relative contrast demonstrated between fat and water density is much lower in xerography than in film recording systems. However, whenever a sharp change in density occurs, the change is intensified on the xerogram by an edge enhancement effect. This effect exaggerates the actual contrast of borders and helps delineate areas of nearly equal x-ray density by accentuating edges. The xerogram has a much wider range of exposure latitude. (Latitude and contrast are reciprocal.) Because the technique depends on edge enhancement rather than natural contrast, the study should be conducted at 55 peak kilovoltage, which is much higher than the peak kilovoltage required for film screen mammography. Xerograms taken with kVp much lower than 50 to 55 result in substantially more radiation to the breast without any advantage in image quality. Xeromammography dosimetry to the breast is approximately 1 rad or less for an entire examination consisting of mediolateral and craniocaudal projections. The average mid-breast dose for a typical xerogram exposure in the BCDDP was 0.37 rad. Xerography should be performed using x rays generated from a tungsten target x-ray tube with 0.2 to 0.3 mm of aluminum filtration. Molybdenum target x-ray tubes that produce a softer x-ray beam are not appropriate for xerography.

The xerographic image contains less overall information than does a film image, but it demonstrates the important features, and the resolution is sufficient to show fine microcalcifications. The final image can be displayed in a positive or a negative mode. The negative mode has some advantage, because it requires less radiation exposure than the positive mode (Figs. 27-16 to 27-18).

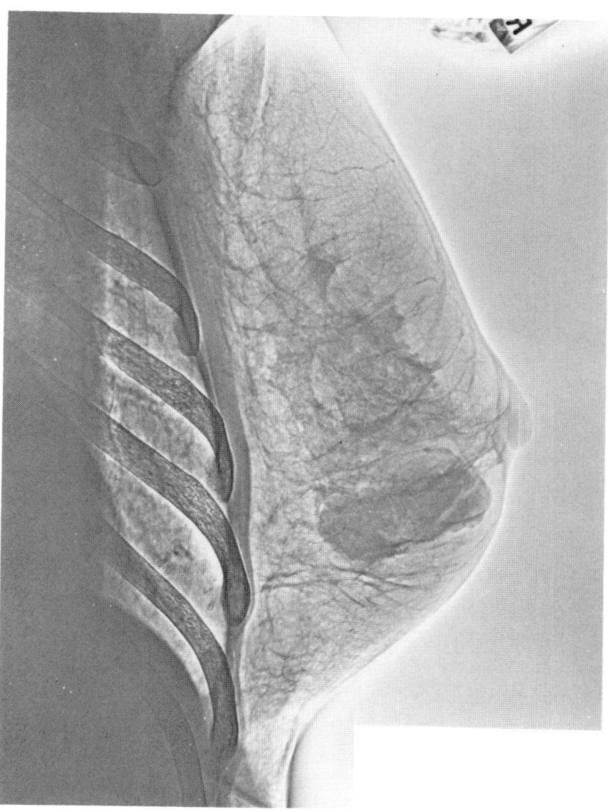

Fig. 27-16. Xerogram illustrating the mediolateral projection of the breast of a 48-year-old woman. Several large cysts are visible in the inferior portion of the breast.

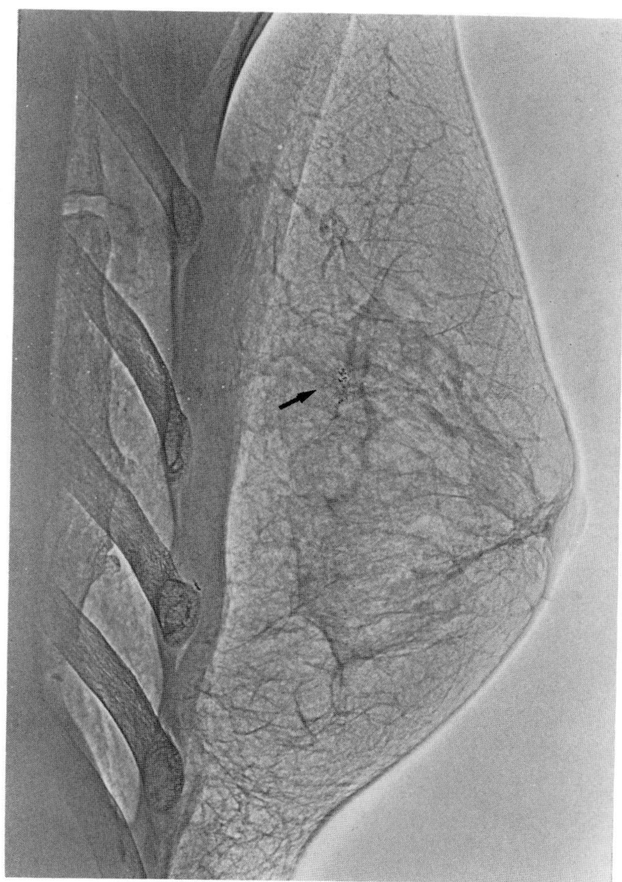

Fig. 27-17. Xerogram demonstrating the mediolateral projection of the breast of a 39-year-old woman. A small cluster of microcalcification (*arrow*) indicates the presence of a carcinoma.

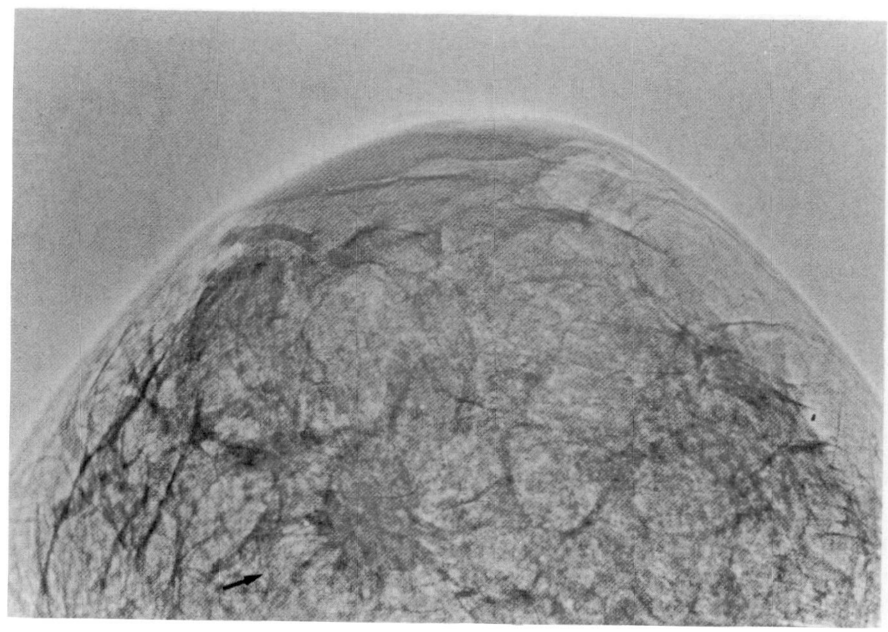

Fig. 27-18. Xerogram demonstrating craniocaudal projection of breast of 51-year-old woman with carcinoma (*arrow*).

FILM SCREEN MAMMOGRAPHY

The most commonly used film screen recording systems available from different manufacturers employ one high-resolution intensifying screen and a single-emulsion fine-grain film. Double-emulsion film screen systems designed for mammography have been developed but are not widely used. The cassettes are designed to achieve a nearly perfect film screen contact, and some cassettes even employ a vacuum to ensure this contact. The current film screen combinations result in a 30- to 150-fold reduction in breast radiation dose as compared with industrial film mammography. Film screen systems can provide excellent images with a total absorbed radiation dose for the examination of well under 1 rad to the breast. For example, the average mid-breast radiation dose from a typical exposure used in film screen mammography in the BCDDP centers was 0.04 rad. Before the successful introduction of fine-detail intensifying screens, industrial-grade nonscreen film or single-emulsion fine-grain nonscreen medical film was required to demonstrate the fine structures of the breast. These older films resulted in a radiation dose to the breast of approximately 4 to 16 rads per examination, and sometimes doses were even higher. Since satisfactory film screen combinations are available, nonscreen films should not be employed except in limited circumstances. Any imaging system, whether film screen or xerographic, that results in a breast dose greater than 1 rad per entire examination is not acceptable.

Although film screen mammography might seem to have more in common with general radiography in terms of using x-ray film, high-quality film screen mammograms cannot be made with standard x-ray equipment. Nearly all of the image contrast on a film screen mammogram is the result of the difference in the attenuation coefficients of fat and water. The maximum difference between fat and water attenuation of the x-ray beam occurs in the low kilovoltage range. With increasing kilovoltage, attenuation coefficients of fat and water become similar and the natural radiographic contrast between these two substances decreases. Film screen mammograms are usually made in the 25 to 30 kilovoltage range. The standard generators found in an x-ray department cannot make reliable exposures at this low kilovoltage. Transformers designed for low kilovoltage are required for film screen mammography.

The standard target material used in x-ray tubes is tungsten. Qualities such as heat tolerance and a smaller percentage of low kilovoltage photons make tungsten a desirable target material for most radiographic applications. However, tungsten is not desirable for film screen mammography. Molybdenum targets are more efficient at producing a low-energy x-ray beam in the kilovoltage appropriate for mammography. Molybdenum target x-ray tubes produce a high percentage of 17.5 keV characteristic molybdenum K-edge x-rays that are ideally suited for soft tissue radiography. With the exception of mammography, molybdenum target x-ray tubes have limited applications in radiology and are entirely undesirable for xeromammography, which is best performed with a tungsten target x-ray tube.

The particular requirements of film screen breast imaging led to the development of dedicated mammography systems. The first such unit was the CGR Senographe introduced in 1969 (Fig. 27-19). Specialized units have many common design features, such as transformers that operate in the low kilovolt range and molybdenum target x-ray tubes. Usually filtration material of 0.03 mm of additional molybdenum (0.5 mm aluminum equivalent) is added to the beam to produce some minimal hardening and to further increase the proportion of 17.5 keV characteristic x-rays. X-ray tubes with small focal spot targets improve geometric sharpness and produce better definition of small structures. The original dedicated units had focal spots of 0.5 to 0.6 mm, and focal spots of 0.3 to 0.4 mm are currently available. Some units are designed for magnification studies, and these units feature target focal spots of 0.1 mm.

It is essential that the anode of the x-ray tube be placed closest to and aligned with the plane of the patient's anterior chest wall and that the cathode end be away from the patient. By orienting the x-ray tube as such, the x-rays that are most parallel to the plane of the chest wall can be projected through the posterior breast (closest to the chest wall) and be included on the image.

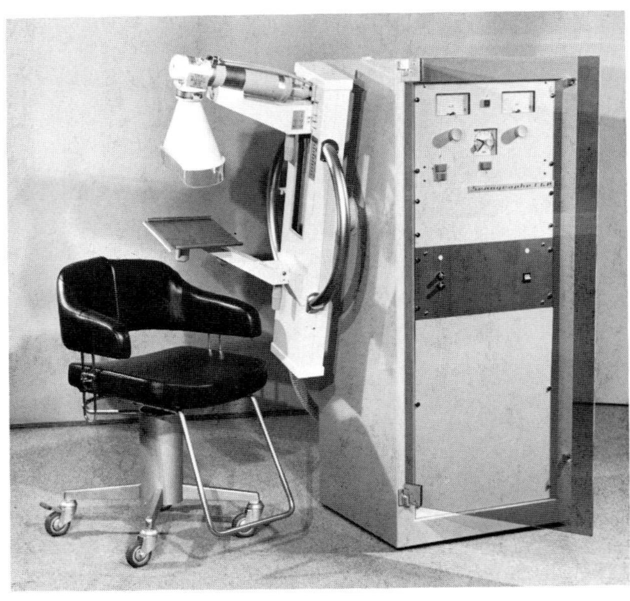

Fig. 27-19. The Senographe by CGR was the first dedicated mammography system.

Compression devices are built into mammographic units. One of the basic problems with breast imaging, particularly with film screen systems, relates to the variation in thickness of the breast from front to back (Fig 27-20). Uniform compression of the entire breast equalizes the great difference of front-to-back thickness. As the maximum thickness of the breast is decreased by compression, exposure time is shortened. In addition to reducing radiation exposure, the compression technique produces a radiograph of more uniform density. Compression pushes all of the contents of the breast closer to the x-ray film, further decreasing geometric distortion. Spreading the breast out over a greater area of the film decreases the summation effects of overlying structures. Compression can also reduce the motion of the breast during relatively long mammographic exposures, and it can enhance the demonstration of any architectural distortion produced by small tumors. The wide latitude of xeromammography allows adequate exposure of the entire breast without the extreme compression necessary for film screen mammography. Compression is still useful to reduce motion, decrease overlap, and enhance recognition of architectural distortion produced by tumors. Compression should be considered an important aid to xeromammography and absolutely essential for film screen mammography.

Some patients may feel considerable discomfort with adequate compression. The patient will be better able to cooperate for the examination and tolerate the compression if she understands why compression is necessary for a satisfactory examination. Some mammographers recommend that patients go on a low-caffeine diet for several days before the mammogram. This is thought to increase some patient's tolerance of compression.

The use of any type of compression requires a firm, nonyielding, film-holding surface on which the breast can be supported. In some units, compression material is attached to the end of the mammography cone, but most units achieve compression by use of an adjustable compression plate attached to the film holding tray. Fig. 27-21 illustrates the effect of compression, focal spot size, and targeted film distance on image sharpness. The target-to-film distance of a dedicated mammography system should be at least 24 inches.

There is considerable variability in the tissue density of breasts of different patients related to the varying amounts of fat-density material and water-density material contained within the breast. The tone and firmness of the breast result from the tone of the supporting suspensory (Cooper's) ligaments and not from the relative proportions of fat and water density tissue. It is not possible to evaluate the relative proportion of fat and water density in the breast based on physical examination of the breast. Therefore accurate exposures in mammography can best be achieved with automatic exposure control. Most dedicated mammography units have an automatic exposure control built into the film holder. As with all automatic exposure systems, it is important to position the thickest part of the breast over the detector so that the exposure does not terminate prematurely.

Dedicated mammography systems all have cones that ensure proper collimation and projection of the useful x-ray beam. These systems are compact and allow for all projections of the breast or axilla with the patient in the standing or seated position. The convenience, speed, and small space required by these units are all advantages, particularly when a large number of patients are to undergo radiography. One perceived disadvantage of the dedicated mammography film screen unit is that the chest wall is not visualized. Some physicians believe this is a drawback because a deeply seated tumor may not be identified. However, with due care, it is usually possible to pull the breast forward into the field of view so that all of the posterior mammary tissue is examined.

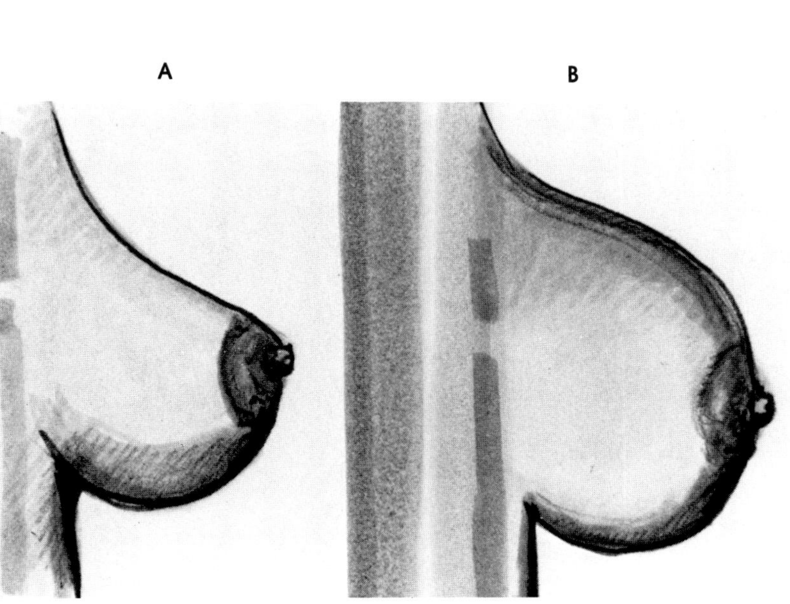

Fig. 27-20. A, Lateral position demonstrating inadequate compression and a drooping breast. **B,** Properly compressed breast shows compression has overcome the effect of gravity. Note the upper portion of the breast bulges outward and the breast does not droop.

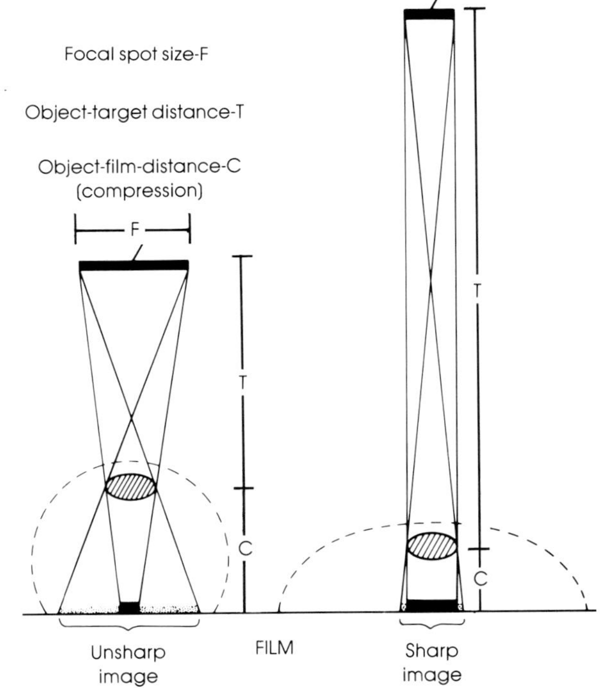

Fig. 27-21. Technical factors affecting image sharpness.

Most mammography systems have moving grids available for reducing the amount of scattered x-radiation reaching the film. Only moving grids are acceptable, because visible grid lines produced by stationary grids will compromise the image quality. The specially designed grids usually have a 5:1 or 6:1 grid ratio.

The use of grids in mammography requires an approximately two-fold increase in the amount of x-radiation required to obtain a properly exposed image. Authorities still debate the merits of routine grid use, contrasting the improved image quality against the increased radiation received by the patient. It is generally accepted, however, that grids do significantly improve image quality in dense breasts (Fig. 27-22) and in breasts that cannot be compressed to 6 cm or less. Grids yield little improvement in image quality when radiographing fatty breasts that can be compressed to 6 cm or less (Fig. 27-23).

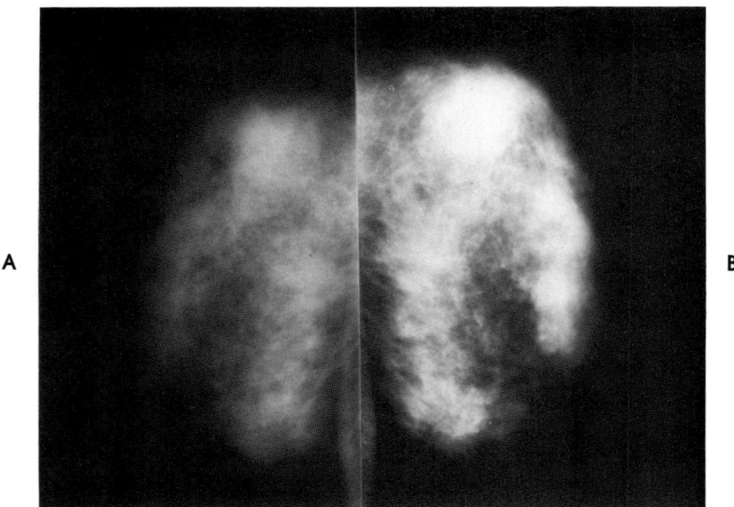

Fig. 27-22. Comparison of lateral breast images of the same dense breast exposed **A,** without a grid, and **B,** using a grid 2 years later. The image using the grid demonstrates much more detail in the breast tissue.

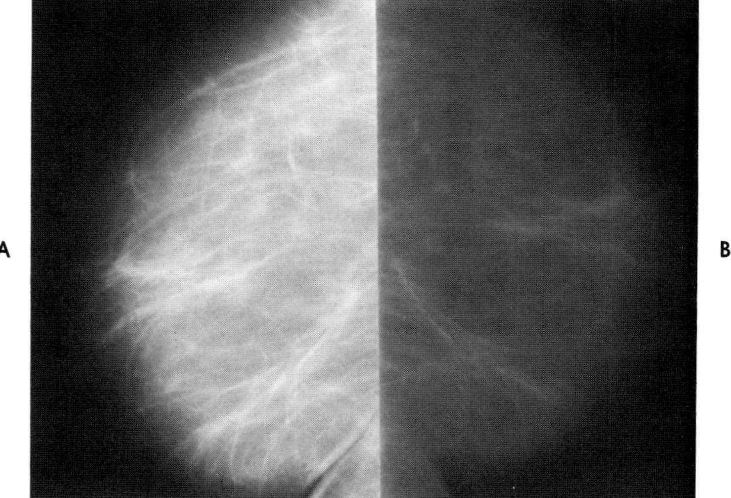

Fig. 27-23. Comparison of lateral breast images of the same fatty breast that was compressed to 6 cm. **A,** was obtained without using a grid, and **B,** was obtained with a grid 2 years later. There is no significant difference in the amount of recorded detail within the breast on the two images.

Some institutions confine the use of grids to breasts that cannot be compressed to less than 6 cm and to breasts that are known to be dense or are shown to be dense after the initial image is reviewed. A grid system that is easily mounted and dismounted makes such flexibility possible.

For any imaging system there must be strict attention to quality assurance. At least once a year a qualified physicist should calibrate the exposure timer's accuracy and reproducibility, the linearity of milliamperage settings, and the uniformity of exposure over the x-ray field. All interlocks need to be checked for proper function, and the unit should be checked for radiation leakage from the x-ray tube housing. At least every 6 months measurements should be taken of the absolute exposures at the breast surface. Measurements of the focal spot size should be taken, the beam quality should be evaluated, and the integrity of the filters should be tested. Exposures of a standard phantom should be made and evaluated at least monthly and preferably at far more frequent intervals. Fig. 27-24 illustrates a standard mammography phantom with which an evaluation of line pair resolution, densitometry, and contrast resolution can be made.

With film screen mammography, close attention must be paid to the temperature of the x-ray processor. The processor must be cleaned at frequent intervals. Single-emulsion film is nonforgiving, and processor insults to the film that would go completely unnoticed with a standard double-emulsion film can severely compromise a mammogram. Xerographic processors also deserve frequent preventive maintenance.

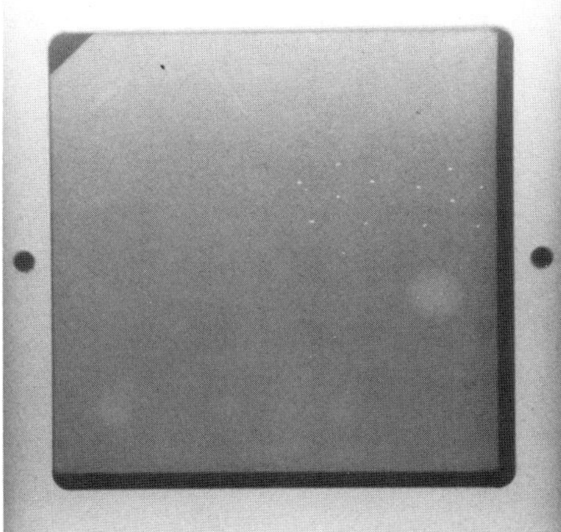

Fig. 27-24. Radiograph of the RMI (Radiation Measurements, Inc.) breast phantom containing a series of fibers, specks, and masses. A minimum of four fibers, three specks, and three masses should be readily visible if the mammography and film processing systems are working properly.

Method of Examination

The patient should be dressed in an open-front gown. The breast must be bared for the examination because the mammogram will record the slightest wrinkle in any cloth covering. Before the breast is radiographed, a careful physical examination is performed, and all biopsy scars, palpable masses, suspicious thickenings, skin abnormalities, and nipple alterations are noted. Both breasts are routinely radiographed in craniocaudal and oblique positions. Sometimes a mediolateral projection is substituted for the oblique position, and occasionally additional positions, including axilla, lateromedial, and modified craniocaudal positions, are useful.

In a symptomatic patient the examination should not be limited to the symptomatic breast. Both breasts should be examined, both for comparison and because significant lesions may be demonstrated in a clinically normal breast.

ROUTINE POSITIONS

In this section, techniques for conducting mammographic examinations on dedicated systems are described.

For each of the two basic breast positions, the breast must be firmly supported and adjusted so that the nipple is directed straightforward and profiled. Film support is used to compress the surface of the breast. This compression tends to spread the breast so that the tissue thickness is more equally distributed over the film and better separation of the glandular elements is achieved. The support also aids in profiling the nipple and in smoothing any wrinkling and puckering of the skin. If the shape of the breast is such that profiling the nipple would cause less of the posterior breast to be included on the image, it is more important to include as much breast as possible on the image than it is to profile the nipple. Positioning of the breast should be performed consistently so that any lesion can be accurately localized in the gland and so that valid comparison can be made between periodic examinations. The identification markers should be placed according to the following standard convention: along the upper border of the breast for the oblique position and the mediolateral projection and along the lateral side of the breast for craniocaudal projections. The marker will always be toward the axilla.

Craniocaudal projection

The patient should stand or be seated on an adjustable stool facing the film holder, which is adjusted to a height sufficient for the breast to lie comfortably on the film. Place the breast on the film, and center it with the nipple in profile. Ensure that the edge of the film cassette is flush against the chest wall under the breast, and instruct the patient to press her thorax against the film holder so that the inferior margin of the breast will be on the film. The ipsilateral (same side) shoulder must be relaxed and pulled slightly inferiorly and posteriorly to permit projection of the lateral quadrants of the breast on the film. Turn the patient's head away from the side being examined (Figs. 27-25 and 27-26).

Select a contoured cone of the size required to completely cover the breast, and place it in the cone mounting bracket. Lower the cone to just below the shoulder level, check the position of the breast, and ask the patient to grip the ring of the positioning assembly. After informing the patient that compression of the breast will be used, bring the cone into contact with the breast, and slowly apply compression. Instruct the patient to indicate when compression becomes uncomfortable. Compression is adequate when palpation of the patient's breasts reveals tenseness of the breast tissue and firmness of the skin. When full compression is achieved, instruct the patient to suspend breathing, and make the exposure.

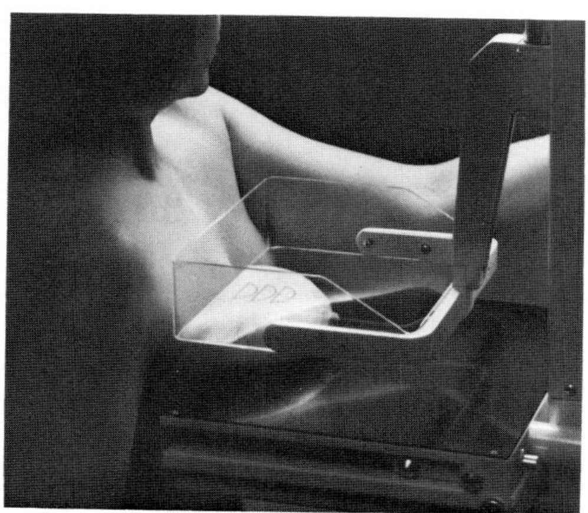

Fig. 27-25. Proper positioning for a craniocaudal projection.

(Courtesy Picker International, Inc.)

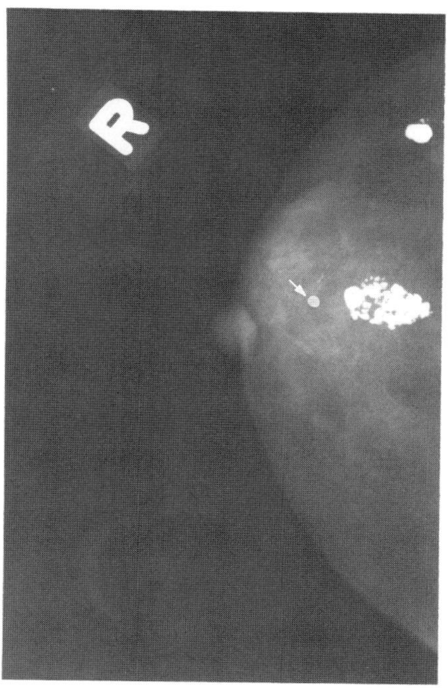

Fig. 27-26. Craniocaudal projection of breast showing several densely calcified fibroadenomas in a 72-year-old woman. *Arrow,* Small cyst or large duct with calcified wall.

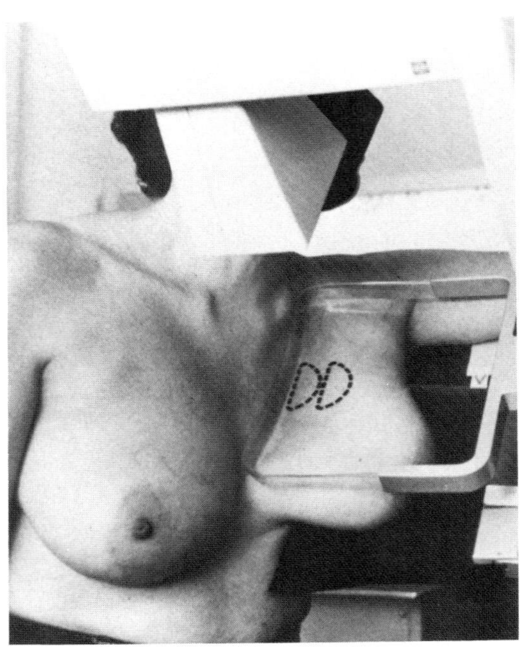

Fig. 27-27. Patient positioned for an oblique breast image.

(Courtesy Eastman Kodak Co.)

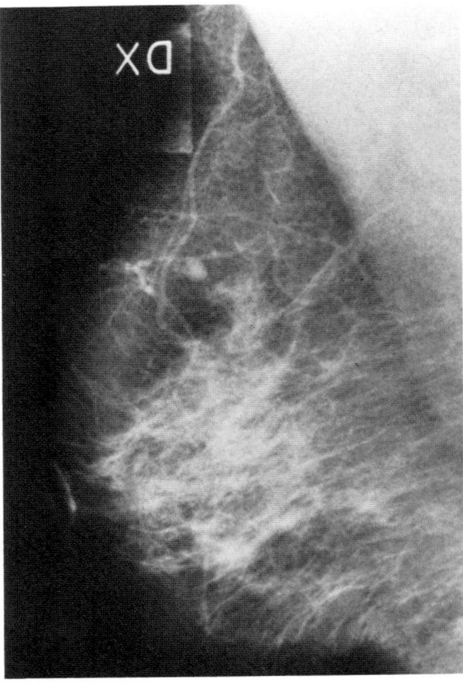

Fig. 27-28. Oblique image encompasses entire breast and part of axilla. The pectoral fold extends inferiorly to the nipple level. Note the small portion of abdomen just inferior to breasts *(arrow)*.

(Courtesy Eastman Kodak Co.)

Oblique position

The second preferred standard position is an oblique position, with the central ray directed from the superomedial to the inferolateral portion of the breast. For this position instruct the patient to raise the ipsilateral arm and rest her hand on her head. Place the film holder as high as possible into the axilla between the pectoral and latissimus dorsi muscles so the film is behind the pectoral fold. With the patient relaxed and the shoulder lowered, turn the patient toward the film holder while gently pulling the breast anteriorly away from the chest and then apply the compression plate. The central ray will pass through the breast at an angle of approximately 45 degrees, but the actual angle will depend on the angle of the pectoral muscle, which varies from patient to patient.

In a properly aligned oblique position (Fig. 27-27), the pectoral fold will extend from the axilla to at least as far as the nipple level of the breast. Additionally, a small portion of abdomen will be projected onto the film just inferior to the breast (Fig. 27-28). Including the abdomen ensures that the patient was as far against the film holder as possible and the maximum amount of posterolateral breast and axilla has been included on the film. The breast is supported by the film holder and the compression plate. The breast will not droop on the image, and the upper contour of the breast will be bulging rather than sagging.

SUPPLEMENTAL POSITIONS

Occasionally additional positions are used to supplement the standard positions.

Mediolateral projection

The mediolateral projection is useful in confirming and localizing abnormalities that are seen in only one of the standard positions.

Upright position. Rotate the tube-film assembly 90 degrees, with the cone placed on the medial side of the breast. Turn the patient slightly to bring the nipple into profile. Instruct the patient to bend slightly forward and to grasp the handgrip on the unit with the ipsilateral hand; gently push the film carrier as high as possible into the axilla. Ask the patient to relax the shoulder. Ensure that the lateral rib margin is pressed firmly against the film cassette. Elevate the dependent breast into its normal form, gently pull the breast forward, and compress it as much as possible between the cassette and the x-ray tube cone. Position the nipple as far laterally toward the film cassette as possible. Demonstration of the retromammary space and the breast lying in close contact with the thoracic walls and ribs is difficult to achieve in this upright lateral position. Pulling the breast forward is essential to bring the posterior breast tissue off the chest wall and into the radiation field (Fig. 27-29).

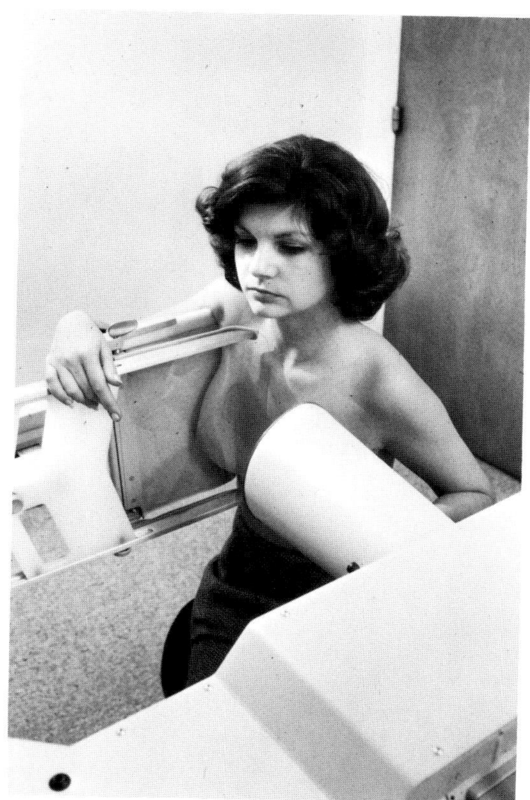

Fig. 27-29. Positioning for upright mediolateral projection.

(Courtesy Picker International.)

Recumbent position. Instruct the patient to lie on her side on the examining table with the arm of the side that is being examined placed as high as possible under the head. Place the cassette as far as possible into the axilla beneath the breast. Elevate the cassette with an adjustable film holder or sponges until the breast is elevated and flattened with the nipple in exact profile. Bring the arm forward until it forms a right angle to the long axis of the body. Flex the forearm, and supinate the hand under the head. Pull the opposite breast and shoulder posteriorly, and position the tube directly against the sternum. Use the tube to compress the breast being examined (Figs. 27-30 and 27-31).

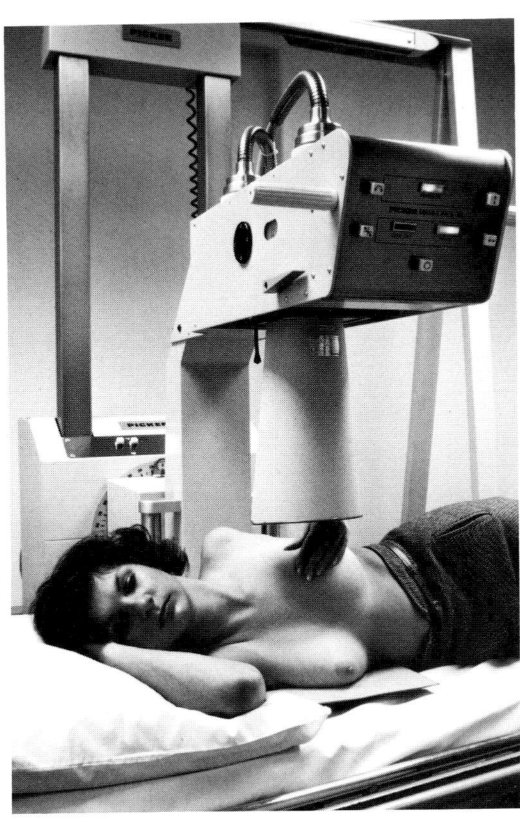

Fig. 27-30. Positioning for supine mediolateral projection.

(Courtesy Picker International.)

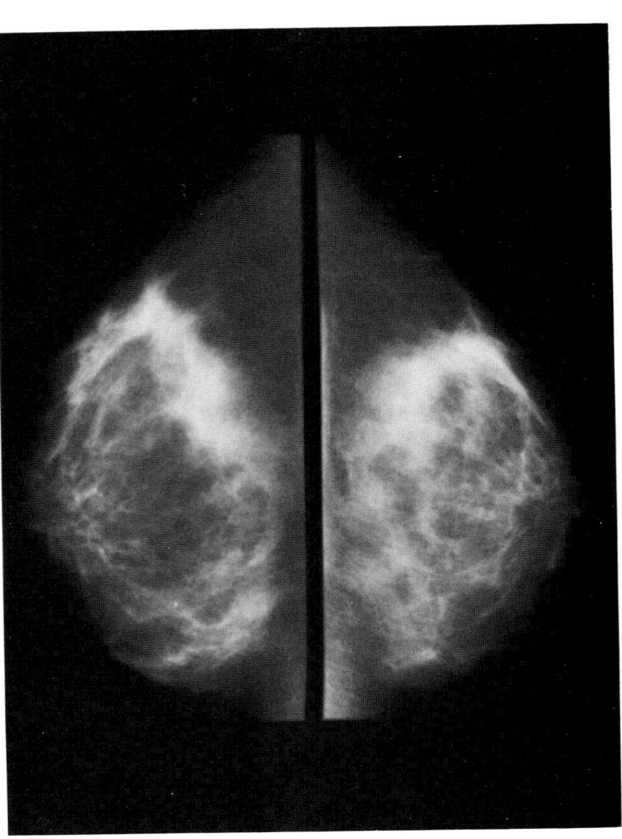

Fig. 27-31. Bilateral mediolateral breast projections. Note the basic bilateral symmetry of breast parenchyma. The tubular structures radiating toward the nipple are dilated ducts.

Lateromedial projection

The lateromedial projection is used to bring abnormalities in the medial part of the breast closer to the film for improved resolution. The film holder and tube are rotated 180 degrees from the mediolateral projection for the same breast. Note that any markers affixed to the film holder will now appear at the bottom of the film. Position the patient so the film holder is against the patient's sternum. Elevate the ipsilateral arm, and center the x-ray tube and film holder midway between the superior and inferior portions of the breast. Have the patient grasp the x-ray tube tower pulling herself forward so the sternum is placed firmly against the edge of the film, and then apply compression (Fig. 27-32).

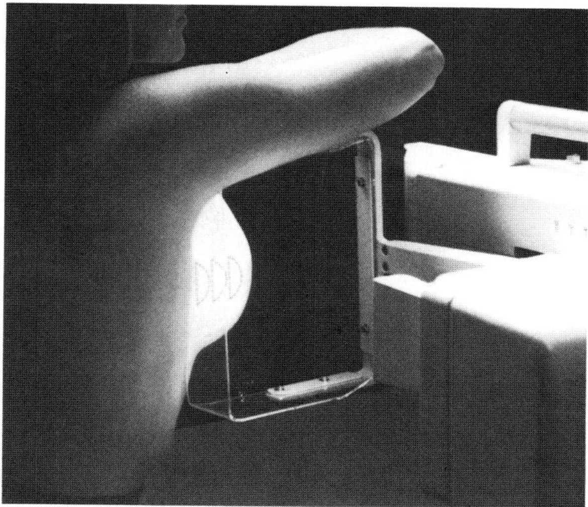

Fig. 27-32. Patient in position for a lateromedial projection. Film holder is against the sternum and the patient is pulling herself towards the x-ray tube tower.

(Courtesy Picker International.)

Axilla position

If it is desirable to evaluate the axillary lymph nodes and the axillary portion of breast tissue, an axilla position can be taken. Depending on the design of the mammography unit, conduct this position in the supine or the upright body position. In the supine position, the upper arm is held at a right angle to the body, the forearm flexed, and the hand placed under the head in supination. Place the film under the axilla in such a way that the upper arm and ribs will be included in the projection. Pull the breast medially, and direct the central ray of the x-ray tube between the head of the humerus and the ribs (Fig. 27-33). Do not use compression in this position. Increase the exposure by approximately 2 kVp.

To demonstrate the axilla in the upright body position, instruct the patient to abduct the arm so that it is perpendicular to the longitudinal axis of the body. Position the patient so the axilla overlies the film and so that the upper arm and ribs will be included in the image. Direct the central ray between the head of the humerus and the ribs (Fig. 27-34).

Modified craniocaudal projection for lateral or medial aspects of breast

Because the anterior thoracic wall curves posteriorly as it extends laterally, and since the edge of the cassette is flat, it is often not possible to project all of the medial and lateral aspects of the breast onto the film during one craniocaudal projection (Fig. 27-35). A modified craniocaudal projection can be taken to accentuate either the medial or lateral portion of the breast. When a questionable abnormality is suspected on the standard images, additional craniocaudal images taken with lateral and medial angulation of the x-ray tube can be helpful.

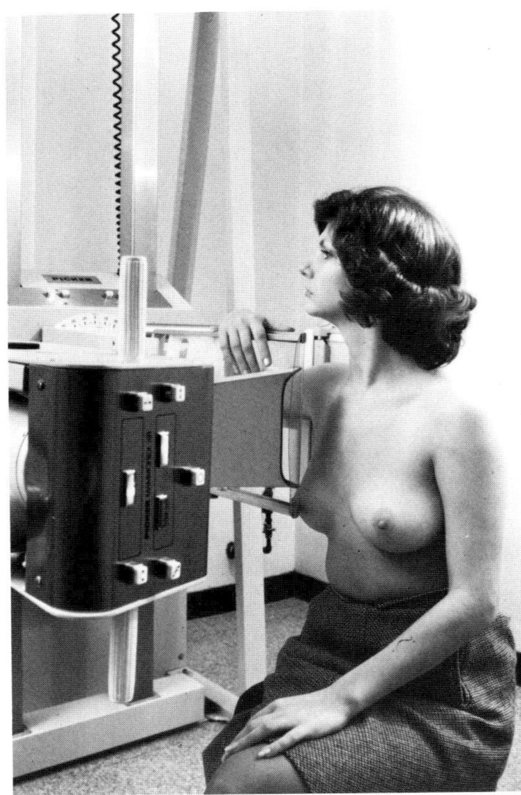

Fig. 27-33. Positioning for axillary portion of breast.

(Courtesy Picker International.)

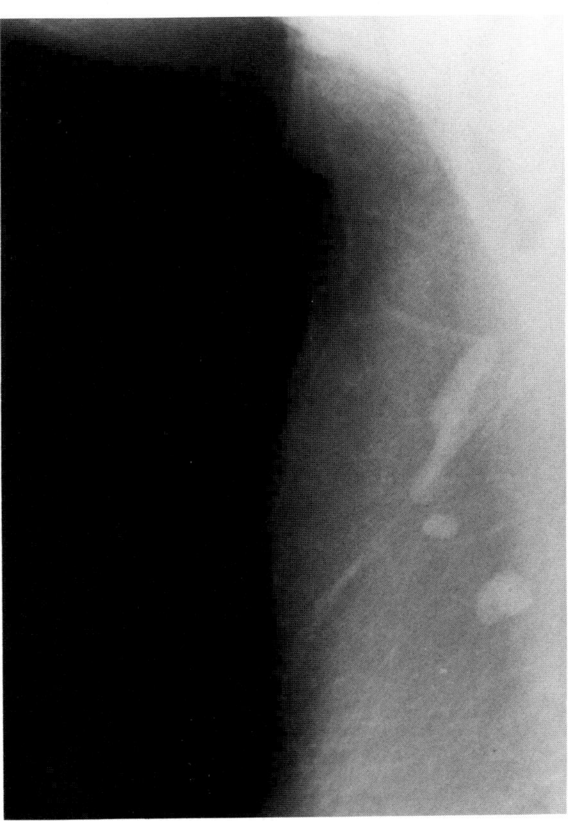

Fig. 27-34. Axillary projection containing several enlarged lymph nodes.

(Courtesy Sylvia L. Cousins, R.T.)

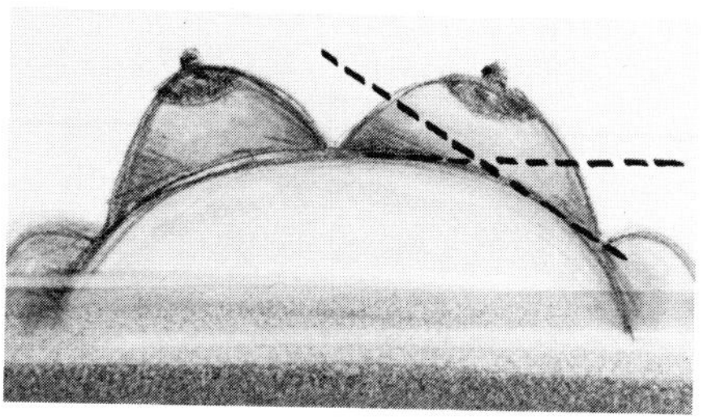

Fig. 27-35. Line drawing illustrating how placement of the flat edge of the film cassette against the curving chest wall will exclude a portion of the breast.

Cleopatra position

Another position that has been developed to demonstrate the lateral aspect of the breast, including the tail, is called the "Cleopatra" position. This position is useful only if a significant amount of breast tissue is present in the tail region (Fig. 27-36). For this position, instruct the seated patient to lean backward and laterally, with the breast support at her side. Rarely, some rotation of the torso is helpful. Ask the patient to use the ipsilateral arm to hold the cassette firmly against the chest wall. Generally, only a slight adjustment of the stool or table height from the craniocaudal position is needed, but some ingenuity is required of the technologist in arranging the breast so the maximum amount of tissue is over the cassette. Compression may be used in the fuller breast, but it can be eliminated in smaller breasts. Direct the central ray vertically; the kilovoltage peak is usually increased by 1 or 2 over that in the craniocaudal technique. This position is beneficial for problem cases in which palpable findings in the tail of the breast cannot be displayed by other methods. Some fullness and elasticity of tissues in the tail region of the breast are required for a successful projection. In addition to illustrating the tail of the breast, the Cleopatra position often demonstrates a portion of the axilla. This is a description of the Cleopatra position as originally described by Goodrich. The term is also used to describe the modified craniocaudal projection accenting the lateral breast.

A

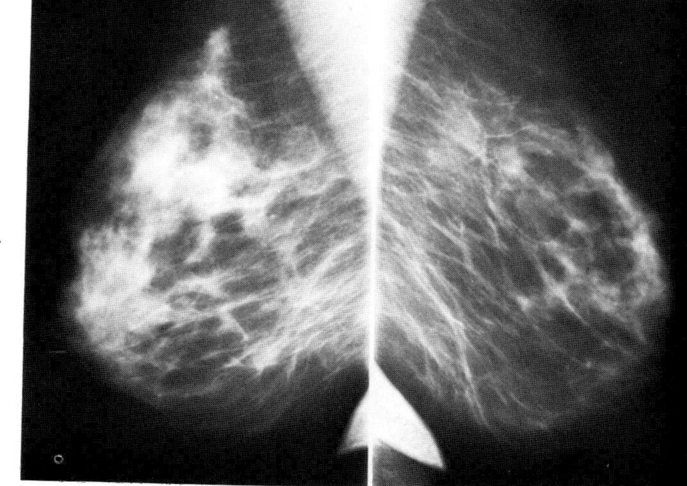

B

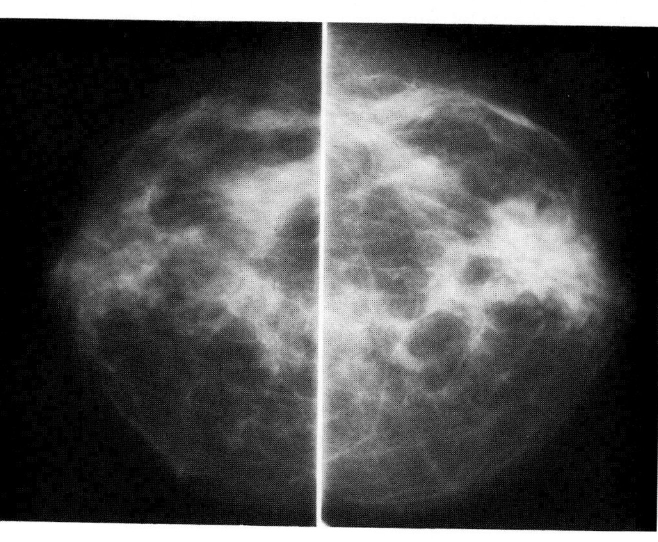

C

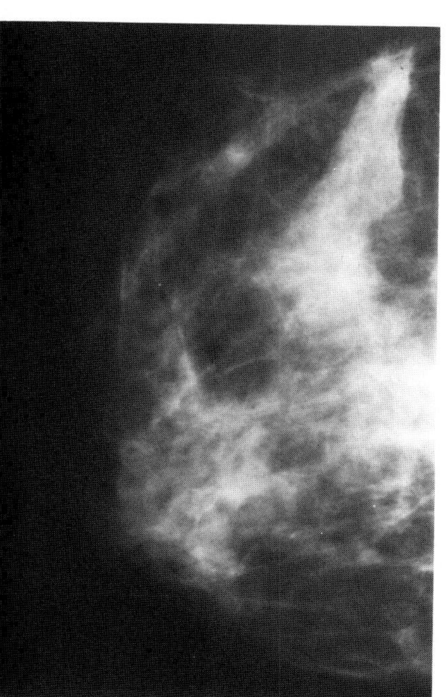

Fig. 27-36. Three images of the same patient. **A,** Oblique position showing a small cancerous mass in the upper posterior breast *(arrow). Arrowhead* shows asymmetrical increased density representing fibrosis and collegenous disposition secondary to the cancer. **B,** Standard craniocaudal projection of right breast does not demonstrate the cancer. **C,** Craniocaudal projection with the film placed under the lateral aspect of the breast demonstrates the cancer *(arrow).*

Examination of medial portion of breast

Have the patient lean forward as far as possible, pressing the sternum against the film holder and supporting herself by grasping the handgrip. Distribute the medial portion of both breasts over the film by pulling the breasts forward and flattening them. Using the smallest cone, position it firmly against the sternum by compressing the parenchyma and skin from above (Fig. 27-37). Instead of combining the medial portions of both breasts on one film, you may choose to project the breasts separately on separate films as described in the modified craniocaudal projection. With the combined projection, the exposure must be manually controlled, since the breasts do not lie over the automatic exposure control detector.

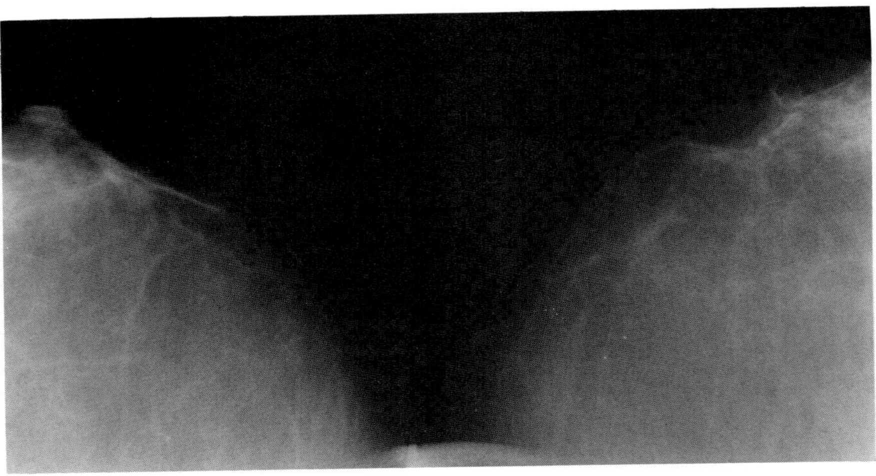

Fig. 27-37. Craniocaudal projection of the medial aspect of both breasts.

(Courtesy Sylvia L. Cousins, R.T.)

MAGNIFICATION TECHNIQUES

If the x-ray tube has a 0.1 mm focal spot target, magnification techniques can be used. Magnification is useful in evaluating the characteristics of breast calcification and the margins of breast masses to determine whether breast lesions are likely to be benign or malignant. If other positions indicate the possible presence of a lesion, magnification may clarify whether a lesion is or is not present.

All magnification techniques require the use of a firm radiolucent device, which elevates the breast above the film holder by increasing the OFD (object-film distance). Increasing the OFD requires using an additional piece of equipment that is attached above the film holder (Figs. 27-38 and 27-39). The amount of magnification is determined by the distance between the breast and the film. The amount of magnification usually ranges from 1.5× to 2× magnification, but is a fixed quantity as determined by the dimension of the magnification surface.

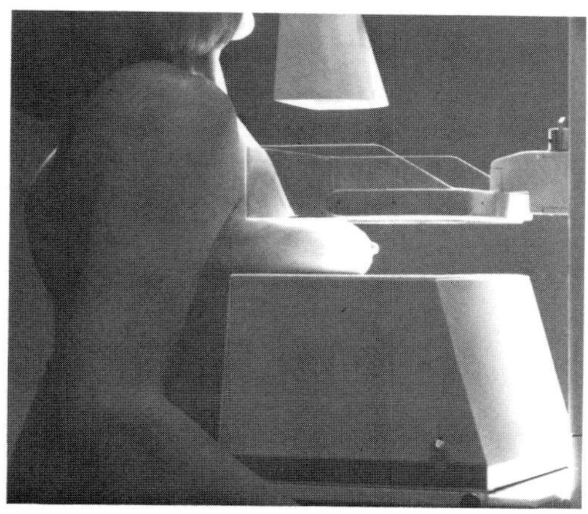

Fig. 27-38. A radiolucent spacer has been placed between the breast and the film holder. This will cause the x-ray image to be enlarged.

(Courtesy Picker International.)

A

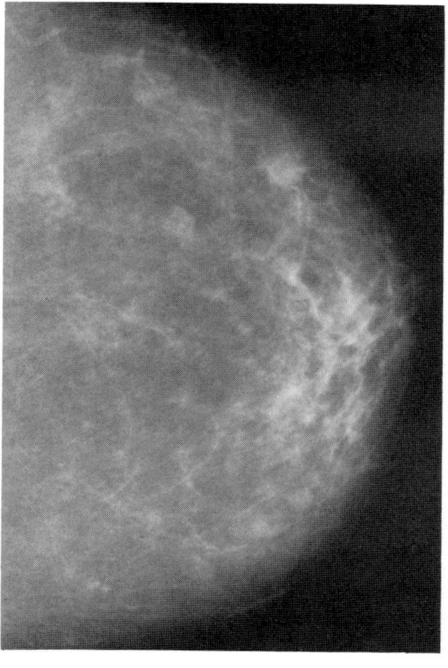

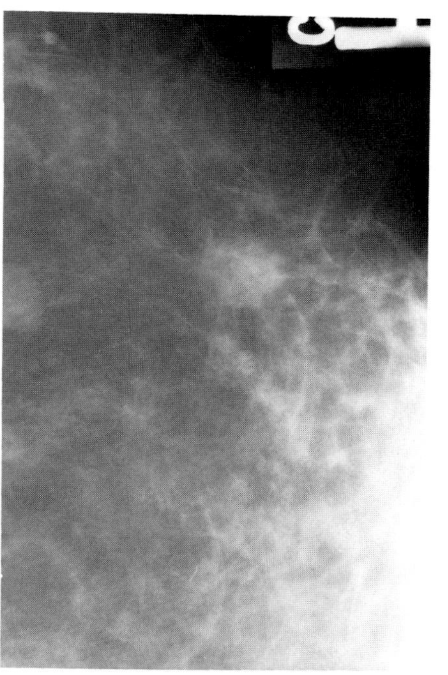

B

Fig. 27-39. A, Craniocaudal projection showing possible lesion in right breast *(arrow).* **B,** Same patient with 2× magnification and convincingly demonstrating a breast mass with irregular margin *(arrow).* Note smooth noninvasive benign lesion *(arrowhead).*

Localization of Nonpalpable Lesions for Biopsy

When mammography identifies a nonpalpable lesion, the radiology team must accurately locate the abnormality for the surgeon so that only a small amount of tissue needs to be removed for microscopic examination and trauma to the breast can be minimized. In this way the maximal amount of normal breast tissue can be preserved unless the biopsy indicates that more extensive surgery is required.

The most popular method of preoperative localization uses a needle that contains a hooked wire. The hook is preformed by folding the tip of the wire back over on itself. The three most common needle-wire designs are the Frank, Kopans, and Homer biopsy guides. With each system, a long needle containing a hooked wire is pushed into the breast so that the tip approximates the lesion. The needle is then withdrawn back over the wire leaving the hooked wire in place. The hook on the end of the wire keeps the wire fastened in the breast tissue (Fig. 27-40).

The surgeon cuts down along the wire and removes the breast tissue around the hooked end of the guide wire. The hooked end of the wire is completely contained within the Kopans and Homer needles (18-gauge). The narrow Frank needle (21-gauge) cannot accommodate the folded wire, so the hook of the wire folds back over the outside of the needle tip. The Frank needle has two minor disadvantages because of the small-diameter design. The needle cannot be pushed directly through the skin and subcutaneous tissue. It is necessary to use a scalpel blade to make a 1 to 2 mm incision in the skin at the site of needle insertion. Because the hook is outside the needle tip, the localization wire cannot be withdrawn and repositioned. The Kopans needle can be inserted without a skin incision and can be repositioned until the needle is pulled back from the end of the wire. In practice, all three systems work well. The localization procedure can be performed several hours before surgery or it can be done as part of an outpatient breast biopsy procedure.

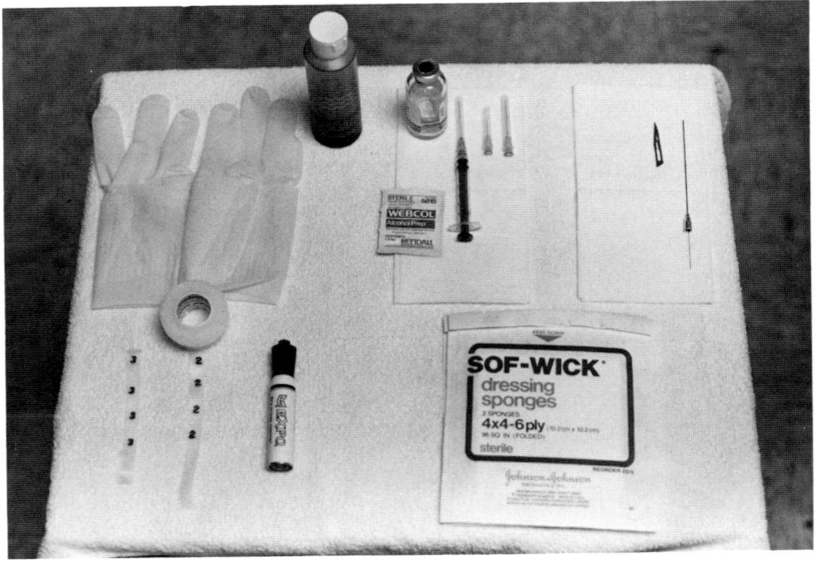

Fig. 27-40. Materials for breast localization procedure: sterile golves, betadine, xylocaine, 5 ml syringe for anesthetic, 25-gauge needle for skin anesthesia, 18-gauge needle, alcohol swab, scalpel blade, a Frank biopsy guide needle containing guide wire, skin markers and tape, magic marker, and sterile gauze.

BREAST LESION LOCALIZATION WITH A SPECIALIZED COMPRESSION PLATE

Many mammography units have an optional compression plate with an opening that can be positioned over a breast lesion and through which a localizing wire and needle can be introduced into the breast. The initial mammogram and the mediolateral projection are reviewed to determine the shortest distance from the skin to the breast lesion; for example, a lesion in the inferior region of the breast would be approached either from the inferior surface of the breast or from the medial or lateral surface, but not from the superior surface. An estimate is also made regarding the approximate depth of the lesion to the closest surface.

The opening in the compression plate may consist of a rectangular cutout with grid markings along two adjacent sides, or it may contain several rows of holes, each of which is large enough to pass the hub of the localization needle (Fig. 27-41). The skin of the breast over the lesion is cleaned with povidone-iodine, and the patient is positioned so the compression plate is as close to the lesion as possible, usually with the x-ray tube oriented along the verified (superior or inferior approach) or horizontal (lateral or medial approach) plane. A preliminary exposure is made using compression (Fig. 27-42). The film is processed without removing the breast from between the compression plate and film holder. The film will show where the lesion lies in relation to the compression plate opening. The localizing needle and guide wire are inserted into the breast perpendicular to the compression plate and parallel to the chest wall directly toward the underlying lesion. The needle is advanced to the estimated depth of the lesion, keeping in mind that it is better to pass beyond the lesion than it is to be short of the lesion. It also must be remembered that the breast is flattened and compressed in the direction of needle travel when the needle is introduced.

With the needle in position, an exposure is made (Fig. 27-43). The compression plate is then released, leaving the wire in place, and an additional image is obtained following a 90-degree shift (Fig. 27-44). From these two radiographs, the position of the end of the needle–wire combination relative to the lesion is determined. If necessary the needle and wire can be repositioned and the exposures repeated. When the needle is satisfactorily placed in the lesion, the needle is withdrawn, leaving the hooked guide wire in place. A gauze bandage is placed over the breast, and the patient is transported to surgery along with the final localization radiographs.

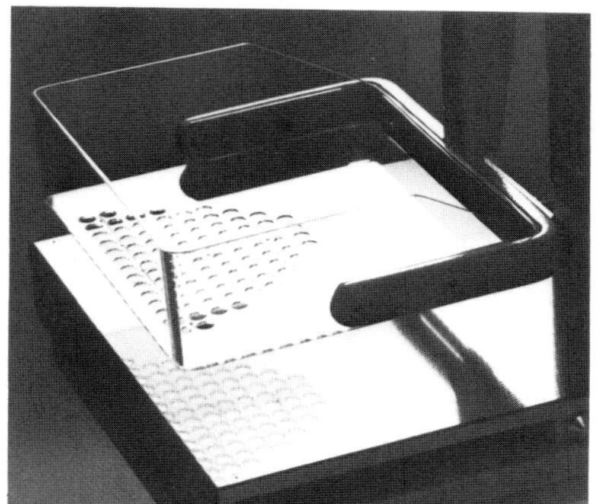

Fig. 27-41. Sample of compression plate with cutouts for introduction of a localization needle.

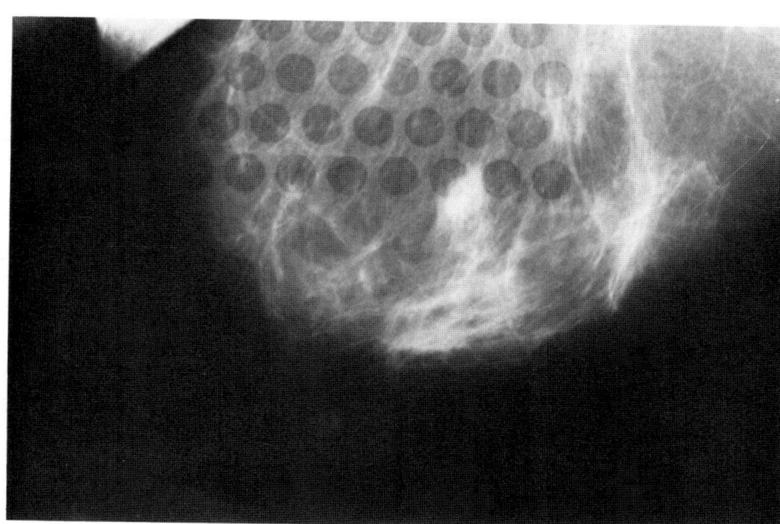

Fig. 27-42. Preliminary exposure in the lateromedial position using the localization compression plate.

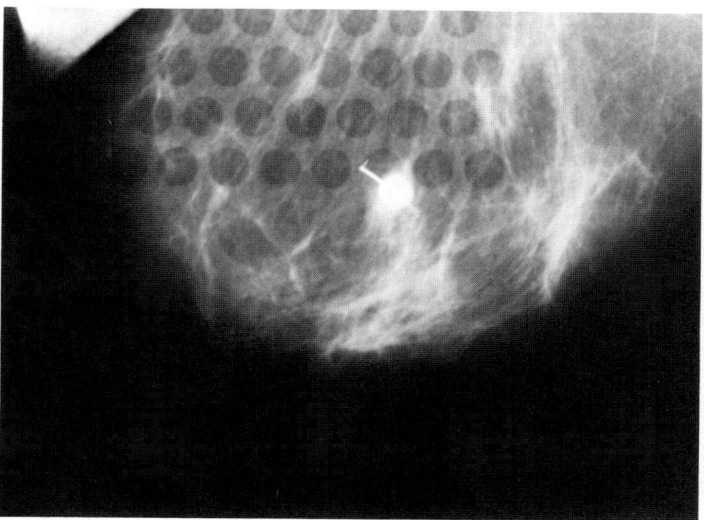

Fig. 27-43. The localizing needle has been advanced through the compression plate towards the lesion.

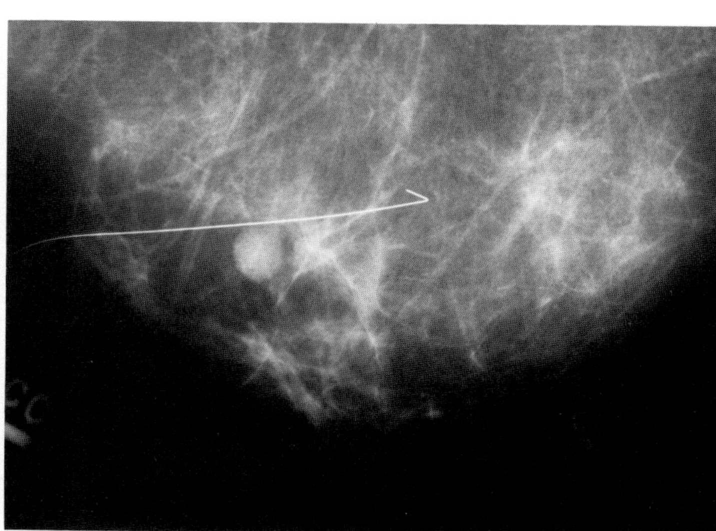

Fig. 27-44. An image obtained after rotating the x-ray tube 90 degrees to obtain the craniocaudal projection shows that the wire passes directly behind the nodule *(arrow)*. This nodule was a benign fibroadenoma.

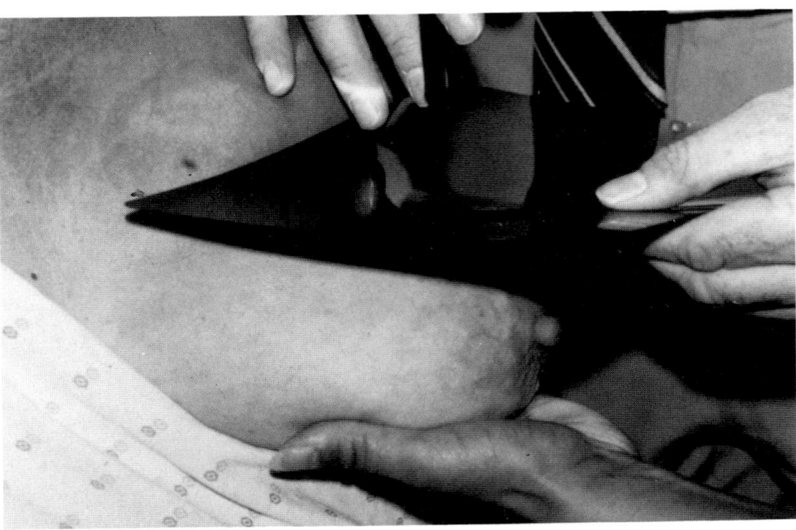

Fig. 27-45. The technologist supports the breast while the physician superimposes the craniocaudal projection mammogram over the breast, used to locate the breast lesion in reference to the skin surface.

BREAST LESION LOCALIZATION WITHOUT A SPECIALIZED COMPRESSION PLATE

Preliminary craniocaudal and mediolateral projections are taken of the abnormal breast. Using these preliminary radiographs, an ink mark is placed on the breast surface relating the position of the lesion in each projection. Taping lead markers to the breast for the preliminary films can aid in relating the position of the lesion on the radiograph to the breast surface in each projection. Because the breast is compressed for the exposures, the breast must approach the compressed position to accurately place the ink marks. The technologist assists by reproducing the compressed position of the breast with her hands while the physician orients the radiograph to the breast and marks the surface of the breast at the appropriate site (Figs. 27-45 and 27-46).

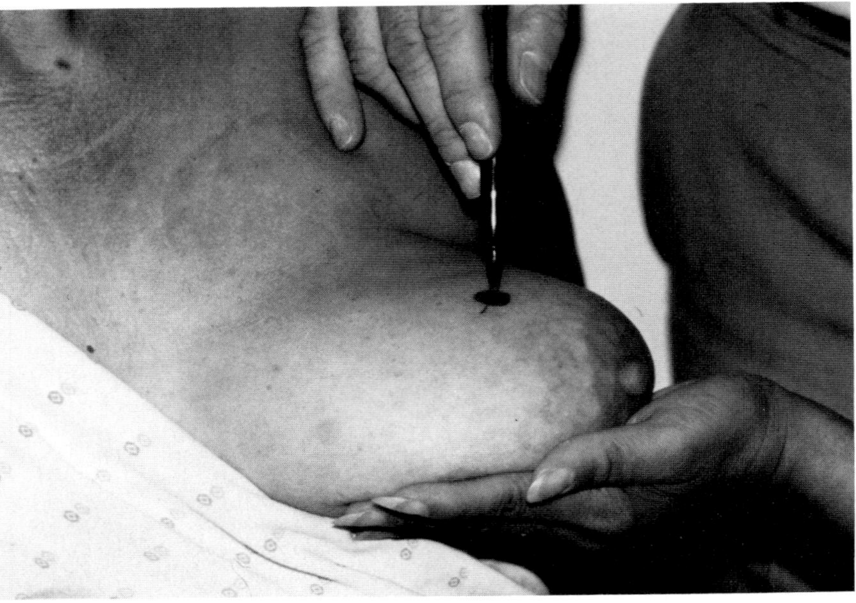

Fig. 27-46. An ink mark is placed on the breast surface directly over the breast lesion, locating the lesion in the superoinferior aspect. The same technique is used to place a mark over the lesion using the mediolateral projection to locate the lesion in the mediolateral aspect.

Triangulation of the two surface marks fixes the three-dimensional location of the lesion within the breast. The needle can be inserted either perpendicular to the chest wall or parallel to the chest wall. The breast is washed with povidone-iodine, and the selected site for needle insertion is anesthetized with lidocaine. The needle is inserted toward the lesion for the predetermined distance (Figs. 27-47 and 27-48). With the Frank system, a preliminary small incision is made in the skin and the needle is withdrawn after insertion, leaving only the guide wire in place. With the Kopans system the needle and wire are left in place. The breast is again radiographed in the craniocaudal and mediolateral projections so the exact site of the wire relative to the lesion can be determined.

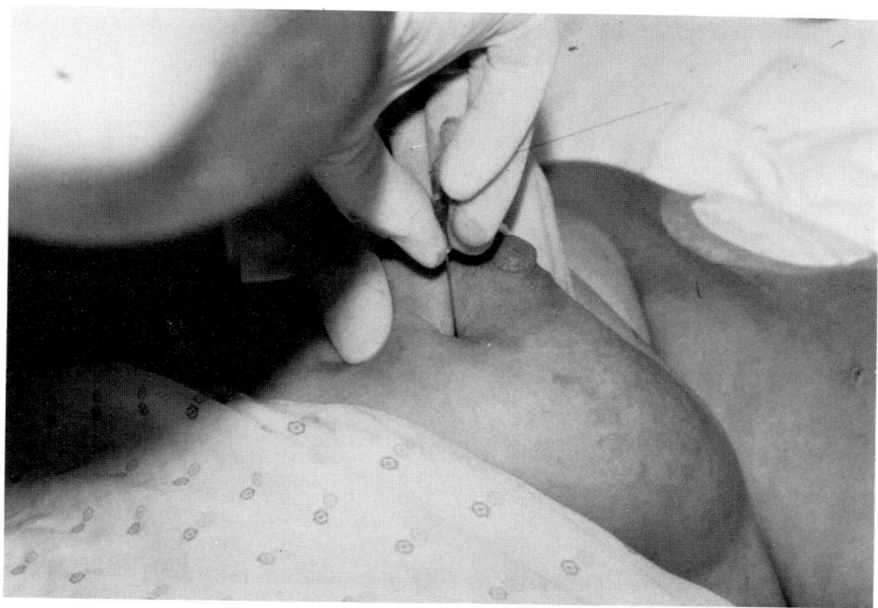

Fig. 27-47. A Frank biopsy needle and guide wire is inserted into the breast perpendicular to the chest wall at a site directly anterior to the lesion. The site and depth of insertion is selected by triangulation using the external skin marks.

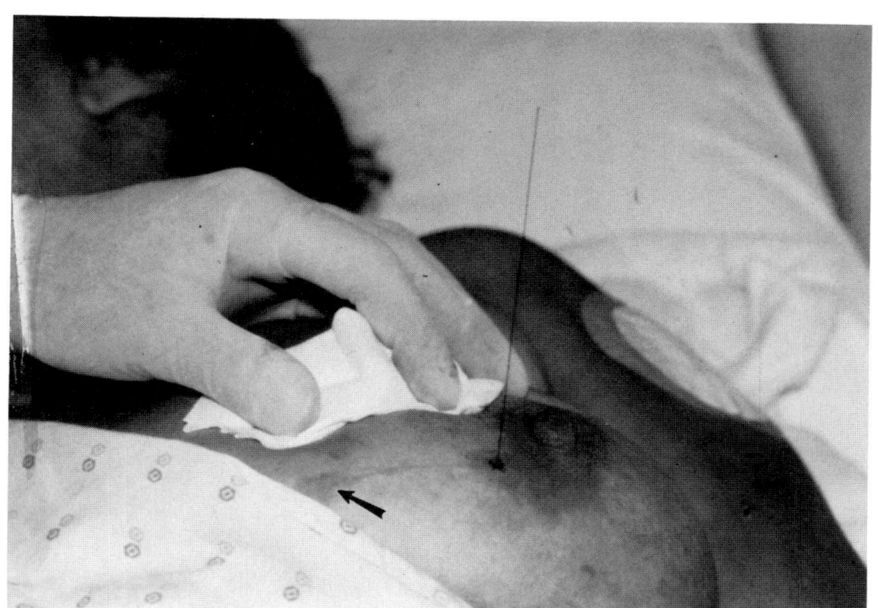

Fig. 27-48. After inserting the needle and gude wire to the depth of the lesion, the needle is removed leaving the guide wire in place. The lateral skin mark used for selecting needle insertion site is seen (*arrow*).

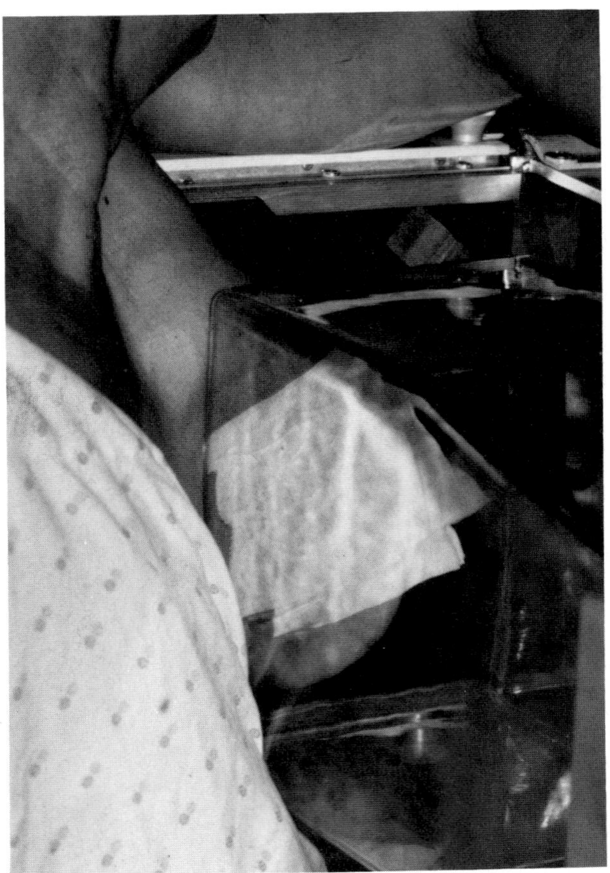

Fig. 27-49. The breast is being radiographed after wire insertion. Wire is under gauze.

The Kopans needle can be repositioned if the original location is unsatisfactory. If the Frank wire position is unsatisfactory, a second wire is introduced. A gauze bandage is placed over the breast, and the patient is referred to the surgeon (Figs. 27-49 and 27-50).

With the Kopans system, some practitioners insert the needle without the wire and, after checking the position, inject 0.3 ml of a colored dye, such as methylene blue. This further helps the surgeon immediately locate the lesion.

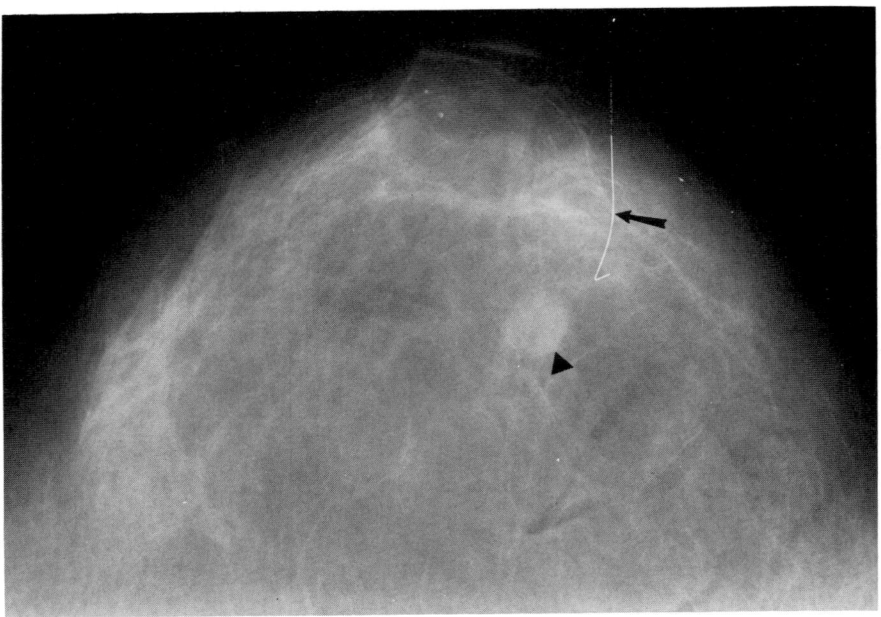

Fig. 27-50. A craniocaudal projection of the breast shows the relationship of the wire (*arrow*) to the nodule (*arrowhead*).

Breast Specimen Radiography

Of equal importance with regard to accurate preoperative localization of the site for excisional biopsy is the need to confirm that the suspected lesion is contained in the tissue removed during the biopsy. Often very small lesions are characterized only by tissue irregularity or minute calcifications that are nonpalpable in the excised specimen and may not be detectable on visual inspection. Specimen radiography is often done in an immediate postexcision procedure while the patient is still under anesthesia. Speed is therefore imperative. The selection of film type, technical factors, and the procedure for handling the specimen must be established ahead of time. The cooperation of the radiologist, technologist, surgeon, and pathologist is a necessity. Extremely fine-grain nonscreen film may be used because exposure to the patient is no longer a factor. Exposure factors used depend on the thickness of the specimen and the film employed (Fig. 27-51).

Examination of Milk Ducts

Occasionally, when a nipple discharge is localized in one of the multiple duct openings on the nipple, the milk duct can be studied with opaque contrast medium. The purpose of the examination is to seek evidence of an intraductal mass as the cause of the discharge.

Equipment and supplies needed for the examination are a sterile hypodermic syringe; a 30-gauge needle with a specially prepared, smooth round tip; a skin cleansing agent; sterile gauze sponges or cotton balls; a waste basin; and an organic, water-soluble, iodinated contrast medium.

After the nipple is cleansed, the round-tipped needle is inserted into the orifice of the duct and the contrast medium is injected. To prevent unnecessary discomfort and possible extravasation, the injection is terminated as soon as the patient experiences a sense of fullness. Usually, less than 1 ml of contrast medium is needed. Occasionally, when ducts are very distended, as much as 3 ml can be used. Immediate radiographs are taken with the patient positioned for the craniocaudal and lateral images (Fig. 27-52). The exposure techniques are the same as in routine mammography. Compression is not employed, because it would expel the contrast medium.

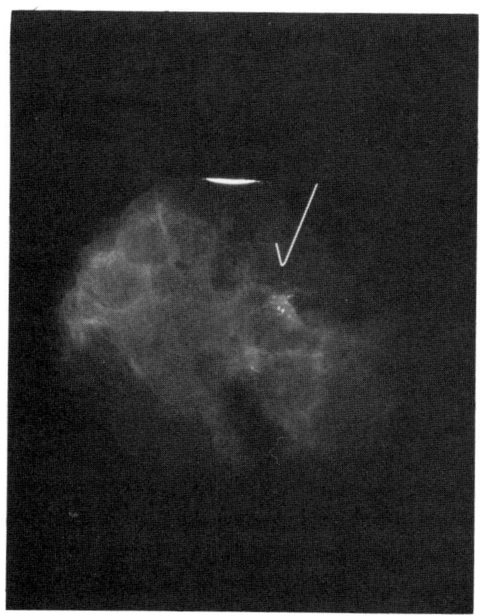

Fig. 27-51. Radiograph of a surgical specimen containing suspicious microcalcifications. This is the noninvasive carcinama illusrated in Fig. 27-2.

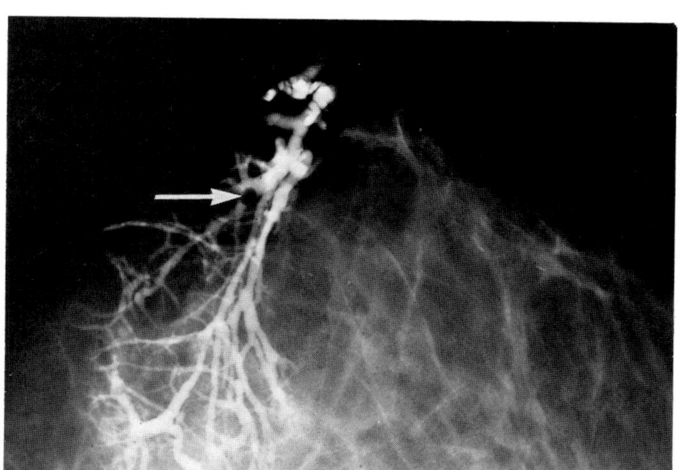

Fig. 27-52. Craniocaudal projection of opacified milk ducts.

Summary

Radiographic examination of the breast is a technically demanding procedure. Success is extremely dependent on the skills of the radiologic technologist, more so than in most other areas of radiology. In addition to skill, the technologist must want to perform good mammography and be willing to work with the patient to allay qualms and obtain cooperation. In the course of taking the patient's history, physically examining the breast, and radiographing the breasts, patients may ask questions about breast disease, breast self-examination, and breast radiography that they have been reluctant to ask of other health professionals. The knowledge, skill, and attitude imparted to the patient may be lifesaving. Although most patients will not have significant breast disease when first examined, the statistics show that over 8% of the patients will develop breast cancer at some time during their life. A positive mammography encounter now may make the patient more willing to undergo mammography in the future. Breast radiography properly done is safe, and at present the application of mammography offers the only hope for significantly reducing the mortality of breast cancer.

Definition of Terms

asymptomatic Without symptoms or evidence of a specific disease.

fatty infiltration A normal process or stage in breast development where increased amounts of fat accumulate around the parenchymal breast tissue. See involution.

film-screen mammography A breast x-ray in which the radiographic densities are recorded on special single-emulsion x-ray film using high-detail intensifying screens.

involution A normal process or stage in the development of the mature breast in which the volume of glandular tissue and supporting connective tissue stroma decreases. The process starts at variable times after the initial maturing of the breast. The process is substantially accelerated by the completion of a pregnancy.

microcalcifications Tiny calcifications found in the breast. Some patterns of microcalcifications are commonly associated with breast cancer; others are rarely associated with cancer.

postpartum mastitis A bacterial infection in the breast appearing after pregnancy, usually as a complication of breast feeding.

radical mastectomy A surgical procedure in which the breast and underlying pectoralis major and pectoralis minor muscles are removed, usually with full removal of lymph nodes from the axilla.

risk versus benefit A comparison of the potential harm from a specific action with the potential benefit to be derived from the action.

screening Testing for evidence of disease in an asymptomatic population.

xeromammogram A breast x-ray study in which the radiographic densities of the breast are reflected in discharges of a charged plate. The discharge pattern is made visible by depositing toner powder on the plate. The powder is transferred to a paper, producing a permanent image. The plate is used again after recharging.

SELECTED BIBLIOGRAPHY

Anderson I, et al: Breast cancer screening with mammography by population-based, randomized trial with mammography as the only screening mode, Radiology 132:273-276, 1979.

Anderson I, et al: Radiographic patterns of the mammary parenchyma; variation with age at examination and age at first birth, Radiology 138:59-62, 1981.

Baker LH: Breast cancer detection demonstration project: five-year summary report, CA 32:194-225, 1982.

Bassett LW, et al: Reduced-dose magnification mammography, Radiology 141:665-670, 1981.

Bassett LW, et al: Breast radiography using the oblique projection, Radiology 149:585-587, 1983.

Bassett LW and Gold RH: The evolution of mammography, AJR 150:493-498, 1988.

Eklund GW, et al: Improved imaging of the augmented breast, AJR 151:469-473, 1988.

Egan RL: Early breast cancer. In Gallager HS, editor: Mammography: a historical perspective, early breast cancer detection and treatment, New York, 1975, John Wiley & Sons, Inc.

Egan RL, et al: Intramammary calcifications without an associated mass in benign and malignant diseases, Radiology 137:1-7, 1980.

Egan RL, et al: Grids in mammography, Radiology 146:359-362, 1983.

Fajardo LL and Westerman BR: Mammography equipment: practiced considerations for the radiologist, Applied Radiol 19(5):12-15, 1990.

Feig SA: Assessment of the hypothetical risk from mammography and evaluation of the potential benefit, Radiol Clin North Am 21:173-183, 1983.

Feig SA: Radiation risk for mammography: is it clinically significant? AJR 143:469-475, 1984.

Feig SA: Mammography equipment: principles, features, selection, Radiol Clin North Am 25:897-911, 1987.

Fox S: Benefit/risk analysis of aggressive mammography screening, Radiology 128:359-365, 1978.

Gisrold JJ, et al: Prebiopsy localization of nonpalpable breast lesions, AJR 143:477-481, 1984.

Goodrich WA: The Cleopatra view in xeromammography, Radiology 128:811-812, 1978.

Hammerstein GR, et al: Absorbed radiation dose in mammography, Radiology 130:485-491, 1979.

Hoeffken W, and Langi M: Mammography: technique, diagnosis, differential diagnosis, results, Philadelphia, 1977, WB Saunders Co.

Homer MJ: Percutaneous localization of breast lesions: experience with the Frank Breast Biopsy Guide, J Can Assoc Radiol 30:238-241, 1979.

Jackson VP, Lex AM and Smith DJ: Patient discomfort during screen-film mammography, Radiology 168:421-423, 1988.

Jensen SR, et al: Wire localization of nonpalpable breast lesions (technical note), Radiology 132:484-485, 1979.

Kimme Smith C, Bassett LW and Gold RH: Evaluation of radiation dose, focal spot, and automatic exposure of newer film-screen mammography units, AJR 149:913-917, 1987.

Kopans DB, et al: Modified needle-hookwire technique to simplify preoperative localization of occult breast lesions (technical note), Radiology 134:781, 1980.

Law J and Kirkpatrick AE: Films, screens and cassettes for mammography, Br J Radiol 62:163-167, 1989.

Linden SS and Sullivan DC: Breast skin calcifications: localization with a stereotactic device, Radiology 171:570-571, 1989.

Loh CK, et al: Improved method of localization of nonpalpable breast lesions (technical note). Radiology 130:244-245, 1979.

Mammography 1982: a statement of The American Cancer Society, CA 32:226-228, 1982.

Martin JE: A demonstration comparing film mammography with the new high sensitivity xeromammography, Radiographics 9:153-168, 1989.

Moskowitz M: Mammographic screening significance of minimal breast cancers, AJR 136:735, 1981.

Moskowitz M: Mammography to screen asymtomatic women for breast cancer, AJR 143:457-459, 1984.

Moskowitz M, et al: Mammographic patterns as markers for high-risk benign breast disease and incident cancers, Radiology 134:293-295, 1980.

Moskowitz M, et al: Evidence of breast cancer mortality reduction aggressive screening in women under age 50, AJR 138:911, 1982.

Muntz EP, et al: Mammography at reduced doses: present performance and future possibilities, AJR 141:665, 1981.

Pennes DR and Homer MJ: Disappearing breast masses caused by compression during mammography, Radiology 165:327-328, 1987.

Sickles EA: Microfocal spot magnification mammography using xeroradiographic and screen-film recording systems, Radiology 131:599-607, 1979.

Sickles EA, et al: Controlled single-blind clinical evaluation of low-dose mammographic screen-film systems, Radiology 130:347-351, 1979.

Stanton L, et al: Study of mammographic exposure and detail visibility using three systems: Xerox 125, Min-R and Zonics XERG, Radiology 132:455-462, 1979.

Tabar L, et al: Screening for breast cancer, the Swedish trial, Radiology 138:219-222, 1981.

Tabar L, et al: Galactography: the diagnostic procedure of choice for nipple discharge, Radiology 149:31, 1983.

Chapter 28

THERMOGRAPHY AND DIAPHANOGRAPHY

JOSEPH FODOR III
JACK C. MALOTT

Thermography is the procedure by which the heat naturally emitted by the body is detected, measured, and imaged. The resultant image—the *thermogram**—is a visualization of the distribution of the heat patterns of the body surface. This heat is naturally emitted as a result of normal body function, disease, or injury. Over the last few years several methods of producing a representation of these heat patterns have been developed.

In "infrared thermography" (the most widely used method of thermography) the heat (infrared) radiation emanating from the skin is detected by a camera in a manner similar to that used in light photography. The infrared radiation is then electronically changed into a signal used to generate an image on a cathode ray tube (typically, a television monitor). This image is then viewed in "real time," and the observations are used to properly adjust the equipment. The real-time image can then be recorded electronically but is most commonly recorded photographically (Fig. 28-1). Polaroid film or another photographic paper is often used to record the image. Recording on transparent film in a manner similar to that used for gamma camera, computed tomography, or ultrasound images may also be used. These images are then used for viewing and interpreting the diagnostic findings.

The above method, in comparison to the following methods, may properly be called *telethermography* since the body heat patterns are detected at some distance (usually a few feet or 1 to 2 meters from the patient's body surface). However, the current practice is to call this method simply *thermography*.

"Liquid crystal thermography" uses certain chemical substances that are painted or otherwise applied to the body

*All italicized terms are defined at the end of this chapter.

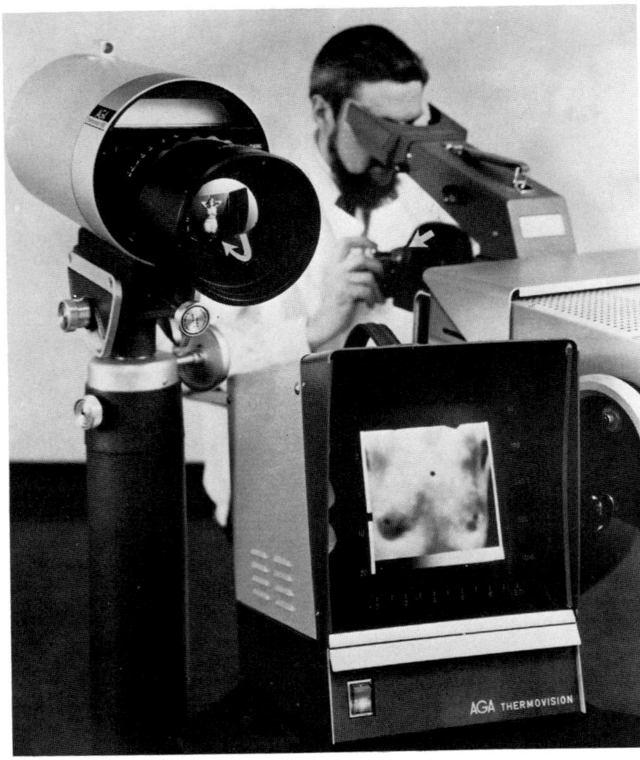

Fig. 28-1. AGA Thermovision unit demonstrating equipment components necessary in thermography. Patient is out of photograph but can be seen reflected in mirror lens of camera *(curved arrow)*. In foreground is "slave unit" that provides enlargement of conventional cathode ray image, which operator is viewing on control panel in background while adjusting controls *(straight arrow)* of camera. Camera attached to control panel records real-time image on cathode ray tube. Larger slave unit shown here is not in general medical use. This arrangement is for direct scan.

(Courtesy AGA Corp.)

surface. These substances change color depending on the local temperature. These color changes can be either observed or photographed.

"Computer-assisted thermography" (judged by some as an inappropriate term since computer assistance may be used in any of these applications) is a method that consists of obtaining multiple local temperature measurements over the body surface. A computer program is then used to determine the likelihood of disease by attempting to recognize specific temperature patterns.

"Microwave thermography" measures and images microwave wavelength radiation emanating from the body. Microwave radiations penetrate better through tissues and thus are thought to give a better representation of the changes in body heat in depth, as compared to the more superficial measurements used in infrared thermography.

Physics

Infrared radiation is an electromagnetic radiation. Thus it shares the characteristics of wave motions and specifically those of electromagnetic radiations. It is part of the same wide spectrum of wavelike radiations that include radio and light waves, ultraviolet rays, x-rays, and cosmic rays. Infrared lies just beyond the red end of the visible spectrum of light and thus has a somewhat longer wavelength and lower energy than light rays. Infrared energy, or heat radiation, is emitted as a function of local temperature. All objects in nature seek to acquire or remain in thermal equilibrium with their surroundings. Thus areas of the skin that are warmer than the surroundings will radiate more infrared rays.

Metabolism generates heat. Local metabolism is often increased in areas of malignant tumor, inflammation, or injury. Circulation and some other body mechanisms contribute to the maintenance of human thermal equilibrium. In the course of these processes, some areas of the skin will be warmer and others cooler. Although heretofore invisible, this spontaneously emitted radiant energy, which is fundamental to all nature, is the physical basis for thermography.

The relationship of temperature to disease has long been recognized as an important factor in medical diagnosis and treatment. The birth of contemporary medical thermography occurred in the early 1950s.

Equipment and Methodology

The relatively new science of thermography developed steadily after the introduction of the medical thermogram, but development has slowed since about 1970 as a result of difficulties in establishing the real value of this procedure and the extremely vigorous development of competing imaging diagnostic methods (such as diagnostic ultrasound, computed tomography, magnetic resonance imaging, and others). Minor advances have been made in the detection systems and the video display chains; liquid crystal thermography, microwave thermography, and computer-assisted thermography have all been developed since 1970.

An excellent historical summary is provided by Gershon-Cohen,[1] one of the early pioneers of thermography. A description and a categorization of the thermographic instruments have been presented by Curcio and Haberman.[2]

[1]Gershon-Cohen J: A short history of medical thermometry, Ann NY Acad Sci 121:4-11, 1964.
[2]Curcio B and Haberman J: Infrared thermography: a review of current medical application, instrumentation and technique, Radiol Techn 42:233-247, 1971.

The input of an infrared imaging system is the radiant energy spontaneously emitted by the patient. The output is the image generated by the resulting electronic signal. The detector converts the heat (infrared) radiation received by the camera into an electronic signal that is then further amplified and processed to eventually produce the image. This image must be sufficiently clear to reveal details of temperature differences and must portray the smallest such differences that might have clinical significance.

In a typical thermogram, temperature is represented in shades of gray. The most frequently used method represents warmer levels of temperature in lighter shades of gray (whiter areas) and cooler levels in darker shades (Fig. 28-2, *A*). Some physicians favor a reversal of this polarity (Fig. 28-2, *B*). Most designs provide both types of polarity at the option of the user. In thermographic imaging, focus, contrast, and brightness must be controlled and adjusted (Fig. 28-3). *Focus* refers to the proper distance of the

A

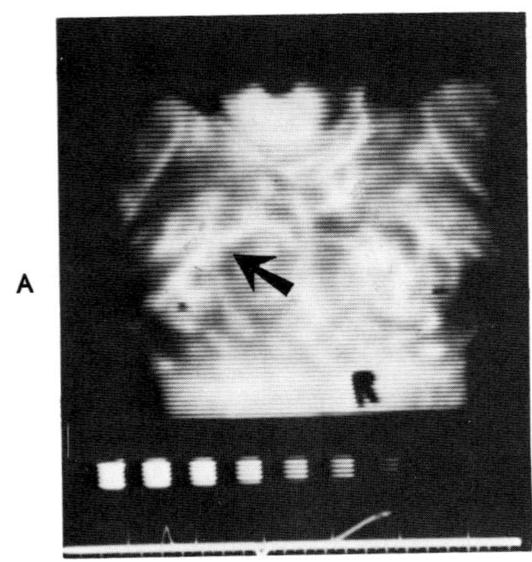

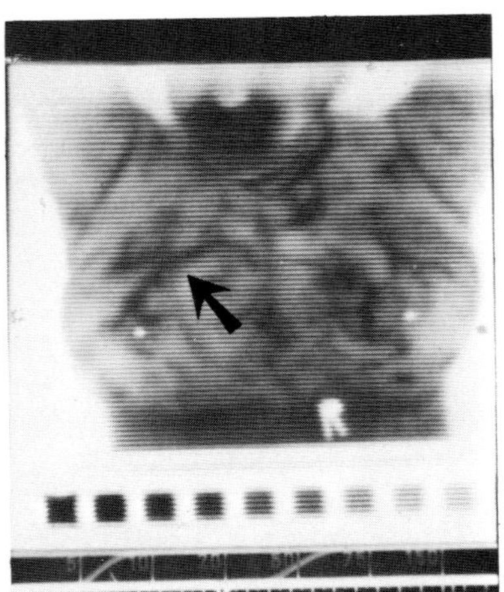

B

Fig. 28-2. Thermograms made with both types of polarity. **A,** Warmer veins appear white. **B,** Same veins appear black.

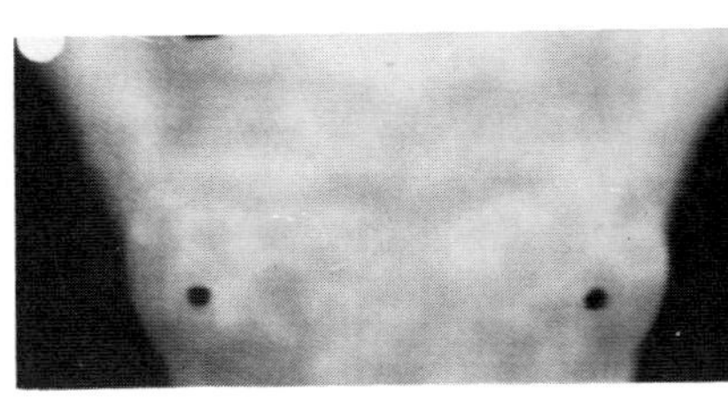

Too little contrast
Range, 6.5°C

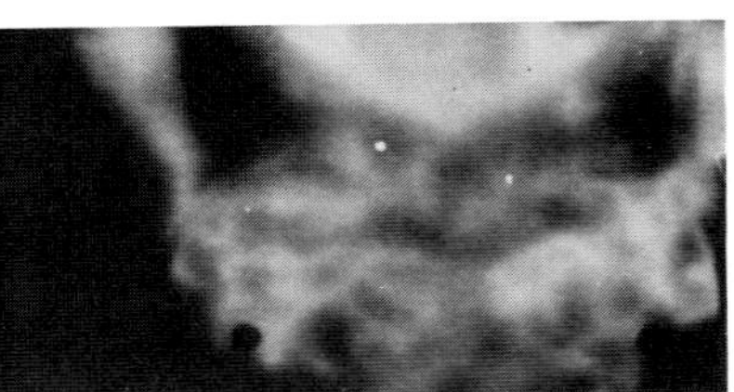

Too much contrast
Range, 4°C

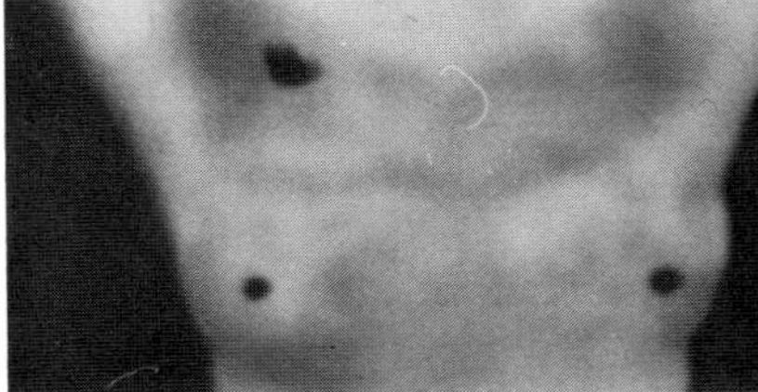

Out of focus
Range, 5.5°C, near correct

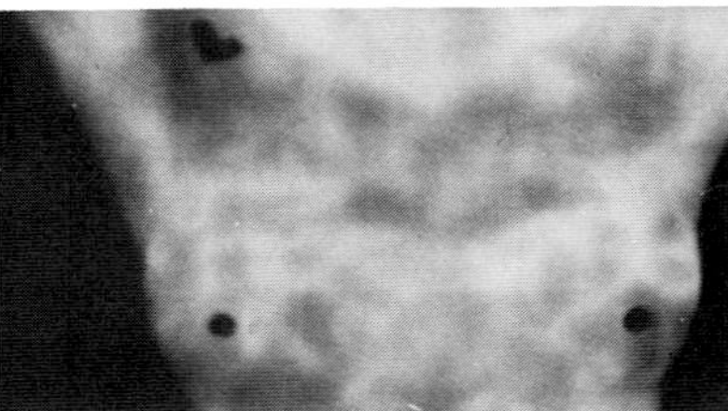

Properly exposed
Range, 5°C

Fig. 28-3. Four thermograms of breasts of same patient illustrate importance of proper focus, contrast, and brightness in obtaining thermal image.

patient from the sensing device and proper adjustment of the lens. *Contrast,* which may also be termed the sensitivity of the particular thermogram, consists of the gradients of tones between black and saturated white displayed on the thermogram. Contrast depicts the range of temperatures, and the sensitivity setting of the instrument should depend on the temperature ranges being emitted by the part examined. *Brightness* relates to the overall lightness or darkness of the thermal image and to the ease with which it can be studied. The most satisfactory brightness for a thermogram is reached when the warmest temperature of the subject approaches, but does not reach, saturated white.

The emitted radiation must be allowed to flow unhampered and unrestricted to the sensing device. The environment in which the patient is examined must be significantly cooler than the surface temperatures of the patient's skin to prevent interference from heat radiation from nearby objects or walls. The patient's clothing must be removed, and the patient is normally required to wait some time for the unclothed area of interest to cool to normal skin temperature. This is because clothing acts as an insulator and allows the temperature of the skin to warm in a more uniform pattern. Additionally, rubbing or scratching of the skin by clothing or other body parts will produce localized elevation of the skin's temperature.

Because infrared radiation travels in a straight line, the patient may be examined by direct scanning, in which case the patient is directly in front of the instrument, or by the use of an angled mirror that will reflect the radiation into the system when the patient is examined in the recumbent position (Fig. 28-4). A body part whose total surface cannot be evaluated in one position must be arranged in several positions to allow evaluation of the entire surface.

In summary, the patient's skin must be uncovered and allowed to come to a normal state of temperature distribution. The patient must be arranged to allow optimum reception of the radiation by the infrared sensing device, and the instrument must be adjusted to receive all temperature information being emitted by the source. Finally, the recording method must accurately record the thermal image demonstrated at the moment (the "real time") of the examination.

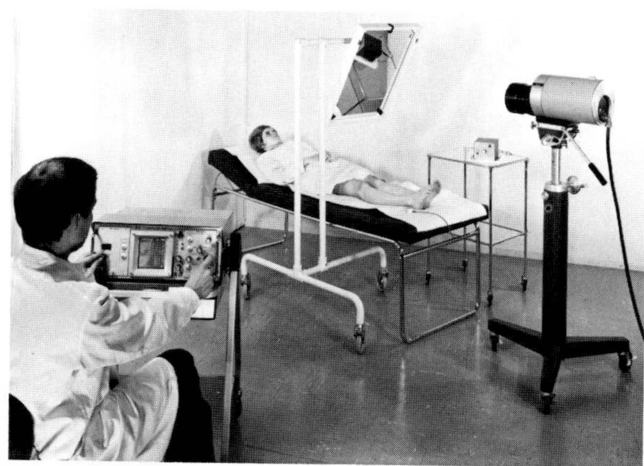

Fig. 28-4. Position of AGA Thermovision for use with reflection mirror. This method is employed when patient can be more conveniently examined in recumbent position. Thermal "real-time" image is displayed on cathode ray tube on control panel.

Selected Clinical Applications

Skin temperatures are the result of normal physiologic processes and disease. They are also influenced by external conditions, such as the temperature of the surroundings, humidity, and evaporation.

BREAST DISEASE

One of the most promising and widely used applications of thermography has been in the detection of breast cancer. It has been widely recognized that a detailed qualitative as well as quantitative study of the thermograms is essential. Comparison of the breast image with the opposite side breast image, with previous thermograms, and with known normal patterns should all be considered in evaluation of the thermographic images (Fig. 28-5). The basic principle of the search for malignant tumor has been to search for areas of elevated temperature and for disturbances of the heat distribution pattern.

The features favoring the use of thermography for this purpose are that (1) the procedure is totally noninvasive and therefore quite safe; (2) no ionizing radiation is used; (3) it is fairly fast, convenient, and, compared to other imaging procedures, inexpensive; and (4) because of the above features, it may be readily repeated for comparison purposes and performed without concern for patient safety.

Unfortunately, and despite this promise, efforts to establish thermography as a tool for breast cancer detection have been unsuccessful.[1,2] Even now, after nearly 2 decades of investigation, the majority opinion is that thermography is not reliable as a tool in screening for early breast cancer. The chief reasons for failure are that it is relatively insensitive in recording some small tumors and that its inability to achieve reliable and consistent interpretation of the images has not been surmounted. There may be hope for improvements in the future, but the lack of diagnostic value has been a real disappointment in view of the anticipated advantages. Nevertheless, the thermographic method cannot be recommended today as a reliable tool of breast cancer detection. Except for institutions continuing investigative work and occasional use in special circumstances, thermography is seldom used. The same conclusions apply to liquid crystal thermography, microwave thermography, and other thermographic methods. When any of these procedures are used in detecting breast disease, one has to constantly guard against the false security brought about by an apparently negative thermogram.

The accuracy of thermography for breast cancer detection has been reported to be only 42%, compared to 57% for physical examination and 91% for mammography.[1] Clearly, x-ray mammography is a diagnostically superior tool compared to thermography. The radiation exposure from mammography has been decreasing and with up-to-date techniques, mammography has a very good risk-versus-benefit ratio (see Chapter 27) and is now the recommended *imaging procedure of choice* for breast cancer detection.[1-4]

[1]Gold RH et al: Breast imaging: state of the art, Invest Radiol 4:298-303, 1988.
[2]Pera A and Freimanis AK: The choice of radiologic procedures in the diagnosis of breast disease, Clin Obstet Gynecol 14(3):635-649, 1987.

[1]Gold RH et al: Breast imaging: state of the art, Invest Radiol 4:298-303, 1988.
[2]Pera A and Freimanis AK: The choice of radiologic procedures in the diagnosis of breast disease, Clin Obstet Gynecol 14(3):635-649, 1987.
[3]Dodd GD: Heat sensing devices and breast cancer detection. In Feig AS and McLelland R, editors: Breast carcinoma: current diagnosis and treatment, New York, 1983, Masson Publishing USA, Inc, pp 207-225.
[4]Sickles EA: Breast thermography. In Feig AS and McLelland R, editors: Breast carcinoma: current diagnosis and treatment, New York, 1983, Masson Publishing USA, Inc, pp 227-231.

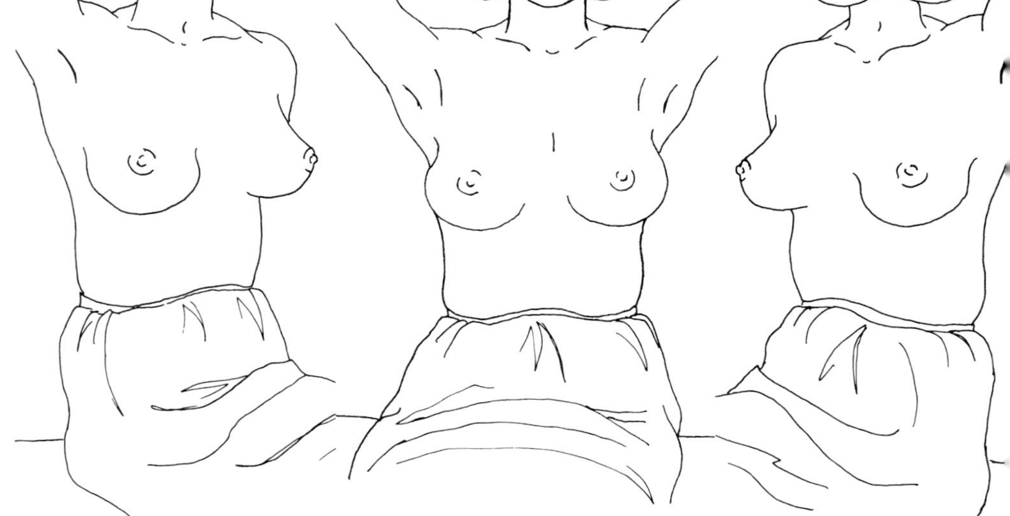

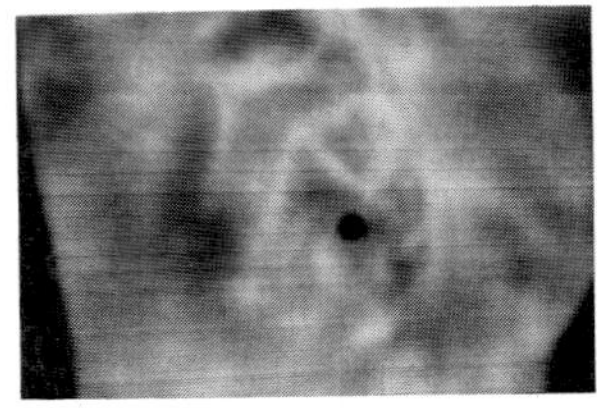

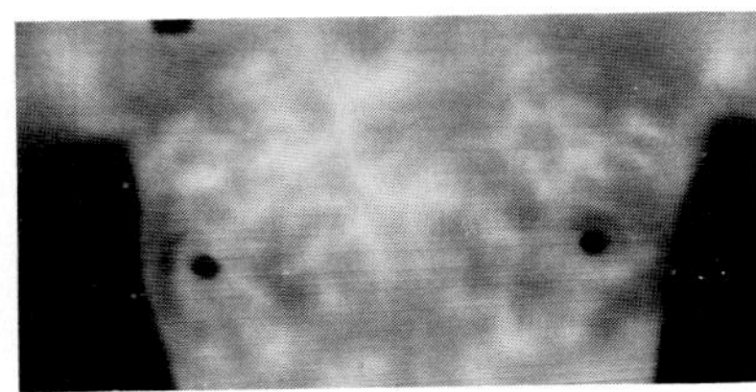

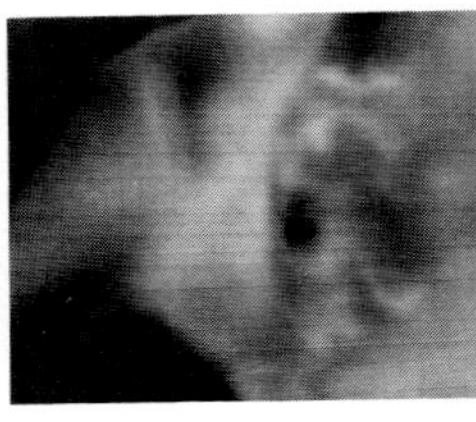

Fig. 28-5. Frontal and oblique positions for routine breast thermography. Frontal position is not sufficient to scan all breast tissue, so that, in addition to frontal surface, the lateral surface of each breast must be turned to sensing device and evaluated separately.

OBSTETRIC APPLICATIONS

Since the placenta is a site of great biologic activity, it is considerably warmer than the surrounding tissues. Therefore thermography can be used for its localization. The advantages of using thermography for localization of the placenta are that it employs no ionizing radiation, it can be used with complete safety to the fetus, and it is not difficult to perform unless the patient is in hard labor.

The patient may be examined in the erect or recumbent position. Scanning is performed under conditions of constant temperature and humidity. All clothing must be removed, and *cross-radiation* must be eliminated by moving the arms well away from the body. Placental studies usually include thermograms made in the frontal and right and left lateral positions.

The placenta, being a warm region, will appear as a light area on the thermogram. Thermography is most accurate in identifying vertical and anteriorly placed placentas (Figs. 28-6 and 28-7). Posteriorly placed placentas are usually so deeply seated that they cannot be imaged by thermography. Thermal scanning does not yield fetal measurements or other details.

Thermography *does not provide exact contours;* thus ultrasound, which is precise and widely available in hospitals throughout the United States, has become the diagnostic modality of choice for placental localization.

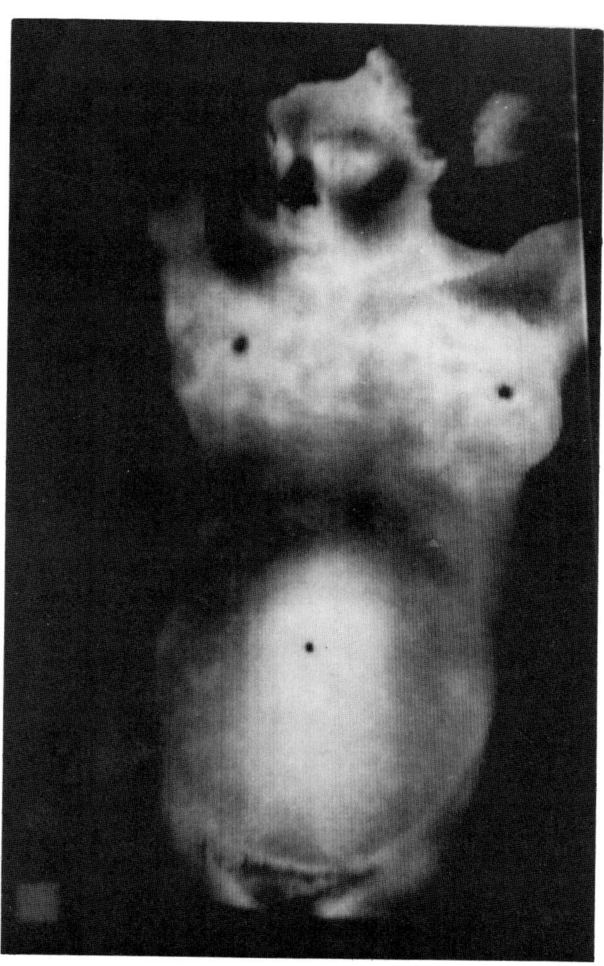

Fig. 28-6. Thermogram of torso of pregnant woman shows large area of increased temperature related to placenta. Breasts also show typically warm appearance associated with increased vascularity and hormonally stimulated physiologic activity of breasts in pregnant state.

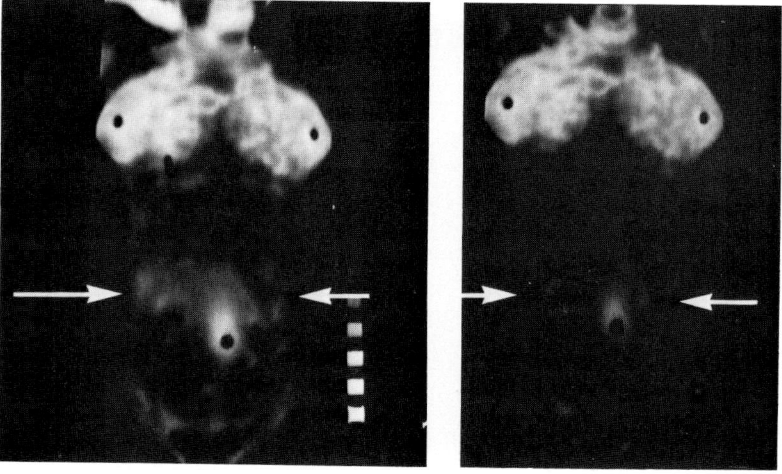

Fig. 28-7. Supine thermogram of 26-year-old woman in last trimester of pregnancy. *White arrows,* High anterior placenta.

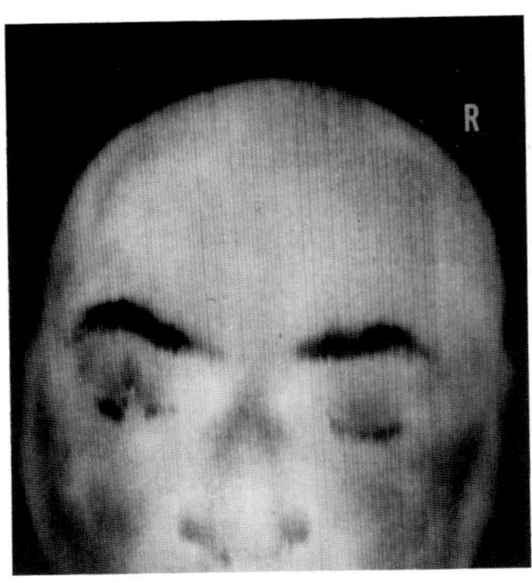

Fig. 28-8. Thermogram of forehead of normal skull shows typical homogeneous appearance.

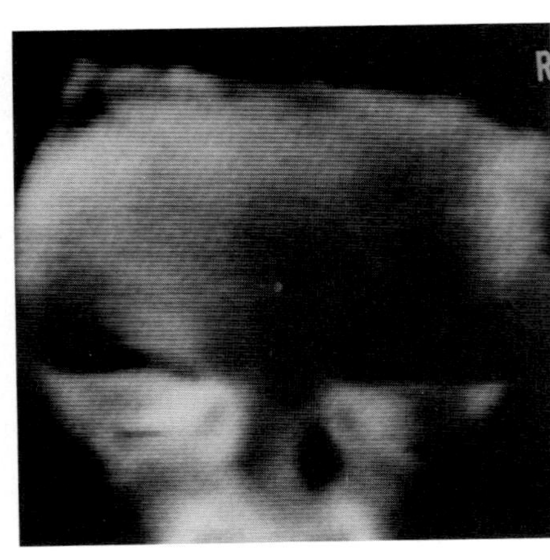

Fig. 28-9. Thermogram of patient with thrombus in right carotid artery. Drop in temperature in right side reflects embarrassment to right internal carotid artery circulation.

OTHER MEDICAL APPLICATIONS

Thermography is employed to study rheumatic and other orthopedic diseases, vascular and cerebrovascular diseases, ophthalmologic disease, and dermatologic diseases (Figs. 28-8 to 28-10). For evaluation of small details, standard roentgenography, angiography, computed x-ray tomography, and ultrasound are superior. Because of the simplicity of the method, thermography as a study of impairment of circulation or innervation still holds considerable promise. Emphasis has recently been placed on the use of thermography to objectively confirm an organic basis for pain. Although a normal thermogram does not exclude organic disease as a cause for pain, a positive (abnormal) thermogram is said to confirm an organic cause for the pain. However, there are no well-documented, controlled studies to prove that these findings are indeed reliable.

Summary

The noninvasive and simple diagnostic thermographic procedure has held much hope, and there may be some future promise. However, other imaging procedures have presently passed thermography in their reliability in producing diagnostic results, as well as in having better sensitivity and specificity. Thermography is presently left with a shrinking field of applications and is recommended only as a screening tool and not as a primary diagnostic device.[1] Research continues, and it is hoped that thermography may find its way back into the field of imaging diagnosis. Its total safety and ease of application certainly make us wish that it would do so.

[1]Handelsman H: Thermography for indications other than breast lesions. Health Technology Assessment Reports, 1989, US Department of Health and Human Services, no. 2, pp 1-31, 1989.

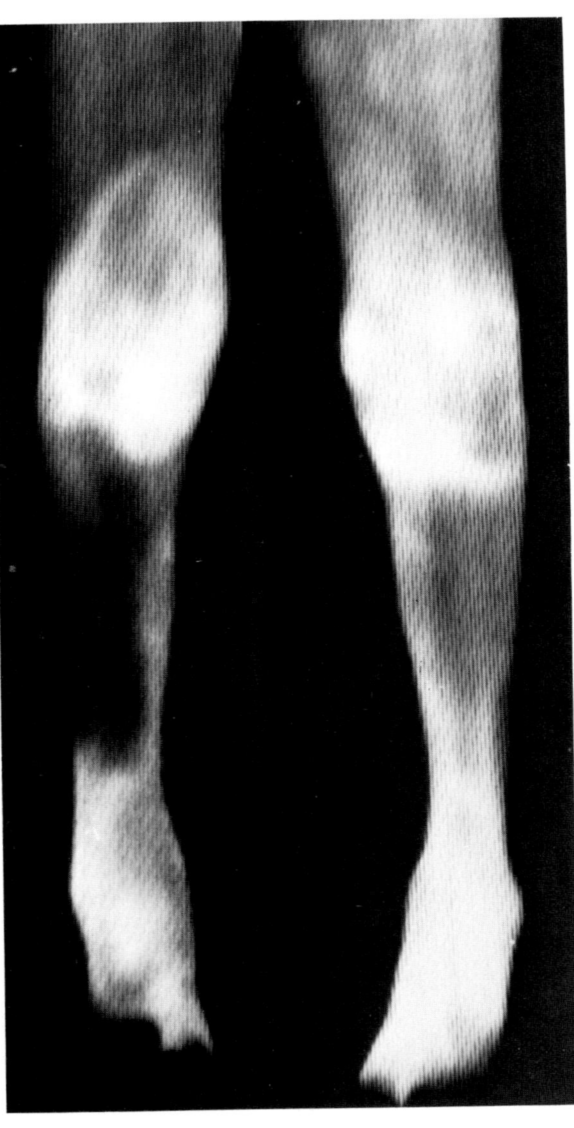

Fig. 28-10. Frontal thermogram of lower extremities of patient with rheumatoid arthritis. Heat is greater over joints. Effects of various therapeutic measures in treatment of arthritis can be monitored by serial thermography.

Diaphanography is a new imaging modality that uses light to examine the breast. Although diaphanography is similar to transillumination, *diaphanography* uses selected wavelengths of light and special imaging equipment. Although the role of diaphanography appears to have a place in the screening and diagnosis of breast disease, it is still under clinical evaluation. Further studies comparing the efficacy of this modality with traditional methods are necessary to define the role of diaphanography in breast examination.

Transillumination is a technique that permits the inspection of a structure's interior by directing light through its exterior wall. Visualization of a structure is dependent on the clarity of the fluids contained, the thickness of the overlying tissue, and the intensity of the transillumination light source, as well as the adaptation of the examiner's eyes.[1] The clinical use of transillumination was first recorded in 1831 by Richard Bright, who used the sun and candles as light sources while reporting an apparent hydrocephalus.[2]

In adults, transillumination has been used to diagnose conditions of the maxillary and frontal sinuses, the breast, and the scrotum. Transillumination has also found many uses in the operative suite, including transventricular illumination for the detection of septal defects, vascular visualization to ensure blood supply, and dacryotransillumination during a dacryocystectomy or dacryocystorhinostomy procedure. Fiberoptic transillumination has also been used in dentistry for the detection of decay and cracks in teeth.

[1]Church S et al: Transillumination in neonatal intensive care: a possible iatrogenic complication, South Med J 74:76, 1981.
[2]McArtor RD et al: Iatrogenic second-degree burn caused by a transilluminator, Pediatrics 63(3):422-423, 1979.

These applications have all used light in the visible spectrum. More recently, transillumination techniques of the breast use other wavelengths of light. This contemporary transillumination technique has been termed *diaphanoscopy* (likened to fluoroscopy for the real-time observation of the image) and *diaphanography* (likened to radiography for the still-framed recorded images). Both terms are derived from the Greek term "dia," meaning through or across, and "phane," meaning shining, thus translating into "shining through." Diaphanography has also been referred to as "transmission spectroscopy" since it is a combination of transillumination light scanning and spectroscopy. The use of light in the visible and infrared spectra coupled with new electronic and sensing systems is responsible for a renaissance in transillumination. Use of these light spectra is said to allow for the differential absorption of infrared and other wavelengths. Recording can be done with infrared-sensitive film and preferably electronic recording devices. Digital recording of the information allows for computerized reconstruction and image analysis.

The efficacy of diaphanography remains under investigation. Since no ionizing radiation is used, transillumination of the breast is an attractive, but as yet unproven, modality for screening for breast cancer. However, transillumination is not without potential complications. Problems with heat from the light source can cause burns although this can be avoided through careful use and appropriate design of the equipment.

Historical Development

Diaphanography, later termed "breast transillumination," was first reported in 1928; however, early instrumentation was plagued with problems in providing enough light intensity. Differentiation between variations in tissues and the ability to distinguish between solid tumors and cysts without producing extreme heat at the patient's skin were not possible. The low-light intensity used required dark adaptation of the operator's eyes and made photography extremely difficult. Additionally, poor contrast made image interpretation subjective and ultimately led to the short-term abandonment of the technique in the 1940s.

In France from 1950 to 1970 improved instrumentation was developed, eliminating the problem of heat from the light source; this allowed improved penetration of the breast and photography of the images. The efficacy of this system was still dependent on the operator's ability, and it appeared that the human eye alone was unable to differentiate the various grades of light absorption needed to distinguish between benign and malignant tumors. This still posed problems, because the film required special developing, which was available only on a limited basis.[1,2]

In recent years new dimensions have been added to the transillumination techniques. The use of selected wavelengths to allow comparison of tissue types, coupled with real-time imaging, has made diaphanography more practical. The use of tissue samples suggests that various wavelengths of light are absorbed differently in the layers of tissue through which the light passes.

In other words, there seem to be different absorptions for light just as there are for x rays. This would mean diaphanography is more than passing light through tissue with the shadows of the internal structures appearing on the surface of the skin. Comparison of the light absorption characteristics of normal and cancerous tissue samples has shown absorption or spectral differences. Unfortunately, cysts filled with blood or another colored material may produce similar changes, and the extent to which other benign lesions produce similar changes is not known. Further, whether small lesions (less than 1 cm or 5 mm) can be regularly detected is also not substantiated.

[1]Carlsen E: Transillumination light scanning, Diagn Imaging, p 28, April 1982.
[2]Ohlsson BS et al: Diaphanography: a method of evaluation of the female breast, World J Surg 4(6):701-706, 1980.

Diaphanography Equipment

The contemporary instrumentation needed for transillumination includes a light source, a light transilluminator, a special electronic camera, digital processing electronics, a television monitor, and a film imaging system. Because light in the infrared spectrum is used, the system must be capable of converting the infrared light to visible light (Fig. 28-11).

The light source must meet two requirements. First, it must not be hot to the skin, and second, it must have wavelengths that penetrate the tissues. These wavelengths range from 600 nm (6000 Å) through the near infrared waves. The transilluminator functions to evenly spread the light via fiberoptics. The transilluminated light is collected by an infrared optical lens system that formats the information into an image. The image is transformed to a raster-scanned or television image. The amplified signal is then available for further processing by analog-to-digital conversion.

The equipment functions by sequentially transmitting light of two different wavelengths through the tissue. The information from the two images is then digitalized and stored in the computer memory. The information is next processed to an algorithm that superimposes the information in the two images pixel by pixel. This is accomplished in real time, providing a single video image that displays the differential information in color and intensity brightness on the monitor. This imaging technique is extremely sensitive to variations in tissue characteristics.

Optical Principles

In performing transillumination studies and viewing these images, an understanding of the optical principles of transillumination is helpful. A lesion near the surface of the skin will show marked absorption of light at the surface of the skin. As the lesion absorbing the light moves deeper in relation to the skin surface, the image is less discernible for several reasons. First, an object further from the surface produces more light scatter interference. Second, the more distant lesion produces a larger halo around the image of the mass; this can be compared with the radiographic problem of penumbra with increased object-film distance.

These problems can be overcome when imaging deep lesions. First, several views can be obtained to bring the lesion as close to the skin as possible. Second, those wavelengths that do not help with differentiation between lesions and normal tissue can be removed from the light source. This is much like filtering the x-ray beam; "white light," which contains all wavelengths, is detrimental to image quality. One last important factor: as the light's wavelength increases, the amount of scattering decreases; therefore wavelengths further into the infrared spectrum should produce more contrast for those lesions deeper in the tissue.

Clinical Applications

The primary application of diaphanography is in the examination of the breast although other soft tissue structures can be evaluated. Diaphanography is still in the investigational stage, and further clinical evaluation of this technology is necessary before there is widespread acceptance (Figs. 28-12 to 28-14).

Several reports on the efficacy of diaphanography have been published in the literature. In these reports the true-positive rate for carcinoma ranged from 20% to 93% and the rate for diagnosing benign lesions ranged from 6% to 36%.

The promising future of diaphanography lies in its ability to detect an occasional cancer as small as 4 to 6 mm. The sensitivity and specificity need to be established by blinded, controlled, prospective trials before the value of diaphanography can be established. Currently, the use of diaphanography in the screening and evaluation of breast disease should not be substituted for established methods of breast examination but used rather as an adjuvant imaging modality on a selective basis.

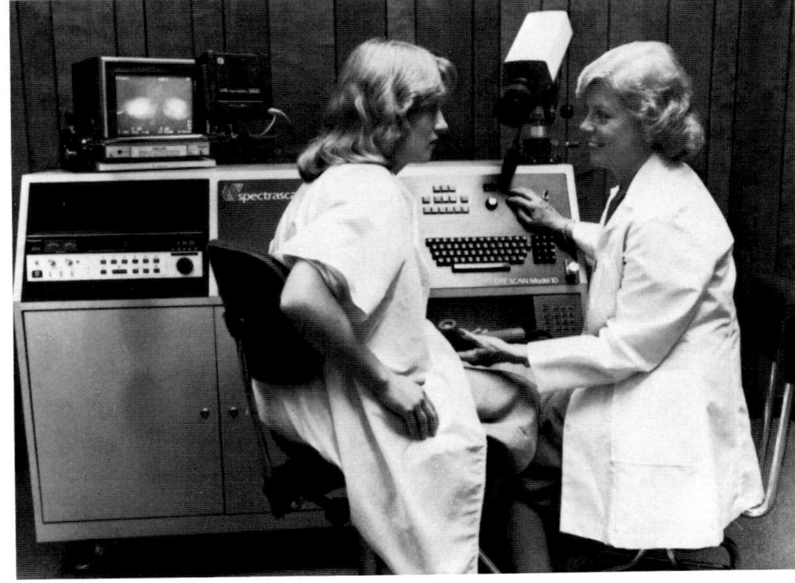

Fig. 28-11. An example of a contemporary diaphanography unit. The light source is held in the operator's hand, and the camera is mounted on the console.

(Courtesy Spectrascan Inc.)

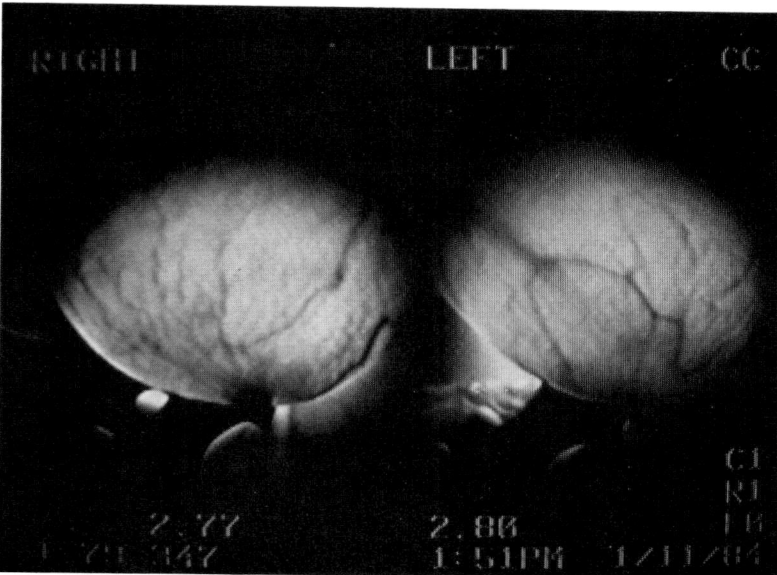

Fig. 28-12. Normal diaphanography study. Vasculature of the breast is demonstrated; note the similar density of both breasts.

(Courtesy Spectrascan Inc.)

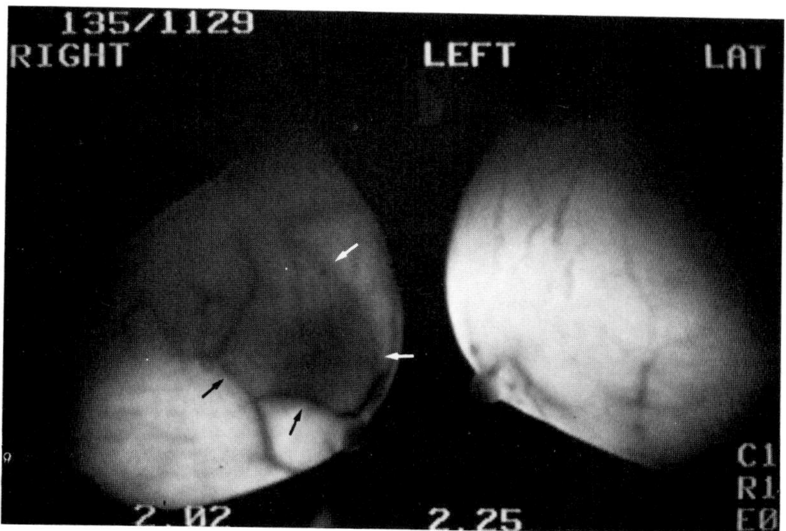

Fig. 28-13. Diaphanography study on a patient with a carcinoma of the right breast. The carcinoma *(arrows)* is demonstrated as an increased density as a result of light being absorbed by the lesion.

(Courtesy Spectrascan Inc.)

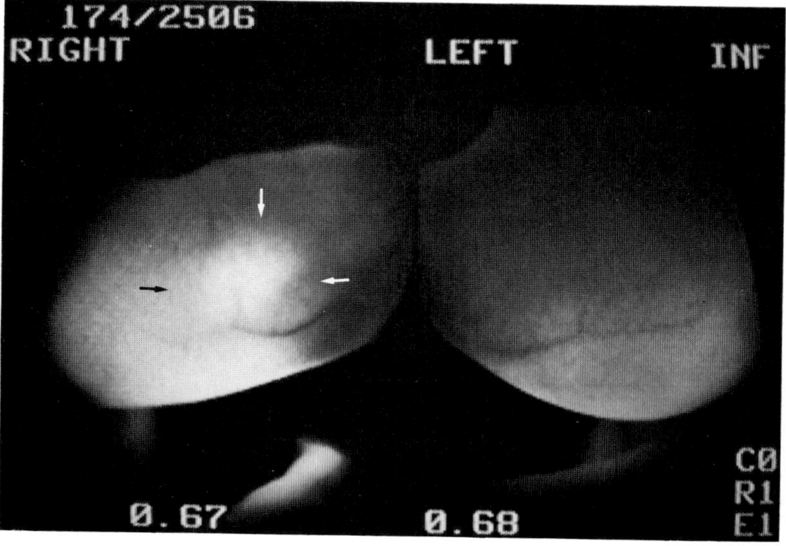

Fig. 28-14. Study on a patient with a cyst in the right breast. The cyst *(arrows)* allows increased transmission of light and appears as a decreased density.

(Courtesy Spectrascan Inc.)

Definition of Terms

brightness The degree of lightness or darkness of the thermographic image.

contrast The range of gray tones on the thermographic image.

cross-radiation Infrared radiation emanating from adjacent body structures.

diaphanography Transillumination using selected light wavelengths and special imaging equipment.

diaphanoscopy Real-time transillumination.

focus Placement of the patient at the proper distance from the sensing device and the proper adjustment of the lens.

infrared radiation Electromagnetic energy between the red visible light waves and the radio waves having wavelengths between 770 nm (7700 Å) and 12,000 nm (120,000 Å).

telethermography Thermogram made at a distance from the patient's body surface.

thermogram A graphic record of variations in body temperature (heat).

thermography Photographically recording the infrared radiation emanating from the patient's body.

transillumination The passage of light through body tissues for purposes of examination. The part being examined is placed between the light source and the examiner.

SELECTED BIBLIOGRAPHY

Thermography

Andersson I et al: Breast cancer screening and mammography: a population based randomized trial with mammography as the only screening mode, Radiology 132:273-276, 1979.

Baer MS and Hetherington: Preliminary report on the use of liquid crystal thermography in podiatry, J Foot Surg 27(5):398-403, 1988.

Baker LH: Breast cancer detection demonstration project: 5 year summary report, CA 32(4):194-225, 1982.

Brooks PG et al: Breast screening in the primary care office: a plea for early detection, J Reprod Med 27(11):685-689, 1983.

Curcio B and Haberman J: Infrared thermography: a review of current medical application, instrumentation and technique, Radiol Technol 42:233-247, 1971.

Dodd GD: Heat sensing devices and breast cancer detection. In Feig AS and McLelland R, editors: Breast carcinoma: current diagnosis and treatment, New York, 1983, Masson Publishing USA, Inc, pp 207-225.

Feig SA et al: Thermography, mammography and clinical examination in breast cancer screening: review of 16,000 studies, Radiology 122:123-127, 1977.

Gautherie M: Improved system for the objective evaluation of breast thermograms, Prog Clin Biol Res 107:897-905, 1982.

Gautherie M, Kotewicz A, and Gueblez P: Accurate and objective evaluation of breast thermograms: basic principles and new advances with special reference to an improved computer assisted scoring system, International Conference on Thermal Assessment of Breast Health, Washington, DC, July 1983.

Gershon-Cohen J: A short history of medical thermometry, Ann NY Acad Sci 121:4-11, 1964.

Gold RH et al: Breast imaging: state of the art, Invest Radiol 4:298-303, 1988.

Haberman JD, Love TJ, and Francis JE: Screening a rural population for breast cancer using thermography and physical examination techniques: methods and results—a preliminary report, Ann NY Acad Sci 335:492-500, 1980.

Handelsman H: Thermography for indications other than breast lesions. Health Technology Assessment Reports, 1989, US Department of Health and Human Services, no. 2, pp 1-31, 1989.

Jones CH et al: Thermography of the female breast: a five year study in relation to the detection and prognosis of cancer, Br J Radiol 48:532-538, 1975.

Kopans DB: Nonmammographic breast imaging techniques: current status and future developments, Clin Obstet Gynecol 25(5):961-970, 1987.

Lawson RN: Thermography: a new tool in the investigation of breast lesions, Can Serv Med J 13:517-521, 1957.

Moskowitz M: Screening for breast cancer: how effective are our tests? CA 33(1):26-39, 1983.

Moskowitz M et al: Lack of efficacy of thermography as a screening tool for minimal and stage 1 breast cancer, N Engl J Med 295:249-252, 1976.

Moskowitz M et al: The potential of liquid crystal thermography in detecting significant mastopathy, Radiology 140:659-662, 1981.

Nyirjesy I: Breast thermography, Clin Obstet Gynecol 25(2):401-408, 1982.

Pera A and Freimanis AK: The choice of radiologic procedures in the diagnosis of breast disease, Clin Obstet Gynecol 14(3):635-649, 1987.

Shapiro S et al: Ten to 14 year effect of screening on breast cancer mortality, JNCI 69(2):349-355, 1982.

Sickles EA: Breast thermography. In Feig AS and McLelland R, editors: Breast carcinoma: current diagnosis and treatment, New York, 1983, Masson Publishing USA, Inc, pp 227-231.

Sterns EE et al: Thermography in breast diagnosis, Cancer 50:323-325, 1982.

Tabar L and Gad A: Screening for breast cancer: the Swedish trial, Radiology 138:219-222, 1981.

Wenth J and Stein MA: Efficacy of breast cancer screening by thermography, Acta Thermographica 0392-0712, pp 76-81, 1983.

Diaphanography

Angquist KA et al: Diaphonoscopy and diaphanography for breast cancer detection in clinical practice, Acta Chir Scand 147:231-238, 1981.

Bartrum RJ et al: Transillumination light scanning to diagnose breast cancer: a feasibility study, AJR 142:409-411, 1984.

Carlsen E: Transillumination light scanning, Diagn Imaging, p 28, April 1982.

Carlsen EN: Transmission spectroscopy: an improvement in light scanning, RNM Images 13(2):23-25, 1983.

Church S et al: Transillumination in neonatal intensive care: a possible iatrogenic complication, South Med J 74:76, 1981.

Cohen SW: Dacryo-transillumination, Am J Ophthalmol 63:427, 1967.

Ersek RA: Mesenteric transillumination for vascular visualization, Surg Gynecol Obstet 152:339, 1981.

Fodor J et al: Diaphanography: transillumination of the breast, Radiol Technol 55(4):97-100, 1984.

Gisvold JJ et al: Comparison of mammography and transillumination light scanning in the detection of breast lesions, AJR 147:191-194, 1986.

Gold RH et al: Breast imaging state-of-the-art, Invest Radiol 21:298-304, 1986.

Gundersen J et al: Diaphanography for assessment of breast changes, Lakartidningen 76:1425-1427, 1979.

Hedley AJ: Breast transillumination using the sinus diaphanograph, Br Med J 283(6291):618-619, 1981.

Holliday HW et al: Breast transillumination using the sinus diaphanograph, Br Med J 283:411, 1981.

Isard HJ: Diaphanography: transillumination of the breast revisited, The Society for the Study Breast Disease Annual Meeting, Philadelphia, 1980.

Kopans DB: Nonmammographic breast imaging techniques: current status and future developments, Radiol Clin North Am 25:961-970, 1987.

Kuhns LR et al: Diagnosis of pneumothorax or pneumomediastinum in the neonate by transillumination, Pediatrics 56:355, 1975.

Martin JE: Breast imaging techniques: mammography, ultrasonography, computed tomography, thermography, and transillumination, Radiol Clin North Am 21(1):149-153, 1983.

McArtor RD et al: Iatrogenic second-degree burn caused by a transilluminator, Pediatrics 63(3):422-423, 1979.

Monsees B et al: Light scan evaluation of nonpalpable breast lesions, Radiology 163:467-470, 1987.

Morgan PP: Trial of electronic diaphanography for detecting breast cancer, Can Med Assoc J 129:686-687, 1983.

Ohlsson BS et al: Diaphanography: a method of evaluation of the female breast, World J Surg 4(6):701-706, 1980.

Pera A and Freimanis AK: The choice of radiologic procedures in the diagnosis of breast disease, Obstet Gynecol Clin North Am 14:635-649, 1987.

Profio AE et al: Scientific basis of breast diaphanography, Med Phys 16:60-65, 1989.

Shurtleff DB et al: Clinical use of transillumination, Arch Dis Child 41:183, 1966.

Sickles EA: Diaphanography. In Feig SA and Mclelland R, editors: Breast carcinoma: current diagnosis and treatment, New York, 1983, Masson Publishing USA, Inc, pp 246-250.

Sickles EA: Breast cancer detection with transillumination and mammography, AJR 142:841-844, 1984.

Spector SL et al: Comparison between transillumination and the roentgenogram in diagnosing paranasal sinus disease, J Allergy Clin Immunol 67:22, 1981.

Thomas BA: Breast transillumination using the sinus diaphanograph, Br Med J 283(6298):1057, 1981.

Watmough DJ: Diaphanography: mechanics responsible for the images, Acta Radiol (Oncol) 21(1):11-15, 1982.

Chapter 29

CENTRAL NERVOUS SYSTEM

NINA KOWALCZYK

For descriptive purposes the central nervous system is divided into two parts: (1) the *brain* (encephalon), which occupies the cranial cavity, and (2) the *spinal cord* (medulla spinalis), which is suspended within the vertebral canal.

The brain is composed of an outer portion of gray matter called the cortex and an inner portion of white matter. The brain consists of the *cerebrum* (telencephalon), the *cerebellum,* and the *brain stem,* which is continuous with the spinal cord (Fig. 29-1). The brain stem consists of the *diencephalon, midbrain* (mesencephalon), *pons,* and *medulla oblongata.* The cerebrum comprises the largest part of the brain and is referred to as the *forebrain.* The stemlike portion that connects the cerebrum to the pons and the cerebellum is termed the *midbrain.* The cerebellum, the pons, and the medulla oblongata make up the *hindbrain.*

A deep cleft, called the longitudinal fissure, separates the cerebrum into *right* and *left hemispheres,* which are closely connected by bands of nerve fibers or commissures. The main commissure between the cerebral hemispheres is the *corpus callosum.* Each cerebral hemisphere contains a fluid-filled cavity called a *lateral ventricle.* At the diencephalon the cerebral hemispheres surround the *third ventricle.* The surface of the cerebral hemispheres is convoluted by many fissures and grooves that mark them into lobes and lobules.

The cerebellum, the largest part of the hindbrain, is separated from the cerebrum by a deep transverse cleft. The hemispheres of the cerebellum are connected by a median constricted area called the *vermis.* The surface of the cerebellum contains numerous transverse fissures that account for its laminated appearance. The tissues between the curved fissures are called *folia.* The pons forms the upper part of the hindbrain, and the medulla, which extends between the pons and the spinal cord, forms the lower part.

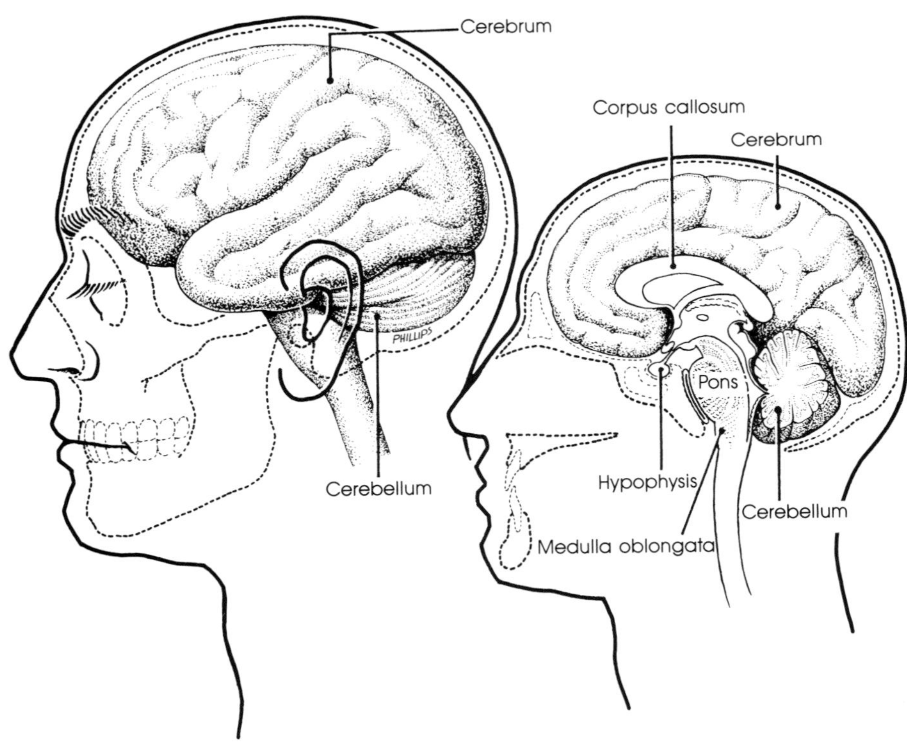

Fig. 29-1. Drawings showing surface and midsection of brain.

The spinal cord is a slender, elongated structure consisting of an inner, gray, cellular substance, which has an H shape on transverse section, and an outer, white, fibrous substance (Figs. 29-2 and 29-3). The cord extends from the brain, being connected to the medulla oblongata at the level of the foramen magnum, to the approximate level of the space between the first and second lumbar vertebrae. The spinal cord ends in a pointed extremity called the *conus medullaris*. A delicate, fibrous strand extending from the conus medullaris attaches the cord to the upper coccygeal segment. There are 31 pairs of spinal nerves, each arising from two roots at the sides of the spinal cord. The nerves are transmitted through the intervertebral and sacral foramina.

The brain and spinal cord are enclosed by three continuous, protective membranes called *meninges*. The inner sheath, called the *pia mater* (L., tender mother), is highly vascular and closely adherent to the underlying brain and cord structure.

The delicate central sheath is called the *arachnoid*. This membrane is separated from the pia mater by a comparatively wide space called the *subarachnoid space,* which is widened in certain areas. These areas of increased width are called cisternae, the widest of which is the *cisterna cerebellomedullaris* (cisterna magna). This cavity is triangular and is situated at the posterosuperior part of the subarachnoid space between the base of the cerebellum and the dorsal surface of the medulla oblongata. The subarachnoid space is continuous with the ventricular system of the brain and communicates with it by way of the *median aperture* (foramen of Magendie) and by *lateral apertures* (foramina of Luschka) located between the cisterna cerebellomedullaris and the fourth ventricle. The ventricles of the brain and the subarachnoid space contain cerebrospinal fluid (CSF). The cisterna cerebellomedullaris is sometimes used as a point of entry into the subarachnoid space.

The outermost sheath, called the *dura mater* (L., hard mother), forms the strong, fibrous covering of the brain and spinal cord. The dura is separated from the arachnoid by the *subdural space* and from the vertebral periosteum by the *epidural space*. These spaces do not communicate with the ventricular system. The dura mater is composed of two layers throughout its cranial portion. The outer (endosteal) layer lines the cranial bones, thus serving as periosteum to their inner surface. The inner (meningeal) layer serves to protect the brain and to support the blood vessels. The meningeal layer also sends out four partitions for the support and protection of the various parts of the brain. The dura mater extends below the spinal cord, to the level of the second sacral segment, to enclose the spinal nerves, which are prolonged inferiorly from the cord to their respective exits. The lower portion of the dura mater is called the *dural sac*.

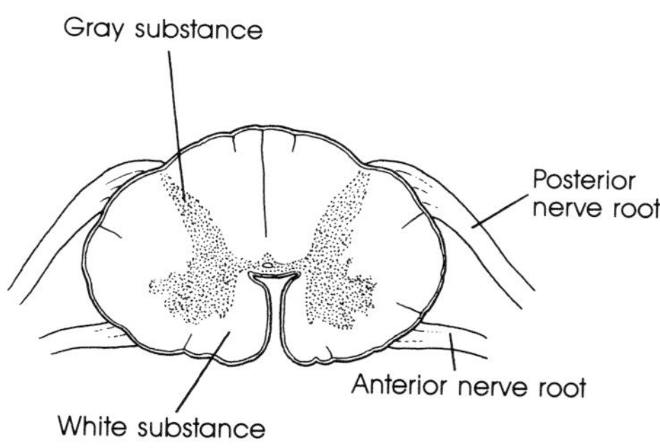

Fig. 29-2. Transverse section of spinal cord.

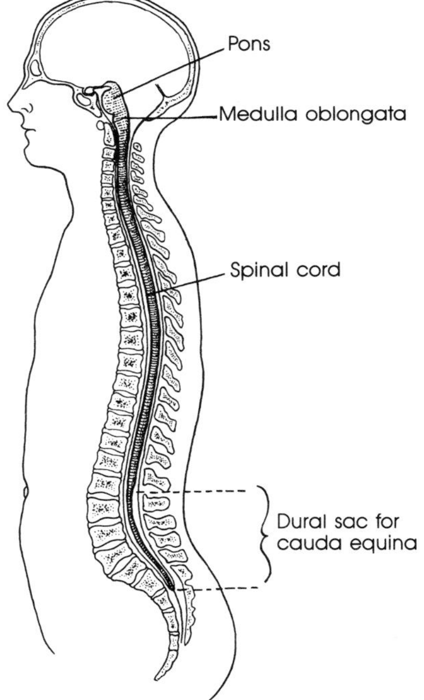

Fig. 29-3. Sagittal section showing spinal cord.

The ventricular system of the brain consists of four irregular, fluid-containing cavities that communicate with each other through connecting channels (Figs. 29-4 to 29-6). The two upper cavities are an identical pair and are simply called *right* and *left lateral ventricles*. They are situated, one on each side of the midsagittal plane, in the inferior, medial part of the corresponding hemisphere of the cerebrum. Radiographic centering for the lateral position of these cavities is 1½ inches (3.7 cm) superior to the level of the external auditory meatuses.

Each lateral ventricle consists of a central portion called the *body* of the cavity. The body is prolonged anteriorly, posteriorly, and inferiorly into hornlike portions that give the ventricle an approximate U shape. The prolonged portions are known as the *anterior* (frontal), the *posterior* (occipital), and the *inferior* (temporal) *horns* (cornua). Each lateral ventricle is connected to the third ventricle by a channel called the *interventricular foramen* (foramen of Monro), through which it communicates directly with the third ventricle and indirectly with the opposite lateral ventricle.

The *third ventricle* is a slitlike cavity with a somewhat quadrilateral shape. It is situated in the midsagittal plane just inferior to the level of the bodies of the lateral ventricles. This cavity extends anteroinferiorly from the pineal gland, which produces a recess in its posterior wall, to the optic chiasm, which produces a recess in its anteroinferior wall. Radiographic centering for the lateral position of the third ventricle is 1 inch (2.5 cm) superior and 1 inch (2.5 cm) anterior to the external auditory meatuses.

The interventricular foramina, one from each lateral ventricle, open into the anterosuperior portion of the third ventricle. The cavity is continuous posteroinferiorly with the fourth ventricle by a passage known as the *cerebral aqueduct* (aqueduct of Sylvius).

The *fourth ventricle* is diamond shaped and is the cavity of the hindbrain. It is also a midline structure located anterior to the cerebellum and posterior to the pons and upper portion of the medulla oblongata. The distal, pointed end of the fourth ventricle is continuous with the central canal of the medulla oblongata. The fourth ventricle communicates with the subarachnoid space via the *median aperture* and the *lateral apertures*, as discussed earlier in this chapter. Radiographic centering for lateral positions of the fourth ventricle is 1 inch (2.5 cm) directly posterior to the level of the external auditory meatuses.

Body of lateral ventricle
Third ventricle
Anterior horn
Posterior horn
Cerebral aqueduct
Interventricular foramen
Inferior horn
Fourth ventricle

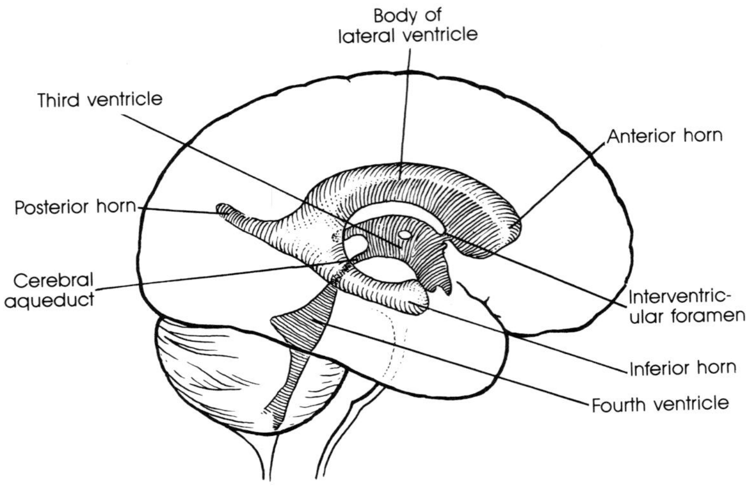

Fig. 29-4. Lateral aspect of cerebral ventricles in relation to surface of brain.

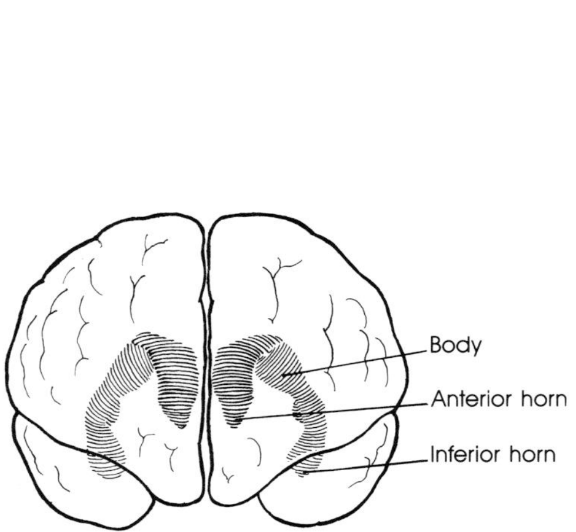

Fig. 29-5. Anterior aspect of lateral cerebral ventricles in relation to surface of brain.

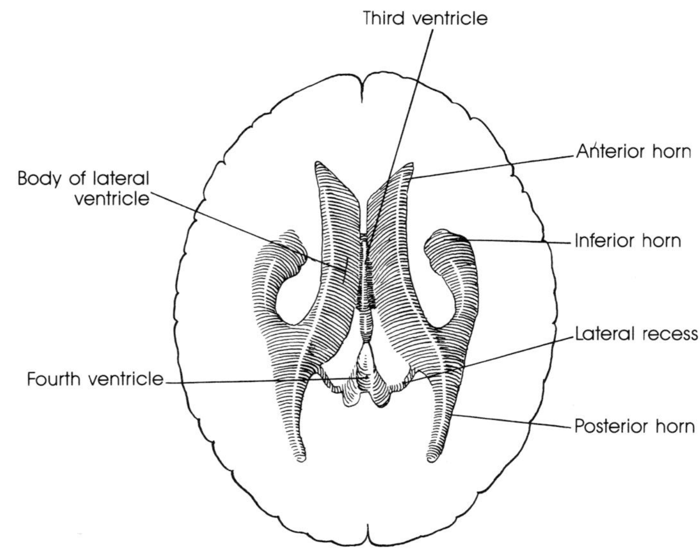

Fig. 29-6. Superior aspect of cerebral ventricles in relation to surface of brain.

Plain Radiographic Examination

Radiographs of the cerebral and visceral cranium and of the vertebral column may be employed to demonstrate bony anatomy. In the case of trauma, radiographs are obtained to detect and characterize bony injury or subluxation or dislocation of the vertebral column and to determine the extent and stability of the bony injury.

When radiographing a traumatized patient with possible central nervous system involvement, a cross-table lateral cervical spine radiograph should be obtained first to rule out fracture or misalignment of the cervical spine. Approximately two thirds of significant spine pathologic conditions can be detected on this initial radiograph. Care must be taken to adequately demonstrate the entire cervical spine, to include the C7-T1 articulation. It may be necessary to pull the patient's arms down while radiographing this region or to employ the Twining method (see Volume 1, p. 318) to fully demonstrate this anatomic region radiographically.

Once the cross-table lateral radiograph has been checked and cleared by a physician, it is necessary to obtain the following cervical spine projections: AP projection, bilateral oblique positions (trauma technique may be necessary), and an AP projection of the dens (odontoid process). A vertebral arch, or pillar position (see volume 1, p. 312) of the cervical spine may be used to provide additional information regarding the posterior portions of the cervical vertebrae.

Multidirectional tomography (see Chapter 26 in this volume) may be used to supplement plain spine radiographs for initial screening purposes. However, tomography has been largely replaced with computed tomography (CT; see Chapter 34 in this volume) in many institutions. Tomography may be employed to demonstrate long, continuous areas of the spine, whereas CT is limited because of the design and reconstruction limitations of the equipment. Disadvantages of tomography include a lack of soft tissue detail and the difficulty in positioning a traumatized patient for lateral tomographic radiographs.

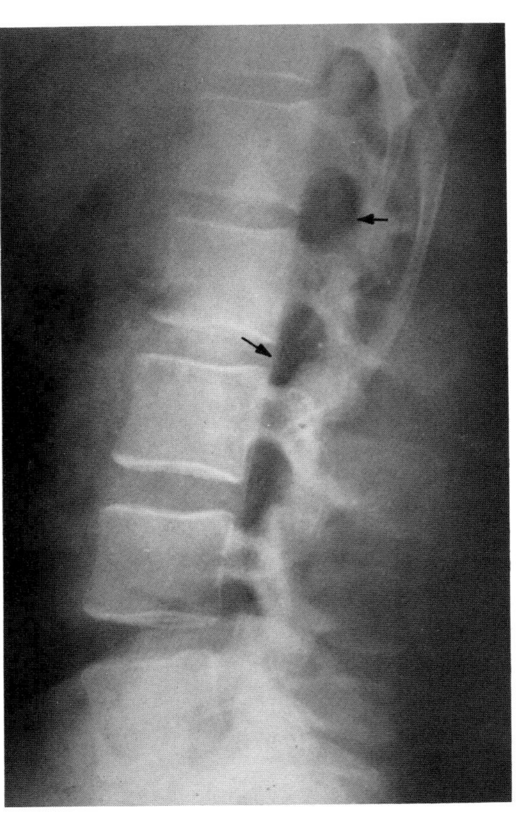

Fig. 29-7. Lateral myelogram showing gas in spinal canal *(arrows)*.

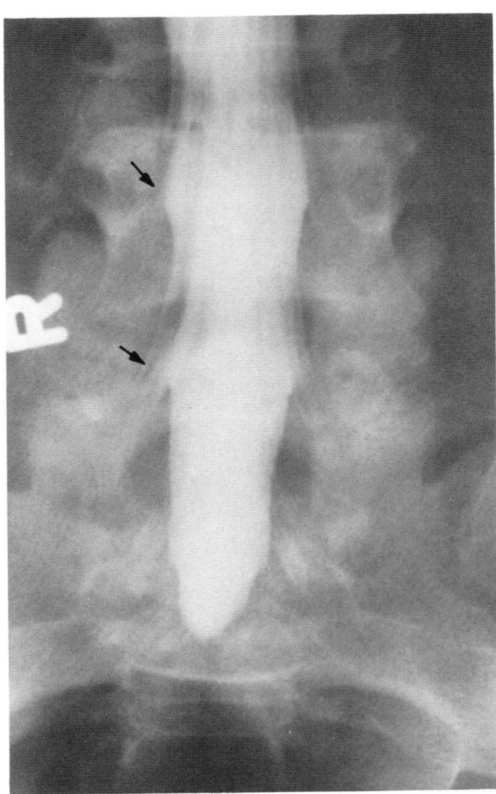

Fig. 29-8. Water-soluble (metrizamide) myelogram showing nerve roots *(arrow)*.

Myelography

Myelography (Gr., *myelos,* marrow; the spinal cord) is the general term applied to radiologic examination of the central nervous system structures situated within the spinal canal. These examinations are performed by introducing a contrast medium into the subarachnoid space by spinal puncture, most commonly at the L2-3 or L3-4 interspace or at the cisterna cerebellomedullaris. Myelography is employed to demonstrate the site and extent of spinal cord lesions such as tumors and encroachment by posterior protrusion of herniated intervertebral disks. These lesions appear radiographically as a deformity in or obstruction of the passage of the column of contrast medium within the subarachnoid space. Contrast agents employed may be either a gaseous medium, termed *gas myelography* (Fig. 29-7), or an opaque medium, termed *opaque myelography* (Fig. 29-8).

CONTRAST MEDIA

Two types of opaque contrast media are currently available for use in myelography: a non–water-soluble iodinated ester and a water-soluble nonionic iodinated contrast agent. Both types of contrast media have advantages and disadvantages.

The non–water-soluble iodinated ester (Pantopaque) was introduced in 1942. It has been used for many years and has proved to be relatively safe for myelography (Fig. 29-9). Disadvantages of this contrast material include poor visualization of the nerve root sheaths and the fact that it must be removed from the subarachnoid space after the completion of the examination.

The first water-soluble nonionic iodinated contrast agent, metrizamide, has been in use since the late 1970s. Following its introduction, it quickly became the medium of choice in many radiology departments. This contrast medium is less viscous than the non–water-soluble iodinated ester, thus providing good visualization of the nerve roots. A water-soluble medium also has the additional advantage of not having to be removed following the examination, since it is readily absorbed by the body. A disadvantage is that it tends to be absorbed quickly; thus radiographs must be taken promptly and accurately. Many physicians use metrizamide only for examination of the thoracic and lumbar areas because research suggests that convulsions may result when the contrast medium reaches the level of the posterior fossa in the skull. Further research has led to the development of "second-generation" water-soluble nonionic iodinated contrast agents: iohexol, iopamidol, and ioversol. These newer contrast agents are associated with fewer side effects than metrizamide and are currently the contrast media of choice when performing myelography.

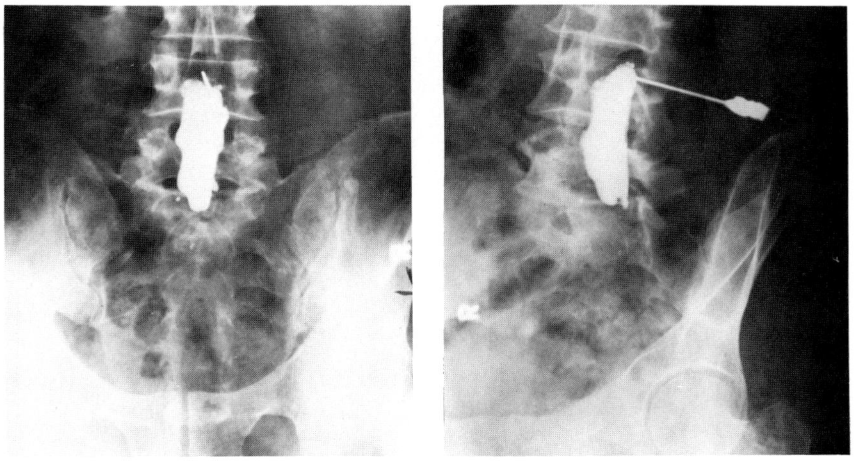

Gas myelography uses air or oxygen. Because of the different weights of gas and opaque contrast agents, they move in opposite directions when the patient is moved. The gas rises as the patient's head is elevated, whereas the opaque medium gravitates downward. Gas myelography is not performed with any regularity at most health care facilities. (For information, see Volume 3, p. 96 of the sixth edition of this atlas.) When used, the gaseous contrast medium is introduced by way of lumbar puncture.

Preparation of examining room

One of the responsibilities of the technologist is the preparation of the examining room before the patient's arrival. The radiographic equipment should be checked, and, since the procedure involves aseptic technique, the table and overhead equipment must be cleaned. The footboard should be attached and the padded shoulder supports placed and ready for adjustment to the patient's height.

Any premedication ordered for the patient is administered by the nursing staff. A representative from the radiology department often calls the patient's nursing service and requests that the ordered premedication be given to coincide with the scheduled time of the myelogram.

The spinal puncture and injection of the contrast medium are performed in the radiology department. This precaution is taken to eliminate the possibility of the medium entering and becoming trapped in the cerebral ventricles and to prevent fragmentation or absorption of the medium as a result of moving the patient. The sterile tray and the nonsterile items required for the spinal puncture and injection of the contrast medium should be ready for convenient placement.

Fig. 29-9. Myelograms with non–water-soluble iodinated contrast medium showing needle in place.

EXAMINATION PROCEDURE

The details of performing the myelogram should be explained to the patient before the examination to reduce the apprehension and to prevent alarm at unexpected maneuvers during the procedure. The patient should be told why there must be repeated and acute changes in the angulation of the examining table (Figs. 29-10 and 29-11) and why the head must be maintained in a fully extended position when the table is tilted to the Trendelenburg position. The patient must be assured of his or her safety when the table is acutely angled, and he or she must be assured that everything possible will be done to avoid causing unnecessary discomfort.

Some physicians prefer to have the patient placed on the table in the prone position for the spinal puncture. Most, however, have the patient adjusted in the lateral position with the spine flexed to widen the interspinous spaces for easier introduction of the needle.

The physician usually withdraws spinal fluid and injects the contrast medium in equal units of exchange for the spinal fluid removed. After the injection has been completed, the traveling of the contrast column is observed fluoroscopically, and the direction of its flow is controlled by varying the angulation of the table. Spot radiographs are taken at the level of any blockage of or distortion in the outline of the contrast column. Conventional radiographic studies, with the central ray directed vertically or horizontally, may be taken as requested by the radiologist. Cross-table radiographs are made with grid-front cassettes or a stationary grid, and they must be closely collimated.

The position of the patient's head must be guarded as the contrast column nears the cervical area to prevent the medium from passing into the cerebral ventricles. Acute extension of the head compresses the cisterna magna and thus prevents further ascent of the medium. Because the cisterna magna is situated posteriorly, neither forward nor lateral flexion of the head will compress the cisternal cavity.

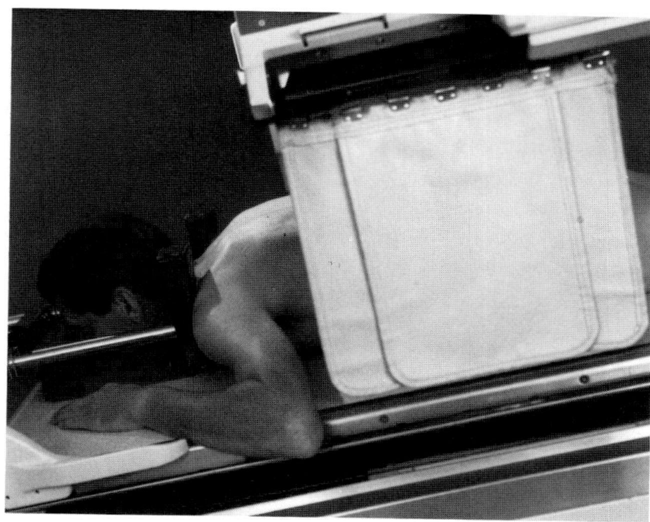

Fig. 29-10. Head of table tilted down.

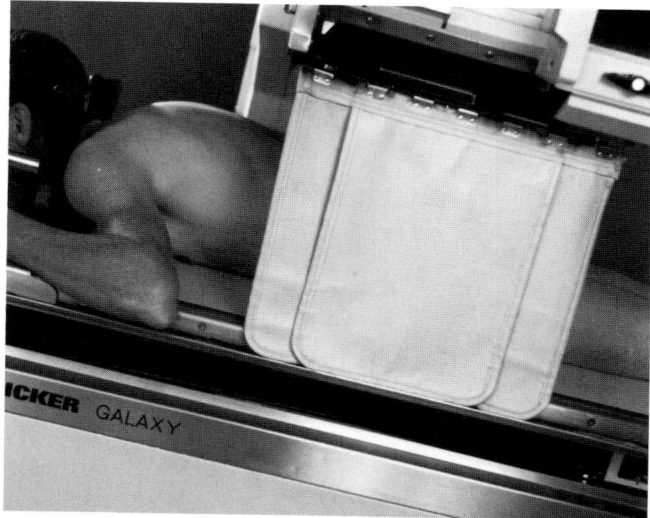

Fig. 29-11. Foot end of table tilted down.

OPAQUE MYELOGRAPHY

Opaque myelography (Figs. 29-12 to 29-17) is performed using sterile conditions under fluoroscopic control. The patient is positioned according to the preference of the examining physician. When using a lumbar puncture approach, the patient may be placed in a prone position, which he or she maintains, or the patient may be adjusted in a lateral position, with the spine flexed for the insertion of the needle, and then turned to the prone position for the examination. If an iodinated ester contrast agent is used, the needle is left in situ for later aspiration of the contrast agent. If this is the case, the needle must be covered with a sterile towel and then protected from accidental bumping by adjusting the height of the image intensifier and securing it in position with the stop-lock device. When a water-soluble contrast agent is employed, the spinal needle may be removed after the instillation of the contrast material.

If a cisternal puncture approach is used, the head of the table may be elevated to prevent leakage of the contrast medium into the ventricular system of the brain. The needle is then removed, regardless of the type of contrast agent utilized, and the head is carefully extended to compress the cisternal cavity. If an iodinated ester contrast agent is employed, withdrawal of the medium requires a second puncture to remove the contrast material.

Opaque myelography is used to determine extrinsic spinal cord compression caused by a herniated disk, bone fragments, or tumors, as well as spinal cord swelling from posttraumatic injury. It is used to evaluate the entire vertebral canal by imaging the dynamic patterns of the cerebrospinal fluid flow, thus demonstrating areas of subarachnoid space narrowing.

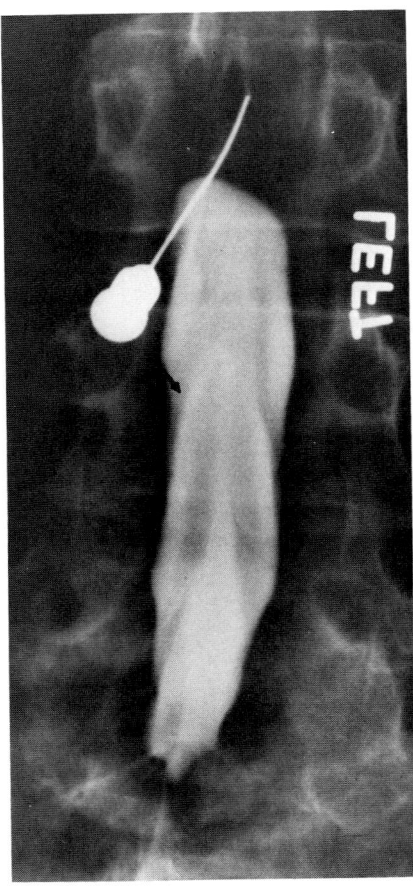

Fig. 29-12. Frontal lumbar myelogram with non–water-soluble iodinated contrast medium, showing axillary pouches and corresponding nerve roots *(arrow)*.

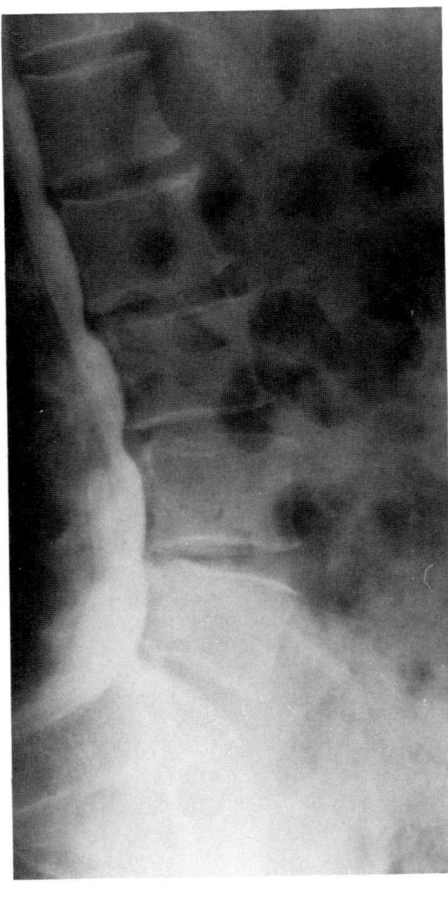

Fig. 29-13. Lateral lumbar myelogram with water-soluble (metrizamide) contrast medium.

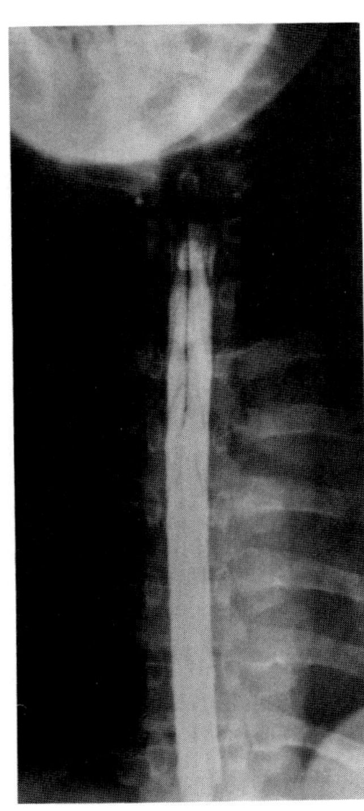

Fig. 29-14. Thoracic myelogram taken in supine position showing anterior spinal vessels and thoracic nerve roots. Isophendylate (Pantopaque), 15 ml, was used.

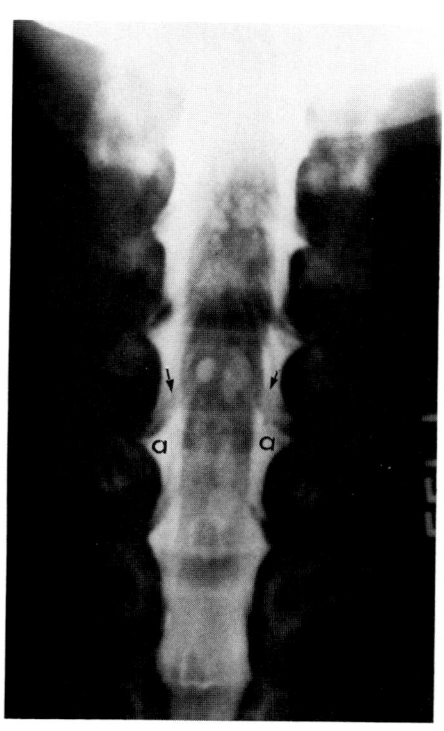

Fig. 29-15. Normal cervical myelogram showing symmetrical nerve roots *(arrows)* and axillary pouches *(a)* on both sides, as well as spinal cord.

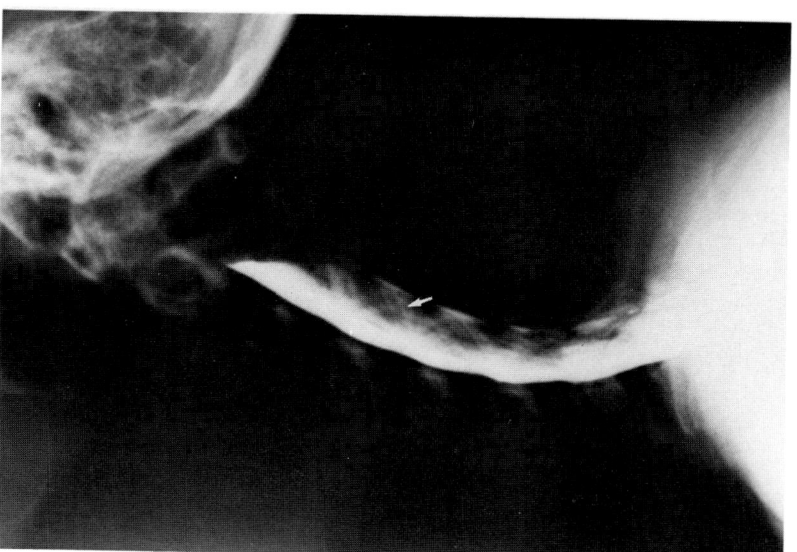

Fig. 29-16. Prone, cross-table lateral radiograph showing dentate ligament and posterior nerve roots *(arrow)*.

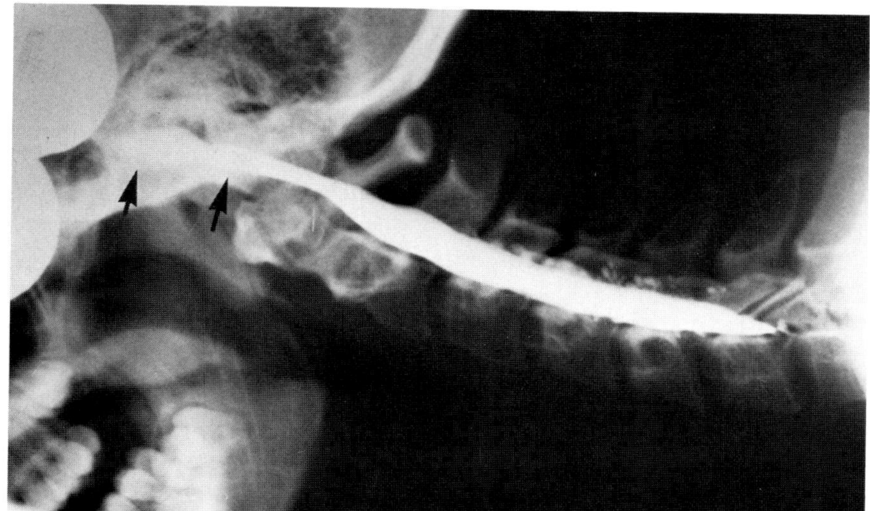

Fig. 29-17. Prone, cross-table lateral radiograph showing contrast medium passing foramen magnum and lying against lower clivus *(arrows)*.

(Courtesy Dr. K.Y. Chynn.)

COMPUTED TOMOGRAPHIC MYELOGRAPHY

Often a myelographic procedure may be followed by a CT examination of the spine (Figs. 29-18 and 29-19). The CT examination is generally limited to specific regions of the spine. If a follow-up CT examination is performed, the myelogram must be performed using a water-soluble contrast material. The use of an iodinated ester contrast agent severely degrades the CT image because of artifacts created by the computer. Water-soluble contrast agents, however, greatly improve the resolution and visibility of structures within the vertebral canal without degrading the imaging of the bony structures of the spine. The CT examination usually follows the myelographic procedure because low concentrations of the water-soluble contrast agent adequately demonstrate opacification of the subarachnoid space because of the high contrast sensitivity of CT.

CT myelography demonstrates the size, shape, and position of the spinal cord and the nerve roots. It is an excellent modality in cases of compressive injuries or in determining the extent of dural tears resulting in extravasation of the cerebrospinal fluid.

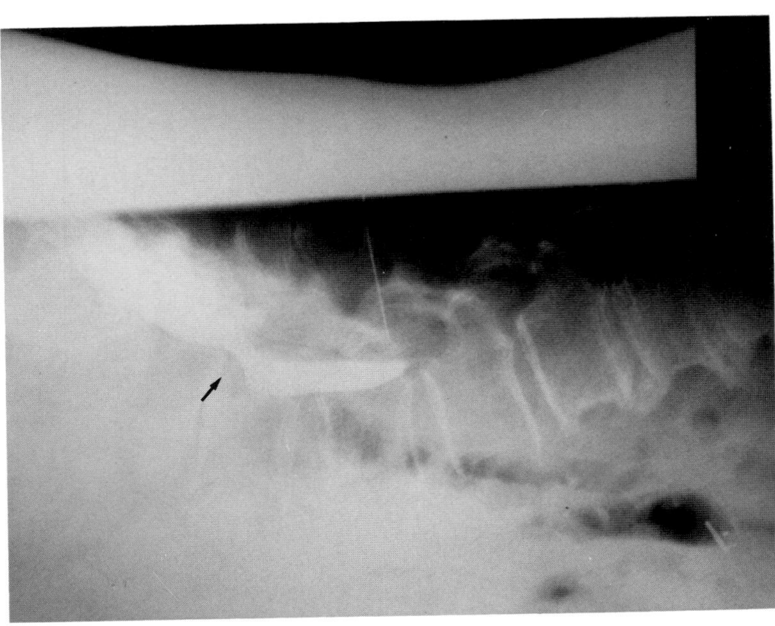

Fig. 29-18. Lumbar opaque myelogram demonstrating subarachnoid space narrowing *(arrow).*

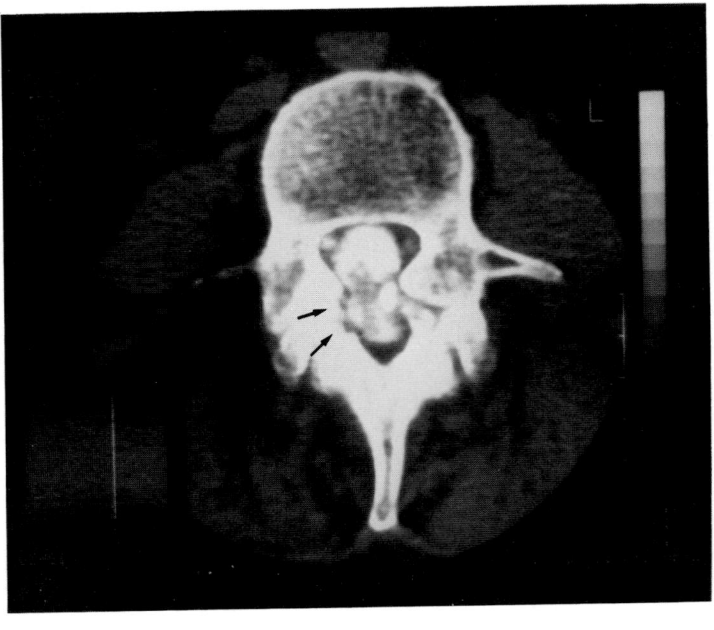

Fig. 29-19. Lumbar CT myelogram demonstrating subarachnoid space narrowing *(arrows).*

Diskography

Diskography and *nucleography* are terms used to denote the radiologic examination of individual intervertebral disks by means of the injection of a small quantity of one of the water-soluble, iodinated media into the center of the disk by way of a double-needle entry. This procedure was introduced by Lindblom[1] in 1950, and it has been further detailed by Cloward[2,3] and by Butt.[4]

Diskography is used in the investigation of internal disk lesions such as rupture of the nucleus pulposus that cannot be demonstrated by myelographic examination (Fig. 29-20). Diskography may be performed separately, or it may be combined with myelography. The patient is given only a local anesthetic so that he will be fully conscious and therefore able to inform the physician as to the location of pain when the needles are inserted and the injection is made.

Except for lidocaine, which is added to and injected with the contrast solution, and a double-needle combination rather than a standard spinal-puncture needle, the instrument setup is the same as for spinal puncture. The double-needle combination consists of an outer, large-bore 20-gauge needle used to perform the spinal puncture and reach the annulus fibrosus of the disk and a longer, fine (26-gauge) needle, which is then passed through the guide needle and advanced to the center of the nucleus pulposus. The needle lengths are usually 2 and 2½ inches for cervical entry and 3½ and 5 inches for lumbar entry. The position of the needles is determined fluoroscopically before the contrast medium is injected.

[1]Lindblom K: Technique and results in myelography and disc puncture, Acta Radiol 34:321-330, 1950.

[2]Cloward RB and Buzaid LL: Discography, AJR 68:552-564, 1952.

[3]Cloward RB: Cervical discography: a contribution to the etiology and mechanism of neck, shoulder, and arm pain, Ann Surg 150:1052-1064, 1959.

[4]Butt WP: Discography—some interesting cases, J Can Assoc Radiol 17:167-175, 1966.

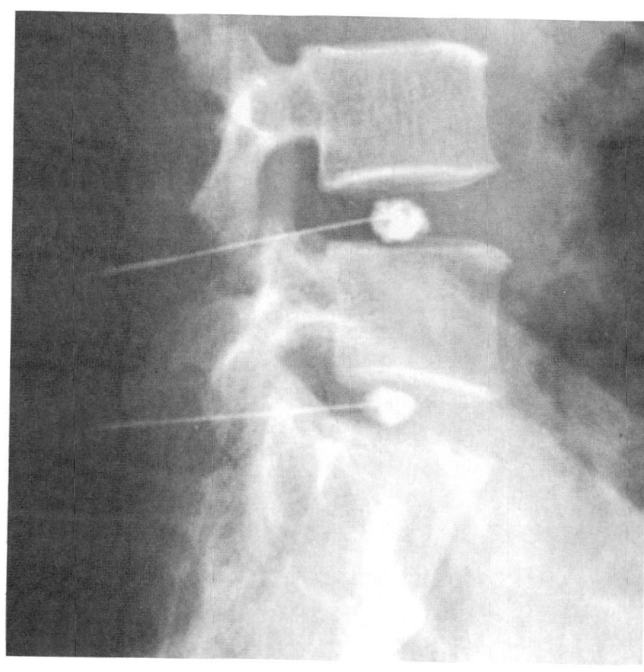

Fig. 29-20. Lumbar diskogram demonstrating normal nucleus pulposus of round contour type.

CERVICAL DISKOGRAPHY

In the absence of biplane equipment, cervical diskography (Figs. 29-21 to 29-26) requires the use of a vertical tabletop grid device to hold a vertically placed film and the use of a mobile unit for cross-table lateral images. The central ray is directed at a cephalic angle of 10 degrees for the AP projection; this angulation is adequate because of the reduction of the lordotic curve caused by elevating the patient's head.

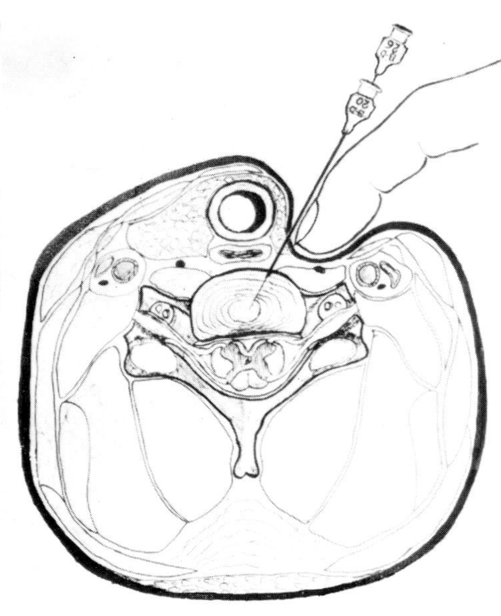

Fig. 29-21. Technique of disk puncture.

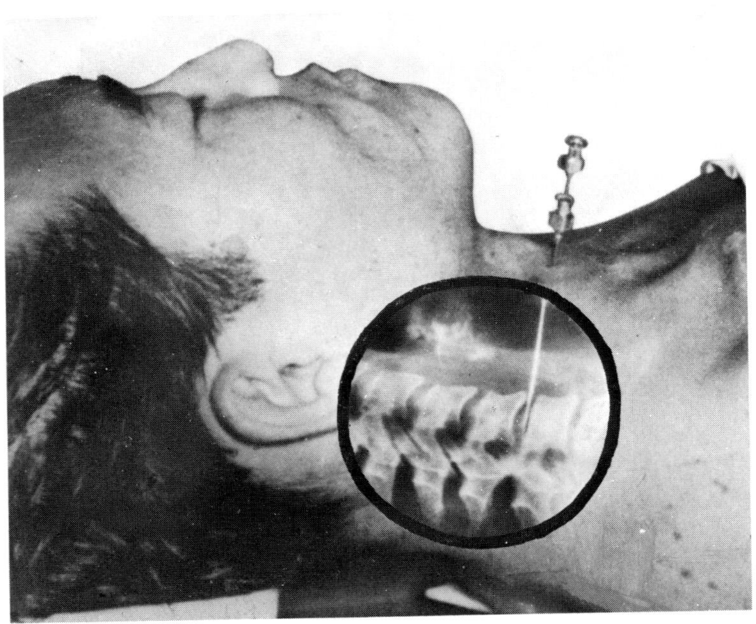

Fig. 29-22. Composite photograph demonstrating cervical diskography.

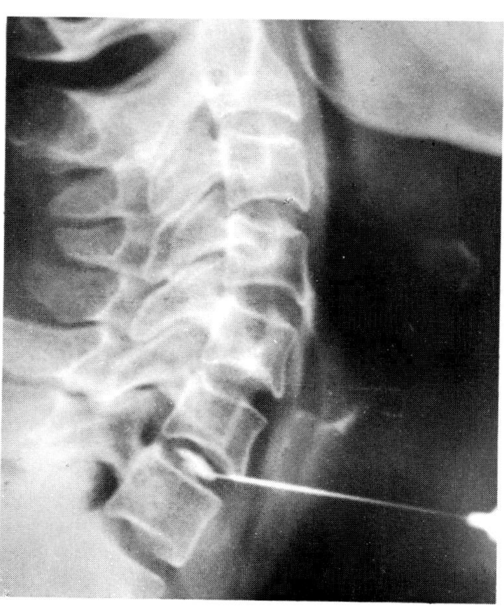

Fig. 29-23. Normal disk (nucleus pulposus).

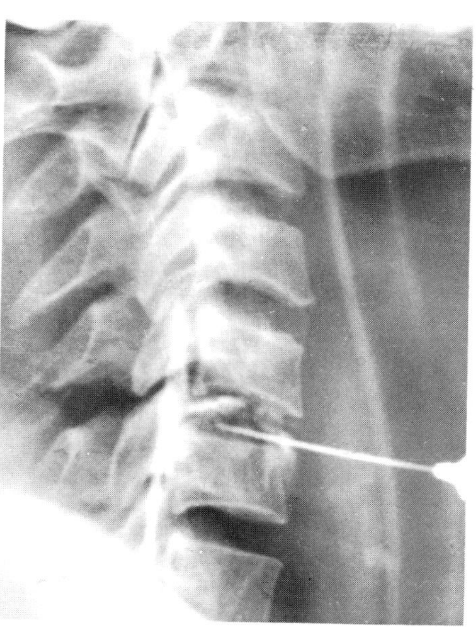

Fig. 29-24. Lacerated disk and fracture dislocation.

(Courtesy Dr. Ralph B. Cloward.)

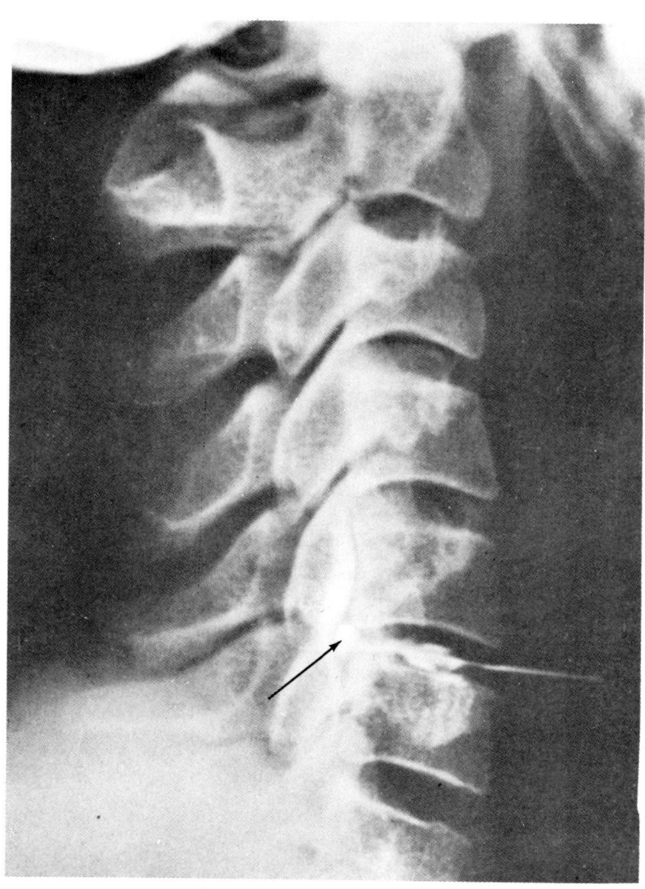

Fig. 29-25. Cervical diskogram showing acute herniation of disk with fragment into spinal canal *(arrow)*.

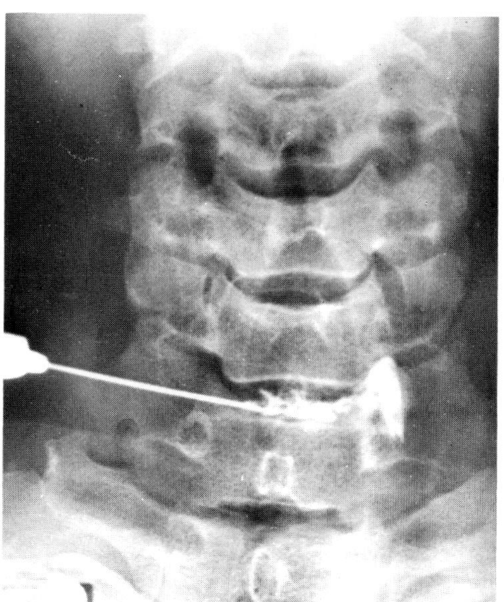

Fig. 29-26. Left lateral disk rupture with sodium diatrizoate (Hypaque) extending beyond disk space.

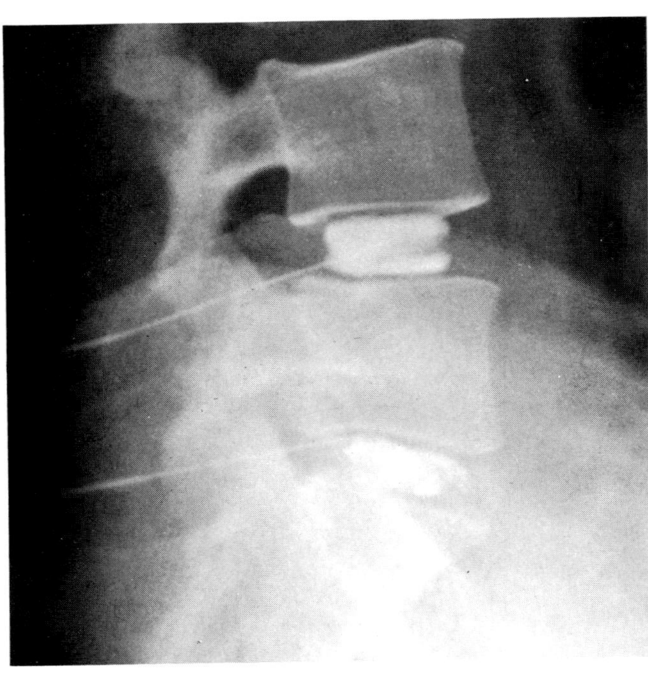

Fig. 29-27. Normal nucleus pulposus of oval or rectangular type.

(Courtesy Dr. Ralph B. Cloward.)

LUMBAR DISKOGRAPHY

For lumbar diskography the patient is placed in the lateral position for the introduction of the needles and the contrast medium and for the first diskogram. A radiolucent support is adjusted under the body so that the long axis of the spine is horizontal.

After the injection of the contrast agent, and with the needles in situ, a direct lateral radiograph is made and inspected. When this study shows that an adequate amount of the medium has been injected, the needles are removed and the puncture site or sites dressed. The patient is then adjusted in the supine position, with the thighs flexed enough to place the back in contact with the table. For the frontal projection of the last two disk spaces, the thighs are flexed to the lithotomy position, and the central ray is then directed at a cephalic angle of 10 to 20 degrees (Figs. 29-27 to 29-29). Last, the patient is placed in the erect position for flexion and extension, weight-bearing, lateral studies of the abdominal disk or disks.

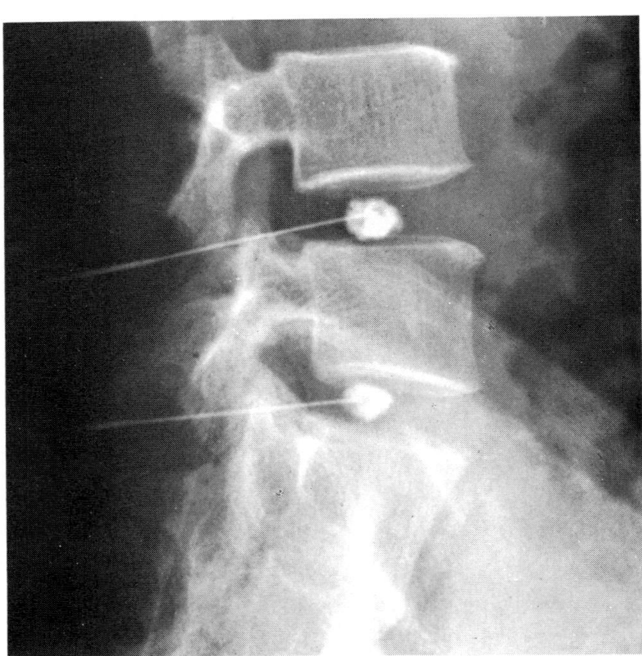

Fig. 29-28. Normal nucleus pulposus of round contour type.

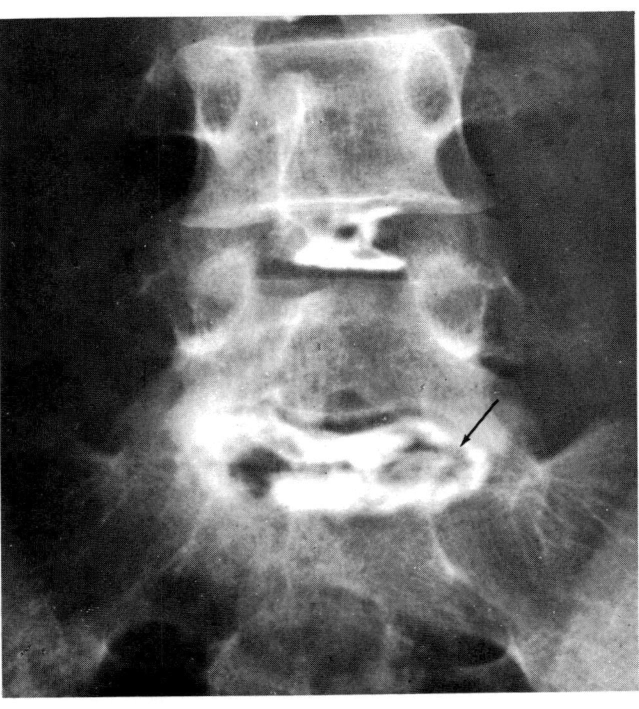

Fig. 29-29. Complete rupture of lumbosacral disk. Contrast solution *(arrow)* fills entire interspace, indicating disorganization of entire annulus fibrosus.

Chemonucleolysis

Begun in the early 1980s, *chemonucleolysis* is an alternative method to conventional laminectomy for the treatment of lumbar herniated nucleus pulposus. This procedure employs a *chymopapain* enzyme, derived from the papaya, to dissolve the herniated disk.

Chemonucleolysis is generally performed after a CT myelogram confirms the presence and location of the herniated nucleus pulposus. The procedure is generally performed in the surgical area under fluoroscopic control. The patient is placed in a lateral position, and an 18-gauge needle is inserted into the nucleus pulposus. Diskography is routinely performed to ensure proper needle placement before the chymopapain injection. Once the enzyme is injected, the needle is kept in place for approximately 5 minutes before being removed.

Chemonucleolysis does not generally result in scarring, which is often associated with a conventional laminectomy procedure. However, posttreatment stiffness and spasm are often associated with chemonucleolysis, especially during the first few weeks after this treatment procedure.

Magnetic Resonance Imaging

The use of magnetic resonance imaging (MRI) in the diagnosis and treatment of central nervous system disorders has increased over the past few years. MRI provides excellent anatomic detail of the brain, spinal cord, and subarachnoid space without the use of contrast agents. MRI also displays excellent visualization of the intervertebral disks and provides good soft tissue contrast resolution. Image reconstruction may be performed in a variety of planes (coronal, sagittal, and axial) to aid in the diagnosis and treatment of a variety of disorders (Figs. 29-30 and 29-31). See Chapter 37 for an in-depth discussion of MR imaging.

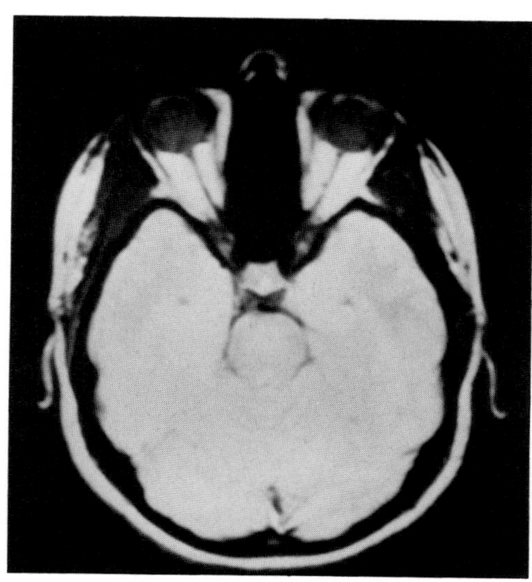

Fig. 29-30. Axial MR section through the brain.

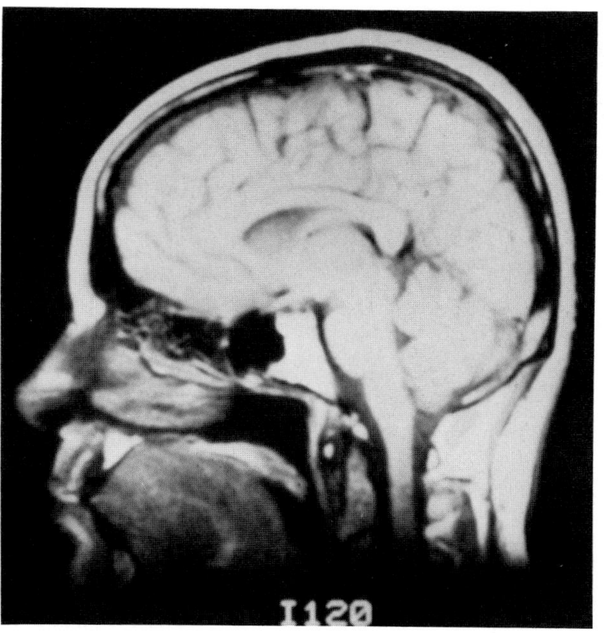

Fig. 29-31. Sagittal MR section through the brain.

Cerebral Pneumonography/ Ventriculography

Since the introduction of CT units, cerebral pneumonography/ventriculography is very rarely performed in radiology departments; thus the discussion included in this chapter has been reduced. For additional information regarding cerebral pneumonography, see the Bibliography in this volume and pp. 872 to 888 in the fourth edition of this atlas.

Cerebral pneumonography is a general term applied to the radiologic examination of the brain by means of the introduction of a gaseous medium into the ventricular system. Because of the radiographic homogeneity of the brain substance and fluid-filled channels, noncalcified lesions of intracranial structures cannot be satisfactorily demonstrated without the use of a contrast agent. A gaseous medium—air, oxygen, or carbon dioxide—is generally used for this purpose in preference to opaque media, because the gases produce less irritation in the ventricular system. In addition, they are readily absorbed in the subarachnoid spaces.

Cerebral pneumonography is employed to demonstrate space-occupying, intracranial lesions as shown by filling defects or deformations in the shadow outline of the gas-filled ventricular system or the subarachnoid cisternae and channels. *Pneumoventriculography* (Fig. 29-32) and *pneumoencephalography* are the two specific terms used, respectively, to denote the direct and indirect routes of injection. These terms also indicate the extent of structural delineation obtained by each injection route.

Direct injection of the gas into the central ventricular system (pneumoventriculography) delineates only the inner, or ventricular, surfaces of the brain. Indirect introduction of the contrast agent by way of the subarachnoid route (pneumoencephalography) delineates the subarachnoid spaces of the brain as well as the ventricular system. Each procedure has specific indications and contraindications, so that the injection route is determined according to the type and location of the intracranial disorder.

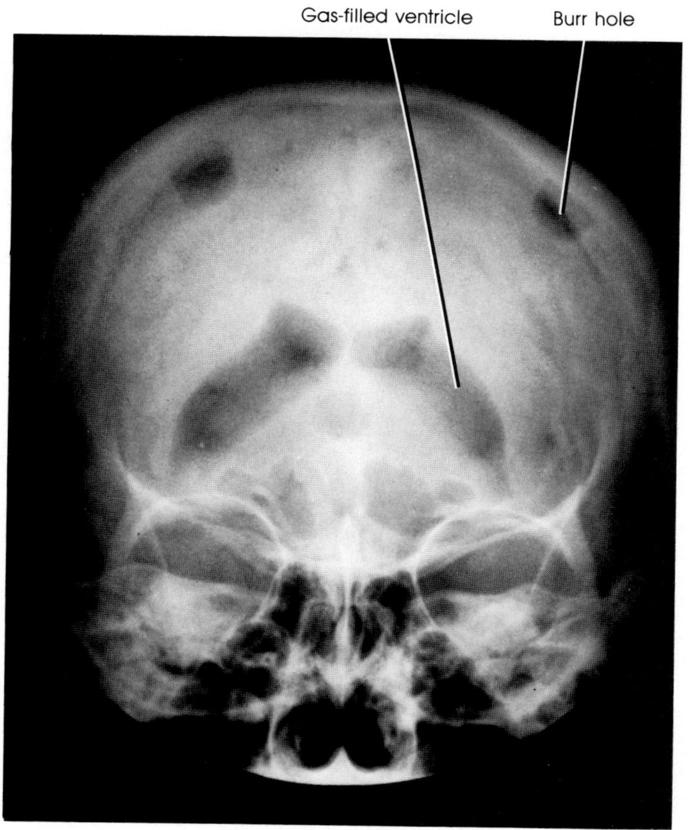

Fig. 29-32. Pneumoventriculogram.

(Courtesy Dr. Ernest H. Wood.)

Stereotactic Surgery

Stereotactic surgery and *stereotrophic surgery* are terms used to denote a highly specialized neurosurgical therapeutic technique for the precise three-dimensional guidance of a slender surgical instrument through a burr hole in the cranium to a predetermined point deep within the brain. The first practical stereotactic instrument was introduced in the late 1940s for use with pneumoencephalography (Fig. 29-33). Stereotactic surgery is used in the treatment of various diseases of the nervous system, some of which cause a loss of control of body movement and some of which cause intractable pain. The most frequent use of this surgical technique may be for the treatment of Parkinson's disease. Other uses are to obtain a biopsy of a deep tumor within the brain and to drain abscesses. Stereotactic surgery is often the preferred method for treatment of such conditions because the diseased structure can be reached and surgically destroyed with a slender, specialized instrument guided through a small burr hole in the cranium, thus eliminating the need for open surgery.

The tip of the surgical instrument must be placed in the target area with an accuracy greater than a 1 mm deviation from the target point. This precise placement requires a specialized instrument guidance system known as a stereotactic frame or stereotactic device (Fig. 29-34). Numerous types of stereotactic devices are currently in use. Basically, they consist of a frame into which the surgeon immobilizes the patient's head with attached fixation screws and that incorporates an external reference system and an adjustable instrument device.

A

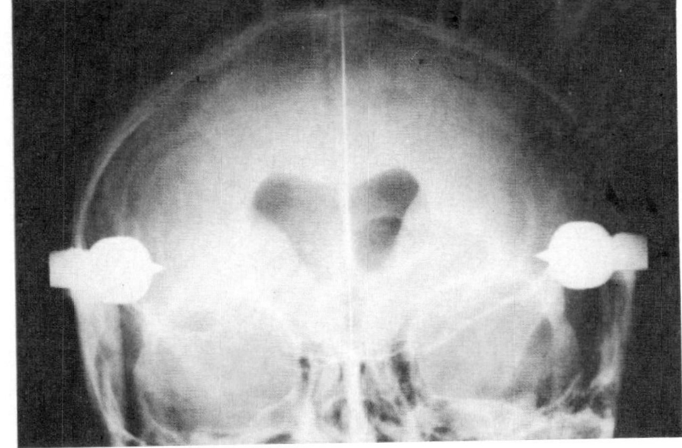

B

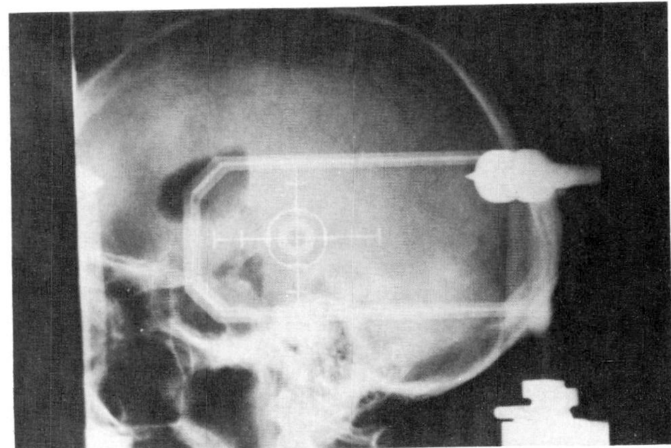

Fig. 29-33. Patient's head fixed in frame. Air has been injected into ventricles, and **A,** frontal, and **B,** centering devices aligned.

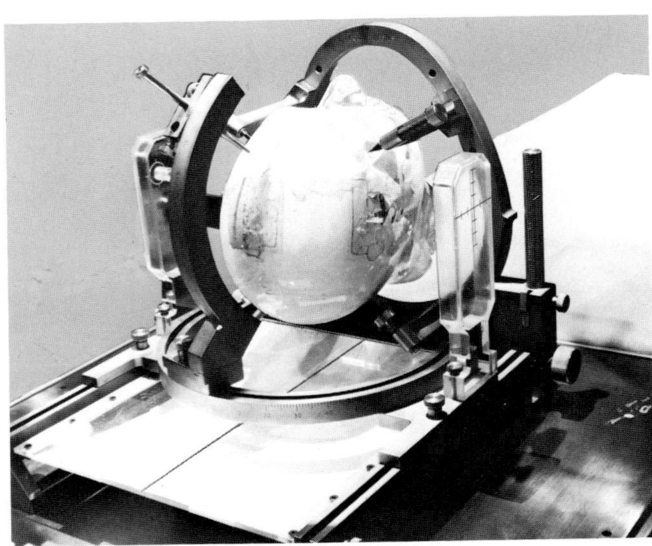

Fig. 29-34. Stereotactic frame with dry skull in place.

(Courtesy Dr. Harold L. Stitt.)

Currently, stereotactic localization is performed with the assistance of CT. Early CT stereotactic devices utilized metal to fix the device to the skull, which resulted in computer-generated artifacts on the CT image. Newer stereotactic devices contain carbon graphite posts and fine metal skull pins surrounded by plastic bushings (Figs. 29-35 and 29-36). Computer programs are available that aid in the guidance of the needle for biopsy procedures. The data processing necessary to determine frame coordinates and probe depth can be performed with a programmable calculator. A software system transforms the two-dimensional coordinates obtained on the CT image to three-dimensional coordinates used by the surgeon. These coordinates are checked using a phantom simulator before the actual surgical procedures is performed.

A metal head ring is fixed to the skull with an attached localizing system consisting of three sets of vertical and diagonal rods. These rods visualize on the CT images and are used to determine spatial relationships. On completion of the CT examination, the patient is transported to the operating room where the localizing rods are removed and replaced by an arc guidance system to allow passage of the surgical instruments. The stereotactic frame is removed following the surgical procedure, and a postoperative CT examination may be performed to check the biopsy site.

The use of MRI in conjunction with stereotactic surgery is still in its infancy. Stereotactic frames must be constructed of nonferromagnetic components and must be constructed so that eddy currents are not induced. The coordinate markers must be constructed of paramagnetic materials that visualize on the MRI. MRI-assisted stereotactic procedures should prove useful for pathologic conditions that do not visualize well on CT images. Additional research into MR applications is currently under investigation.

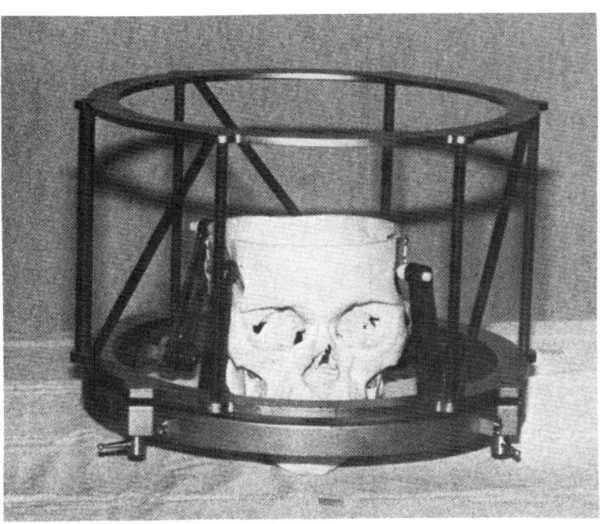

Fig. 29-35. Localizing system attached to head ring.

(From Haaga JR: Computed tomography, St Louis, 1983, The CV Mosby Co.)

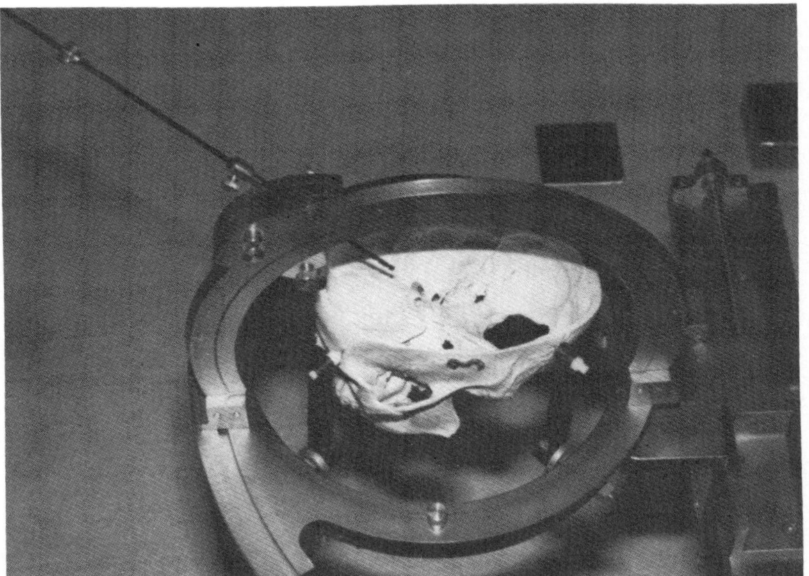

Fig. 29-36. Stereotactic instrument arc guidance system.

(From Haaga JR: Computed tomography, St Louis, 1983, The CV Mosby Co.)

SELECTED BIBLIOGRAPHY

Brown RA, Roberts TS, and Osborn AB: Stereotaxic frame and computer software for CT-directed neurosurgical localization, Invest Radiol 15:308-312, 1980.

Cooper PR and Cohen W: Evaluation of cervical spinal injuries with metrizamide myelography–CT scanning, J Neurosurg 61:281-289, 1984.

Donovon-Post MJ et al: Spinal infection: evaluation with MR imaging and interoperative ultrasound, Radiology 169:765-771, 1988.

Gehweiler JA, Osborn RL, and Becker RF: The radiology of vertebral trauma, Philadelphia, 1980, WB Saunders Co.

Haaga JR and Alfidi RJ: Computed tomography of the whole body, ed 2, St Louis, 1988, The CV Mosby Co, vols. I and II.

Javid MJ: Signs and symptoms after chemonucleolysis: a detailed evaluation of 214 worker's compensation and noncompensation patients, Spine 13:1428-1437, 1988.

Katirji MB, Agrawal R, and Kantra TA: The human cervical myotomes: an anatomical correlation between electromyography and CT/myelography, Muscle Nerve 11:1070-1073, 1988.

Lemansky E: Contrast agents used for myelography: an historical perspective, Radiol Technol 60:489-496, 1989.

Maravilla KR, Cooper PR, and Sklar FH: The influence of thin section tomography on the treatment of cervical spine injuries, Radiology 127:131-139, 1978.

Marymount JV and Shapiro WM: Vertebral hemangioma associated with spinal cord compression, South Med J 81:1586-1587, 1988.

Russin LD and Guinto FC: Multidirectional tomography in cervical spine injury, J Neurosurg 45:9-11, 1976.

Zee CS et al: MR imaging of neurocysticercosis, J Comput Assist Tomogr 12:927-934, 1988.

Chapter 30

CIRCULATORY SYSTEM

MICHAEL G. BRUCKNER

The circulatory system comprises two complex systems of intimately associated vessels through which fluid is transported throughout the body in a continuous, unidirectional flow. The major portion of the circulatory system transports blood and is called the *blood-vascular system** (Fig. 30-1). The minor portion, called the *lymphatic system,* collects from the tissue spaces the fluid that is filtered out of the blood vessels and conveys it back to the blood-vascular system. The fluid conveyed by the lymphatic system is called *lymph*. Together, the blood-vascular and lymphatic systems carry oxygen and nutritive material to the tissues and collect and transport carbon dioxide and other waste products of metabolism from the tissues to the organs of excretion: the skin, the lungs, the liver, and the kidneys.

*All italicized words are defined at the end of this chapter.

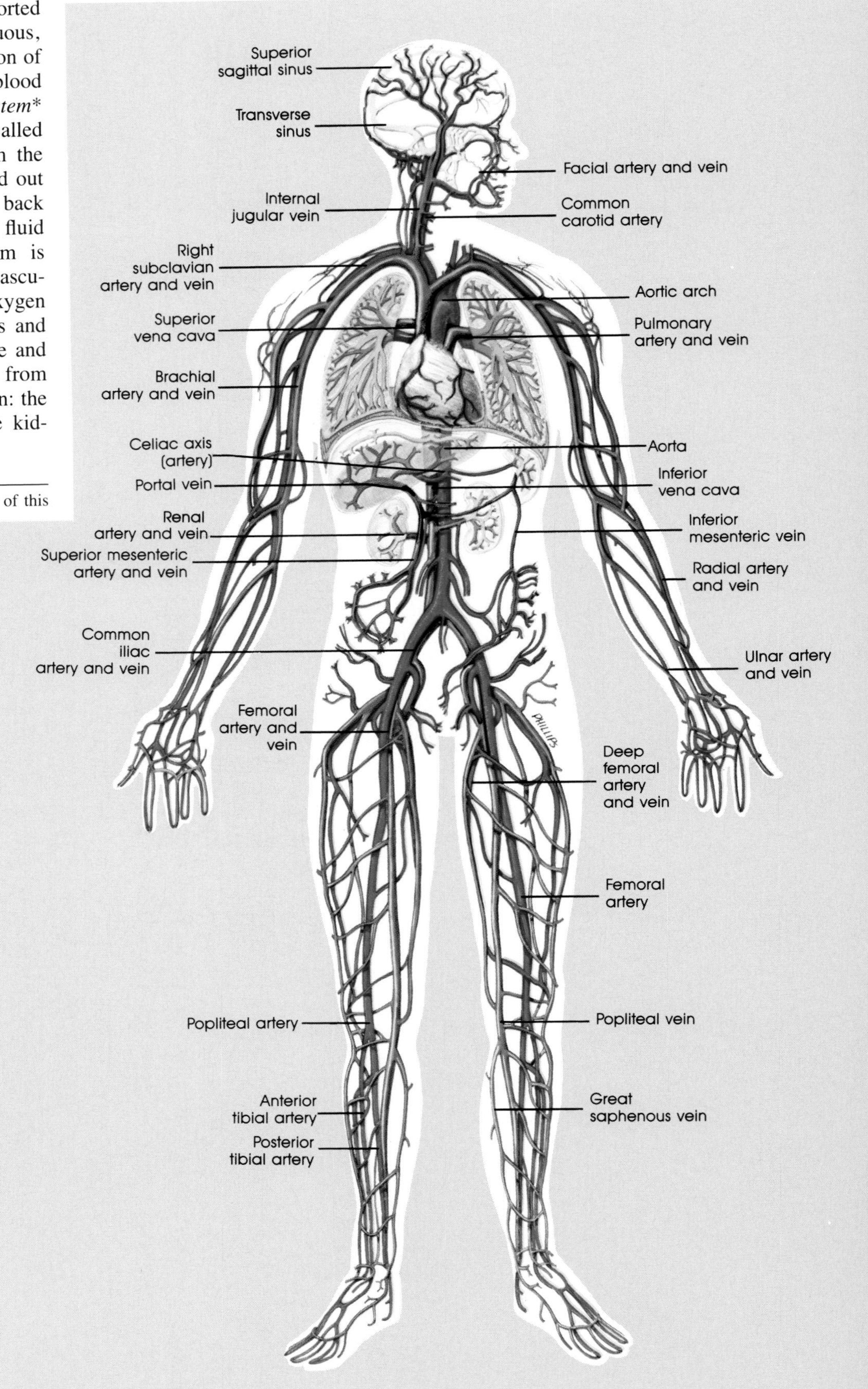

Fig. 30-1. Major arteries and veins. *Red,* arterial; *blue,* venous; *purple,* portal.

Blood-Vascular System

The blood-vascular system consists of the heart and two circulatory systems that branch out from and return blood back to the heart. One of these systems traverses the lungs to discharge carbon dioxide and take up oxygen for delivery to the remainder of the body tissues; this system of vessels is known as the *pulmonary circulation*. The second system branches throughout the body to the various organs and tissues and is called the *systemic circulation*. The heart serves as a pumping mechanism to keep the blood in constant circulation throughout the vast system of blood vessels. Arteries convey the blood *away* from the heart. Veins convey the blood back *toward* the heart for redistribution.

From the main trunk vessels arising at the heart—the *pulmonary artery* for the pulmonary circulation and the *aorta* for the systemic circulation—the arteries progressively diminish in size as they divide and subdivide along their course, finally ending in minute branches called *arterioles*. The arterioles divide to form the capillary vessels, and the branching process is then reversed: the capillaries unite to form *venules,* the beginning branches of the veins, which in turn unite and reunite to form larger and larger vessels as they approach the heart. The pulmonary veins end in four trunks opening into the heart, two trunk veins leading from each lung. The systemic veins are arranged in a superficial set and in a deep set with which the superficial veins communicate; both sets converge toward a common trunk vein. The systemic veins end in two large vessels opening into the heart: the *superior vena cava* leads from the upper portion of the body, and the *inferior vena cava* leads from the lower portion.

The capillaries connect the arterioles and venules to form networks that pervade most organs and all other tissues supplied with blood. The capillary vessels have exceedingly thin walls through which the essential functions of the blood-vascular system take place—the blood constituents are filtered out, and the waste products of cell activity are absorbed. The exchange takes place through the medium of *tissue fluid,* which is derived from the blood plasma and is drained off by the lymphatic system for return to the blood-vascular system. The tissue fluid undergoes modification in the lymphatic system and is then called *lymph*.

The *heart* is the central organ of the blood-vascular system and functions solely as a pump to keep the blood in circulation. It is shaped somewhat like a cone and measures approximately 12 cm in length, 9 cm in width, and 6 cm in depth. It is situated obliquely in the middle mediastinum, largely to the left of the midsagittal plane. The base of the heart is directed superiorly, posteriorly, and to the right. Its apex rests on the diaphragm and against the anterior chest wall and is directed anteriorly, inferiorly, and to the left.

The muscular wall of the heart is called the *myocardium,* and, because of the force required to drive blood through the extensive systemic vessels, it is about three times as thick on the left side as on the right. The membrane that lines the heart interior is called the *endocardium*. The heart is enclosed in the double-walled *pericardial sac,* the exterior wall being fibrous. The thin, closely adherent membrane that covers the heart is referred to as the *epicardium* or, because it also serves as the serous inner wall of the pericardial sac, the *visceral pericardium*. The narrow, fluid-containing space between the two walls of the sac is called the *pericardial cavity*.

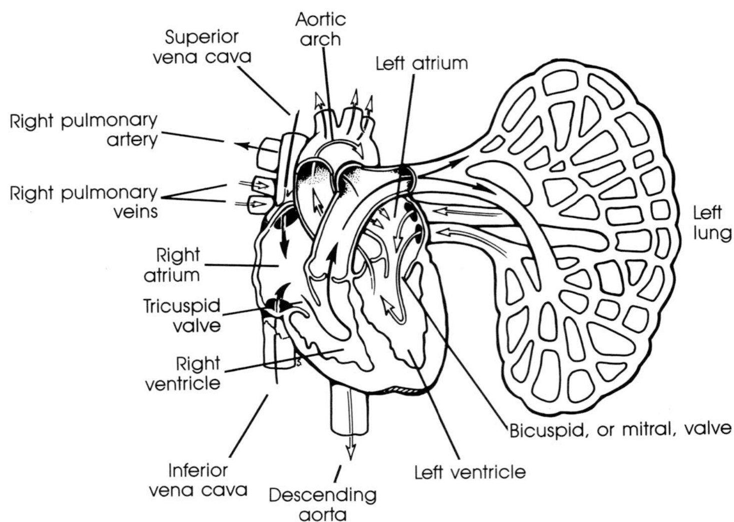

Fig. 30-2. The heart and great vessels. *Black arrows* indicate deoxygenated blood flow. *White arrows* indicate oxygenated blood flow.

The cavity of the heart is divided by septa into right and left halves, and each half is subdivided by a constriction into two cavities, or chambers. The two upper chambers are called *atria,* and each *atrium* consists of a principal cavity and of a lesser one called the *auricula*. The two lower chambers of the heart are called *ventricles*. The opening between the right atrium and the right ventricle is controlled by the *tricuspid valve,* and the opening between the left atrium and the left ventricle is controlled by the *bicuspid,* or *mitral, valve*. The atria function as receiving chambers, and the ventricles as distributing chambers. The right side of the heart handles the venous, or deoxygenated, blood, and the left side handles the arterial, or oxygenated, blood. The left ventricle pumps oxygenated blood through the *aortic valve* into the aorta. The right ventricle pumps deoxygenated blood through the *pulmonary valve* into the pulmonary artery. The pulmonary veins, two right and two left, open into the left atrium. The superior and inferior venae cavae open into the right atrium (Fig. 30-2).

Blood is supplied to the myocardium by the *right* and *left coronary arteries*. They arise in the aortic sinus immediately superior to the aortic valve. Most of the cardiac veins drain into the *coronary sinus* on the posterior aspect of the heart, which drains into the right atrium (Figs. 30-3 and 30-4).

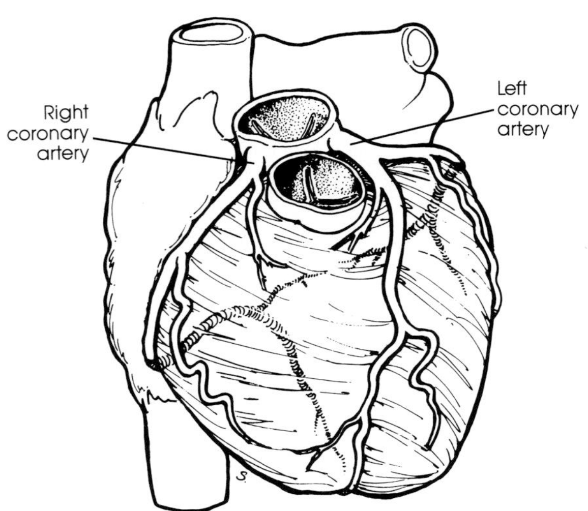

Fig. 30-3. Anterior view of coronary arteries.

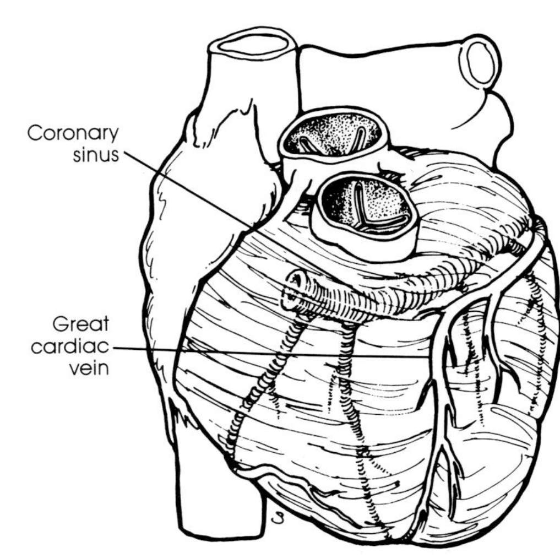

Fig. 30-4. Anterior view of coronary veins.

The *aorta* arises from the superior portion of the left ventricle and passes superiorly and to the right for a short distance. It then arches posteriorly and to the left and descends along the left side of the vertebral column to the level of the fourth lumbar vertebra, where it divides into the right and left *common iliac arteries*. The common iliac arteries diverge from each other as they pass to the level of the lumbosacral junction, where each ends by dividing into the *internal iliac,* or *hypogastric, artery* and the *external iliac artery*. The internal iliac artery passes into the pelvis. The external iliac artery passes to a point about midway between the anterior superior iliac spine and the pubic symphysis and then enters the thigh to become the *femoral artery*.

The arteries are usually named according to their location. The several portions of the aorta—the *ascending aorta,* the *arch* of the aorta, and the *descending aorta*—are described according to direction. The last division, the descending aorta, has thoracic and abdominal portions. The systemic arteries branch out, treelike, from the aorta to all parts of the body except the lungs. The systemic veins usually lie parallel to their respective arteries and are given the same names.

Each organ has its own vascular circuit that, arising from the trunk artery, leads back to the trunk vein for return to the heart. The veins returning blood from the abdominal viscera do not join the systemic venous system directly but rather join to form the *portal vein,* which drains into the liver. After the blood is processed in the liver it flows via the *hepatic vein* into the inferior vena cava.

The *pulmonary artery,* the main trunk of the pulmonary circulation, arises from the right ventricle of the heart, passes superiorly and posteriorly for a distance of about 5 cm, and then divides into two branches, the *right* and *left pulmonary arteries*. These vessels enter the root of the respective lung and, following the course of the bronchi, divide and subdivide to form a dense network of capillaries surrounding the alveoli of the lungs. Through the thin walls of the capillaries, the blood discharges carbon dioxide and absorbs oxygen from the air contained in the alveoli. The oxygenated blood passes onward through the *pulmonary veins* for return to the heart. In the pulmonary circulation, the deoxygenated blood is transported by the arteries, and the oxygenated blood is transported by the veins.

As shown in Fig. 30-5, the oxygenated (arterial) blood leaves the left ventricle by way of the aorta and is carried through the arteries to all parts of the body except the lungs. The deoxygenated (venous) blood is collected by the veins and returned to the right atrium, through the superior vena cava from the upper part of the body and through the inferior vena cava from the lower part of the body. This circuit, from the left ventricle to the right atrium, is called the *systemic circulation*. The venous blood passes from the right atrium into the right ventricle and out through the pulmonary artery and its branches to the lungs. After being oxygenated in the capillaries of the lungs, the blood is conveyed to the left atrium of the heart through the pulmonary veins. The circuit from the right ventricle to the left atrium is called the *pulmonary circulation*. The pathway of venous drainage from the abdominal viscera to the liver is called the *portal system*.

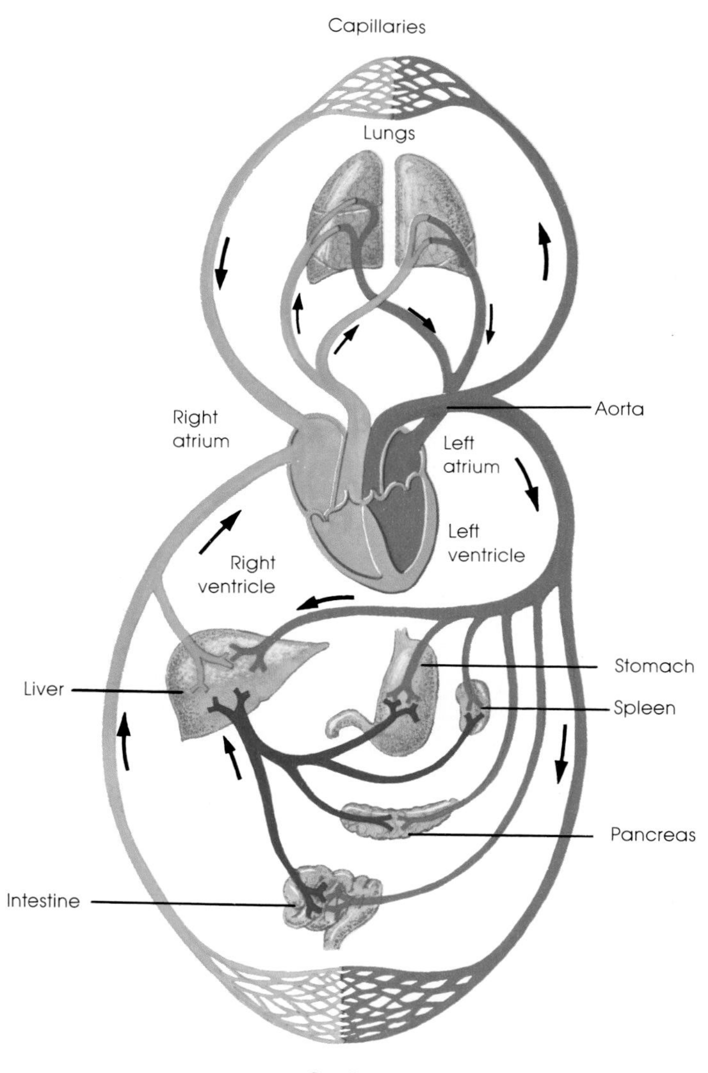

Fig. 30-5. The pulmonary, systemic, and portal circulation, depicting oxygenated (orange), deoxygenated (blue), and nutrient-rich (brown) blood.

The heart contracts (systole) in pumping blood into the arteries and relaxes or dilates (diastole) in receiving blood from the veins. One phase of contraction (referred to as the *heartbeat*) and one phase of dilation are called a *cardiac cycle*. In the average adult one cycle lasts 8/10 second. However, the *heart rate*, or number of pulsations per minute, varies with size, age, and sex, being faster in small persons, young individuals, and females. The heart rate is also increased with exercise, food, and emotional disturbances.

The velocity of blood circulation varies with the rate and intensity of the heartbeat, as well as in the different portions of the system in accordance with their distance from the initial pressure of the intermittent waves of blood issuing from the heart. The speed of flow is thus highest in the large arteries arising at or near the heart because these vessels receive the full force of each wave of blood pumped out of the heart. The arterial walls expand during the pressure of receiving each wave. They then rhythmically contract, gradually diminishing the pressure of the advancing wave from point to point until the flow of blood is normally reduced to a steady, nonpulsating stream through the capillaries and veins. The *beat*, or contraction and expansion of an artery, which may be felt with the fingers at a number of points, is called the *pulse*.

It has been calculated that a complete circulation of the blood through both the systemic and pulmonary circuits, from a given point and back again, requires about 23 seconds and an average of 27 heartbeats. In certain contrast examinations of the cardiovascular system, tests are made on each subject to determine the circulation time from the point of injection of the contrast medium to the site of interest. The circulation time is influenced by body position, that is, whether the patient is erect or recumbent.

Lymphatic System

The lymphatic system consists of an elaborate arrangement of closed vessels that collect fluid from the tissue spaces and transport it to the blood-vascular system. Almost all lymphatic vessels are arranged in two sets—a superficial set that lies immediately under the skin and accompanies the superficial veins and a deep set that accompanies the deep blood vessels and with which the superficial lymphatics communicate (Fig. 30-6). Unlike the blood-vascular system, the lymphatic system has no pumping mechanism. The conducting vessels are richly supplied with valves to prevent backflow, whereas the movement of the lymph through the system is believed to be maintained largely by extrinsic pressure from the surrounding organs and muscles.

The lymphatic system begins in complex networks of thin-walled, absorbent capillaries situated in the various organs and tissues. The capillaries unite to form larger vessels, which in turn form networks and unite to become still larger vessels as they approach the terminal collecting trunks. The terminal trunks communicate with the blood-vascular system.

The lymphatic vessels are small in caliber and have delicate, transparent walls. Along their course the collecting vessels pass through one or more nodular structures called lymph nodes. The nodes occur singly but are usually arranged in chains or groups of 2 to 20. The nodes are situated so that they form strategically placed centers toward which the conducting vessels converge. The nodes vary from the size of a pinhead to the size of an almond or larger. They may be spherical, oval, or kidney shaped. Each node has a hilum through which the arteries enter and veins and efferent lymph vessels emerge; the afferent lymph vessels do not enter at the hilum. In addition to the lymphatic capillaries, blood vessels, and supporting structures, each lymph node contains masses, or follicles, of lymphocytes that are arranged around its circumference and from which cords of cells extend through the medullary portion of the node.

A number of conducting channels, here called afferent lymph vessels, enter the node opposite the hilum and break into wide capillaries that surround the lymph follicles and form a canal known as the peripheral or marginal lymph sinus. The network of capillaries continues into the medullary portion of the node, widens to form medullary sinuses, and then collects into several efferent vessels that leave the node at the hilum. The conducting vessels may pass through several nodes along their course, each time undergoing the process of widening into sinuses. Lymphocytes, a variety of white blood cells formed in the lymph nodes, are added to the lymph while it is in the nodes. It is thought that a majority of the lymph is here absorbed by the venous system and that only a small part is passed on through the conducting vessels.

The absorption and interchange of tissue fluids and of cells take place through the thin walls of the capillaries. The lymph passes from the beginning capillaries through the conducting vessels, which eventually empty their contents into terminal lymph trunks for conveyance to the blood-vascular system. The main terminal trunk of the lymphatic system, the lower, dilated portion of which is known as the cisterna chyli, is called the *thoracic duct*. This duct receives the lymphatic drainage from all parts of the body below the diaphragm and from the left half of the body above the diaphragm. The thoracic duct extends from the level of the second lumbar vertebra to the base of the neck, where it ends by opening into the venous system at the junction of the left subclavian and internal jugular veins. Three terminal collecting trunks—the right jugular, the subclavian, and the bronchomediastinal trunks—receive the lymphatic drainage from the right half of the body above the diaphragm. These vessels open into the right subclavian vein separately or occasionally after uniting to form a common trunk called the right lymphatic duct.

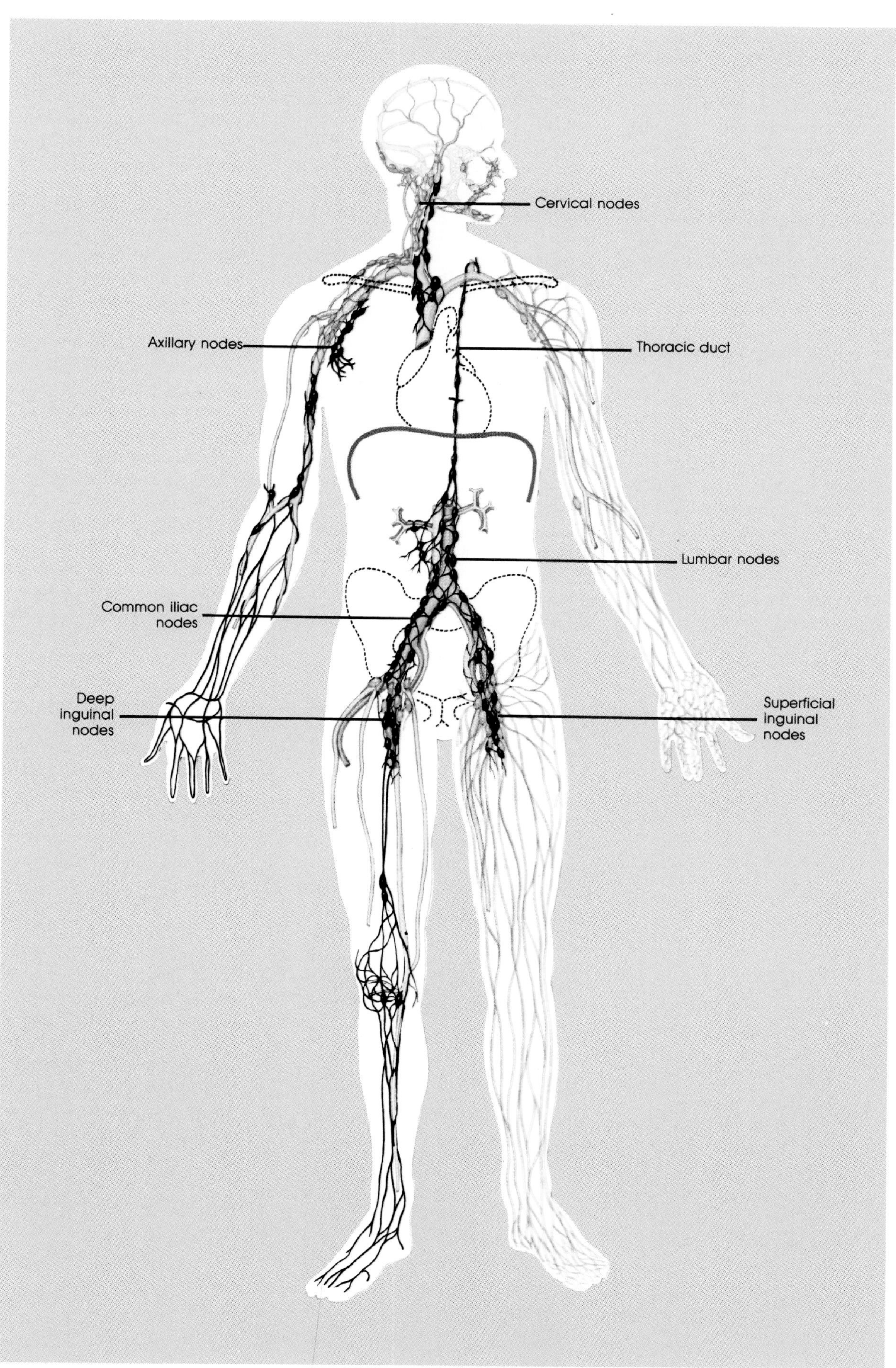

Fig. 30-6. Lymphatic system.

Blood vessels are not normally visualized in conventional radiography because no natural contrast exists between them and the other adjacent soft tissues of the body. Therefore it is necessary to fill vessels with a radiopaque contrast medium to delineate them for radiography. *Angiography* is a general term that describes the radiologic examination of vascular structures within the body after the introduction of an iodinated contrast medium.

The diagnostic visceral and peripheral angiography procedures identified in this chapter can be categorized generally as either *arteriography* or *venography*. Examinations are more precisely named for the specific blood vessel opacified and for the method of injection. For example, for intravenous digital vascular imaging of the right renal artery, a contrast medium is injected into a vein but images are obtained of the renal artery (see Chapter 36). Producing images of the right renal artery by injecting a contrast medium directly into the artery is accomplished by performing a selective right renal arteriogram.

Angiography is used mainly to identify the anatomy or pathologic process of the vessels being studied. For example, the lower extremity venogram, probably the most common of all angiograms, is usually performed to determine if deep venous *thrombosis* is the cause of a patient's leg swelling or pain. Chronic cramping leg pain following physical exertion, a condition known as claudication, may prompt a physician to order an arteriogram of the lower extremities to determine if *atherosclerosis* is diminishing the blood supply to the leg muscles. Detection of a *stenosis*, most often caused by atherosclerosis, is the purpose of many arteriograms. Detecting and verifying the existence and exact position of an *aneurysm* are the purposes of cerebral angiography (which is presented in the next section of this chapter). Although most angiographic examinations are performed to investigate anatomic variances, some evaluate the motion of the part. Certain cardiac catheterization procedures (see Chapter 31), for example, visualize the interior anatomy of the heart and the motion of the cardiac valves. Other vascular examinations evaluate suspected tumors by opacifying the organ of concern. Angiography for therapeutic rather than diagnostic purposes is discussed in a later section of this chapter.

The broad term *angiography* also encompasses examinations involving other vessels of the body. For example, lymphangiography is discussed in a later section of this chapter and cholangiography is described in Volume 2, Chapter 16.

HISTORICAL DEVELOPMENT

Angiography was conceived just 10 weeks after the announcement of Roentgen's discovery when, in January 1896, Haschek and Lindenthal announced that they had produced a radiograph demonstrating the blood vessels of an amputated hand using Teichman's mixture, a thick emulsion of chalk, as the contrast agent. The potential for this new type of examination to delineate vascular anatomy was immediately recognized. The advancement of angiography was hindered by a lack of suitable contrast media and by a lack of low-risk techniques to deliver the contrast medium to the desired location. By the 1920s researchers had used sodium iodide as a contrast medium to produce lower extremity studies that were comparable in quality to studies seen in modern angiography. However, limitations still existed. Until the 1950s, contrast medium was most commonly injected through a needle that punctured the vessel or through a ureteral catheter that passed into the body through a surgically exposed peripheral vessel. Then in 1952, shortly after the development of a flexible thin-walled catheter, Seldinger announced a *percutaneous* method of catheter introduction. The Seldinger technique eliminated the surgical risk associated with the exposure of tissues and made a much smaller wound (see catheterization section of this chapter for a description).

Early angiograms consisted of single radiographs or the visualization of vessels by fluoroscopy. Because the advantage of serial filming was recognized, cassette changers, roll film changers, cut film changers, and cine and serial spot-filming devices were developed. Pumps to inject contrast media were also developed to allow more rapid and precise control of injection rates and volumes than was possible by hand. Early mechanical injectors were powered by pressurized gas, and the injection rate was a function of the pressure setting. Electrically powered automatic injectors were subsequently developed that allowed the injection rate to be set directly.

CONTRAST MEDIA

A wide variety of opaque contrast media are used in angiographic studies. All materials currently in use are organic iodine solutions. Although usually tolerated, the injection of iodinated contrast medium causes undesirable consequences. Iodinated contrast medium is filtered out of the bloodstream by the kidneys but is nephrotoxic. It causes physiologic cardiovascular side effects including peripheral vasodilation, blood pressure decrease, and cardiotoxicity. It also produces an uncomfortable burning sensation in muscular artery branches and nausea in roughly 1 out of 10 patients. Most significantly, the injection of iodinated contrast medium may invoke allergic reactions. They may be minor, such as hives or a slight difficulty in breathing, and not require any treatment, or they may be severe and require immediate medical intervention. Severe reactions are characterized by a state of shock in which the patient exhibits shallow breathing and a high pulse rate and may lose consciousness. Historically, 1 out of every 14,000 patients suffers a severe allergic reaction. The administration of contrast medium is clearly one of the significant risks in angiography.

At the kilovoltages used in angiography, iodine is slightly more radiopaque, atom for atom, than lead. The iodine is incorporated into water-soluble molecules formed as tri-iodinated benzene rings. These molecules vary in exact composition. Some forms are organic salts that dissociate in solution and are therefore ionic. The iodinated anion is diatrizoate or iothalamate. The radiolucent cation is meglumine, sodium, or a combination of both. These ionic forms yield two particles in solution for every three iodine atoms (a 3:2 ratio) and are six to eight times as osmolar as plasma. Other tri-iodinated benzene rings are created as nonionic molecules. These forms have three iodine atoms on each particle in solution (a 3:1 ratio) because they do not dissociate and are only two to three times as osmolar as plasma. Studies indicate that these properties of nonionic contrast media result in decreased chemotoxicity to the kidneys. Nonionic contrast media also cause decreased physiologic cardiovascular side effects, less sensations, and less allergic reactions. They are, however, much more expensive than ionic media.

One form of ionic contrast medium is a dimer; two benzene rings are bonded together as the anion. This results in six iodine atoms for every two particles in solution, which yields the same 3:1 ratio as a nonionic contrast medium. The ionic dimer has advantages over the ionic monomeric molecule but lacks some of the properties of the nonionic molecule.

All forms of iodinated contrast media are available in a variety of iodine concentrations. The agents of higher contrast are more opaque. Typically, 30% iodine concentrations are used for cerebral and extremity arteriography, whereas 35% concentrations are used for visceral angiography. Peripheral venography may be performed with 30% or lower concentrations. The ionic agents of higher concentration and the nonionic agents are more viscous and produce greater resistance in the catheter during injection. The choice of contrast medium may vary with the patient and is usually made by the examining physician.

INJECTION TECHNIQUES

Contrast medium may be introduced into a vessel through a "direct stick," which is simply the process of placing a needle tip into the desired vessel and injecting through the needle. This technique is acceptable in limited situations. A flush injection through a catheter involves placing the catheter tip into a large proximal vessel so that the vessel and its major branches are opacified. In a selective injection the catheter tip is positioned into a specific artery orifice so that only that artery is injected. This has the advantage of more densely opacifying the vessel and of limiting the superimposition of vessels.

Contrast medium may be injected by hand with a syringe, but ideally an automatic injector is used. The major advantage of an automatic injector is to control the injection of a known quantity of the contrast medium during a predetermined period. Automatic injectors have controls to set the injection rate, injection volume, and the maximum pressure to be allowed to occur inside a catheter or other injection pathway. Another useful feature is a control to set a time interval during which the injector gradually achieves the set injection rate. This may prevent a catheter or needle from being dislodged by whiplash.

Because the opacifying contrast medium is often carried away from the area of interest by blood flow, the injection and filming of the opacified vessels usually occur simultaneously. The injector, therefore, is often electronically connected to the rapid filming equipment to coordinate the timing between the injector and filming. Such accurate timing is required when the filming is to commence slightly before or after the injection begins.

EQUIPMENT

Most angiograms record flowing contrast medium in a series of radiographs, which requires rapid *film changers* and/or cinefluorography devices. Less complex angiographic procedures such as peripheral arteriography and venography may be performed with a conventional Bucky tray.

A number of rapid film changers are available from different manufacturers. All these devices move the film and permit exposures at intervals of a fraction of a second; one device is capable of changing as many as 12 films per second, although most film changers have a maximum speed of six films or fewer per second. Some film changers use cut film, whereas others use roll film. These rapid film changers transport films from a supply magazine to a position between screens that come into close contact with the film during exposure and then retract so the film can be transported into a receiving magazine. Cut film changers that can move twenty or thirty 14 × 14 inch (35 × 35 cm) films are common. Rapid film changers may be used either singularly or in combination at right angles to obtain simultaneous frontal and lateral images of the vascular system under investigation with one injection of contrast medium. This arrangement of units is called a biplane rapid film changer.

Lower extremity angiograms are the most likely to use cassette changers. Cassette changers specialized for these procedures move large cassettes containing 11 × 48 inch (30 × 120 cm), or 14 × 51 inch (35 × 130 cm) film, depending on the manufacturer, into and out of the exposure field. Because these devices move heavy objects, they operate at slower maximum speeds, usually one film per second.

Cinefluorography apparatus essentially consists of a movie camera that photographs the output phosphor of an image-intensification system. Almost all image-intensification devices used for vascular procedures include television monitoring. Such equipment allows angiographic examinations to be viewed on a television screen and simultaneously videotaped in conjunction with obtaining the cine recording.

A cine camera uses 16 or 35 mm roll film and usually can achieve sequential exposure rates of up to 60 frames or more per second, with the resultant true motion picture radiography. These cameras use 16 or 35 mm film rather than the larger "true" size of film used in rapid film changers. The photographic resolution achieved with cine units is not as great as that seen with rapid film changers. However, many more events can be photographed with the cine attachment, and dynamic function can be more satisfactorily evaluated with cinefluorography.

Serial radiographic filming requires large focal spot x-ray tubes capable of withstanding a high heat load. Magnification studies, however, require fractional focus tubes with focal spot sizes of between 0.1 and 0.3 mm. X-ray tubes may have to be specialized to satisfy these extreme demands.

Rapid serial filming also necessitates radiographic generators with high-power output. Since short exposure times are needed to compensate for all patient motion, the generators must be capable of producing high-milliampere output. The combination of high kilowatt-rated generators and rare earth film-screen technology significantly aids in decreasing the radiation dose to the patient while producing radiographs of improved quality with the added advantage of prolonging the life of such high-powered generators and x-ray tubes.

A comprehensive angiographic room contains a great amount of equipment other than specifically radiologic devices. Monitoring systems record patient electrocardiographic data and blood pressure readings from within vessels. Emergency equipment may include resuscitators, a defibrillator for the heart, and anesthesia apparatus. The technologist must be familiar with the use of each piece of equipment (Fig. 30-7).

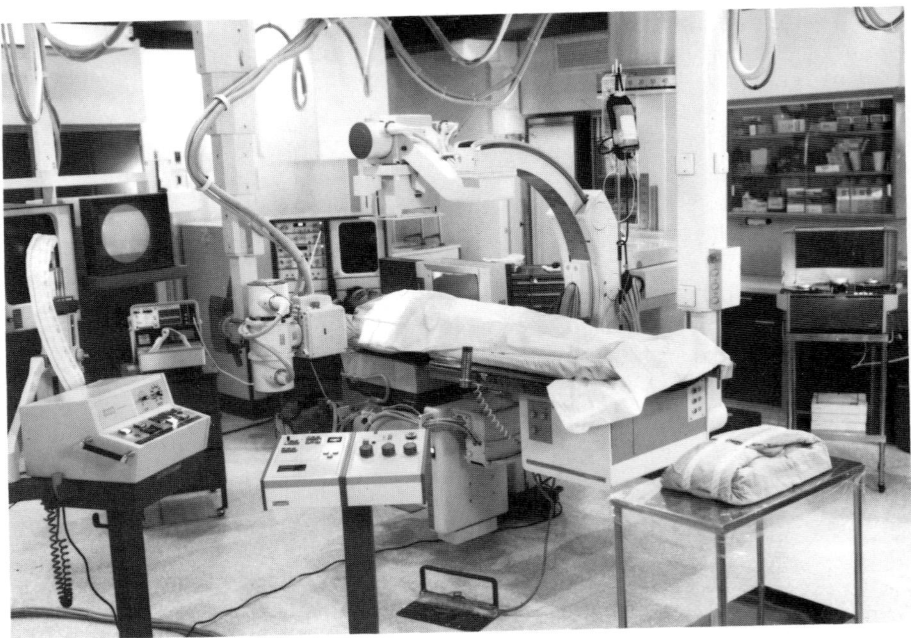

Fig. 30-7. Angiographic suite demonstrating equipment used to perform vascular procedures.

Circulatory system

FILM PROGRAMMING

Film programming is the task of controlling the rate and number of serial exposures made with a film changer. This is accomplished either through manipulation of the device intimately associated to the *film changer* known as the film programmer or through a combination of precisely patterning films in the film changer's supply magazine and setting the film programmer to operate the film changer at specific rates for specific amounts of time. Film programmers instruct the film changers at which rate to cycle, but every cycle does not necessarily transport and expose a film. When two film changers operate together for simultaneous *biplane* imaging, exposures in both planes cannot be made at the same moment because scatter radiation would fog the films; yet biplane changers must cycle exactly together so that synchronization can be electronically controlled. Therefore it is necessary to alternate the cycles that transport film in the two planes. In the first cycle, even though both changers are cycling, only one changer is allowed to transport and expose a film. In the second cycle, the changer that transported film in the first cycle will be allowed to cycle empty while the other changer transports and exposes a film. This process of changers alternating between transporting and not transporting film during opposite cycles must continue throughout the series. The maximum exposure rate of a film changer operated in the biplane mode is one half of its maximum cycle rate because only every other cycle transports and exposes a film.

The most sophisticated film programmers automatically control the alternating of film in the biplane mode. The technologist selects single-plane or biplane mode and enters the number of exposures to be made in each second interval of the series. With less sophisticated programming systems the technologist has control of the cycle rate and rate duration but must manually select which cycles will transport film. For a biplane program with manually loaded equipment, the film supply magazine for the AP changer is loaded with film in the odd-numbered spaces. The even-numbered spaces are left empty. The lateral film supply magazine is loaded in the even-numbered spaces. The film programmer must then be set to cycle the changers at a rate double to the film rate for each plane. The rate duration, however, remains the same. The time interval in which the film remains motionless for exposure must be known for every cycle rate so that a cycle rate with a motionlessness interval less than the radiographic exposure time can be selected.

Fig. 30-8. Seldinger technique.

(Illustrated by Ron G. Boisvert, M.S.M.I.)

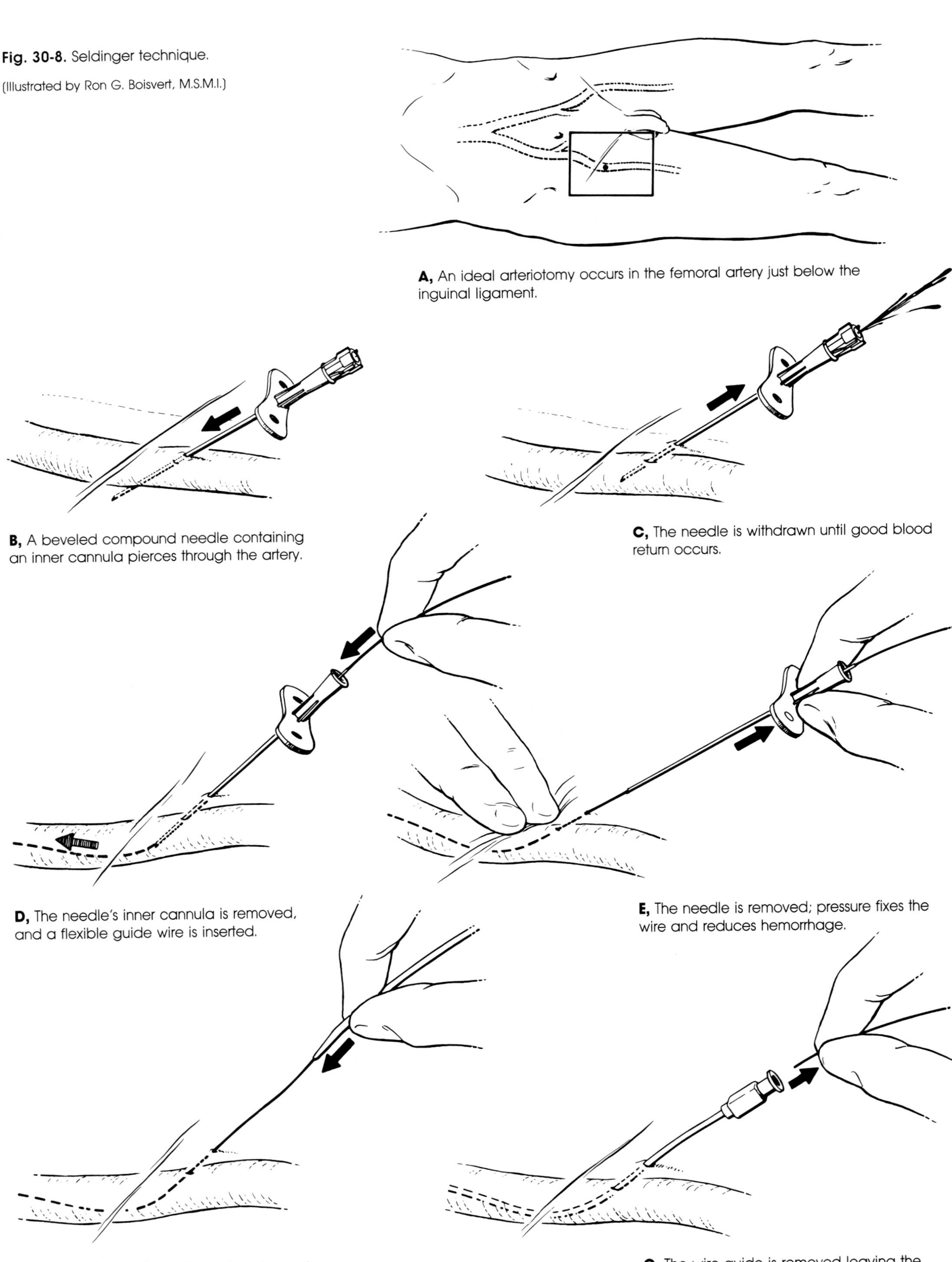

A, An ideal arteriotomy occurs in the femoral artery just below the inguinal ligament.

B, A beveled compound needle containing an inner cannula pierces through the artery.

C, The needle is withdrawn until good blood return occurs.

D, The needle's inner cannula is removed, and a flexible guide wire is inserted.

E, The needle is removed; pressure fixes the wire and reduces hemorrhage.

F, The catheter is slipped over the wire and into the artery.

G, The wire guide is removed leaving the catheter in the artery.

CATHETERIZATION

Catheterization for filling vessels with contrast media is a technique that is preferred over the injection of the media through a needle. The advantages of catheterization are that the risk of *extravasation* is reduced, most body parts can be reached for selective injection, the patient can be positioned as needed, and the catheter can be safely left in the body while radiographs are being examined. The femoral, axillary, and brachial arteries are the ones most frequently catheterized. The femoral site is preferred because it is associated with the least risks.

The most widely used method of catheterization is the modern Seldinger technique; the steps of which are described in Fig. 30-8. It is performed under sterile conditions. The catheterization site is suitably cleaned and then surgically draped. The conscious patient is given local anesthesia at the catheterization site.

With this percutaneous technique an arteriotomy or venotomy is no larger than the catheter itself. Hemorrhage, therefore, is minimized. Usually the patient can resume normal activity within 24 hours. The risk of infection is lower than in surgical procedures because tissues are not exposed.

After a catheter is introduced into the blood-vascular system, it can be maneuvered by pushing, pulling, and turning the part of the catheter still outside the patient so that the part of the catheter inside the patient travels to a specific location. The wire is sometimes positioned inside the catheter to help manipulate and guide the catheter to the desired location. Whenever the wire is removed from the catheter, the catheter is infused with sterile solution to help prevent clot formation. Infusing the catheter and assisting the physician in the catheterization process may be the technologist's responsibility.

When the examination is complete, the catheter or needle is removed. Pressure is applied to the site until hemorrhage ceases. Blood flow through the vessel, however, is maintained. The physician often prescribes complete patient bed rest and orders to be alert for the development of a *hematoma*.

When the peripheral artery sites are unavailable, a catheter may sometimes be introduced into the aorta using the translumbar approach. For this technique the patient is positioned prone and a special catheter introducer system is inserted percutaneously through the posterolateral aspect of the back and directed superiorly so that the catheter enters the aorta around the T11 to T12 level. This method is used primarily for aortography and rarely for selective studies.

Catheters are produced in various forms, each with a particular advantage in shape, maneuverability, or maximum injection rate (Fig. 30-9). Angiographic catheters are made of pliable plastic that allows them to straighten for insertion over the wire guide. They normally reassume their original shape after the wire guide is withdrawn. The reverse-curve catheter, which has a bend of 180 degrees a few centimeters from the tip, usually requires manipulation from the angiographer to resume its original shape. Catheters with a bent tip are designed for maneuverability into artery origins for selective injections. They may have only an end hole, or they may have two additional side holes near the tip. The side holes stabilize the catheter tip by reducing the whiplash that occurs from the rapid ejection of contrast medium from the end hole. Some catheters have multiple side holes to facilitate high injection rates but are used only in large vascular structures for flush injections. A "pigtail" catheter is a special multiple side hole catheter that has a circular tip to further reduce the amount of contrast that exits the end hole. Common angiographic catheters range in size from 4 Fr. (0.05 inch) to 7 Fr. (0.09 inch), although even smaller or larger sizes may be used. Most have inner lumens allowing them to be inserted over wire guides ranging from 0.032 to 0.038 inches in size.

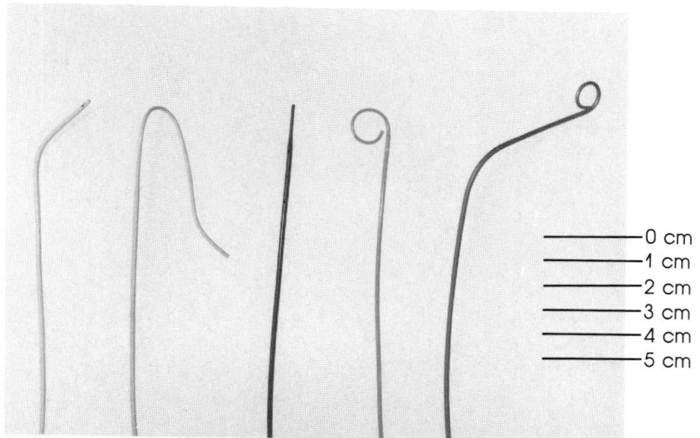

Fig. 30-9. Selected catheter shapes used for angiography.

PATIENT CARE

Before the initiation of an angiographic procedure it is appropriate to explain the process and the potential complications to the patient. Written consent is often obtained after such an explanation. Potential complications include a vasovagal reaction; stroke; bleeding at the catheterization site; nerve, blood vessel, or tissue damage; and an allergic reaction to the contrast medium. Bleeding at the arteriotomy or venotomy site is usually easily controlled with pressure to the site. Blood vessel and tissue damage may require a surgical procedure to correct. A vasovagal reaction is characterized by sweating and nausea caused by a drop in blood pressure. The patient's legs should be elevated, and intravenous fluids may be administered to help restore blood pressure. Minor allergic reactions to iodinated contrast media, such as hives and congestion, are usually controlled with medications and may not require any treatment. Severe allergic reactions may result in shock, which is characterized by shallow breathing, high pulse rate, and possibly loss of consciousness. The examining physician must be immediately notified of any change in patient status. Of course, angiography is performed only if the benefits of the examination outweigh the risks.

Patients are usually restricted to clear liquid intake and routine medications before undergoing angiography. Adequate hydration from liquid intake may minimize damage to the kidneys from iodinated contrast media. Solid food intake is restricted so that the chance of aspiration from the nausea that occurs in 10% of patients from iodinated contrast media is reduced. Contraindications to the examination will be determined by physicians and include previous severe allergic reaction to iodinated contrast media, severely impaired renal function, impaired blood clotting factors, and the inability to undergo a surgical procedure or general anesthesia.

Because general anesthesia is more of a risk than most angiographic procedures, adult patients are usually conscious for the examination. Just before the procedure, most are given a sedative to reduce anxiety and discomfort. Thoughtful communication from the technologist and physician will also calm and reassure the patient. It is important that either the technologist or physician warn the patient about the sensations that the contrast medium will cause and the noise produced by the filming equipment. This information also reduces the patient's anxiety and helps ensure a good radiographic series free from patient motion.

ANGIOGRAPHIC TEAM

The angiographic team consists of the physician, usually a radiologist, the radiologic technologist, and other specialists such as an anesthetist and a nurse.

The technologist often assists in performing procedures that require sterile technique and may be responsible for operating monitoring devices and emergency equipment, in addition to operating the radiographic equipment. When the technologist is required to operate the supporting apparatus, he must be provided adequate directions for proper use of the equipment. Instruction in patient care techniques and sterile procedure, however, is included in the basic preparation of the radiographer.

Visceral Angiography

AORTOGRAPHY

The most satisfactory method for visualizing the aorta is achieved by placing a catheter into the aorta at the desired level. This is usually accomplished with the Seldinger technique from the right or left femoral artery sites using a multiple side hole catheter. Aortography is usually accomplished with the patient in the supine position for simultaneous frontal and lateral imaging with the central ray perpendicular to the film. Translumbar catheter introduction is an alternative for aortography and requires that the patient is in the prone position.

Thoracic aortography

Thoracic aortography may be performed to rule out an aortic aneurysm, for *aortic dissection,* or to evaluate congenital or postsurgical conditions. Biplane film changers are recommended so that frontal and lateral images may be obtained with one contrast medium injection. Lateral images require that the patient's arms be moved superiorly to move them out of the view. For best results the lateral source-to-image distance (SID) is increased, usually to 60 inches, so that magnification is reduced. If biplane equipment is not available, a single-plane 45-degree RPO (right AP oblique) or LAO (left PA oblique) position will often produce an adequate study of the aorta. With all positions, the central ray is directed to the center of the chest at the level of T6. This should allow visualization of the entire thoracic aorta including the proximal brachiocephalic vessels.

Injection of contrast medium is made at rates ranging from 25 to 35 ml/sec for a total volume of 50 to 70 ml. Filming must begin simultaneously. Exposures are made in each plane at rates ranging from one and one-half to three exposures per second for 3 to 4 seconds and then may slow to one film or less per second for an additional 3 to 5 seconds. The exposures are made at the end of suspended inhalation (Figs. 30-10 and 30-11).

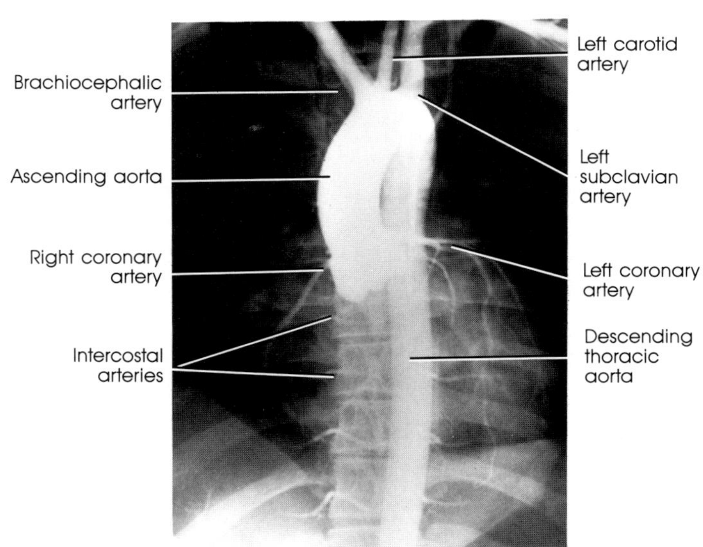

Fig. 30-10. AP projection of thoracic aorta that also demonstrates right and left coronary arteries.

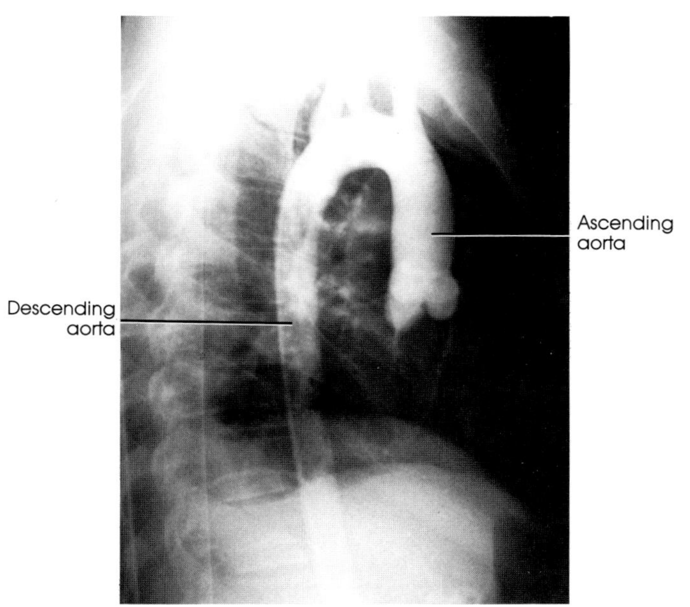

Fig. 30-11. Lateral position of thoracic aorta.

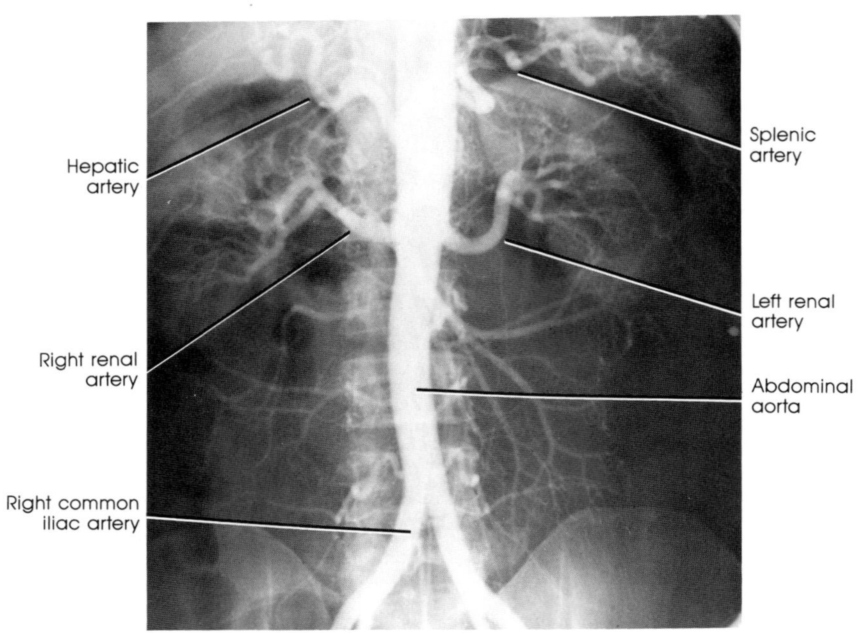

Fig. 30-12. AP projection of abdominal aorta.

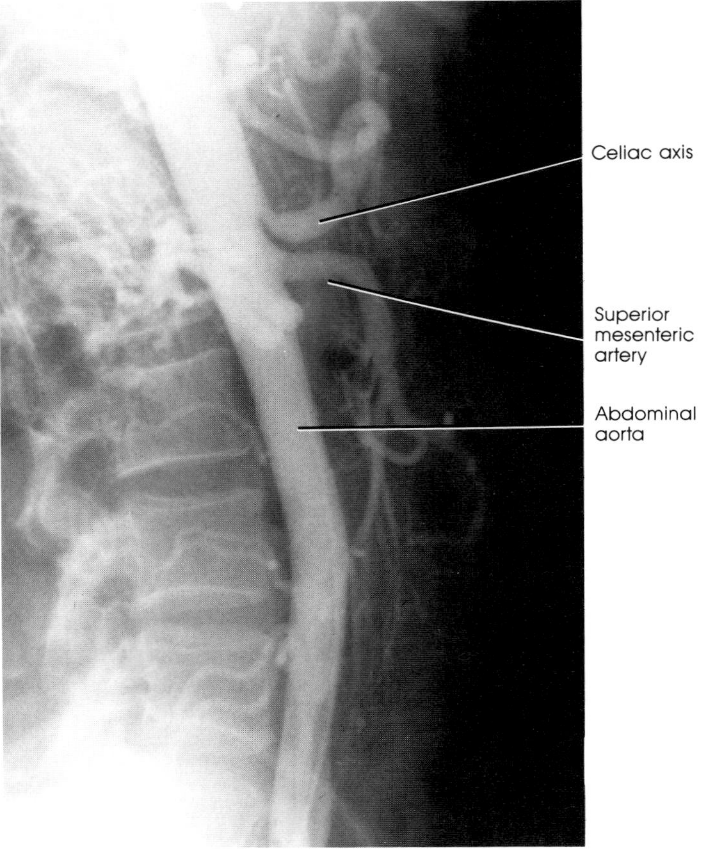

Fig. 30-13. Lateral position of abdominal aorta.

Abdominal aortography

Abdominal aortography may be performed to evaluate abdominal aortic aneurysm, occlusion, or atherosclerotic disease. Simultaneous AP and lateral images are recommended. For the lateral position the patient's arms must be moved superiorly to move them out of the image field, and the field is usually collimated in the anteroposterior aspect. The central ray is usually directed at the level of L2 so that the aorta is visualized from the diaphragm to the aortic bifurcation. The AP projection will best demonstrate the renal artery origins, the aortic bifurcation, and the course and general condition of all of the abdominal visceral branches, whereas the lateral position best demonstrates the celiac and superior mesenteric artery origins. Representative injection and film programs are 25 ml/sec for 60 ml total volume and two films per second for 4 seconds followed by one film per second for 4 seconds in each plane. Exposures begin simultaneously with the beginning of the injection and at the end of suspended expiration (Figs. 30-12 and 30-13).

Pulmonary Arteriography

Under fluoroscopic control, a catheter is passed from a peripheral vein through the vena cava and right side of the heart and into the pulmonary arteries. This technique is usually employed for a selective injection, and the examination is primarily performed for the evaluation of embolic disease.

Simultaneous AP and lateral images of the supine patient are recommended for this procedure. The suggested SID for the lateral position is 60 inches. The patient's arms must be moved superiorly to move them out of the field of view. When biplane projections are not possible, a single-plane 35-degree RAO (right PA oblique) or LPO (left AP oblique) position usually achieves satisfactory results for both the right and left pulmonary arteriograms. The central ray is directed perpendicularly to the film for all of these radiographs. A compensating (trough) filter can be used on the AP projection to obtain a radiograph with more uniform density between the vertebrae and the lungs. In studies of the pulmonary arteries, lengthening the time of the filming program reveals the opacified left atrium, left ventricle, and thoracic aorta. Representative injection and film programs are 25 ml/sec for 50 ml total volume and two to four films per second for 4 seconds followed by one film per second for an additional 4 seconds in each plane (Figs. 30-14 to 30-17).

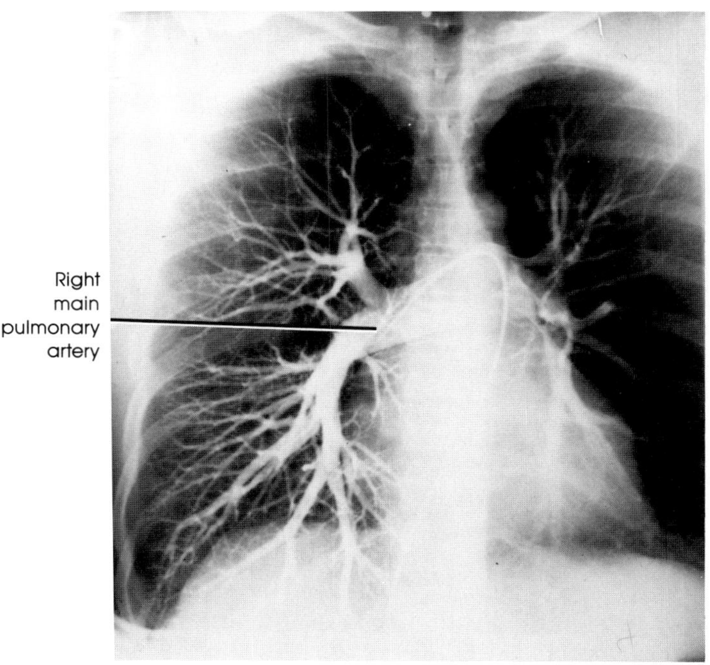

Fig. 30-14. AP projection of right main pulmonary artery during early phase of injection.

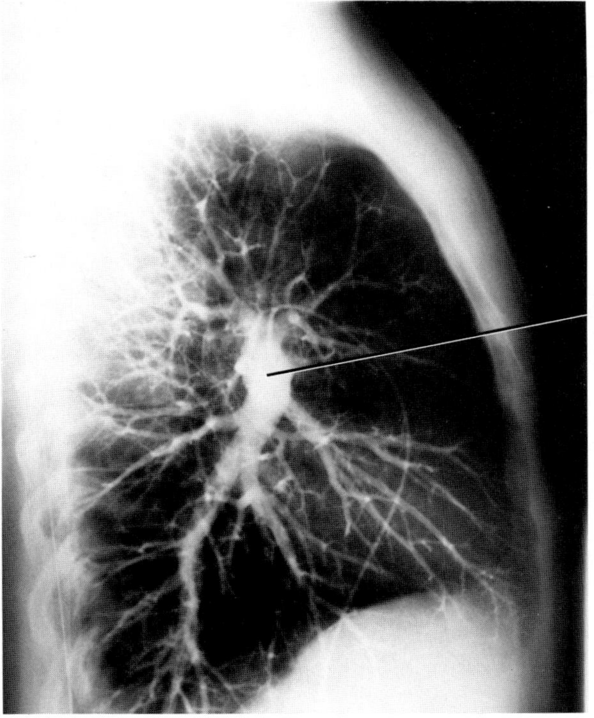

Fig. 30-15. Lateral position of right pulmonary artery during early phase of injection.

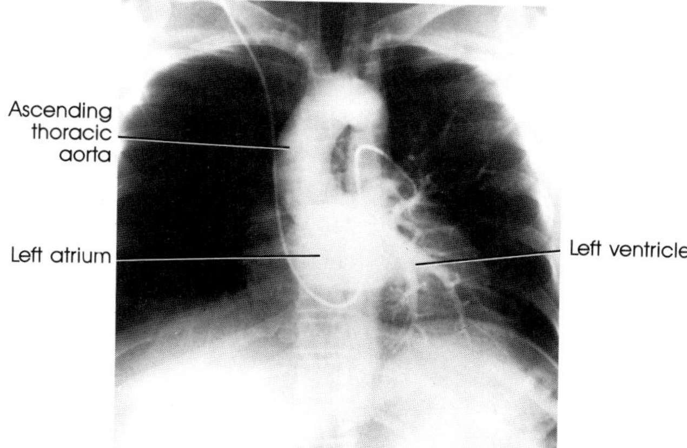

Fig. 30-16. Late-phase AP pulmonary arteriogram demonstrates left atrium, left ventricle, and thoracic aorta.

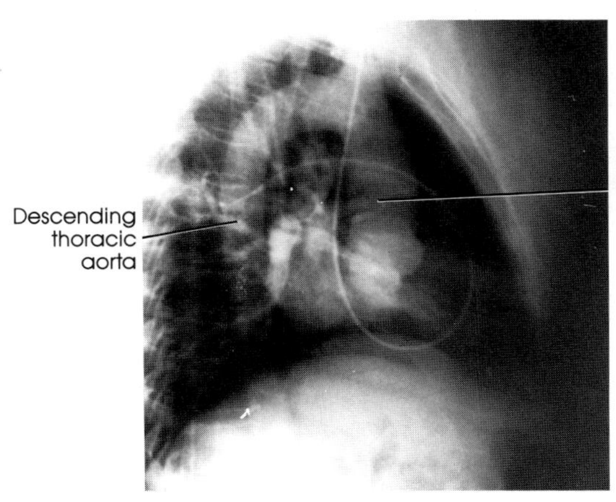

Fig. 30-17. Lateral position in late phase of filming pulmonary artery injection.

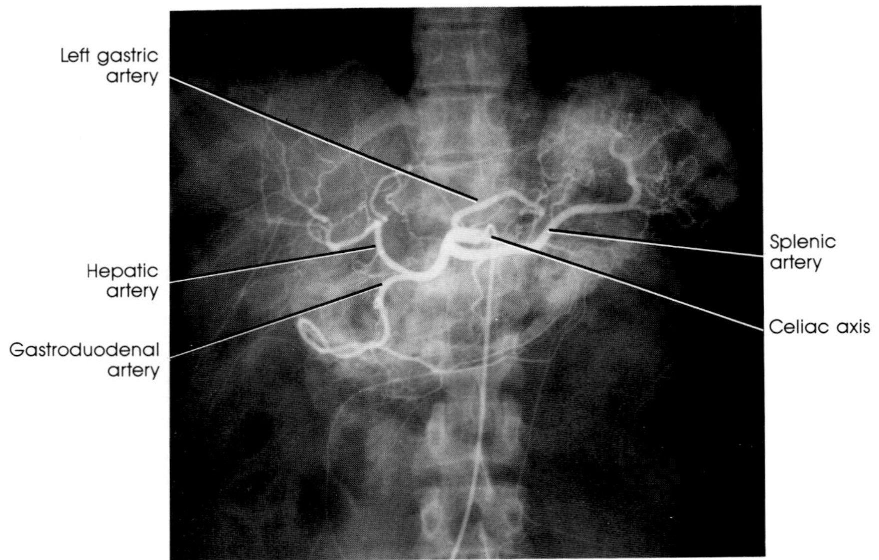

Fig. 30-18. Selective AP celiac arteriogram.

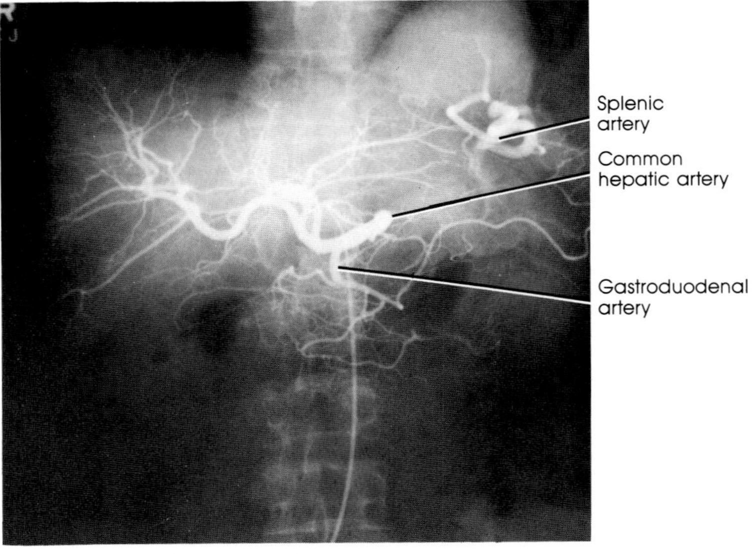

Fig. 30-19. Superselective hepatic arteriogram with overflow into splenic artery.

SELECTIVE ABDOMINAL VISCERAL ARTERIOGRAPHIC STUDIES

Abdominal visceral arteriographic studies are usually performed to rule out atherosclerotic disease, thrombosis, embolization, occlusion, or bleeding or to visualize tumor vascularity. The Seldinger technique is the preferred approach. An appropriately shaped catheter is introduced, usually at the femoral artery site, and advanced into the orifice of the desired artery.

Each of these selective studies is initially accomplished with the patient in the supine position for single-plane frontal projections and the central ray directed perpendicularly to the film. A preliminary radiograph usually is obtained to establish optimum exposure and positioning. Oblique positions may be necessary for improved visualization or to avoid superimposition of vessels. Radiographs for all abdominal visceral studies are obtained during suspended expiration.

The following are various types of selective abdominal visceral arteriograms.

Celiac arteriogram

The celiac artery normally arises from the aorta at the level of T12 and carries blood to the stomach, liver, spleen, and pancreas. For the angiographic examination the patient is centered to the film, and the central ray is directed to L1 (Fig. 30-18). Representative injection and film programs are 10 ml/sec for 40 ml total volume and two films per second for 5 seconds followed by one film per second for 5 seconds.

Hepatic arteriogram

The common hepatic artery branches from the right side of the celiac artery and supplies circulation to the liver, gastroduodenum, and pancreas. The patient is positioned to place the upper and right margins of the liver at the respective margins of the film (Fig. 30-19). Representative injection and film programs are 8 ml/sec for 40 ml total volume and two films per second for 5 seconds followed by one film per second for 5 seconds.

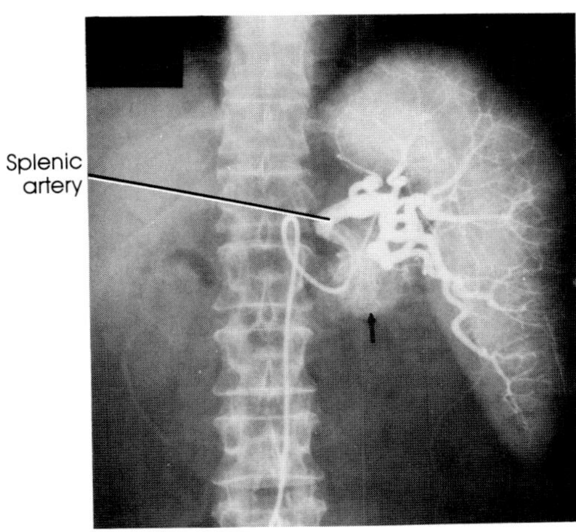

Fig. 30-20. Superselective splenic arteriogram with moderately enlarged spleen. *Arrow,* Tail of pancreas.

Splenic arteriogram

The splenic artery branches from the left side of the celiac artery and supplies blood to the spleen and pancreas. The patient is positioned to place the left and upper margins of the spleen at the respective margins of the film (Figs. 30-20 and 30-21). Extending the length of the filming sequence will often allow adequate visualization of the portal system on the later radiographs. Splenic artery injection is, in fact, the common method of demonstrating the portal venous system. For demonstration of the portal vein, the patient is centered to the film. Representative injection and film programs for a standard splenic arteriogram are 8 ml/sec for 40 ml total volume and two films per second for 5 seconds followed by one film per second for 5 seconds. Representative programs for portal vein visualization are 8 ml/sec for 80 ml total volume and one film per second for 20 seconds.

Superior mesenteric arteriogram

The superior mesenteric artery (SMA) supplies blood to the small intestine and the ascending and transverse colon. It arises at about the level of L1 and descends to L5-S1. To demonstrate the SMA, the patient is centered to the midline of the table, and the central ray is directed to the level of L3 (Fig. 30-22). Representative injection and filming programs are 8 ml/sec for 40 ml total volume and two films per second for 5 seconds followed by one film per second for 5 seconds. When attempting to visualize bleeding sites, the filming may be conducted at one film per second for 18 seconds. Use of an increased injection volume and an extended filming sequence will optimize visualization of the mesenteric and portal veins.

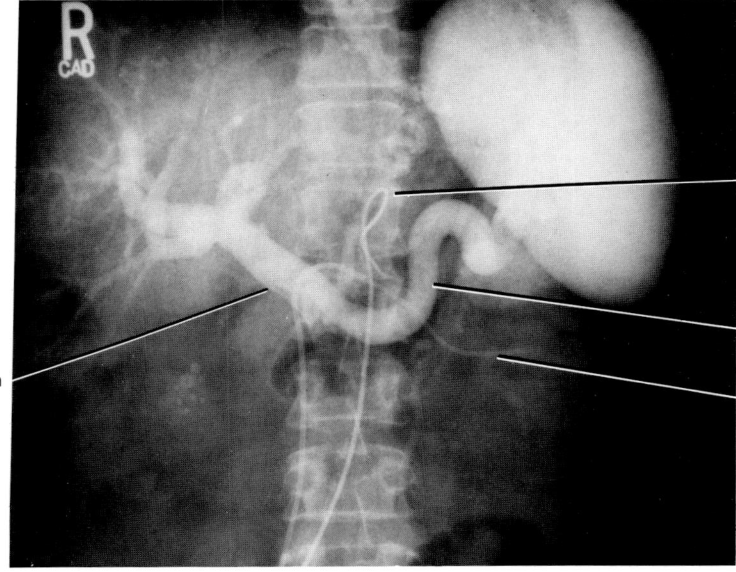

Fig. 30-21. Late-phase splenic arteriogram demonstrating portal system.

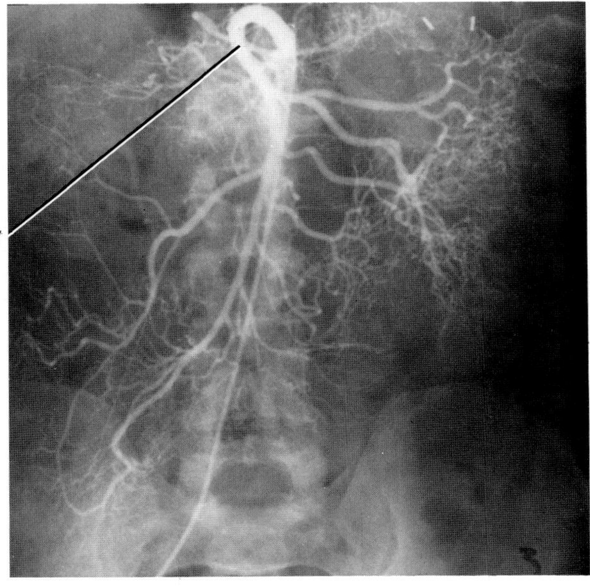

Fig. 30-22. Selective superior mesenteric arteriogram.

Inferior mesenteric arteriogram

The inferior mesenteric artery (IMA) supplies blood to the splenic flexure, the descending colon, and the retrosigmoid area. It arises from the left side of the aorta at about the level of L3 and descends into the pelvis. The best visualization of the IMA results from a 15-degree RAO (right PA oblique) or LPO (left AP oblique) position that places the descending colon and rectum at the left and inferior margins of the film (Fig. 30-23). A representative injection program is 3 ml/sec for 15 ml total volume. Filming is the same as that performed for the SMA.

Renal arteriogram

The renal arteries arise from the right and left side of the aorta between L1 and L2 and supply blood to the respective kidneys. It is helpful to check the patient's intravenous pyelogram or renal flush arteriogram for the exact size and location of the kidneys before performing this selective study. This step enables the radiographer to collimate precisely to the kidney being studied and ensures exact centering of the patient and central ray.

For a right renal arteriogram the patient is positioned so that the central ray enters at the level of L2 midway between the center of the spine and the patient's right side. In the position for a selective left renal arteriogram, the central ray usually enters at the level of L1 and midway between the center of the spine and the patient's left side (Figs. 30-24 and 30-25). A renal flush arteriogram may be accomplished by injecting 25 ml/sec for 40 ml total volume through a multiple side hole catheter positioned in the aorta at the level of the renal arteries. A representative selective injection is 8 ml/sec for 12 ml total volume. Filming for both methods of injections is commonly three to six films per second for 2 to 3 seconds followed by nephrogram films, perhaps only one or two, made between 5 and 10 seconds after the beginning of the injection.

• • •

Other arteries branching from the aorta may be selectively studied to demonstrate the anatomy and possible pathologic condition. The positioning for these procedures depends on the area to be studied and on the surrounding structures.

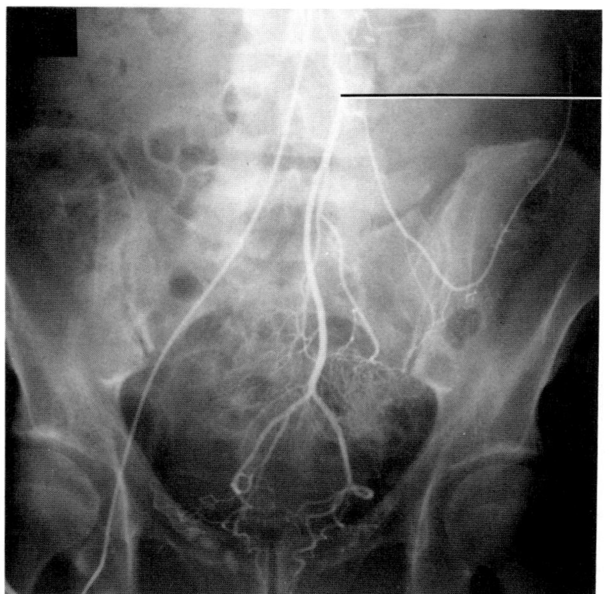

Fig. 30-23. Selective inferior mesenteric arteriogram.

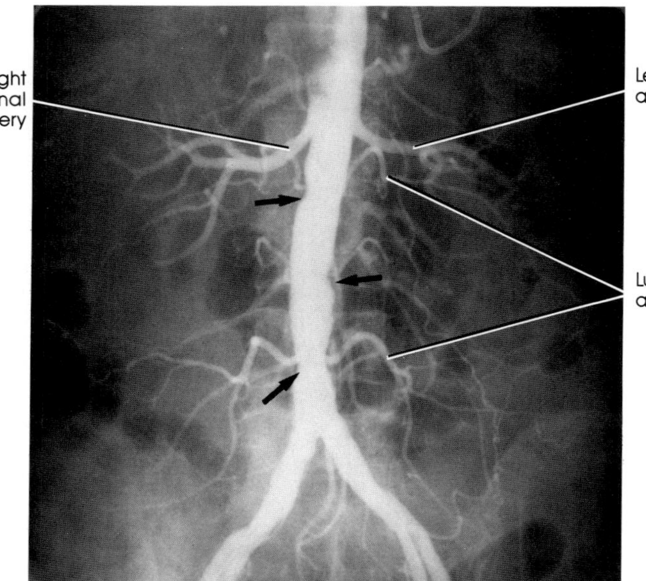

Fig. 30-24. Renal flush arteriogram showing atherosclerotic changes in the aorta *(arrows).*

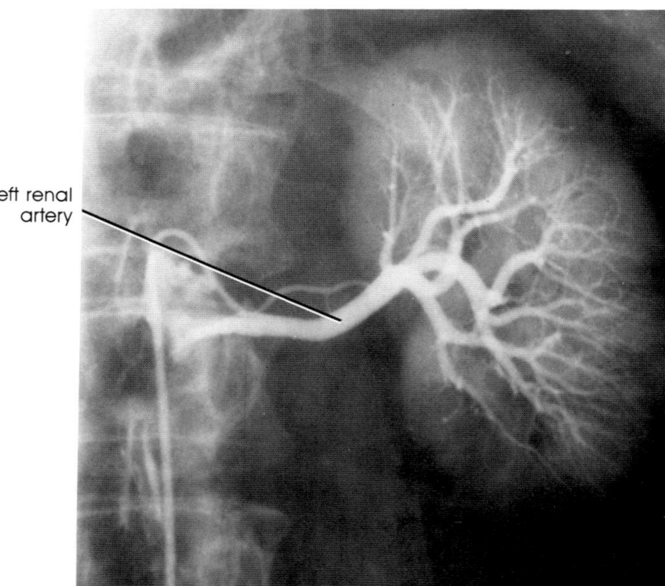

Fig. 30-25. Selective left renal arteriogram in early arterial phase.

Central Venography

Blood in veins flows proximally. Injection into a central venous structure may not opacify the peripheral veins that *anastomose* to it. However, the position of peripheral veins can be indirectly documented by the filling defect from unopacified blood in the opacified central vein. The patient is positioned supine for either a single-plane frontal projection or biplane projections. Lateral positions should be obtained at increased SID, if possible, to reduce magnification, and require that the patient's arms be moved out of the view. Collimation to the long axis of the vena cava will improve image quality but may prevent visualization of peripheral or collateral veins.

Superior vena cavogram

A superior vena cavogram is performed primarily to rule out the existence of thrombus or the occlusion of the superior vena cava. Injection may be made through a needle or angiographic catheter introduced into a vein in an antecubital fossa, although superior opacification results from injection through a catheter positioned in the axillary or subclavian vein. Radiographs should include the opacified subclavian vein, the upper central chest including the superior vena cava, and the right atrium (Fig. 30-26). The injection program depends mostly on whether a needle, angiographic catheter, or regular catheter is used. A representative program for a catheter injection is 10 to 15 ml/sec for 30 to 50 ml total volume. Radiographs are produced in both planes, if desired, at a rate of one or two films per second for 5 to 10 seconds and are made at the end of suspended inspiration.

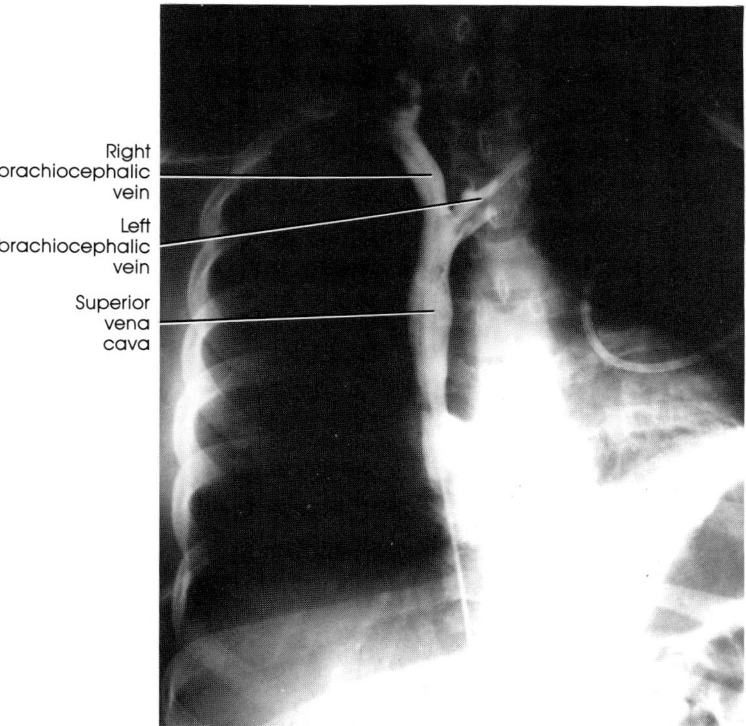

Fig. 30-26. Frontal projection of superior vena cava.

Inferior vena cavogram

An inferior vena cavogram is performed primarily to rule out the existence of thrombus or the occlusion of the inferior vena cava. Injection is usually made through a multiple side hole catheter inserted through the femoral vein and positioned in the common iliac vein or the inferior aspect of the inferior vena cava. Radiographs may need to include the opacified vasculature from the catheter tip to the right atrium (Figs. 30-27 and 30-28). Representative injection and film programs are 25 ml/sec for 50 ml total volume and two films per second for 4 to 8 seconds in both planes. Filming begins at the end of suspended expiration.

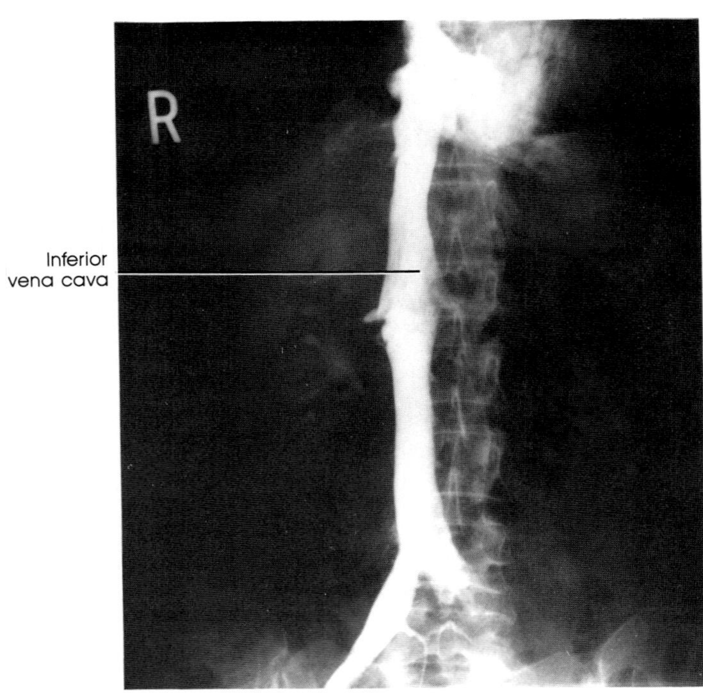

Fig. 30-27. Frontal projection of inferior vena cava.

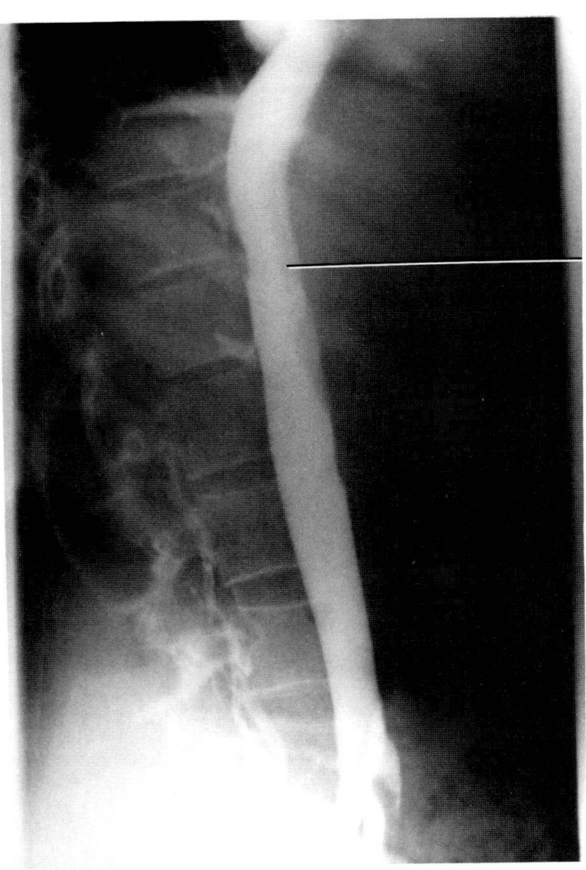

Fig. 30-28. Lateral position of inferior vena cava.

Selective Visceral Venography

The visceral veins are often visualized by extending the filming program of the corresponding visceral artery injection. For example, the veins that drain the small bowel are normally visualized by extending the filming program of a superior mesenteric arteriogram. Portal venography can be performed by injecting the portal vein directly from a percutaneous anterior abdominal wall approach, but it is usually accomplished by late-phase filming of a splenic artery injection. Some visceral veins are catheterized, however, for optimum visualization, blood sampling, or blood pressure measurements obtained through the catheter.

Hepatic venogram

A hepatic venogram is usually performed to rule out stenosis or thrombosis of the hepatic vein. The hepatic vein is also catheterized to obtain pressure measurements from the liver interior. The hepatic vein courses slightly superiorly and to the left out of the liver and carries blood from the liver to the inferior vena cava. (The portal vein carries nutrient-rich blood from the other organs of digestion to the liver.) The hepatic vein is most easily catheterized from an upper extremity vein approach, but a femoral vein approach may also be used. The patient is positioned supine for frontal radiographs that include the liver tissue and the extreme upper inferior vena cava (Fig. 30-29). Representative injection and film programs are 10 ml/sec for 30 ml total volume and one film per second for 8 seconds. Films are made at the end of suspended expiration.

Renal venogram

A renal venogram is usually performed to rule out thrombosis of the renal vein. The renal vein is also catheterized for blood sampling, usually to measure the production of renin, an enzyme produced by the kidney when it lacks adequate blood supply. The renal vein is most easily catheterized from an upper extremity vein approach, but a femoral vein approach may also be used. The patient is positioned supine for single-plane frontal radiography. The selected kidney is centered to the film, and the field is collimated to include the kidney and area of the inferior vena cava (Fig. 30-30). Representative injection and filming programs are 8 ml/sec for 16 ml total volume and two films per second for 4 seconds. Films are made at the end of suspended expiration.

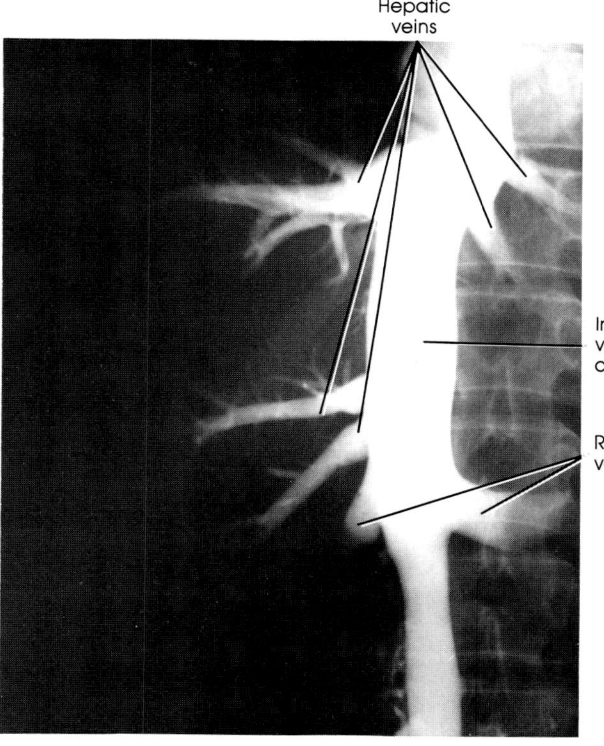

Fig. 30-29. Hepatic vein visualization from inferior vena caval injection overflow.

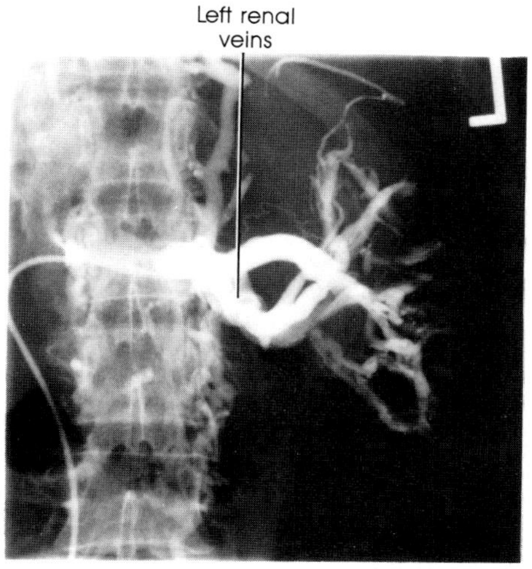

Left renal veins

Fig. 30-30. PA projection of selective left renal venogram.

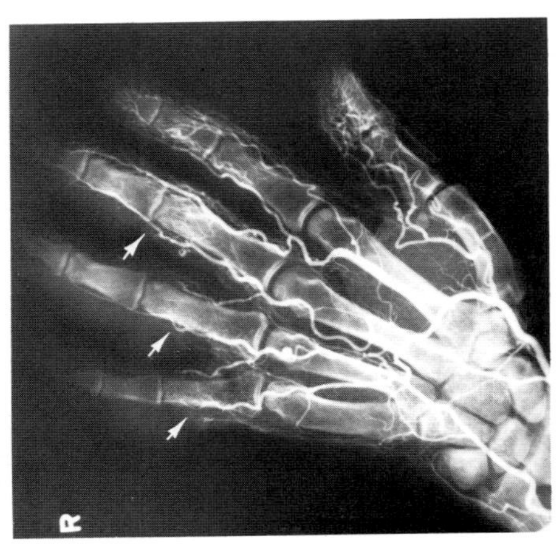

Fig. 30-31. Right hand arteriogram (2:1 magnification), showing severe arterio-occlusive disease *(arrows)* affecting digits after cold-temperature injury.

Peripheral Angiography

Upper limb arteriograms

Upper limb (extremity) arteriograms are most often performed to evaluate traumatic injury or an arteriovenous shunt created for renal dialysis. They are usually obtained by using the Seldinger technique to introduce a catheter, usually at a femoral artery site, and positioning it for selective injection into the subclavian artery. The contrast medium may also be injected at a more distal site through a catheter or needle. The area to be radiographed may therefore be just a hand or other selected part of the arm, or it may include the entire upper limb and thorax. The equipment available and the condition of the patient control the filming procedure. The recommended projection is a true AP with the arm extended and the hand supinated. Hand arteriograms may be obtained in the AP or the PA arm position (Figs. 30-31 and 30-32). The injection and filming programs depend on the equipment used. Injection varies from around 3 or 4 ml/sec through a large needle positioned distally to around 10 ml/sec through a proximally positioned catheter. Filming using a long film cassette changer may be performed with 1- or 2-second delays between exposures. A representative program for a rapid film changer may be two films per second for 5 seconds followed by one film per second for 5 seconds.

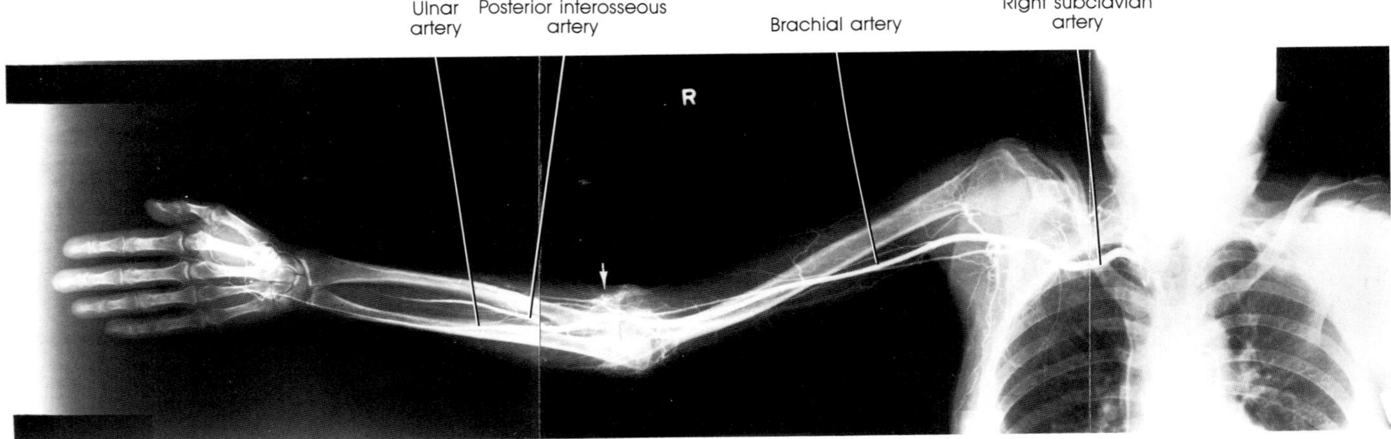

Fig. 30-32. Right upper limb arteriogram showing iatrogenic occlusion of radial artery *(arrow)*.

Upper limb venograms

Upper limb (extremity) venograms are most often performed to look for thrombosis. The contrast medium is injected through a needle or catheter into a superficial vein at the elbow or wrist. The radiographs should cover the vasculature from the wrist or elbow to the superior vena cava. The patient position selected may be determined by fluoroscopy, or the patient may be positioned for an AP projection with the hand supinated. The projection and filming sequence depend on the location of the injection site and the limitations and condition of the patient and equipment (Fig. 30-33). If the injection and filling of veins are observed with a fluoroscopic spot film device, radiographs can be exposed as the vessels opacify. If a Bucky tray or film changer is used, a series of films with a delay of a few seconds between exposures is normally obtained. Injections may be made by hand, or an automatic injector may be set to deliver a total of 40 to 80 ml at a rate of 1 to 4 ml/sec, depending on whether a needle or catheter is used. If the study is performed with the patient supine, tourniquets positioned proximal to the wrist and elbow are required to force the contrast medium into the deep veins.

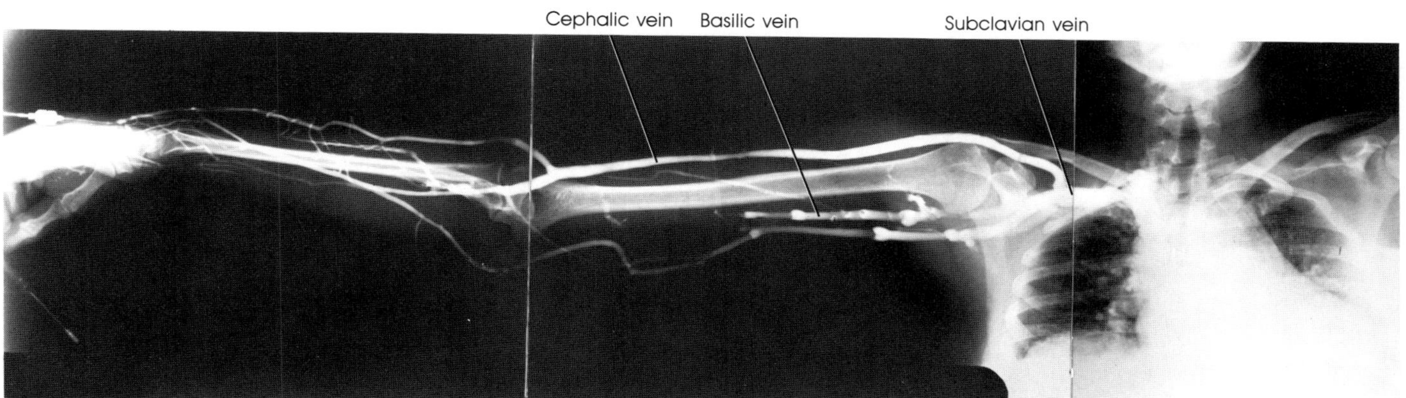

Fig. 30-33. Normal right upper limb venogram.

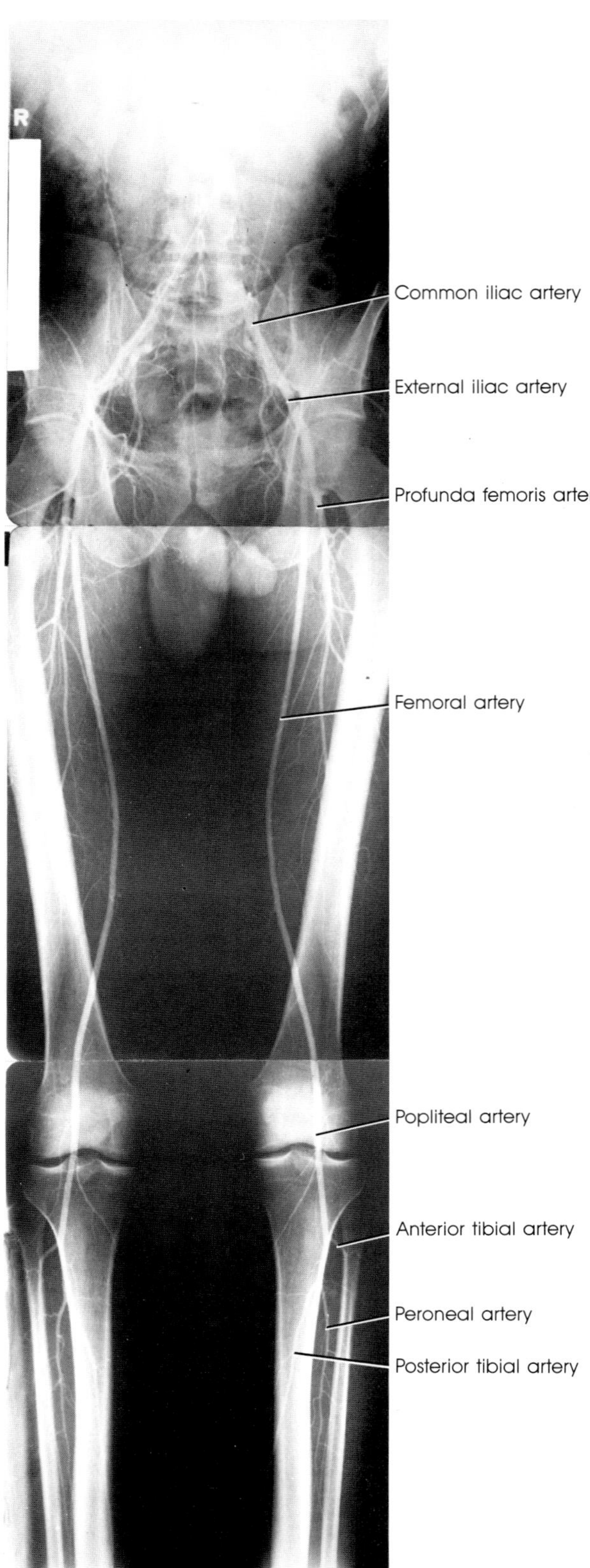

Fig. 30-34. Normal aortofemoral arteriogram in late arterial phase.

Aortofemoral arteriograms

Aortofemoral arteriograms are usually performed to determine if atherosclerotic disease is the cause of *claudication*. A catheter is usually introduced into a femoral artery using the Seldinger technique. The catheter tip is positioned superior to the aortic bifurcation so that bilateral arteriograms are simultaneously obtained. When only one leg is to be examined, the catheter tip is placed below the bifurcation, or the contrast medium is injected through a needle placed in the femoral artery. For a bilateral examination the patient is positioned supine for single-plane frontal radiographs and centered to the midline of the film changer to include the area from the renal arteries to the ankles. The patient may be positioned prone for a translumbar catheterization. For either patient position, the legs should be internally rotated 30 degrees. For best results a cassette changer with 120 cm long film is used. If the cassette changer is not available, the radiographs obtained must overlap to ensure coverage of all vasculature. Such overlapping radiographs can be produced automatically by specialized moving tables. Films of the opacified lower abdominal aorta and aortic bifurcation should be made with the patient in suspended expiration. Film programs will vary and are set based on the predicted rate of flow through the long arterial course of the lower extremity. Flow through normal arteries may take as little as 10 seconds, whereas flow through severely diseased arteries may take 30 seconds or more. A representative injection program designed to create a long bolus of contrast medium is 13 ml/sec for 80 ml total volume (Fig. 30-34).

Examinations of a specific area of the leg (e.g., popliteal fossa or foot) are occasionally performed. For these procedures the preferred injection site is usually the femoral artery. AP, lateral, or both images may be obtained with the patient centered to the designated area.

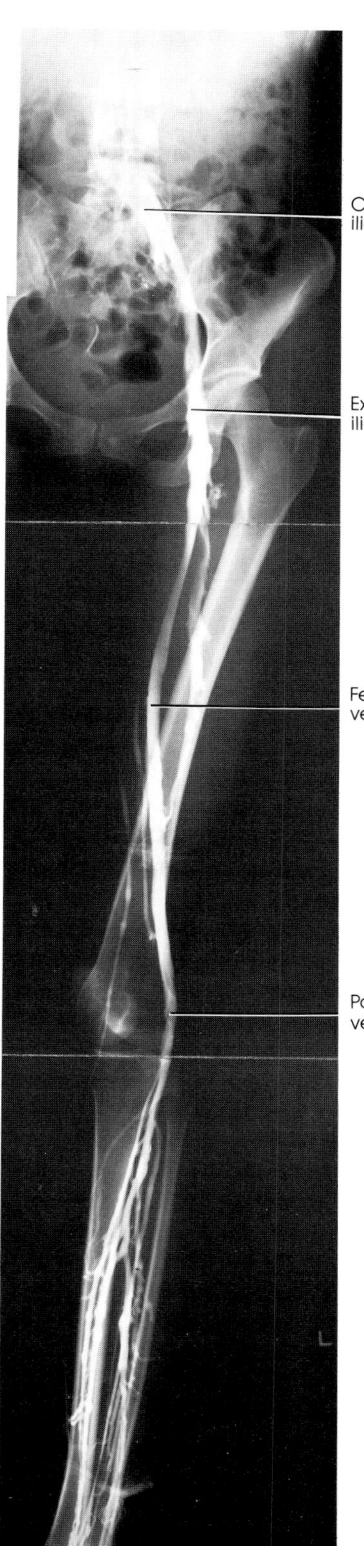

Fig. 30-35. Normal left lower limb venogram.

Lower limb venograms

Lower limb (extremity) venograms are common and are usually performed to rule out thrombosis of the deep veins of the leg. These venograms are usually obtained by making an injection through a needle placed directly into a superficial vein in the foot. It is preferred that radiographs be obtained with the patient on a tilt table in a semierect position at a minimum angle of 45 degrees. Filming begins at the ankle and proceeds superiorly to include the inferior vena cava as the injection continues. Exact positioning is often determined with fluoroscopic aid. Without fluoroscopy, AP projections with the leg internally rotated 30 degrees are usually obtained to include the entire area of interest (Fig. 30-35). Lateral positions may also be taken if needed. If filming is performed with the patient supine, tourniquets must be applied just proximal to the ankle and knee to force filling of the deep veins in the leg. Serial radiographs obtained with a Bucky tray or film changer are usually exposed 5 to 10 seconds apart. Injections may be made by hand, or an automatic injector may be set to deliver 1 or 2 ml/sec for a total of 50 to 100 ml.

• • •

In all angiographic procedures, precise methods must be followed, and the sequence of filming and injection must be determined in consultation with the physician. As in all surgical procedures, great care must be exercised to ensure that sterile techniques are strictly maintained. Precise positioning of the patient is also essential so that the desired body part will be adequately demonstrated. It is imperative that careful and complete cooperation be maintained among the physician, the radiologic technologist, and the patient to obtain radiographs with the maximum amount of diagnostic information.

Angiography in the Future

Visceral and peripheral angiography is a dynamic profession that challenges angiographers to keep abreast with new techniques and equipment. New diagnostic modalities that reduce or eliminate irradiation may be developed that will possibly replace some current angiographic procedures. Some diagnostic information, however, can only be obtained through conventional angiographic methods. Angiography will, therefore, continue to examine vasculature and, through therapeutic procedures, provide beneficial treatment to the body.

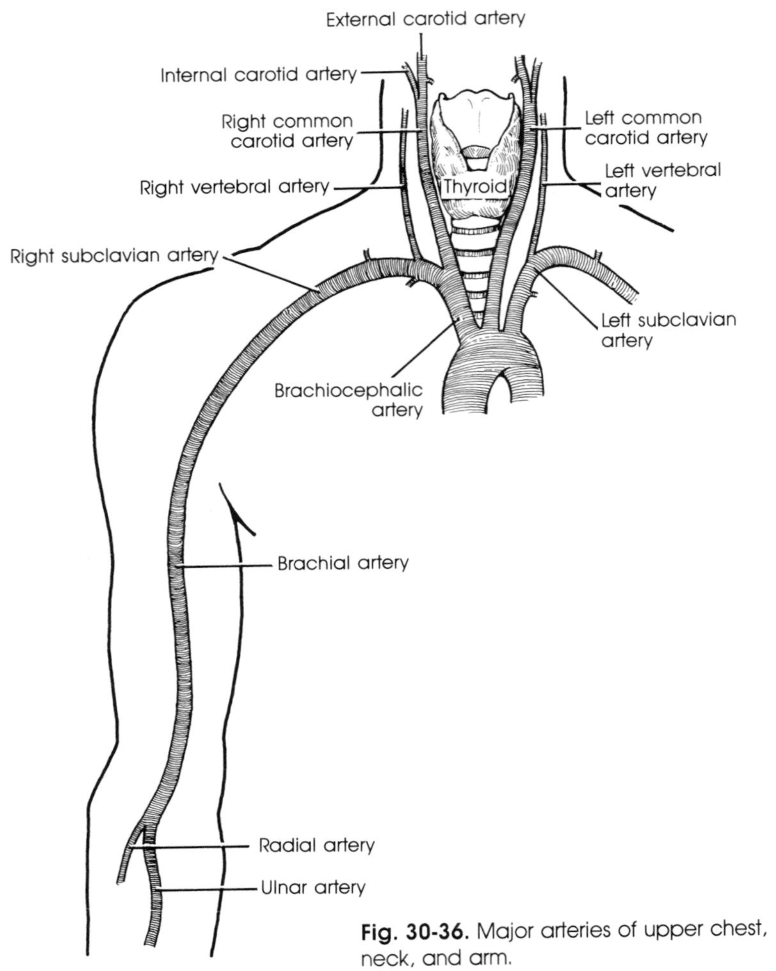

Fig. 30-36. Major arteries of upper chest, neck, and arm.

Cerebral angiography is the term used to denote radiologic examinations of the blood vessels of the brain by means of injecting the vessels with a radiopaque contrast medium. The procedure was introduced by Egas Moniz[1] in 1927. It is performed to investigate intracranial *aneurysms* or other vascular *lesions* and to demonstrate tumor masses, which are shown by displacement of the normal cerebrovascular pattern or by the tumor's circulation.

The brain is supplied by four trunk vessels: the right and left common carotid arteries, which supply the anterior circulation, and the right and left vertebral arteries, which supply the posterior circulation. These paired arteries branch from the arch of the aorta and ascend through the neck, as shown in Fig. 30-36.

The left common carotid artery originates directly from the aortic arch. The right common carotid artery arises with the right subclavian artery about 1½ inches (3.7 cm) higher at the *bifurcation* of the brachiocephalic artery (Fig. 30-37). The left subclavian artery originates directly from the arch of the aorta. The vertebral arteries arise from the subclavian arteries. *Anomalies* in the origin of these vessels are common.

Each common carotid artery passes superiorly and somewhat laterally alongside the trachea and larynx to the level of C4, where each divides into internal and external carotid arteries. The latter vessel contributes to the supply of the *meninges* but not to that of the intracerebral circulation. The internal carotid artery enters the cranium through the carotid foramen and then bifurcates into the anterior and middle cerebral arteries. They, in turn, branch and rebranch to supply the anterior circulation of the respective hemisphere of the brain (Fig. 30-38).

The vertebral arteries ascend through the cervical transverse foramina and then pass medially to enter the cranium through the foramen magnum. The vertebral arteries unite to form the basilar artery, which, after a short superior course along the posterior surface of the dorsum sellae, bifurcates into the right and left posterior cerebral arteries. The blood supply to the posterior fossa (cerebellum) originates from the vertebral and basilar arteries (Fig. 30-39).

A

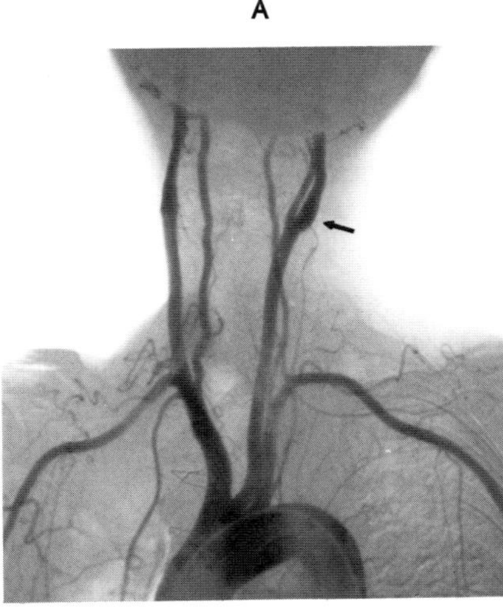

B

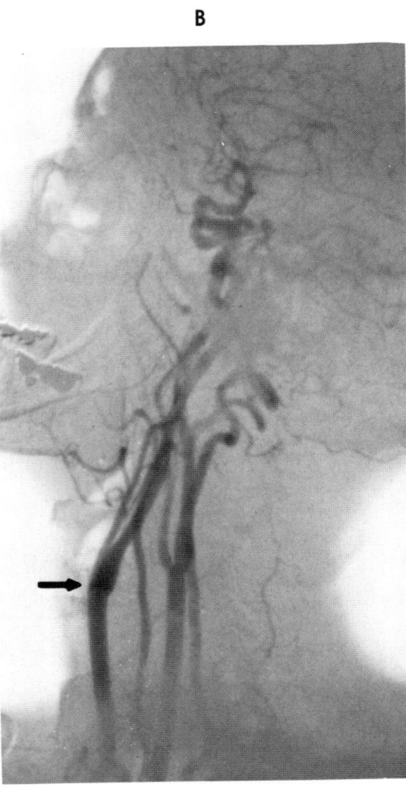

Fig. 30-37. Photographic subtraction AP, **A,** and lateral, **B,** oblique of aortic arch with patient in RPO (right AP oblique) position. Note excellent visualization of extracranial brachiocephalic arteries. *Arrow,* Normal left common carotid bifurcation.

[1]Egas Moniz AC: L'encéphalographie artérielle, son importance dans la localisation des tumeurs cérébrales, Rev Neurol 2:72-90, 1927.

The anterior and posterior cerebral arteries are connected by communicating arteries at the level of the midbrain to form the circulus arteriosus, commonly known as the *circle of Willis*. The anterior communicating artery forms an anastomosis between the anterior cerebral arteries. The right and left posterior communicating arteries each form an anastomosis between the internal carotid artery and the posterior cerebral artery on their side of the cerebral circulation.

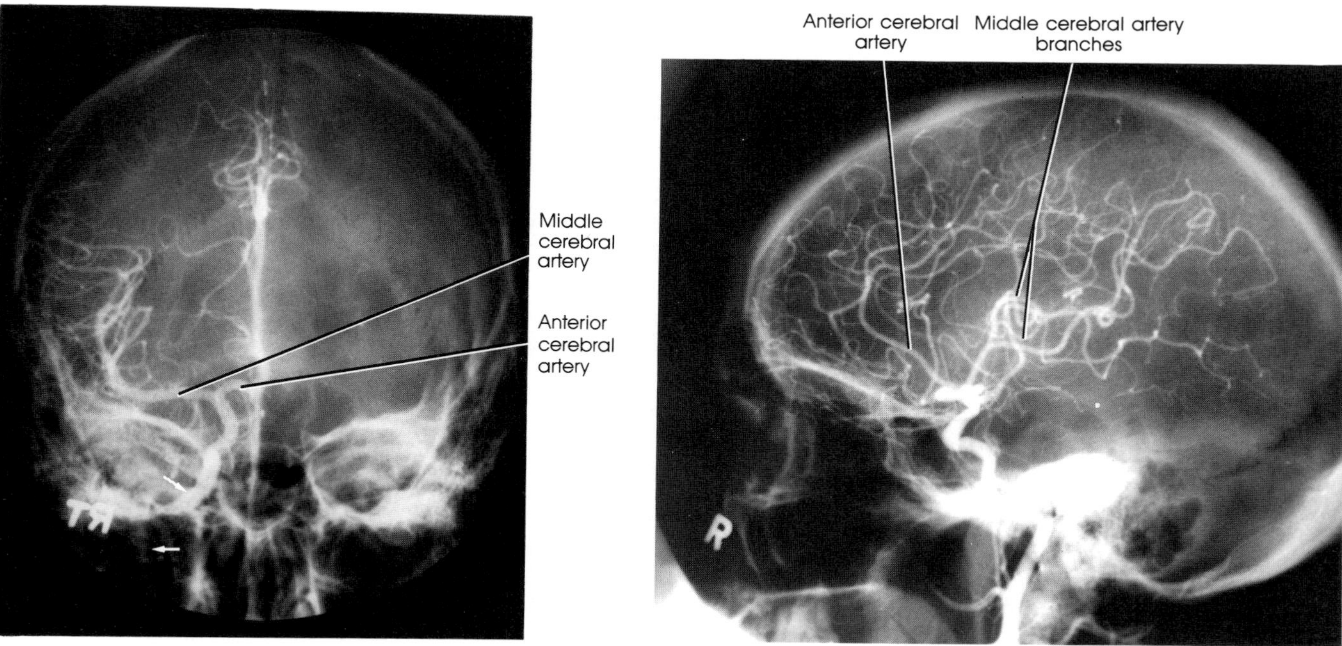

Fig. 30-38. Carotid arteriogram showing internal carotid artery *(arrows)* and anterior cerebral blood circulation.

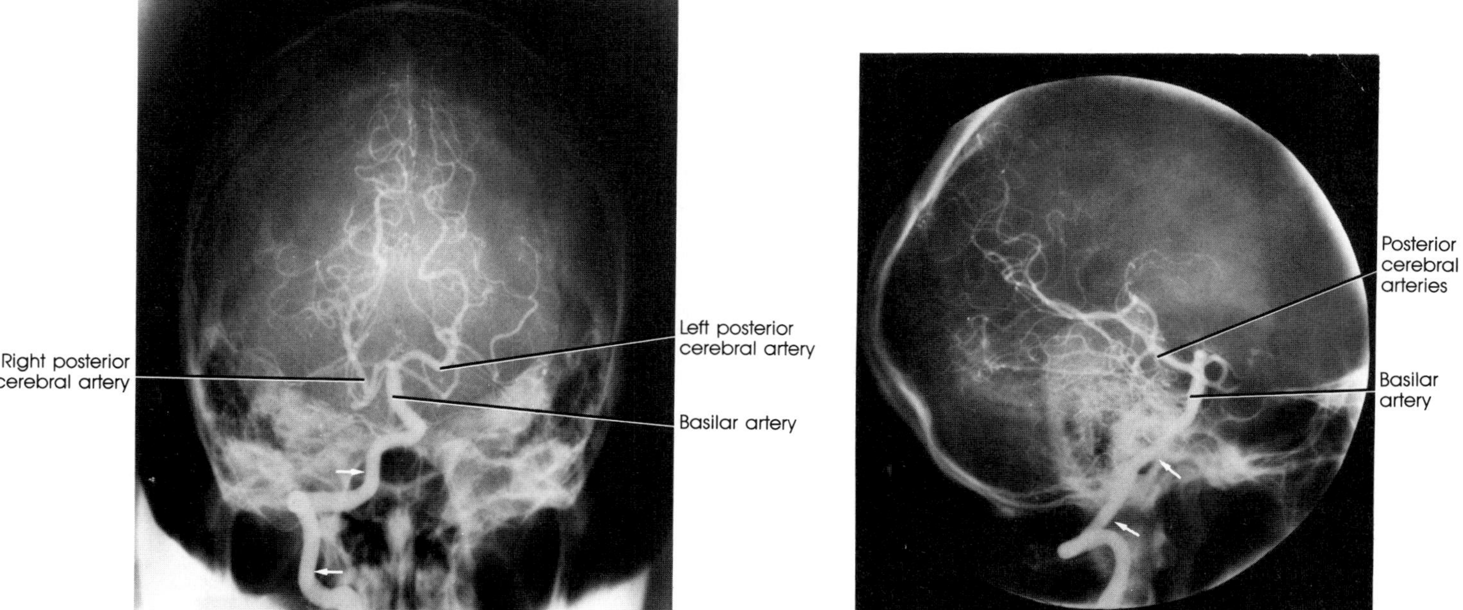

Fig. 30-39. Vertebral arteriogram showing vertebral artery *(arrows)* and posterior cerebral blood circulation.

TECHNIQUE

Cerebral angiography should be performed only in facilities equipped to produce studies of high technical quality with minimum risk to the patient. The ability to obtain rapid-sequence biplane radiographs with automatic injection represents the minimum standard. This equipment is available in all major medical centers and in most large community hospitals.

Access to the *brachiocephalic* and cerebral vessels is almost universally accomplished by catheterization from the femoral artery (Fig. 30-40). If this route is blocked by previous surgical procedures such as aortofemoral bypass grafting or intrinsic atherosclerotic disease, catheterization from a brachial or axillary artery approach is frequently employed. The entire intracerebral circulation can also be visualized by direct puncture and injection of the left common carotid artery and a right retrograde brachial artery injection. This technique is associated with a higher complication rate and significantly more discomfort to the patient. Selective catheterization techniques also allow the study of internal and external carotid circulations separately, which is useful in delineating the blood supply of some forms of cerebral tumors and vascular malformations.

The final position of the catheter depends on the information sought from the angiographic study. When atherosclerotic disease of the brachiocephalic vessels is being evaluated, an injection of the aortic arch with filming of the extracranial portion of these vessels is an appropriate way to begin. Selective studies depend on fluoroscopic positioning of an appropriate catheter in a stable but *nonocclusive* position in the proximal segment of the carotid or vertebral artery of interest.

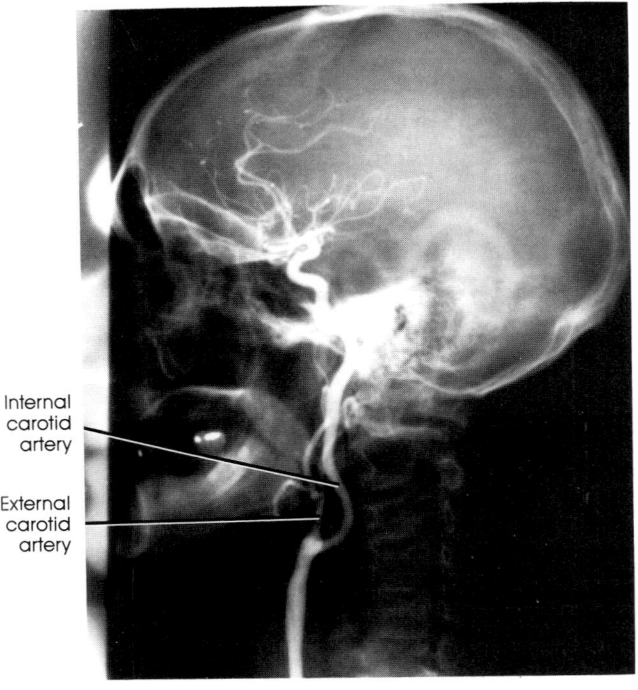

Fig. 30-40. Lateral intracranial and extracranial carotid arteriogram with catheter in right common carotid artery orifice by way of femoral artery catheterization.

CIRCULATION TIME AND FILMING PROGRAM

According to the estimation of Egas Moniz,[1] only 3 seconds is the usual time required for the blood to circulate from the internal carotid artery to the jugular vein, the circulation time being slightly prolonged by the injected contrast solution. Greitz,[2] who measured the cerebral circulation time as "the time between the points of maximum concentration [of contrast medium] in the carotid siphon and in the parietal veins," found a normal mean value of 4.13 seconds. Thus *time* is a highly important factor in cerebral angiography.

Certain pathologic conditions significantly alter the cerebral circulation time. *Arteriovenous malformations* shorten the transit time, and increased intracranial pressure or arterial spasm may cause a considerable delay.

[1]Egas Moniz AC: L'angiographie cérébrale, Paris, 1934, Masson & Cie.

[2]Greitz T: A radiologic study of the brain circulation by rapid serial angiography of the carotid artery, Acta Radiol Suppl 140, 1956.

A standard radiographic program should include a radiograph taken before the arrival of contrast material to serve as a subtraction mask (see discussion of the photographic subtraction technique at the end of this chapter) and rapid-sequence films at one and one-half to three films per second in the AP and lateral planes during the early, or arterial, phase (first 1½ to 2½ seconds) (Fig. 30-41). After the arterial phase, filming may be slowed to one film per second for the capillary, or parenchymal, phase (Fig. 30-42) and maintained at one film per second or every other second for the venous phase (Fig. 30-43) of the angiogram. The entire program should cover 7 to 10 seconds depending on the preference of the angiographer. The filming program must be tailored to demonstrate the suspected pathologic condition.

Injection rates and volumes through the catheter are coupled with the filming program, usually by automatic means. Injections at rates of 5 to 9 ml/sec for 1 to 2 seconds are most often employed in the cerebral vessels, with variations dependent on vessel size and the patient's circulatory status.

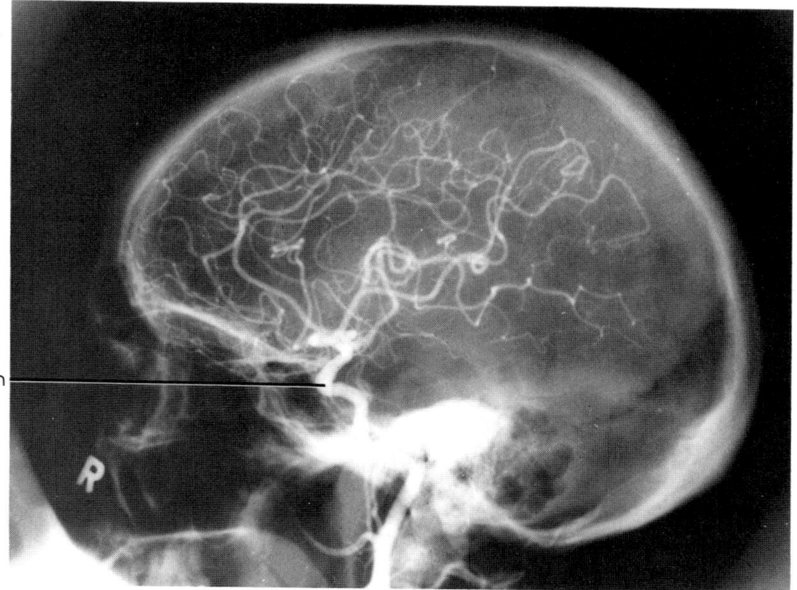

Fig. 30-41. Arterial phase of percutaneous carotid circulation.

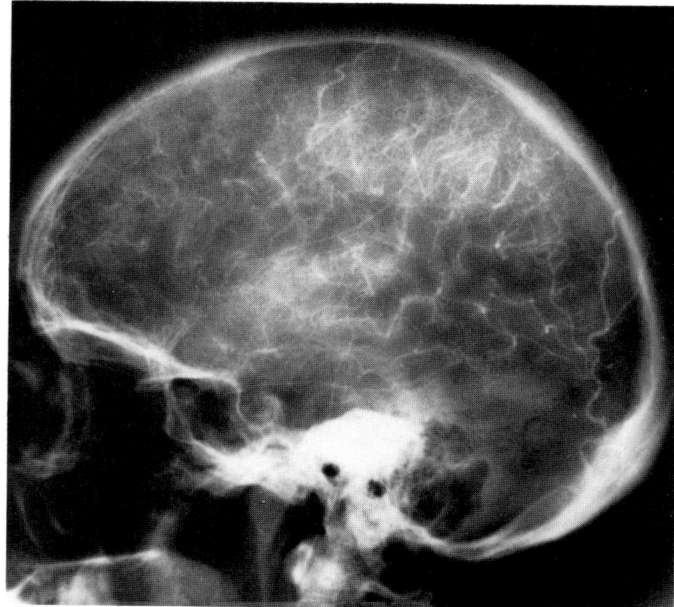

Fig. 30-42. Capillary phase of percutaneous carotid circulation.

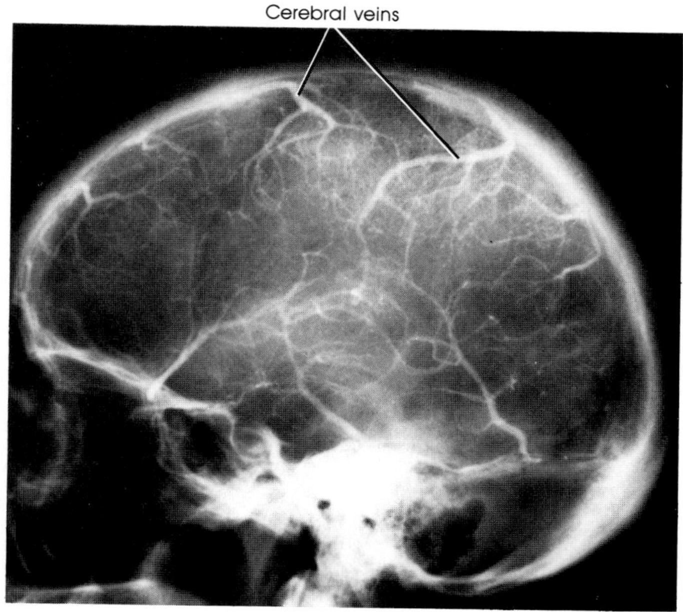

Fig. 30-43. Venous phase of circulation.

(Courtesy Dr. John A. Goree.)

EQUIPMENT

Rapid-sequence biplane filming with mechanically or electronically coupled automatic injection is used almost universally in cerebral angiography. Magnification in one or both planes is also frequently employed (Figs. 30-44 to 30-46). Fractional focal spot x-ray tubes of 0.3 mm or less are necessary for direct radiographic magnification techniques. A threefold or greater linear magnification is possible with a significant increase in resolution of fine vessel detail.

The selection of a fractional focal spot necessitates the use of low milliamperage. Short exposure time is maintained by the use of the air gap rather than the grid to control scatter radiation. For a 2:1 magnification study using a 100 cm source-to-image distance (SID), both the focal spot and the film changer are positioned 50 cm from the area of interest. A 3:1 magnification study using a 100 cm SID is accomplished by placing the focal spot 33 cm from the area of interest and the film changer 67 cm from the area of interest.

Special training and experience are necessary to use this sophisticated and expensive equipment. The operational and filming capabilities of cerebral angiographic units are diverse and vary considerably according to the manufacturer. However, routine maintenance of all equipment is essential to ensure reliable performance. Careful attention to maintenance and other details by technical and professional staff members is necessary to prevent unnecessary delay in completing studies and inconvenient downtime.

Collimating to the area of the head and neck is essential for improving image quality in the nonmagnified study. The standard tube collimator may be used for this purpose, or lead cutout diaphragms may be additionally positioned on the collimator. These diaphragms may have openings in the shape of a circle or a "keyhole." Keyhole diaphragm openings are rounded in the area of the cranium and taper inward in the area of the neck. The frontal and lateral keyhole diaphragms are each designed to resemble the shape of the head and neck in their respective views.

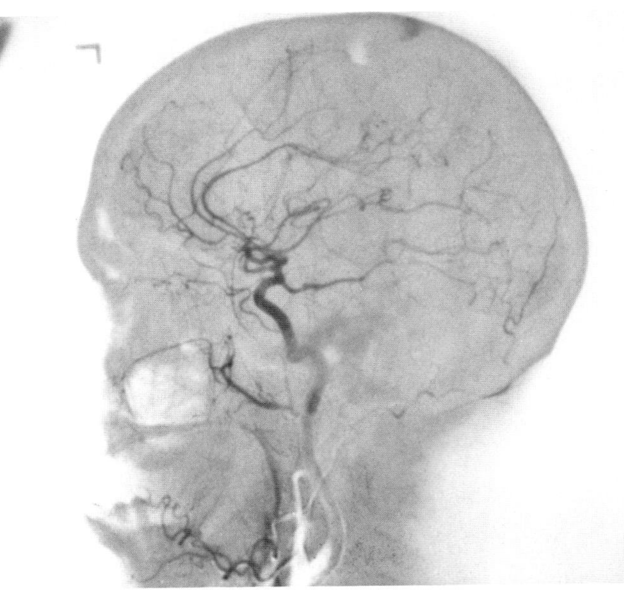

Fig. 30-44. Nonmagnified, photographically subtracted, normal lateral selective common carotid arteriogram.

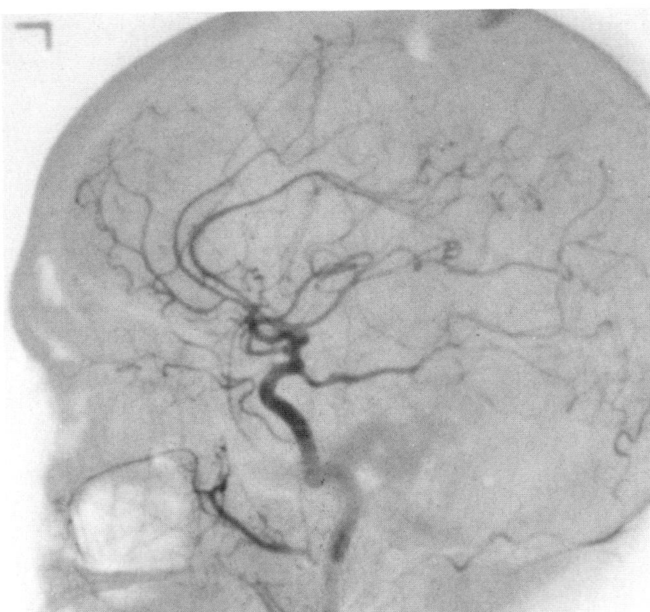

Fig. 30-45. 2:1 magnified, photographically subtracted, normal lateral selective common carotid arteriogram.

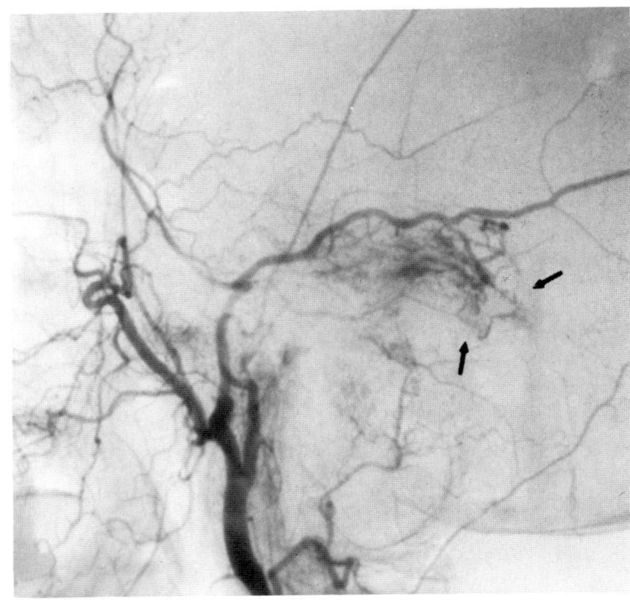

Fig. 30-46. 3:1 magnified, photographically subtracted, lateral selective external carotid arteriogram. *Arrows* indicate visualization of fine tumor neovascularity.

PREPARATION OF PATIENT

Other than withholding the preceding meal, preliminary preparation of the patient depends on his condition and is accordingly determined by the radiologist and the referring physician. Whenever possible, adult patients are examined under local anesthesia in conjunction with sedation. Adequate sedation minimizes the intensity of the burning pain felt along the course of the injected vessel and in the areas supplied by it during the rapid injections of the iodinated medium. The sedative has the further advantage of lessening the possibility of a reaction resulting in reflex movement during initial arterial filming at or before the end of each injection. It is imperative that the conscious patient receive a careful explanation of what to expect during the examination and what is expected of him. This explanation is essential for the successful completion of the examination.

PREPARATION OF EXAMINING ROOM

It cannot be said too often that radiographic examining rooms and every item in them should be as scrupulously clean as any other room used for medical purposes. The room should be fully prepared, with every item needed or likely to be needed on hand before the patient is admitted. Cleanliness and advance preparation are of vital importance in examinations that must be carried out under aseptic conditions.

The radiographic machine and all working parts of the equipment should be checked, and the controls adjusted for the exposure technique to be employed. Identification markers and all accessories should be conveniently located. Compression and restraining bands should be ready for application. Immobilization of the head by suitable strapping must be adapted to the type of equipment employed. Arrangements should be made for immediate processing of the films as the examination proceeds.

The sterile and nonsterile items required for the introduction of the contrast medium vary according to the method of injection. The supplies specified by the radiologist for each procedure should be listed in the angiographic procedure book. Sterile trays or packs, set up to specifications, can usually be obtained from the central sterile-supply room. Otherwise, it is the responsibility of a qualified member of the technologic staff to prepare them. Extra sterile supplies should always be on hand in case of an accident. Preparation of the room includes having life-supporting emergency equipment immediately available.

RADIATION PROTECTION

As in all radiographic examinations, the patient is protected by filtration totaling not less than 2.5 mm of aluminum, by sharp restriction of the beam of radiation to the area being examined, and by avoidance of repeat exposures. In angiography each repeated exposure necessitates a repeated injection of the iodinated compound. For this reason, only skilled and specifically trained technologists should be assigned to take part in these examinations.

Angiography suites should be designed to allow observation of the patient at all times as well as to provide adequate protection to the physician and x-ray personnel. These goals are usually accomplished with leaded glass observation windows.

POSITION OF PATIENT

All cerebral angiographic injection methods require that the patient be placed in the supine position for the entire examination. Regardless of whether the patient is awake, suitable supports should be placed under points of strain—the small of the back, the knees, and the ankles—and the patient should be covered according to room temperature. Wrist restraints and compression bands across the body are applied as indicated by the patient's condition.

When the catheter is in place, there is little danger of unseating it during positioning. However, care must still be exercised to prevent excessive patient motion, especially with extremely selective studies.

POSITION OF HEAD

The centering and angulation of the central ray required for the demonstration of the anterior circulation differ from that required for the demonstration of the posterior circulation, but the same head position is used for the basic AP and lateral images of both regions. For the initial right-angle studies, the head must be elevated on a radiolucent support so that it is centered for horizontally projected lateral representations. The head is then adjusted to place its midsagittal plane *exactly perpendicular* to the headrest and consequently *exactly parallel* with the laterally placed film changer. The *infraorbitomeatal line* is placed perpendicular to the horizontal plane when positioning is accomplished manually.

The central ray angulation for caudally inclined AP and AP oblique positions may be based from the vertically placed infraorbitomeatal line, or the central ray may be adjusted so that it is parallel to the floor of the anterior fossa, as indicated by a line extending from the supraorbital margin to a point 2 cm superior to the external auditory meatus. In some angiographic suites, fluoroscopy can be used to determine the final position of the head and the angulation of the central ray required to achieve the desired view.

The literature on cerebral angiography contains numerous position variations concerning the degree of central ray angulation, the base from which it should be angled or the line that it should parallel, and the degree of part rotation for oblique studies. The most frequently employed images, and reasonably standard specifications for obtaining them, have been selected for inclusion in this chapter.

The number of radiographs required for satisfactory delineation of a lesion depends on the nature and location of the lesion. Oblique positions and/or variations in central ray angulation are taken to separate the shadows of vessels that overlap in the basic positions and to evaluate any existing abnormality.

Aortic Arch Angiogram

An aortic arch angiogram is most commonly performed to visualize atherosclerotic or occlusive disease of the extracranial brachiocephalic arteries. A multiple side hole catheter is positioned in the arch of the aorta so that the subsequent injection fills all of the vessels simultaneously.

For best results, simultaneous biplane oblique positions are produced so that superimposition of vessels is minimized. The patient is placed in an RPO (right AP oblique) position on the tabletop, with the midsagittal plane of the head either perpendicular to the frontal film changer or in an RPO (right AP oblique) position. This patient position opens the aortic arch in the frontal oblique image and frees the carotid and vertebral arteries from superimposition in the lateral oblique image. The patient's chin usually needs to be raised to superimpose the inferior margin of the mandible onto the occiput so that as much of the neck as possible is exposed in the frontal radiograph. The patient's shoulders must also be moved inferiorly so that they are removed as much as possible from the lateral view.

Offset biplane film changers are preferred for this procedure. The lateral film changer is positioned approximately 15 cm superiorly to the frontal changer so that the lateral position exposes the head and neck while the frontal projection exposes the neck and upper chest. For the frontal projection, the central ray is directed perpendicularly to the center of the film and enters the patient at a level 3 cm superior to the sternal angle. The central ray for the lateral position is directed perpendicularly to the midline of the vertically oriented grid and usually enters the patient a few centimeters inferior to the angle of the mandible. The lateral field is collimated in the anteroposterior aspect (see Fig. 30-37).

A representative injection program for an aortic arch examination is 30 to 35 ml/sec for a total volume of 60 to 70 ml. A representative film program is two to three films per second in each plane for 4 seconds. Because subtraction films are frequently produced from aortic arch angiograms, it is important that the initial films are exposed before the injection begins. An alternative film program exposes one film in each plane, pauses 1 second as the injection begins, and then continues with two to three films per second for 3 seconds.

Positioning

ANTERIOR CIRCULATION PROJECTIONS

Lateral position

The patient's head is elevated on a suitable support so that it is centered to the vertically placed film. The head is extended enough to place the infraorbitomeatal line perpendicular to the horizontal; it is then adjusted to place the midsagittal plane *exactly* vertical and thereby parallel with the plane of the film. Immobilization must be adapted to the type of equipment being employed.

Lateral positions of the anterior, or carotid, circulation are made with the central ray directed horizontally to a point slightly cranial to the auricle and midway between the forehead and the occiput. This centering allows for variation (Figs. 30-47 to 30-49).

For assistance in identifying the cerebral vessels in these and the following radiographs, please see Fig. 30-72 at the end of this section of this chapter.

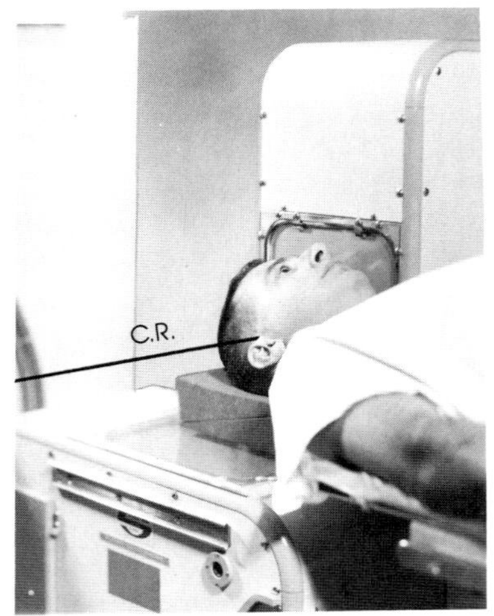

Fig. 30-47. Lateral cerebral angiogram.

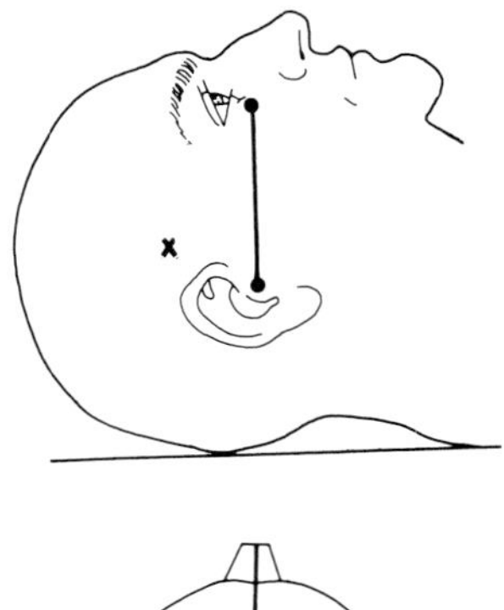

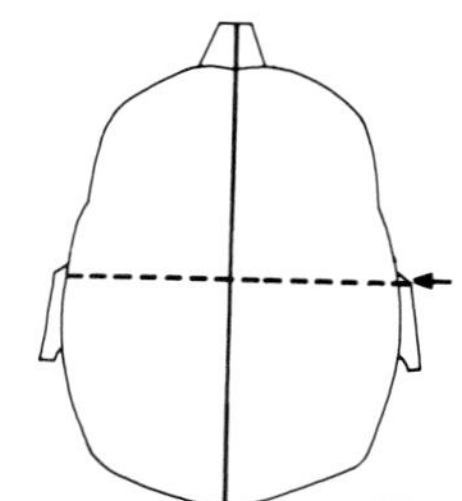

Fig. 30-48. Lateral projection.

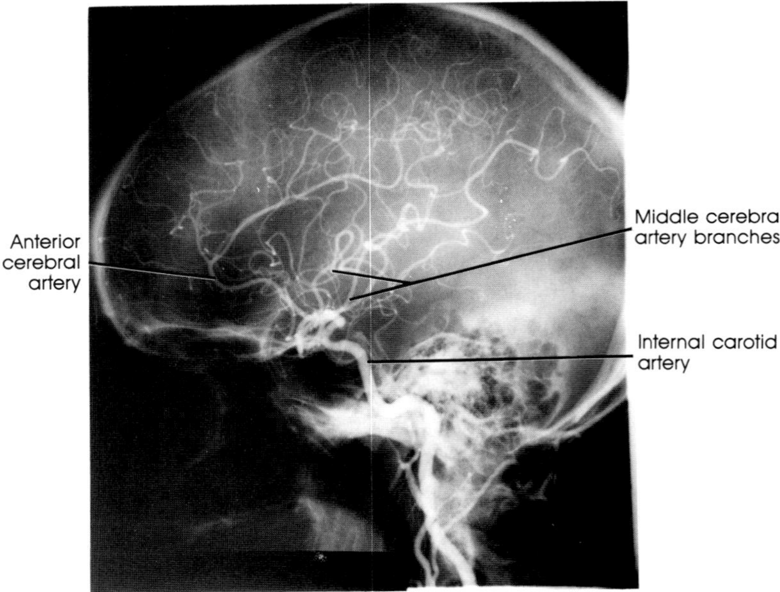

Fig. 30-49. Lateral position demonstrating anterior circulation.

(Courtesy Joyce Torzewski, R.T.)

AP supraorbital position

Unless simultaneous biplane images are being made, the support is removed, and the head is rested directly on the table for frontal studies. The head is adjusted so that its midsagittal plane is centered over and *exactly* perpendicular to the midline of the grid and so that it is extended enough to place the infraorbitomeatal line vertically. The head is then immobilized.

The aim in this radiograph is to superimpose the supraorbital margins on the superior margin of the petrous ridges so that the vessels are projected above the floor of the anterior cranial fossa. This result is achieved in a majority of patients by directing the central ray along a line passing 2 cm superior to and parallel with a line extending from the supraorbital margin to a point 2 cm superior to the external auditory meatus; the latter line coincides with the floor of the anterior fossa (Figs. 30-50 to 30-52).

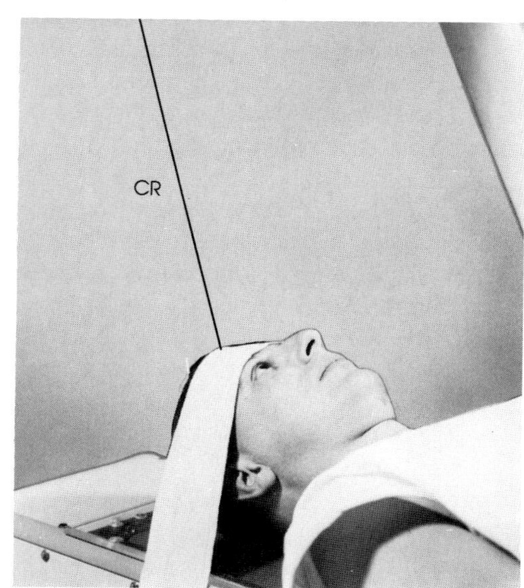

Fig. 30-50. Supraorbital carotid.

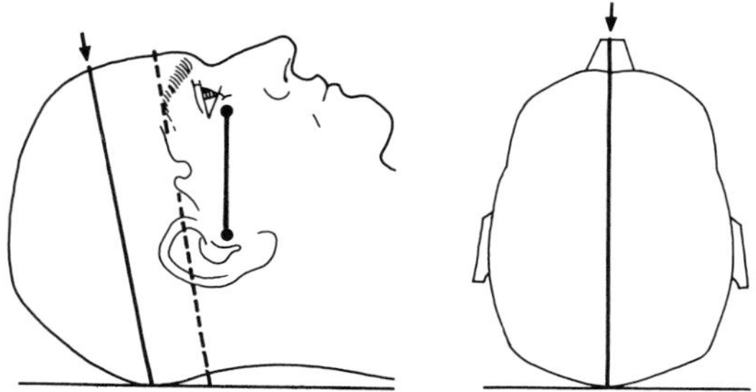

Fig. 30-51. AP supraorbital.

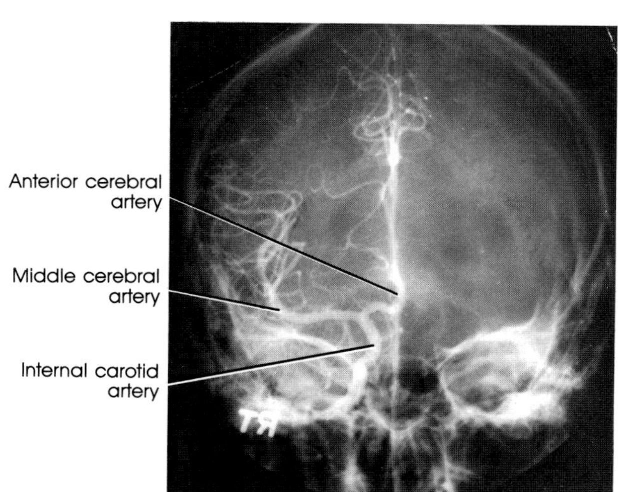

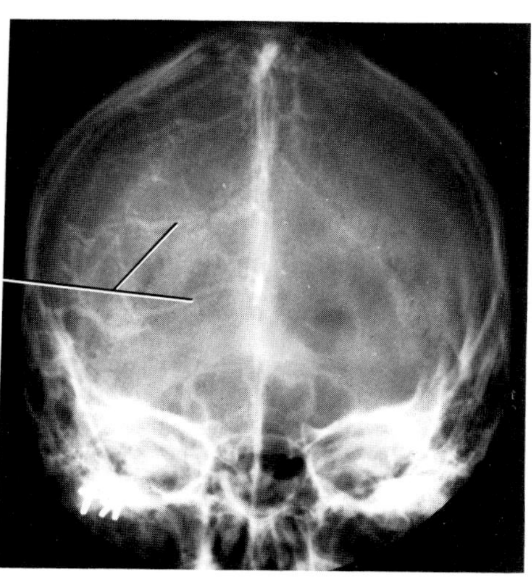

Fig. 30-52. Serial percutaneous carotid angiograms: *left,* arterial and, *right,* venous phases of circulation.

Aortic arch angiogram

Supraorbital oblique position

For demonstration of the region of the anterior communicating artery, the preceding head position is maintained, except that it is rotated approximately 30 degrees away from the injected side. The central ray is directed as for the direct supraorbital position (Figs. 30-53 and 30-54).

AP transorbital position

The AP transorbital position demonstrates the middle cerebral artery and its main branches within the orbital shadow.

The head is adjusted in the basic AP position. The central ray is directed through the midorbits at an average angle of 20 degrees cephalad; it should coincide with a line passing through the center of the orbit and a point about 2 cm superior to the auricle of the ear (Figs. 30-55 and 30-56).

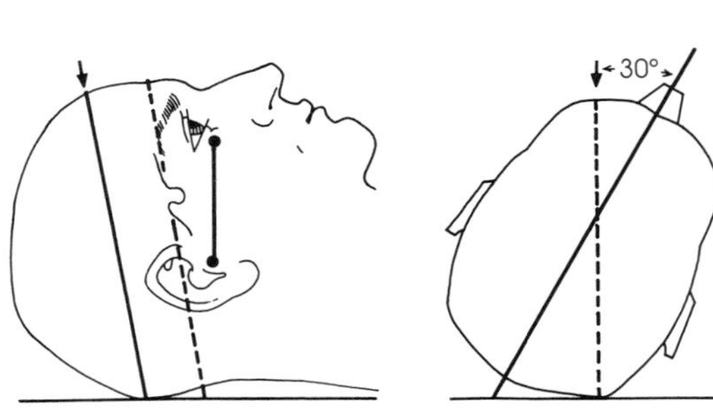

Fig. 30-53. AP supraorbital oblique.

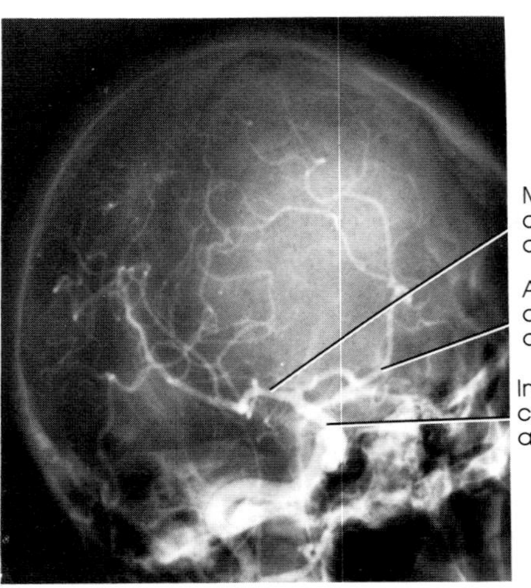

Fig. 30-54. AP supraorbital oblique carotid arteriogram.

(Courtesy Dr. John A. Goree.)

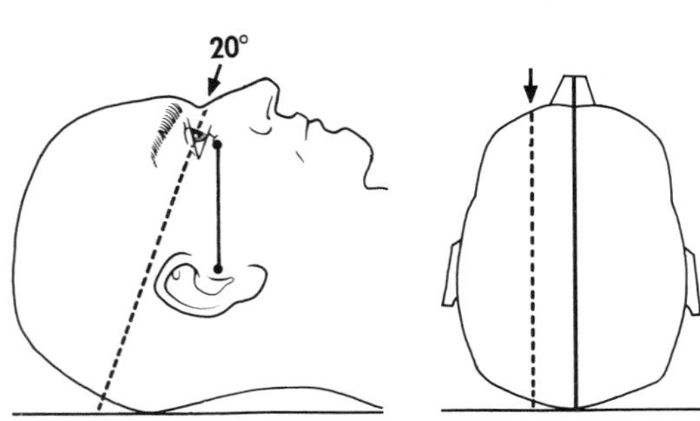

Fig. 30-55. AP transorbital position.

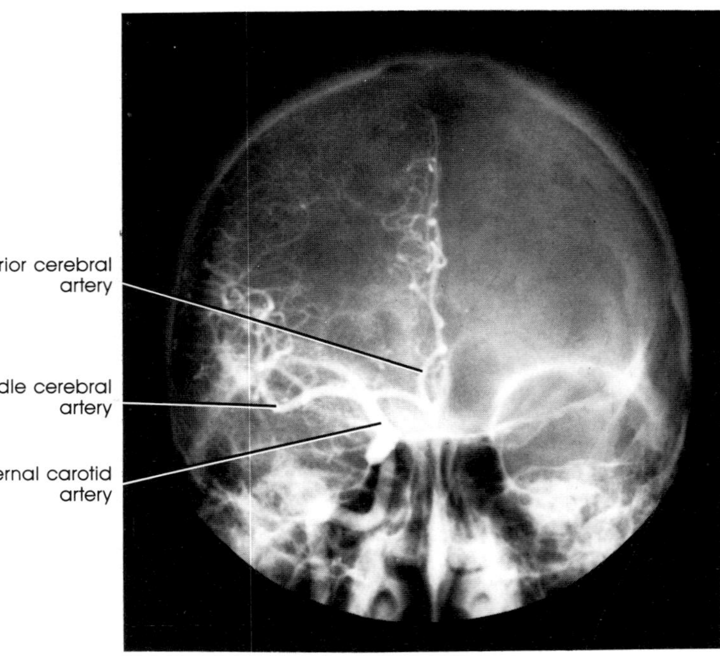

Fig. 30-56. Percutaneous carotid arteriogram: AP transorbital.

Oblique transorbital position

The oblique transorbital position demonstrates the internal carotid bifurcation and the anterior communicating and middle cerebral arteries within the orbital shadow.

From the basic AP transorbital position, the head is rotated approximately 30 degrees away from the injected side. The central ray is angled as for the direct AP transorbital position and centered to the midorbit of the uppermost side (Figs. 30-57 and 30-58).

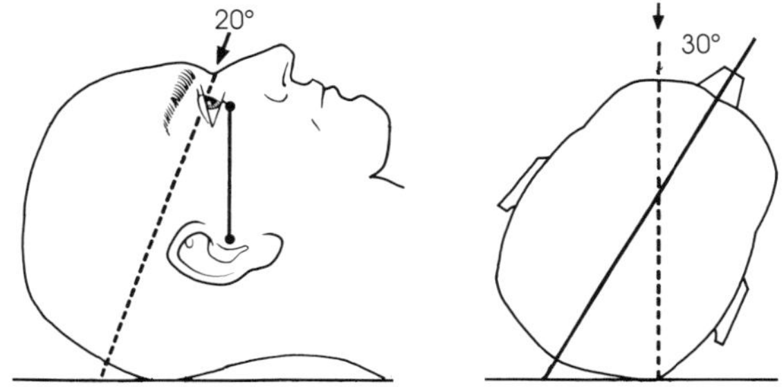

Fig. 30-57. Oblique transorbital position.

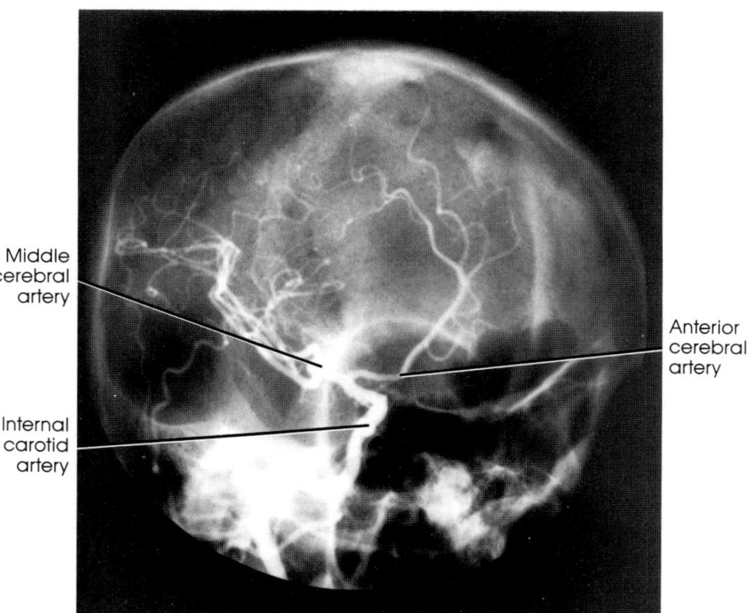

Fig. 30-58. Percutaneous carotid arteriogram: transorbital oblique.

(Courtesy Dr. John A. Goree.)

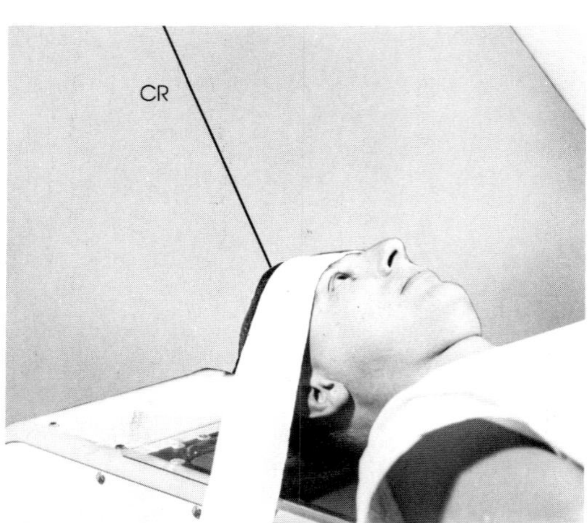

Fig. 30-59. AP axial position.

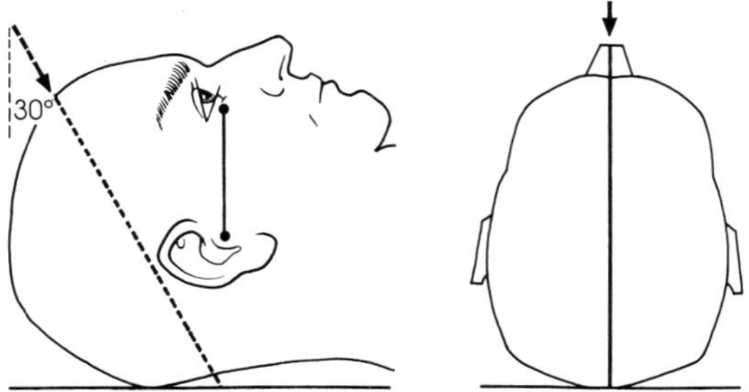

Fig. 30-60. AP axial position.

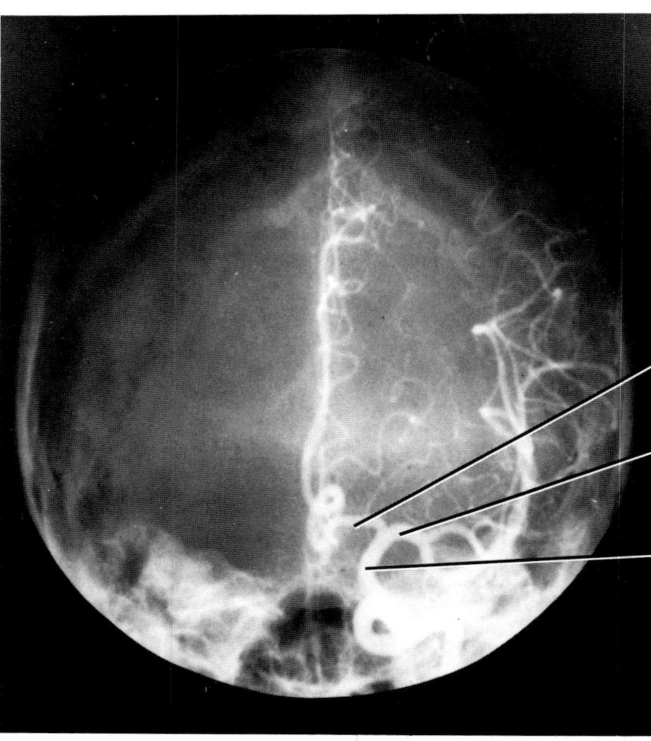

Fig. 30-61. Percutaneous carotid arteriogram: AP axial position.

AP axial positions

AP axial and/or AP axial oblique positions are used in carotid angiography, when indicated, for further evaluation of vessel displacement or of aneurysms.

1. For an AP axial position, the head is adjusted in the basic position. The central ray is directed to the region of the hairline at an average angle of 30 degrees caudad; it exits at the level of the external auditory meatus (Figs. 30-59 to 30-61).

2. For an AP axial oblique position, the head is rotated 35 to 45 degrees away from the injected side. The central ray is angled as for the AP axial position (Figs. 30-62 and 30-63).

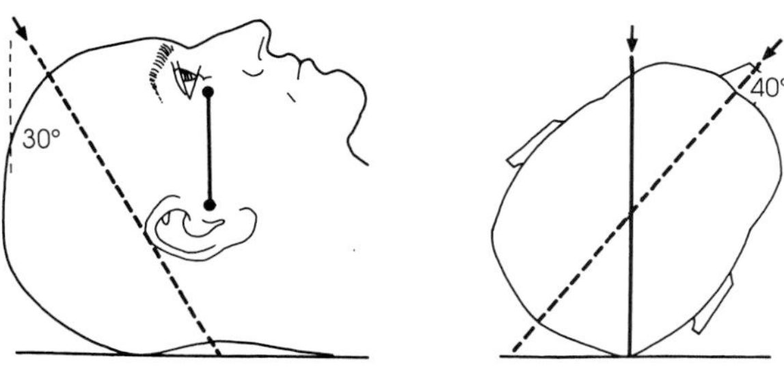

Fig. 30-62. AP axial oblique position.

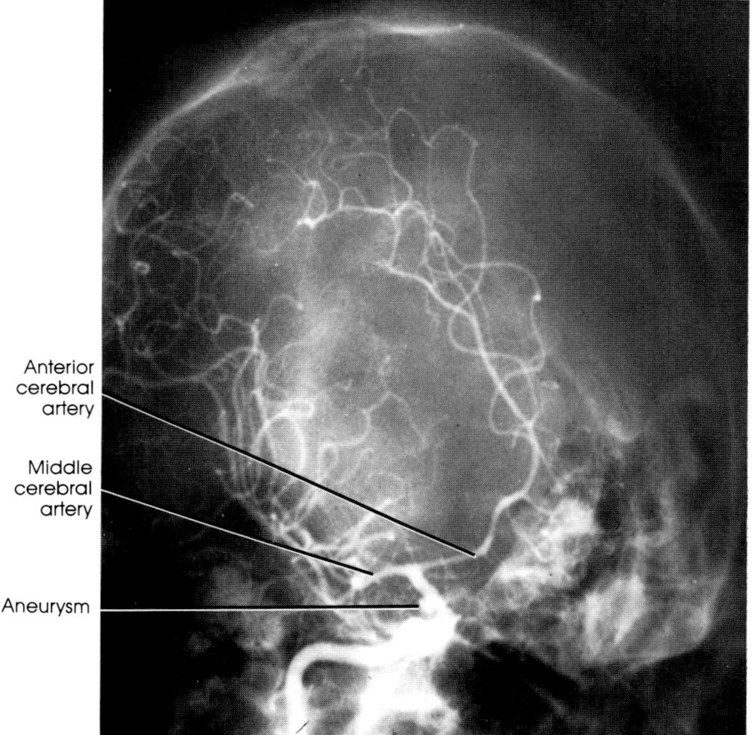

Fig. 30-63. Percutaneous carotid arteriogram: AP axial oblique position showing small internal carotid artery aneurysm at posterior communicating junction.

(Courtesy Dr. John A. Goree.)

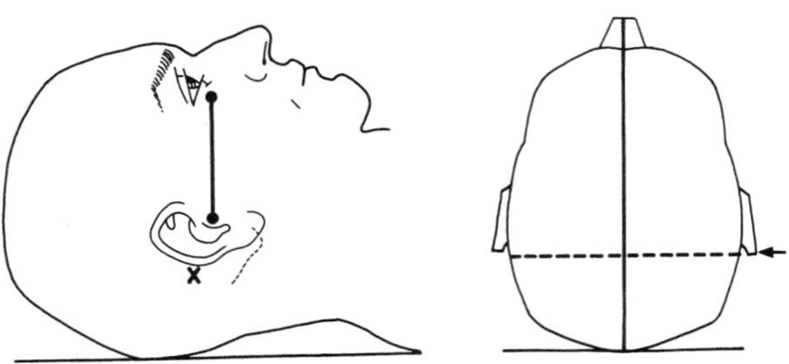

Fig. 30-64. Lateral position for posterior circulation.

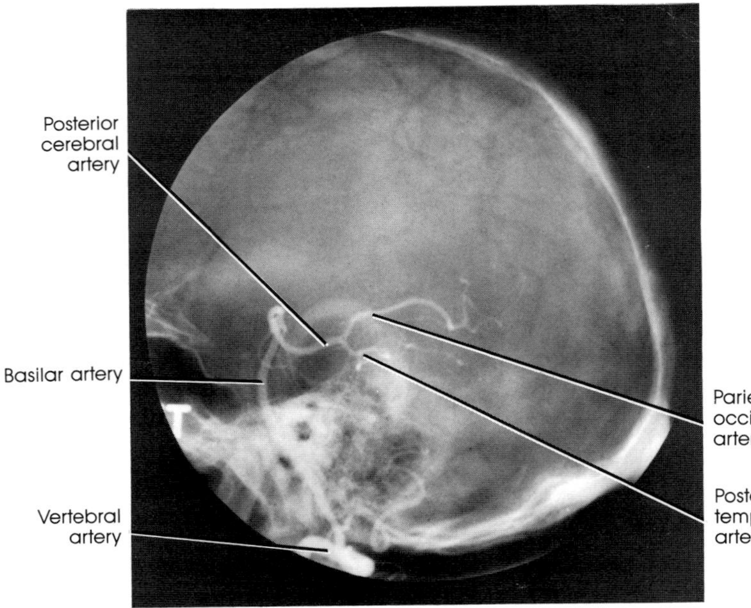

Fig. 30-65. Lateral in early arterial phase showing vertebral artery and posterior vascular structures.

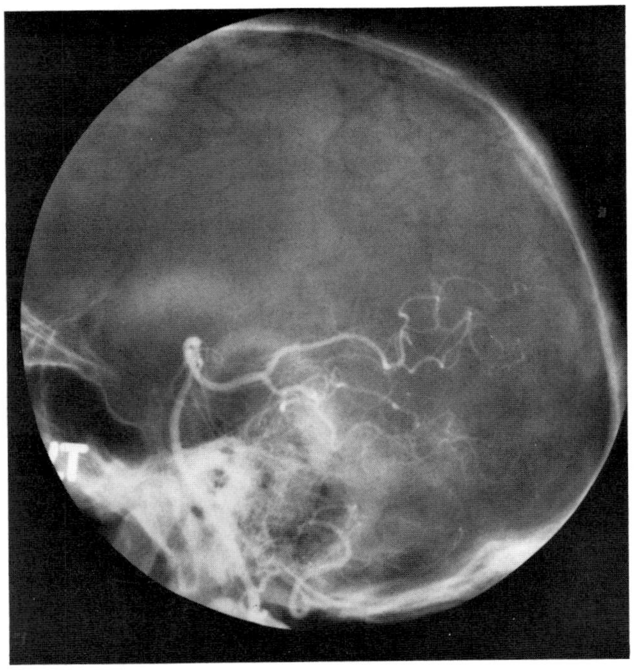

Fig. 30-66. Later arterial phase.

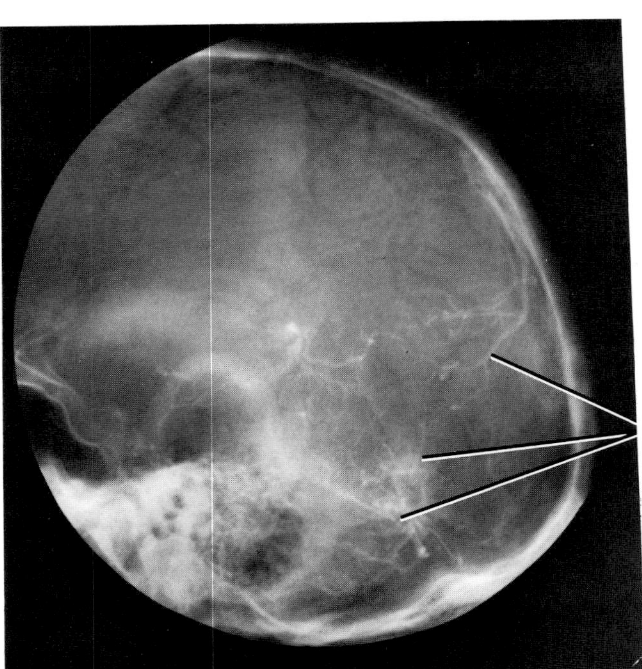

Fig. 30-67. Venous phase. Contrast medium for above serial angiograms was introduced by percutaneous retrograde injection into left brachial artery.

POSTERIOR CIRCULATION PROJECTIONS

Lateral position

The patient's head is elevated on a suitable support so that it is centered to the vertically placed film. It is extended enough to place the infraorbitomeatal line perpendicular to the horizontal plane and is then adjusted to place the midsagittal plane *exactly* vertical and thereby parallel with the plane of the film. The head must be rigidly immobilized.

Lateral positions of the posterior, or vertebral, circulation are made with the central ray directed horizontally to the mastoid process at a point about 1 cm superior to and 2 cm posterior to the external auditory meatus.

The exposure field can be restricted to the middle and posterior fossae for lateral studies of the posterior circulation, the inclusion of the entire skull being neither necessary nor, from the standpoint of optimum technique, desirable (Figs. 30-64 to 30-67).

AP axial position

Except for simultaneous biplane positions, the support is removed and the head is rested directly on the table for frontal studies. The head is adjusted so that its midsagittal plane is centered over, and is exactly perpendicular to, the midline of the grid, and the head is extended enough so that the infraorbitomeatal line is vertical. The head is then immobilized.

The central ray is directed to the region of the hairline at an angle of 30 to 35 degrees caudad; it exits at the level of the external auditory meatuses. In this view the shadows of the supraorbital margins are positioned approximately 2 cm below the superior margins of the petrous ridges (Figs. 30-68 and 30-69).

Submentovertical projection

A modified submentovertical projection is sometimes employed in the investigation of the posterior circulation. It is also used for the anterior circulation when a middle fossa lesion is suspected.

The success of this position depends on the patient's ability to hyperextend the neck and maintain this position for the time required for a filming sequence. This position may not be possible for elderly patients with cervical degenerative arthritis (Figs. 30-70 and 30-71). Fig. 30-72, showing the intracerebral circulation, is shown on the following page.

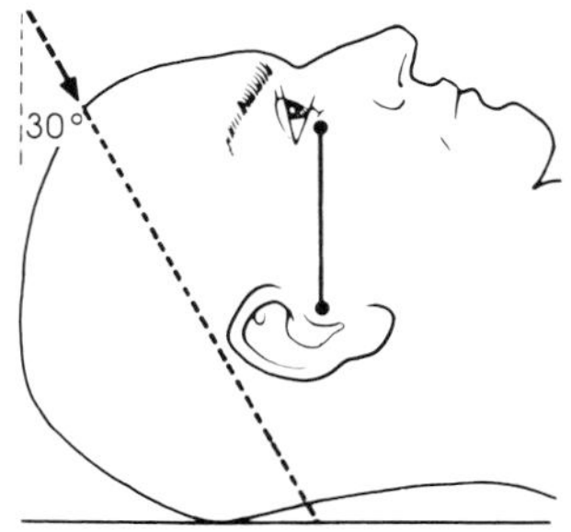

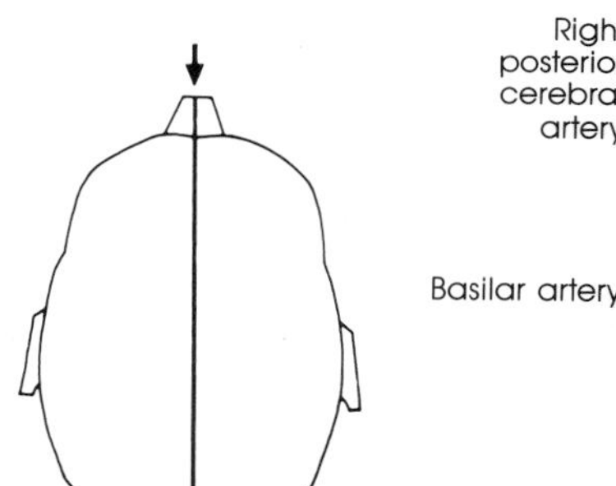

Fig. 30-68. AP axial position for posterior circulation.

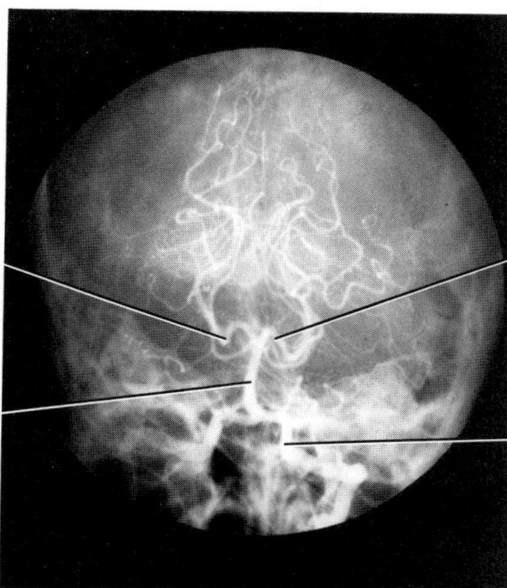
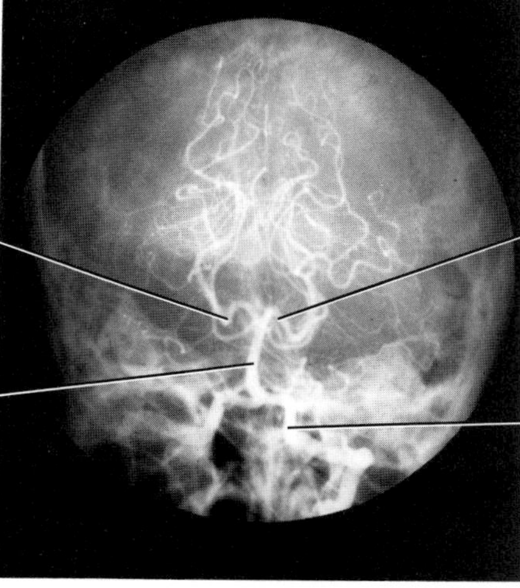

Fig. 30-69. AP axial: arterial phase of posterior circulation.

(Courtesy Dr. John A. Goree.)

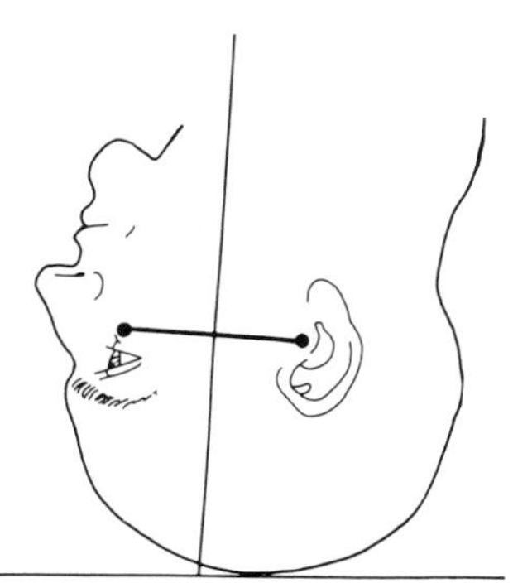

Fig. 30-70. Submentovertical projection.

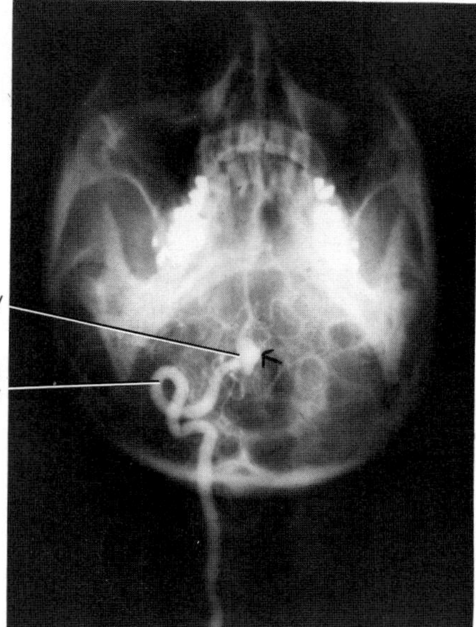

Fig. 30-71. Transaxillary selective right vertebral arteriogram: basal projection showing excellent opacification of right vertebral artery and aneurysm *(arrow)* at vertebrobasilar junction.

(Courtesy Dr. K.Y. Chynn.)

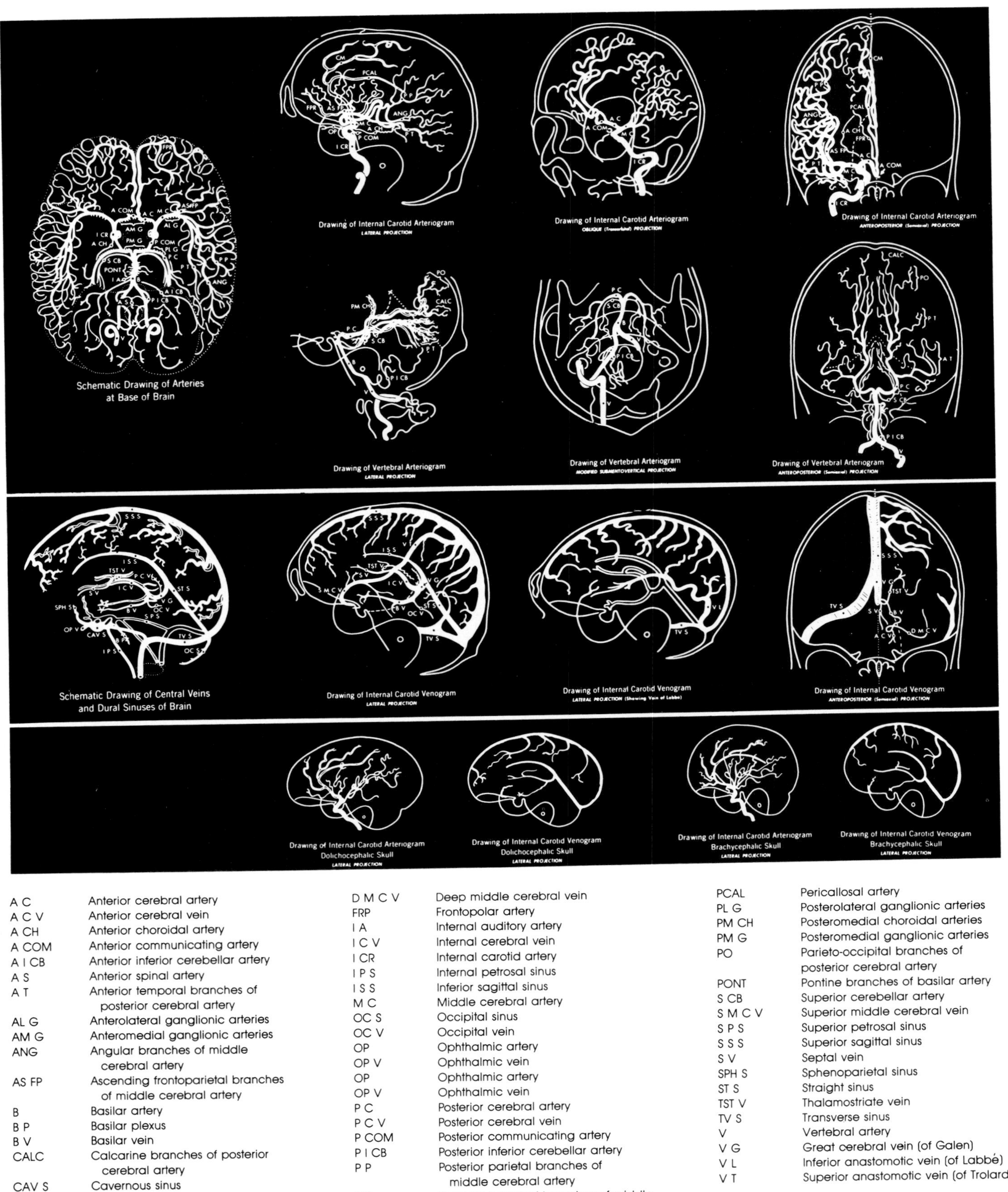

A C — Anterior cerebral artery
A C V — Anterior cerebral vein
A CH — Anterior choroidal artery
A COM — Anterior communicating artery
A I CB — Anterior inferior cerebellar artery
A S — Anterior spinal artery
A T — Anterior temporal branches of posterior cerebral artery
AL G — Anterolateral ganglionic arteries
AM G — Anteromedial ganglionic arteries
ANG — Angular branches of middle cerebral artery
AS FP — Ascending frontoparietal branches of middle cerebral artery
B — Basilar artery
B P — Basilar plexus
B V — Basilar vein
CALC — Calcarine branches of posterior cerebral artery
CAV S — Cavernous sinus
CM — Callosomarginal artery
D M C V — Deep middle cerebral vein
FRP — Frontopolar artery
I A — Internal auditory artery
I C V — Internal cerebral vein
I CR — Internal carotid artery
I P S — Internal petrosal sinus
I S S — Inferior sagittal sinus
M C — Middle cerebral artery
OC S — Occipital sinus
OC V — Occipital vein
OP — Ophthalmic artery
OP V — Ophthalmic vein
OP — Ophthalmic artery
OP V — Ophthalmic vein
P C — Posterior cerebral artery
P C V — Posterior cerebral vein
P COM — Posterior communicating artery
P I CB — Posterior inferior cerebellar artery
P P — Posterior parietal branches of middle cerebral artery
P T — Posterior temporal branches of middle and posterior cerebral arteries
PCAL — Pericallosal artery
PL G — Posterolateral ganglionic arteries
PM CH — Posteromedial choroidal arteries
PM G — Posteromedial ganglionic arteries
PO — Parieto-occipital branches of posterior cerebral artery
PONT — Pontine branches of basilar artery
S CB — Superior cerebellar artery
S M C V — Superior middle cerebral vein
S P S — Superior petrosal sinus
S S S — Superior sagittal sinus
S V — Septal vein
SPH S — Sphenoparietal sinus
ST S — Straight sinus
TST V — Thalamostriate vein
TV S — Transverse sinus
V — Vertebral artery
V G — Great cerebral vein (of Galen)
V L — Inferior anastomotic vein (of Labbé)
V T — Superior anastomotic vein (of Trolard)

Anatomic terms used are based on *Nomina Anatomica* wherever possible; otherwise terms employed are those usually referred to in anatomic texts. From Bean, B.C.: A chart of the intracerebral circulation, ed 2, Med. Radiogr. Photogr. 34:25, 1958; courtesy Dr. Berton C. Bean and Eastman Kodak Co.

Fig. 30-72. Intracerebral circulation.

Interventional radiology is a process that intervenes, or interferes, with the course of a disease process or other medical condition. It has a therapeutic, rather than diagnostic, purpose. Since its conception in the early 1960s, the realm of interventional radiology has become so vast and sophisticated that periodicals struggle to keep abreast of the rapidly advancing specialty.

Interventional radiology allows the angiographer, a specially trained radiologist, to assume an important role in the management and reduction of disease in many patients. In most cases the interventional procedure has helped reduce the length of a patient's stay in the hospital and helped some patients avoid surgery, lowering medical costs for those patients.

All interventional radiologic procedures must include two integral processes. The first process is the interventional or medical side of the procedure where the highly skilled radiologist uses needles, catheters, and special medical devices (e.g., occluding coils, guide wires) to produce an improvement in the process of the patient. The second process involves using fluoroscopy and radiography for guiding and documenting the progress of the steps taken during the first process. The radiologic technologist, specially trained in the angiographic and interventional laboratory, has a very important role in assisting the angiographer in the interventional procedures.

In the succeeding pages, the interventional procedures more frequently performed are described. The selected bibliography at the end of this chapter provides a listing of more detailed information.

Percutaneous Transluminal Angioplasty

Percutaneous transluminal angioplasty (PTA) is a therapeutic radiologic procedure designed to dilate or reopen stenotic or occluded areas within a vessel using a catheter introduced by the Seldinger technique. PTA was first described by Dotter and Judkins[1] in 1964 using a coaxial catheter method. The first step in this method is passing a wire guide through the narrowed area of a vessel. Then a smaller catheter is passed over the wire guide through the *stenosis* to begin the dilation process. Finally, a larger catheter is passed over the smaller catheter positioned through the stenosis to cause further dilation (Fig. 30-73). Although this method can achieve dilation of stenoses, it has the significant disadvantage of creating an arteriotomy as large as the dilating catheters.

In 1974 Gruntzig and Hopff[1] introduced the double-lumen balloon-tipped catheter. One lumen allows the passage of a wire guide and fluids through the catheter. The other lumen communicates with a balloon at the distal end of the catheter that, when inflated, expands to a size much larger than the catheter. These catheters are available in sizes ranging from 4.5 to 9 Fr. with attached balloons varying in length and expanding to diameters of 2 to 20 mm or more (Fig. 30-74).

Fig. 30-75 illustrates the process of balloon angioplasty. Of course, the stenosis is initially identified on a previously conducted angiogram. The balloon diameter used for a procedure is often the measured diameter of the normal artery adjacent to the stenosis. The angioplasty procedure is often conducted at the same time through the same catheterization site as the initial diagnostic examination. After the wire guide is positioned across the stenosis, the angio-

[1]Dotter CT and Judkins MP: Transluminal treatment of arteriosclerotic obstruction: description of a new technique and preliminary report of its application, Circulation 30:654-670, 1964.

[1]Gruntzig A and Hopff H: Perkutane rekanalisation chronischer arterieller Verschlusse mit einem neuen dilatationskatheter; modifikation der Dotter-Technik, Deutsch Med Wochenschr 99:2502-2511, 1974.

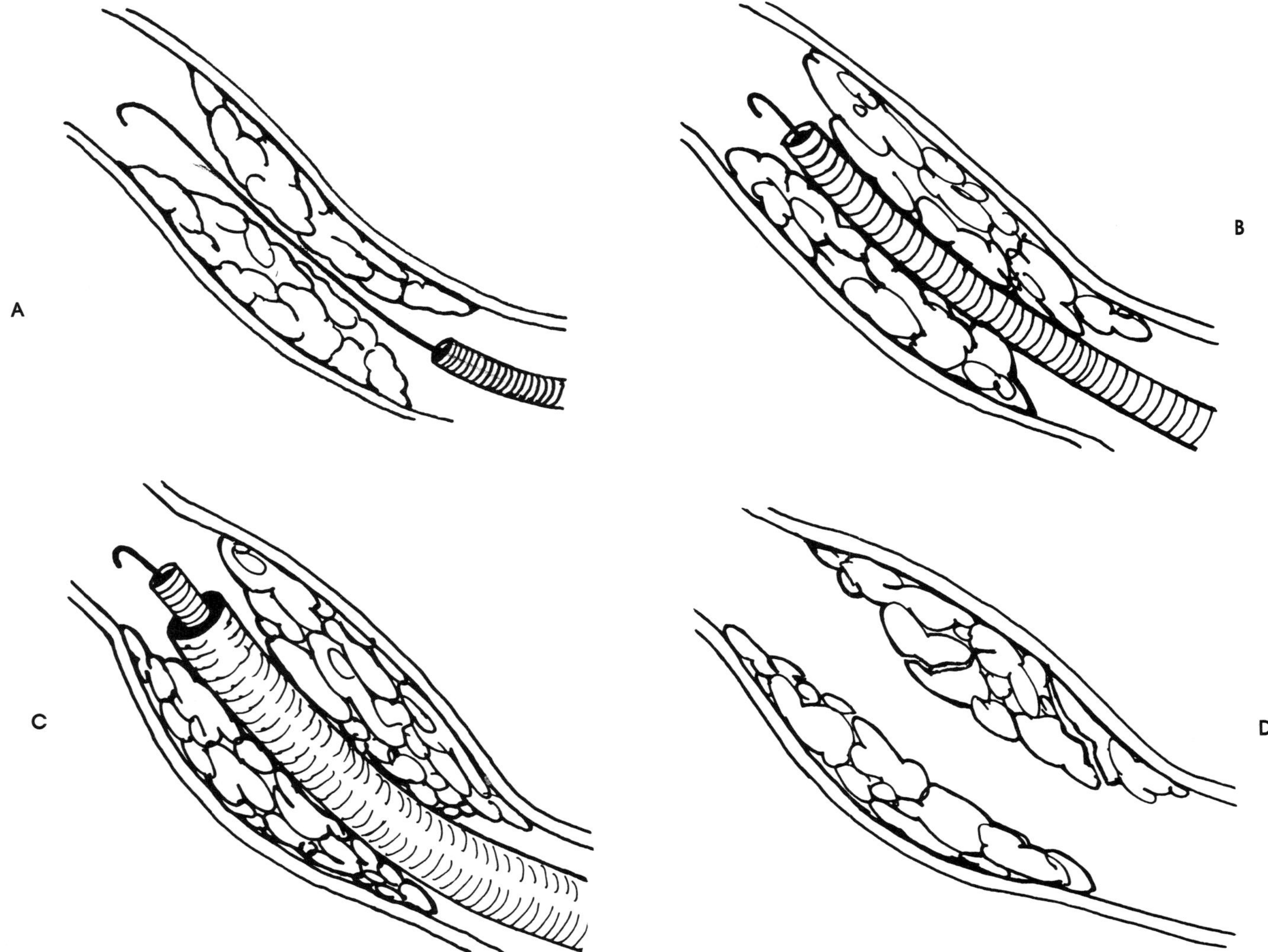

Fig. 30-73. Coaxial angioplasty of atherosclerotic stenosis. **A,** Wire guide advanced through stenosis. **B,** Small catheter advanced through stenosis. **C,** Large catheter advanced through stenosis. **D,** Postangioplasty stenotic area.

(Illustrated by Stephen G. Moon, M.S., and David R. Schumick, B.S.)

graphic catheter is removed over the wire guide and the balloon-tipped catheter is introduced and directed by the wire guide through the stenosis. The balloon is usually inflated with a dilated contrast medium mixture for 15 to 45 seconds, depending on the degree of stenosis and the particular vessel being treated. The balloon is then deflated and repositioned or withdrawn from the lesion. Contrast medium can then be injected through the angioplasty catheter for a repeat angiogram. Success of the angioplasty procedure may be additionally determined by comparing transcatheter blood pressure measurements from a location distal and a location proximal to the lesion site. Nearly equal pressures indicate a reopened stenosis.

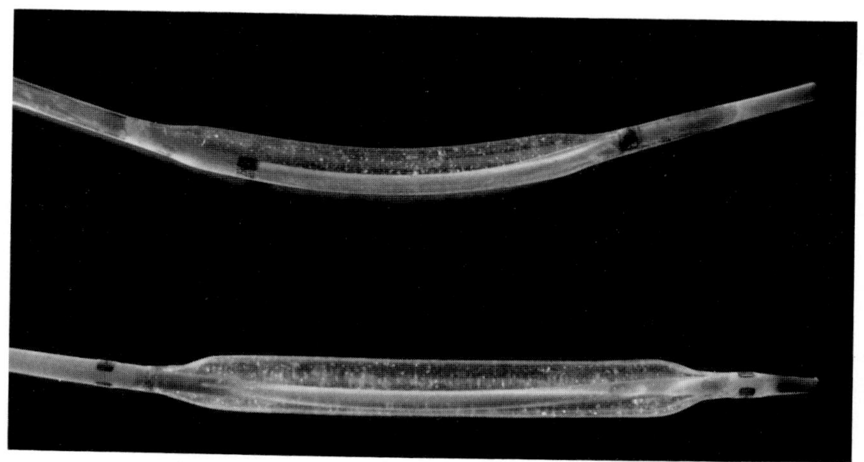

Fig. 30-74. Magnified view of balloon angioplasty catheter deflated *(above)* and inflated *(below)*.

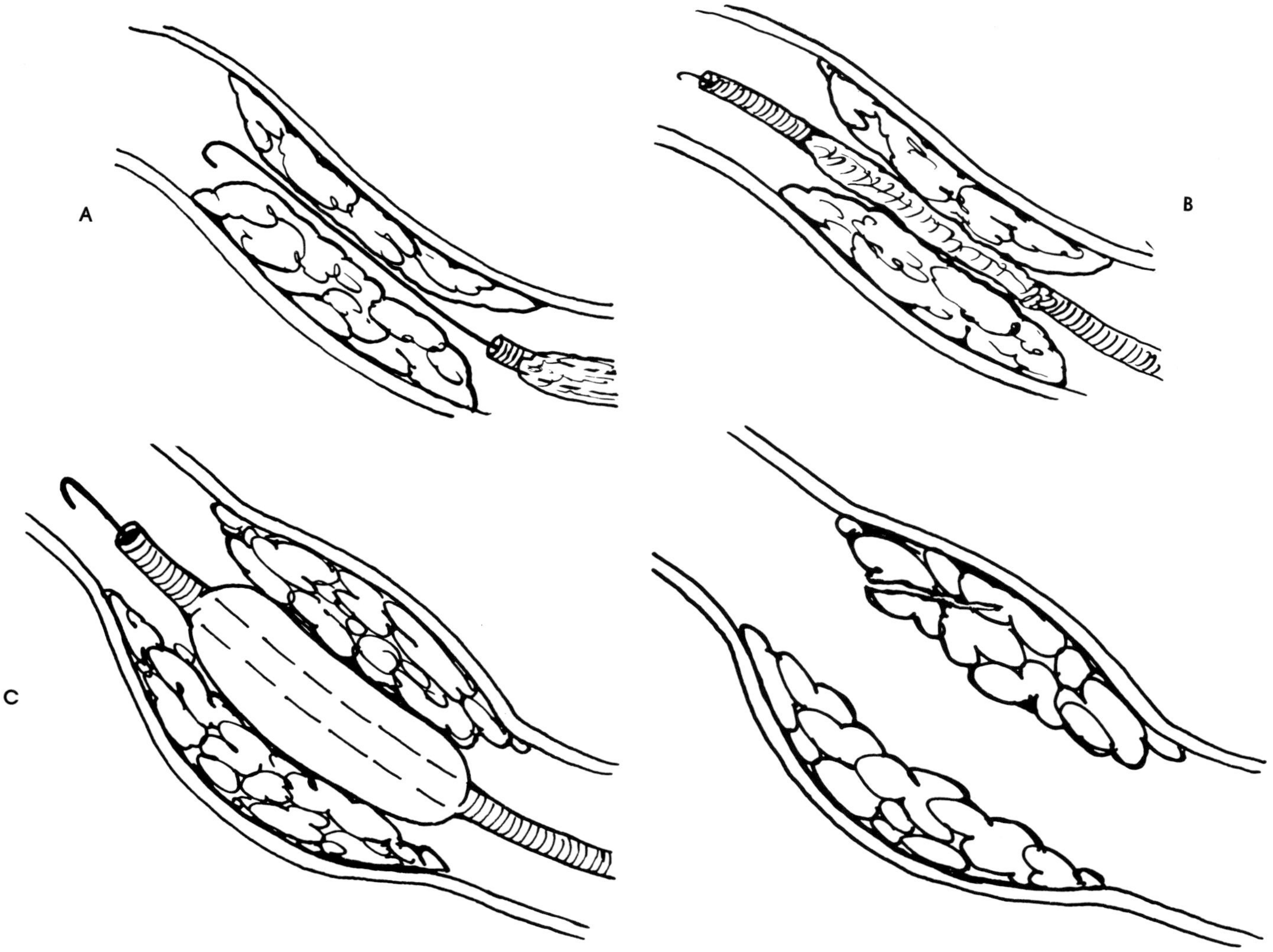

Fig. 30-75. Balloon angioplasty of atherosclerotic stenosis. **A,** Wire guide advanced through stenosis. **B,** Balloon across stenosis. **C,** Balloon inflated. **D,** Postangioplasty stenotic area.

(Illustrated by Stephen G. Moon, M.S., and David R. Schumick, B.S.)

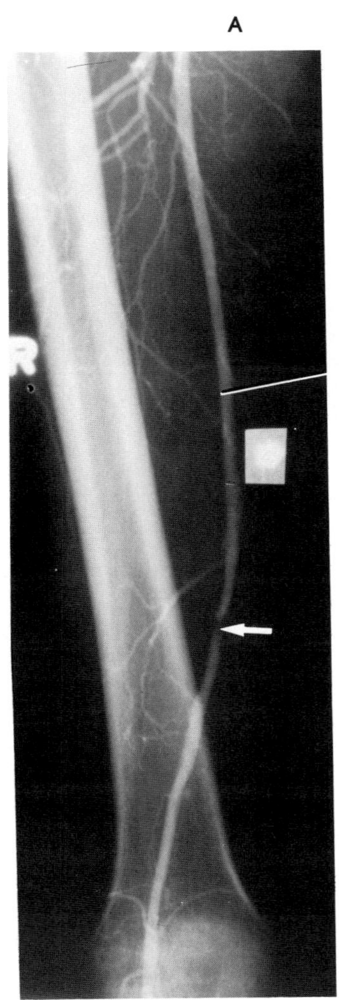

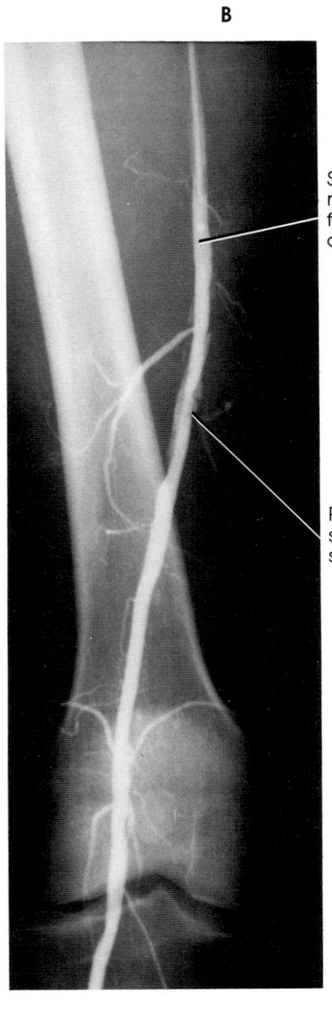

Fig. 30-76. Femoral arteriogram: **A,** denotes stenosis *(arrow)* and, **B,** postangioplasty femoral arteriogram.

Transluminal angioplasty can be performed in virtually any vessel that can be reached percutaneously with a catheter. It is most commonly performed in the renal, iliac, and femoral arteries, and the procedure is primarily used for therapy within an artery (Figs. 30-76 and 30-77). In 1978, however, Molnar and Stockum[1] described the use of balloon angioplasty for dilation of strictures within the biliary system (Fig. 30-78). Balloon angioplasty is also conducted in venous structures and in the ureteral and gastrointestinal tracts.

Balloon angioplasty has been used successfully to manage various diseases that cause arterial narrowing. The most common form of arterial stenosis treated by transluminal angioplasty is caused by atherosclerosis. Dotter and Judkins speculated that this atheromatous mass was soft and inelastic and therefore could be compressed against the artery wall. The success of coaxial and balloon method angioplasty was initially attributed to enlargement of the arterial lumen because of compression of the atherosclerotic plaque. Later research showed, however, that the plaque does not compress. If plaque surrounds the inner diameter of the artery, it cracks at its thinnest portion

[1]Molnar W and Stockum AE: Transhepatic dilatation of choledochoenterostomy strictures, Radiology 129:59, 1978.

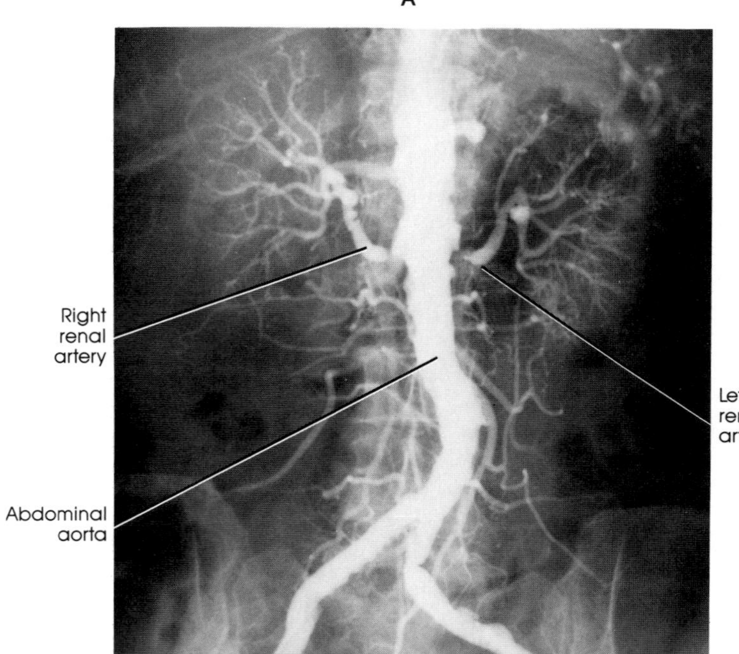

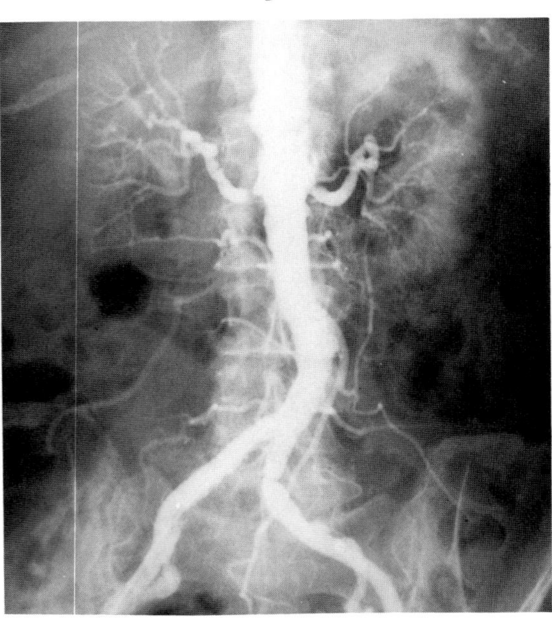

Fig. 30-77. **A,** Renal flush angiogram showing bilateral renal artery stenosis and, **B,** angiogram showing improved postangioplasty left renal artery.

as the lumen is expanded. Continued expansion cracks the arterial wall's inner layer, the intima, then stretches and tears the middle layer, the media, and finally stretches the outer layer, the adventitia. The arterial lumen is increased by permanently enlarging the artery's outer diameter. Restenosis, when it occurs, is usually caused by deposits of new plaque, not arterial wall collapse.

In addition to balloon angioplasty, other angioplasty technologies treat atherosclerotic disease. Some of these technologies involve the use of lasers. In laser-tipped angioplasty, laser energy is directed through a special catheter and pulsed at the atheromatous mass to vaporize it. It leaves a smooth, carbonized surface up to 5 mm in diameter, which is somewhat larger than the catheter tip. In thermal angioplasty a laser-heated probe is advanced through an atheroma to recanalize the vessel lumen. It also creates a smoother surface than balloon angioplasty, resulting in less restenosis at the lesion site. Sometimes, a balloon angioplasty procedure follows lumen recanalization to further expand the vessel lumen.

Percutaneous atherectomy is an angioplasty technology that removes an atheroma by cutting it. The Kensey catheter system has a blunt cam at the distal tip of the catheter that rotates at speeds up to 100,000 rpm. A fluid mixture is infused through the catheter as the cam rotates, creating a radial fluid spray. Together, the rotating cam and fluid spray cut and recirculate atherosclerotic material until it is micropulverized, while sparing normal tissue. A balloon angioplasty procedure frequently follows lumen restoration by this method. The Simpson atherectomy catheter has, at its distal end, a cylindrically shaped chamber called the housing with an opening along one side called the housing window. Opposite the housing window is a balloon that, when inflated, presses the atheromatous mass into the window. A round, rotating cutter is then advanced through the housing to cut the atheroma, which is collected in the distal housing chamber. The balloon is then deflated, and the housing window is rotated 90 degrees in the vessel. The procedure is repeated until the atheroma has been removed circumferentially from the vessel lumen.

A final possibility for percutaneous treatment of vessel stenoses is the placement of vascular stents. A vascular stent is a wire or plastic cylinder that is introduced through a catheter system and positioned across a stenosis to keep the narrowed area spread apart. These devices permanently remain in the vessel.

The success of PTA in the management of atherosclerosis has made it a significant alternative to surgical procedures as a treatment for this disease. PTA is not indicated in all cases, however. Long segments of occlusion, for example, may be best treated by surgery. PTA has a lower risk than surgery but is not risk free. Generally, patients must be able to tolerate the surgical procedure that may be required to repair vessel damage that could be caused by PTA. Unsuccessful attempts of transluminal angioplasty procedures rarely prevent, or complicate, any necessary subsequent surgery. In selected cases the procedure is effective and almost painless and can be repeated as often as necessary with no apparent increase in risk to the patient. The recovery time is often no longer than the time required to stabilize the arteriotomy site, usually a matter of hours, and general anesthesia is normally not required. Therefore the length of the hospital stay and the cost to the patient are reduced.

Although most PTA procedures occur in the radiology angiographic laboratory, angioplasty involving the arteries of the heart is generally performed in a more specialized laboratory. Percutaneous transluminal coronary angioplasty (PTCA) takes place in the cardiac catheterization laboratory because of the possibility of potentially serious cardiac complications. (See Chapter 31 for further information on PTCA.)

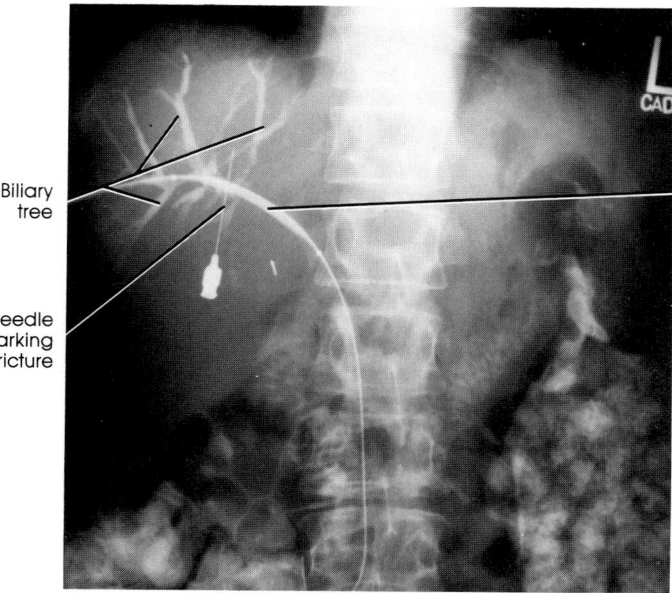

Fig. 30-78. Radiograph showing balloon catheter in common bile duct.

Transcatheter Embolization

Transcatheter embolization was first discovered by Nusbaum and Baum[1] in 1963 when they found that active bleeding in various areas of the body could be demonstrated with angiography. *Extravasated* blood when mixed with injected contrast media appears as a collection of small "pools" at the bleeding site. They later discovered that this bleeding could be adequately managed through angiographic procedures.

Transcatheter embolization involves the therapeutic introduction of various substances to occlude or drastically reduce the blood flow within a vessel. The three main purposes for embolization are (1) to stop active bleeding sites, (2) to end blood flow to diseased or malformed areas (i.e., tumors or arteriovenous malformations), and (3) to stop or reduce blood flow to a particular area of the body before surgery.

[1]Nusbaum M and Baum S: Radiographic demonstration of unknown sites of gastrointestinal bleeding, Surg Forum 14:374-375, 1963.

Patient condition and the situation must be considered when choosing an embolizing agent. The radiologist in consultation with the attending physician will usually identify the appropriate agent to be used. Embolizing agents must be administered with care to assure that they flow to the predetermined vessel. Once given, *they cannot be retrieved and their effects are irreversible*. Many types of embolizing agents exist, and their use depends on whether the occlusion is to be temporary or permanent. Table 30-1 lists some of the most widely used agents.

When the occlusion is to be temporary, for example in gastrointestinal bleeding, occlusion need only be sustained until adequate *hemostasis* occurs. Gelfoam, which is a spongelike substance that can be formed into large or small pledgets, may be used and injected into the vessel. After each Gelfoam injection, however, contrast medium injections should follow to check the progress of the occlusion. After satisfactory embolization occurs, the Gelfoam will remain intact for a number of days.

Table 30-1. Embolization agents

Permanent	Temporary
Ivalon (polyvinyl alcohol)	Gelfoam
Silicone beads	Microfibrillar collagen (Avitene)
Gianturco stainless steel coils	Vasoconstrictors (vasopressin, Pitressin)
Detachable balloons	

Vasoconstricting drugs can be used to temporarily reduce blood flow. Although vasoconstrictors, such as vasopressin (Pitressin), do not function as emboli, they drastically constrict the vessels, which results in hemostasis.

When permanent occlusion is desired, as in trauma to the pelvis that causes hemorrhage or when vascular tumors are supplied by large vessels, the Gianturco stainless steel coil is most widely used for occlusion. This coil (Fig. 30-79) is simply a looped segment of guide wire with dacron fibers attached that functions to produce *thrombogenesis*. These coils

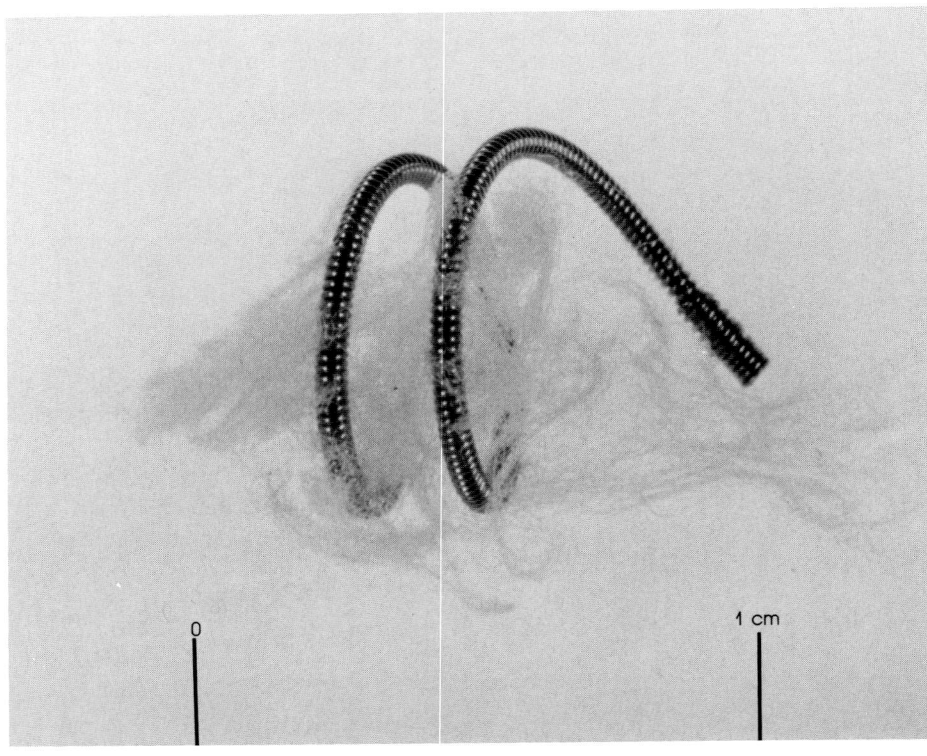

Fig. 30-79. Gianturco stainless steel occluding coil (magnified).

are initially straight and are easily introduced into a catheter that has been placed into the desired vessel. The coil is then pushed out of the catheter tip with a wire guide. The coil assumes its looping shape immediately as it enters the bloodstream. It is important that the catheter tip be specifically placed in the vessel so the coil will "spring" into precisely the desired area. Numerous coils can be "stacked" as needed to occlude the vessel.

An indication for this type of embolization is shown in the arteriogram in Fig. 30-80 where a large vascular tumor is demonstrated in the upper and middle portions of the right kidney. A significant reduction of surgical bleeding was noted in a subsequent *nephrectomy* because of the embolization therapy (Fig. 30-81).

Transcatheter embolization has also been used in the *cerebral vasculature* of the brain. *Arteriovenous malformations* within the cerebral vasculature can be managed with the use of silicone beads or tissue adhesives. Very small catheters (2 or 3 Fr.) are passed through a larger catheter that is positioned in the internal carotid artery. The smaller catheter is then manipulated into the appropriate cerebral vessel and the embolic material injected through it until sufficient embolization occurs.

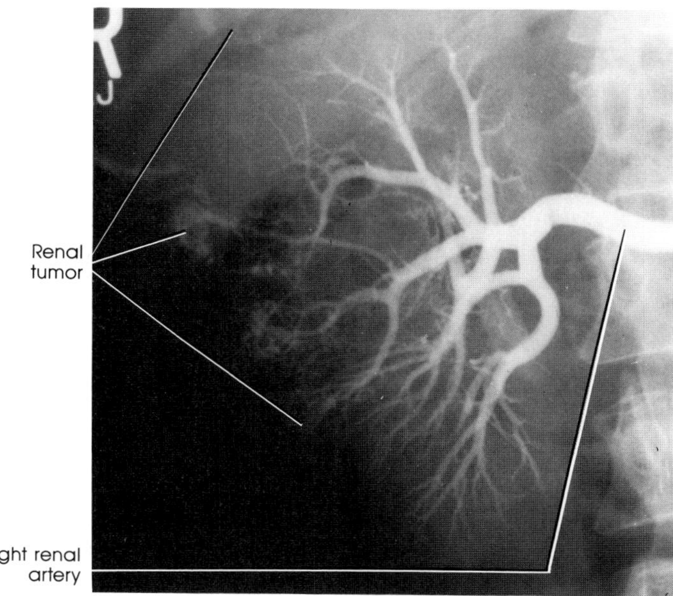

Fig. 30-80. Selective right renal arteriogram.

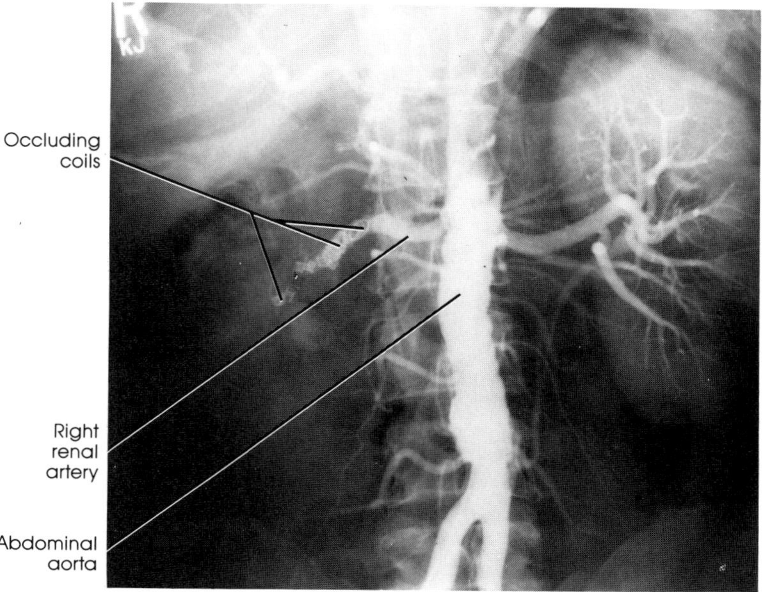

Fig. 30-81. Postembolization renal flush angiogram on same patient as in Fig. 30-80.

Percutaneous Nephrostomy Tube Placement and Related Procedures

Nephrostomy tube drainage is indicated in the patient who has some type of ureteral or bladder blockage that causes *hydronephrosis*. If urine cannot be eliminated from the kidney, renal failure with necrosis to the kidney will occur.

A nephrostomy tube is a catheter that has multiple side holes at the distal end through which urine can enter. The urine will drain into a bag connected to the proximal end of the catheter outside the patient's body. These catheters range in size from 8 to 24 Fr. and are usually about 30 cm in length. Nephrostomy tubes are also placed in patients with kidney stones to facilitate subsequent passage of ultrasonic lithotripsy catheters through the tract from the flank to the renal pelvis created by the nephrostomy tube.

The renal pelvis must be opacified to provide a target for percutaneous nephrostomy tube placement. A percutaneous nephrostogram may be performed to accomplish this. For this procedure the patient is positioned prone or in an anterior oblique position on the tabletop. The patient's back and posterolateral aspect of the affected side are prepared and surgically draped. Following the administration of a local anesthetic, a 7-inch thin-wall cannula needle is passed through the back under fluoroscopic control and the cannula is removed. The needle is examined for drainage of urine. When urine returns through the needle, the needle is injected with contrast medium to opacify the renal pelvis.

A particular calyx of the opacified renal pelvis is often selected as the target for the nephrostomy tube placement. Following administration of a local anesthetic a 7-inch cannula needle is then inserted through the posterolateral aspect of the back and directed toward the renal pelvis. A fluoroscopic C arm offers a distinct advantage for this process. The C arm can be obliqued to match the angle between the needle insertion site and the target. The needle can then be advanced directly toward the target visualized on the fluoroscopic monitor. The C arm is then obliqued 90 degrees from this angle to see if the needle tip has reached the renal pelvis or calyx. When the needle tip has entered the desired target, a wire guide is passed through the needle into the renal pelvis and is then maneuvered into the proximal ureter for additional support. The needle is then removed, the tract dilated, and the drainage catheter is passed over the wire guide and into the renal pelvis. The pigtail end of the catheter must be placed well within the renal pelvis and not outside the kidney itself or in the proximal ureter (Figs. 30-82 and 30-83). The catheter's position is maintained by attaching it to a fixation disk or other device that is then sutured or taped to the body wall. A dressing is applied over the entry site. Either the fixation device or the dressing must prevent the catheter from becoming kinked, which would prevent drainage out through the catheter. Periodic antegrade nephrostograms may be performed by injecting the drainage catheter to evaluate anatomy and the functionality of the catheter.

Nephrostomy tubes may be placed for temporary or permanent external drainage of urine. Nephrostomy tubes that are left in place for a long time need to be exchanged periodically for new ones. A wire guide is inserted through the existing catheter, and the catheter is removed, leaving the wire guide in place. A new nephrostomy tube is then passed over the wire guide and positioned in the renal

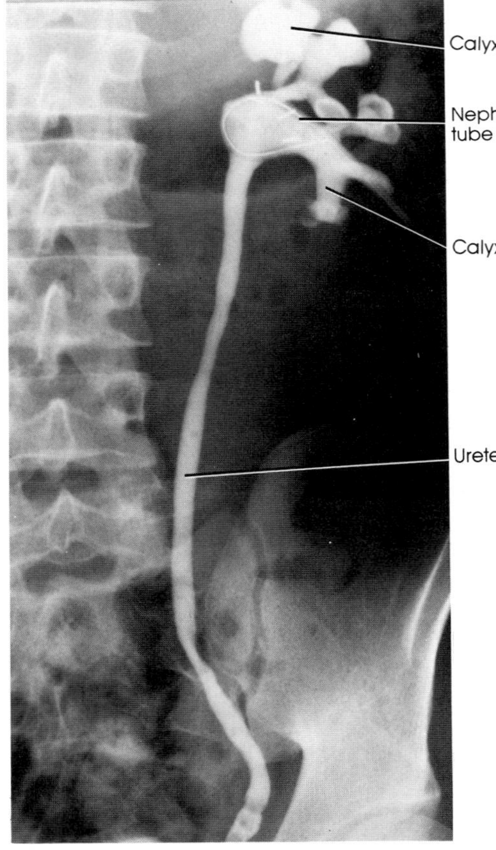

Fig. 30-82. Nephrostogram through Coop Loop drainage tube.

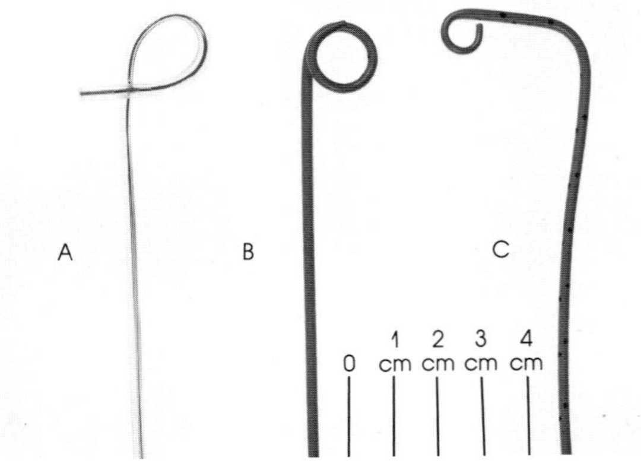

Fig. 30-83. Drainage catheters: **A,** Coop Loop nephrostomy catheter; **B,** Vance nephrostomy catheter; and, **C,** Ring biliary drainage catheter.

pelvis. Nephrostomy tubes can be permanently removed by simply pulling them out. The tract from the body wall to the renal pelvis usually closes in a day or so without complication.

In addition to nephrostomy tube placement, other *uroradiologic* procedures occur in the angiographic and interventional laboratory. *Percutaneous nephrolithotomy* offers the patient an alternative to surgical removal of kidney stones. Only stones that are relatively small can be removed by this method. Large stones may require surgery or ultrasonic lithotripsy for removal. The percutaneous nephrolithotomy procedure begins like a nephrostomy tube placement. After a wire is passed into the renal pelvis and ureter, a large tract is formed by using dilators or a balloon-tipped catheter. Then a sheath large enough to facilitate removal of the stone is placed between the renal pelvis and body wall. A stone basket or other retrieval catheter is introduced through the tract and manipulated to grasp the stone (Figs. 30-84 and 30-85). The stone is removed by withdrawing the retrieval catheter as it grasps the stone. The sheath is then also withdrawn, and a nephrostomy tube is placed in the renal pelvis to drain urine and any blood resulting from trauma from the procedure. The nephrostomy tube is eventually removed.

Angioplasty of stenoses in the ureteral system, renal cyst puncture with drainage, and percutaneous antegrade ureteral stent placement are additional procedures. A ureteral stent is a double-ended pigtail catheter that is passed into the ureter and remains inside the body, with one end placed into the renal pelvis and the other into the bladder (Fig. 30-86). This catheter is used when a constriction of the ureter or ureterovesicular junction is present, blocking the drainage of urine from the renal pelvis. The stent has multiple side holes at both pigtail ends that allow urine to drain into one end and exit the other end. The stent provides an internal passageway for urine across the area of blockage. Usually a nephrostomy tube is initially placed to provide access to the renal pelvis and to allow a tract to form in the body. At a later time a wire guide is passed through the nephrostomy tube and down the ureter into the bladder. The nephrostomy tube is removed and the stent is inserted over the wire guide using a catheter-like pusher. Usually a nephrostomy tube is replaced to provide external drainage until it is known that the stent is providing internal drainage. These stents can usually be removed through the urethra by a cystoscopic procedure.

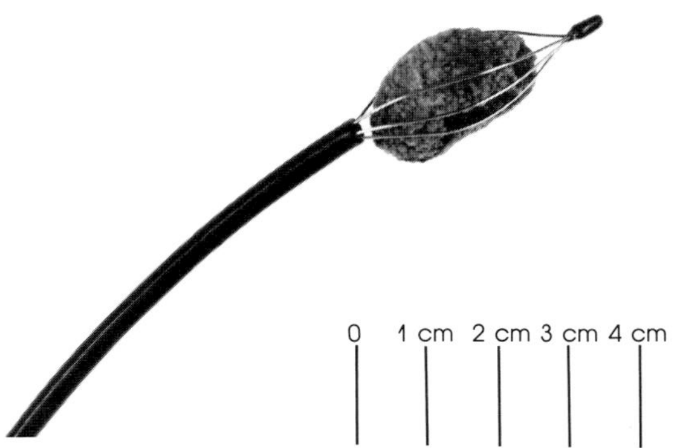

Fig. 30-84. Retrieval catheter and basket with large renal stone.

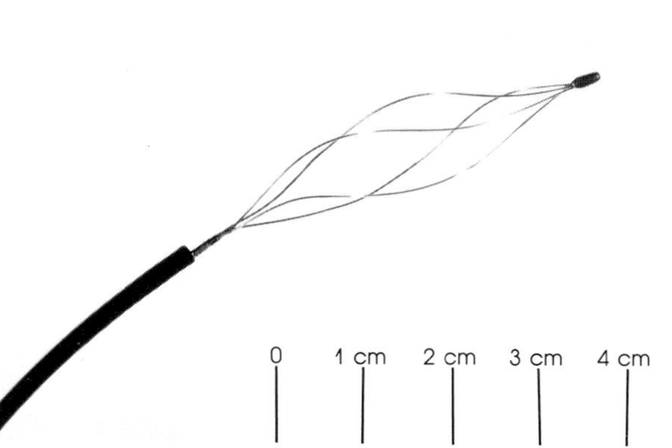

Fig. 30-85. Retrieval catheter with stone basket extended.

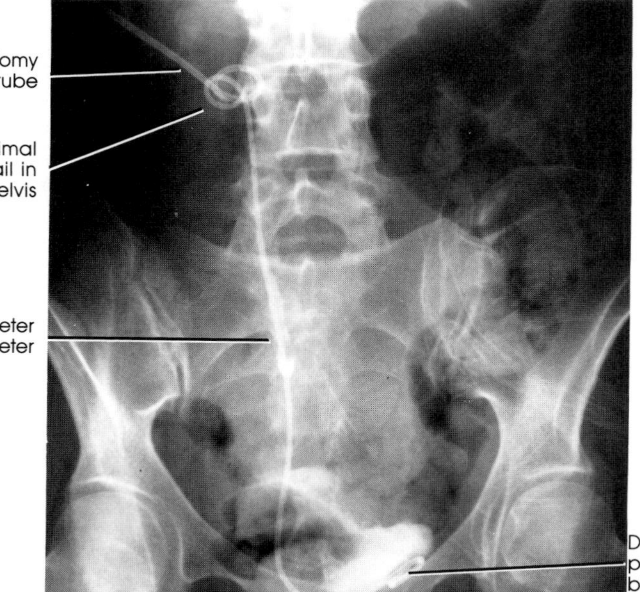

Fig. 30-86. Postplacement radiograph of ureteral stent.

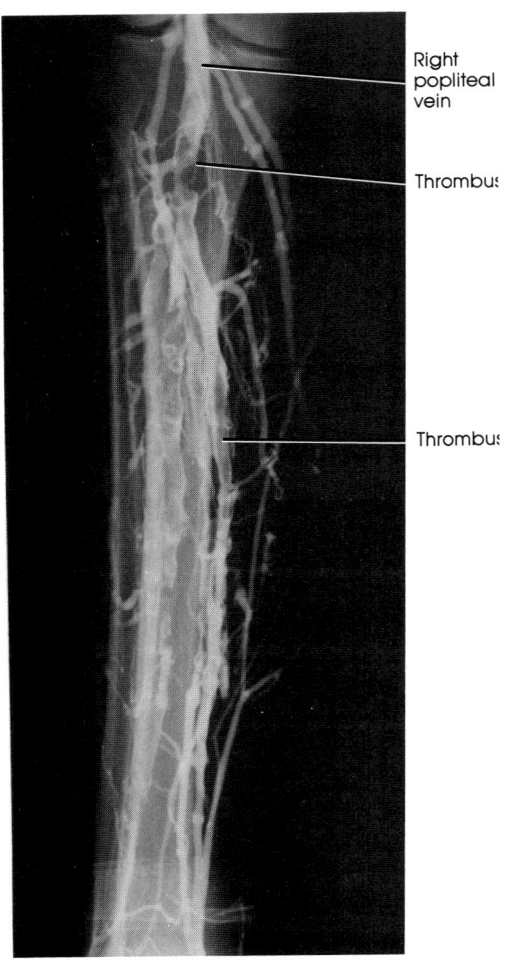

Fig. 30-87. Lower limb venogram.

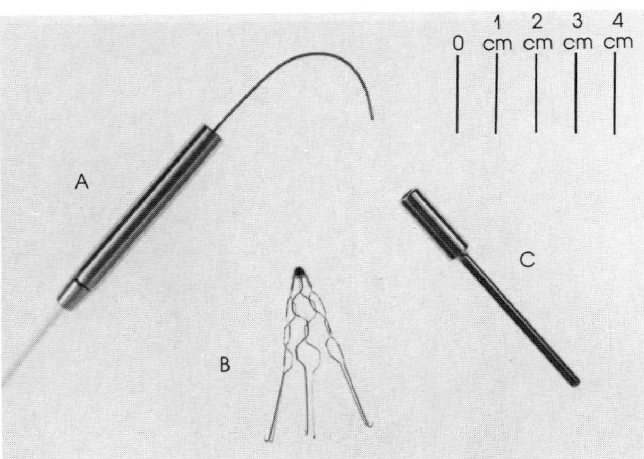

Fig. 30-88. A, Distal end of introducer catheter with guide wire. **B,** Greenfield vena cava filter. **C,** Loader device.

Inferior Vena Caval Filter Placement

As discussed earlier in this chapter, pulmonary angiography primarily evaluates embolic disease of the lungs. A pulmonary embolus is usually a blood clot, but it does not form in the lungs. Instead, it forms as a *thrombus,* usually in the deep veins of the leg (Fig. 30-87). When such a thrombus becomes dislodged and migrates, it is called an *embolus*. An embolus originating in the leg may migrate through the inferior vena cava and right side of the heart and finally lodge in the pulmonary arteries. A filter can be percutaneously placed in the inferior vena cava to trap such an embolus.

Lower limb vein thrombosis is not necessarily an indication for inferior vena caval filter placement. Normally, blood-thinning medications are administered to treat deep vein thrombosis. When such anticoagulant therapy is contraindicated because of hemorrhaging or the risk of hemorrhaging, filter placement may be indicated. The filter placement itself has associated risks. They include thrombosis of the vein through which the filter is introduced and caval thrombosis, but these risks are normally not life threatening after the placement of a filter. It is important to note that inferior vena caval filter placement is not a treatment for deep venous thrombosis of the leg but a therapy intended to reduce the chance of pulmonary embolism.

Inferior vena caval filters are available in a variety of forms. All of these filters are initially compact inside an introducer catheter device and assume their functional shape as they are released (Fig. 30-88). The introducers are passed through sheaths ranging in size from 9 to 29 Fr.

The filters are made of inert metals and most are designed for permanent placement. The Kimray-Greenfield filter is composed of eight legs joined at the apex to form a conical shape. Each leg has a hook on the end that engages the wall of the vena cava. The LGM filter is similar to the Kimray-Greenfield filter, but each leg ends with a side rail that is parallel to the wall of the vena cava. The side rails have barbs to hold the filter in place. The Gianturco-Roehm bird's nest filter consists of a bundle of fine wire anchored on each end by hook wire struts. The Gunther filter has four anchoring struts inferiorly and a spiral basket superiorly. The Simon Nitinol filter is made of a wire that has thermal memory. This allows the device, which is very compact in its introducer, to achieve a completely different shape when placed in the body temperature environment of the vena cava. Inferiorly, it has six struts resembling a Kimray-Greenfield filter, and, superiorly, it has seven overlapping pedals for additional clot-trapping capability. The Amplatz filter consists of 12 struts joined at the inferior aspect to form an inverted cone shape. The Amplatz and Gunther filters are removable. They have a hook on the bottom that allows them to be grasped by a catheter snare device and removed percutaneously. They must be removed within about 10 days, or they will become permanently attached to the vena caval endothelium. Inferior vena caval filter development is changing rapidly, and new designs will certainly become available.

The filters are percutaneously inserted through a femoral or jugular vein, usually for placement in the inferior vena cava just inferior to the renal veins. Placement inferior to the renal veins is important to avoid risking renal vein thrombosis. An inferior vena cavogram is performed using the Seldinger technique, usually from the right femoral vein approach. The inferior vena cavogram defines the anatomy, including the level of the renal veins, and rules out the presence of a thrombus (Fig. 30-89). A filter insertion from the jugular approach may be indicated if a thrombus is present in the inferior vena cava. The filter insertion site, usually the right femoral vein site from the inferior vena cavogram, is dilated to accommodate the filter introducer. After the filter is placed, the introducing system is removed and external compression is applied to the venotomy site until hemorrhage ceases. A postplacement plain radiograph is obtained to document the location of the filter (Fig. 30-90).

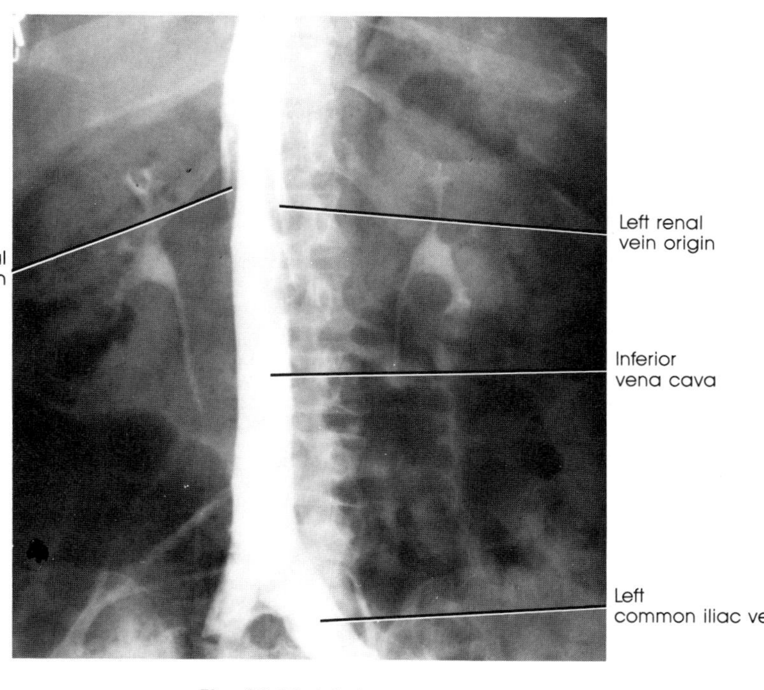

Fig. 30-89. Inferior vena cavogram.

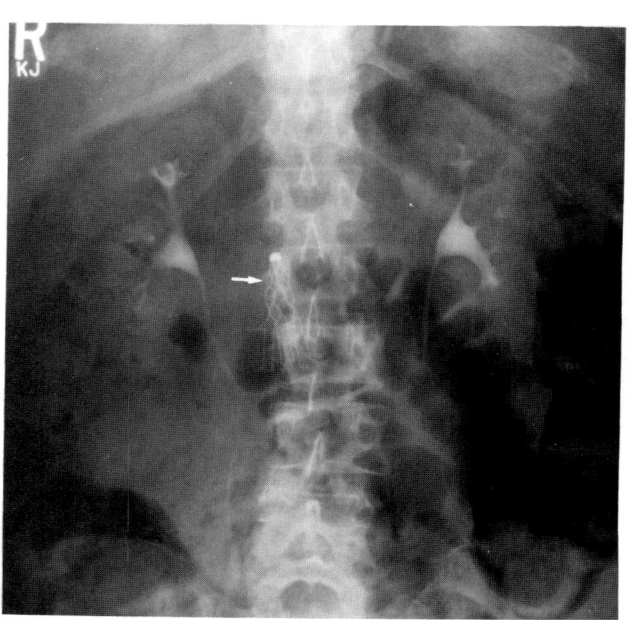

Fig. 30-90. Postplacement radiograph showing vena cava filter in place *(arrow)*.

Other Procedures

When an arteriogram demonstrates thrombosis, the procedure may be continued for thrombolytic therapy. Blood clot–dissolving medications can be infused through an angiographic catheter positioned against the thrombus. Special infusion catheters that have side holes may be manipulated directly into the clot. Periodic repeat arteriograms evaluate the progress of lysis. The catheter may need to be advanced under fluoroscopic control to keep it against or in the clot as lysis progresses.

Catheters can also be used to percutaneously remove foreign bodies, such as catheter fragments, from vasculature. A variety of snares are available for this purpose. The snare catheter is introduced using the Seldinger technique and manipulated under fluoroscopic control to grasp the foreign body. Then the snare and foreign body are withdrawn as a unit.

Interventional radiologic procedures are also performed in the biliary system and include biliary drainage and biliary stone removal. For more information see the section on the biliary tract in Volume 2, Chapter 16 of this atlas.

Interventional Radiology: Present and Future

Interventional procedures bring therapeutic capabilities into the hands of the radiologist. Procedures that are done initially for diagnosis can be extended, using the same basic techniques, to perform therapeutic processes. New equipment is continuously becoming available to improve techniques and broaden the scope of percutaneous intervention. Although use of the catheter for angiographic diagnosis may wane, its ability to provide therapy percutaneously ensures a future for angiography.

Lymphography is a general term applied to radiologic examinations of the lymph vessels and nodes (Figs. 30-91 and 30-92) after they have been opacified by an injected iodinated contrast medium. The study of the lymph vessels, which may be called *lymphangiography,* is carried out within the first hour after injection of the contrast material. The study of the lymph nodes, which may be called *lymphadenography,* is made 24 hours after injection of the contrast medium. The lymph vessels empty the contrast agent within a few hours. The nodes normally retain the contrast substance for 3 to 4 weeks. Abnormal nodes may retain the medium for several months, so that delayed lymphadenograms may be made, as indicated, without further injection.

PURPOSE

The primary indication for lymphography is to assess the clinical extent of lymphomas. Lymphography may also be indicated in patients in whom there is clinical evidence of obstruction or other impairment of the lymphatic system.

CONTRAST MEDIA

Lymphography is currently performed with the use of an iodinated oil contrast medium and by the direct-injection technique developed by Kinmonth, Harper, and Taylor.[1] A water-soluble, iodinated contrast medium may be used to delineate the lymphatic vessels and nodes of the limbs, but these agents are miscible with lymph and undergo dilution, and they diffuse out through the lymphatic walls so rapidly that they cannot be used to study the proximal lymphatics.

The oily contrast medium currently employed is ethiodized oil (Ethiodol). This agent affords opacification of the lymphatic vessels for several hours after the injection. The lymph nodes are outlined on the studies of the vessels, but their internal structure does not become optimally opacified until about 24 hours later.

[1]Kinmonth JB, Harper RAK, and Taylor GW: Lymphangiography by radiologic methods, J Fac Radiologists 6:217-223, 1955.

DYE SUBSTANCE

Ordinarily the peripheral lymphatic vessels cannot be easily identified because of their small size and lack of color. For identification of the lymphatic vessels on the dorsum of the feet and hands, a blue dye that is selectively absorbed by the lymphatics is injected subcutaneously into the first and second interdigital web spaces about 15 minutes before the examination. The dyes frequently used for this purpose are 11% patent blue violet and 4% sky blue.

Following patent blue violet injection, the patient's urine and skin will be tinted blue. This condition disappears within a few hours.

PRECAUTIONS

As in any procedure involving injection of foreign materials, untoward reactions must be anticipated. The patient must be observed closely, and appropriate medications and resuscitation equipment must be nearby.

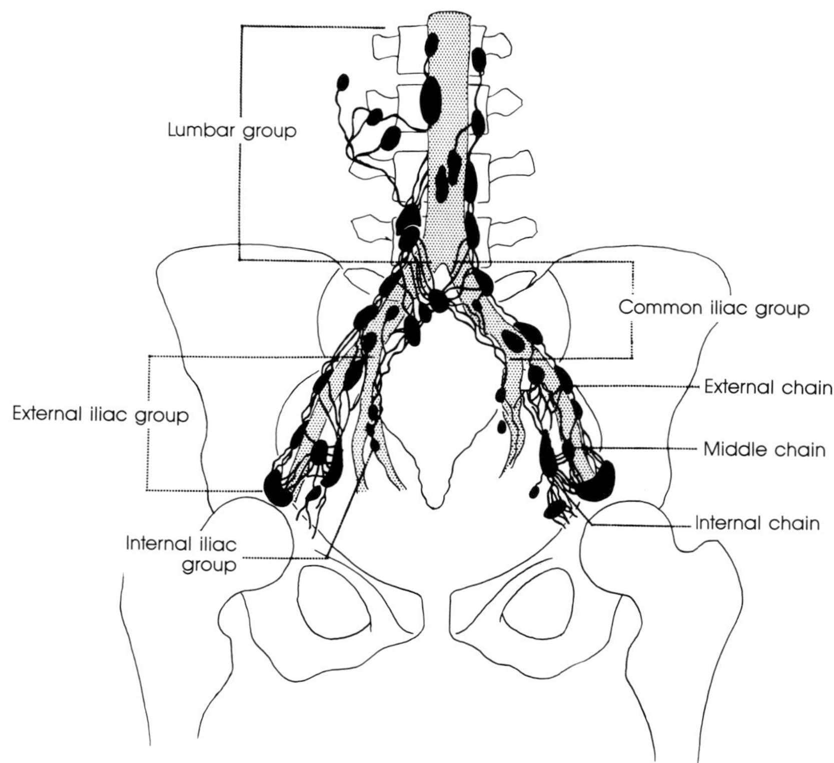

Fig. 30-91. Iliopelvic-aortic lymphatic system (after Cuneo and Marcille). Anterior projection.

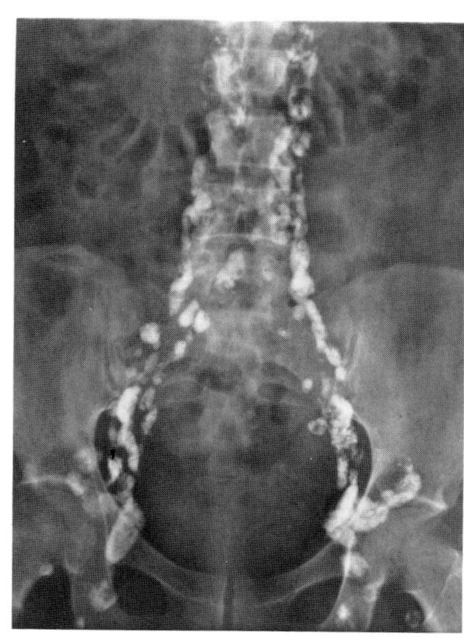

Fig. 30-92. AP projection of iliopelvic-abdominoaortic lymph nodes.

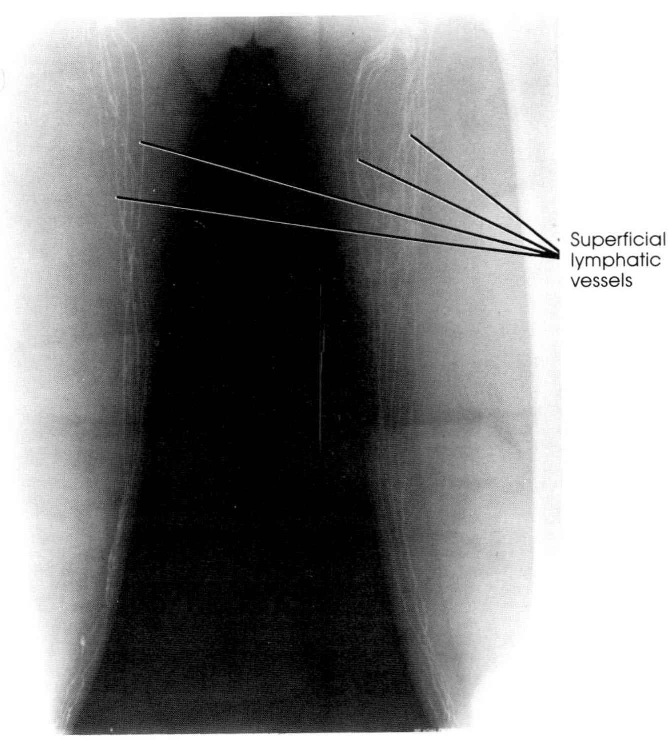

Fig. 30-93. Superficial lymphatics of thigh taken 10 minutes after completion of dorsal pedal lymphatic injection.

INJECTION SITES

Lymphography is limited to easily accessible injection sites—the lymphatics of the feet and of the hands. Most examinations are performed by injection of the lymphatics of the feet. This injection route provides visualization of the lymphatic structures of the lower limb, the groin, the iliopelvic-abdominoaortic region, and the thoracic duct. Injection of the lymphatics of the hand provides visualization of the upper limb and of the axillary, infraclavicular, and supraclavicular regions.

FILMING PROCEDURE

Radiographs are made within the first hour after completion of the injection for the demonstration of the lymph vessels (Fig. 30-93). A second series of radiographs, which may include tomographic studies, is made 24 hours later to demonstrate the lymph nodes.

The exposure factors employed for lymphographic studies are the same as those used for bone studies of the respective region.

Tomography and magnification radiography are other techniques sometimes required to obtain better delineation of the opacified lymph nodes.

Lymphatic Injection of Feet

Preceding the examination, the feet must be thoroughly washed, and the areas about the sites of injection must be shaved. The patient is placed in the supine position for the injection procedure and is so kept until the lymphangiographic studies have been completed. The injection need not be made in a radiographic examining room; it may be carried out in an operating room, and the patient may be on a padded stretcher, ready for conveyance to the radiology department.

Both feet are surgically cleansed and draped. The blue dye is injected subcutaneously into the first and second interdigital web spaces of each foot to stain the lymph for identification of the lymphatic vessels. The dye may be mixed with a local anesthetic to minimize the pain of the injections.

About 15 minutes after the injection of the blue dye, a local anesthetic (1% lidocaine) is injected subcutaneously in an amount sufficient to distend the tissues overlying the body of the first metatarsal, which is the site of cutdown for exposure and cannulation of the lymphatic vessel. A small (2 cm), longitudinal incision is made over the body of the first metatarsal immediately lateral to the extensor tendon of the great toe. (Some physicians advocate a transverse incision at this site.) The dye-filled lymphatic vessel is seen as a fine blue vessel in the subcutaneous tissue. The vessel is dissected free of surrounding tissue and is then cannulated with a 27- or 30-gauge needle connected to polyethylene tubing. The needle is tied securely in the vessel, and the tubing is connected to the syringe containing the contrast medium. An automatic injection device is used. A total of 6 ml of the contrast medium is slowly injected into each lower limb over a period of 30 minutes.

Confirmation that the injection is intralymphatic and not intravenous may be determined fluoroscopically or radiographically. After completion of the injection, the needle is removed, the overlying skin incision closed with interrupted silk sutures, and a dressing applied. The lymphatic vessel is not ligated or disturbed in any way. The patient, still in the supine position, is prepared for filming (Fig. 30-94).

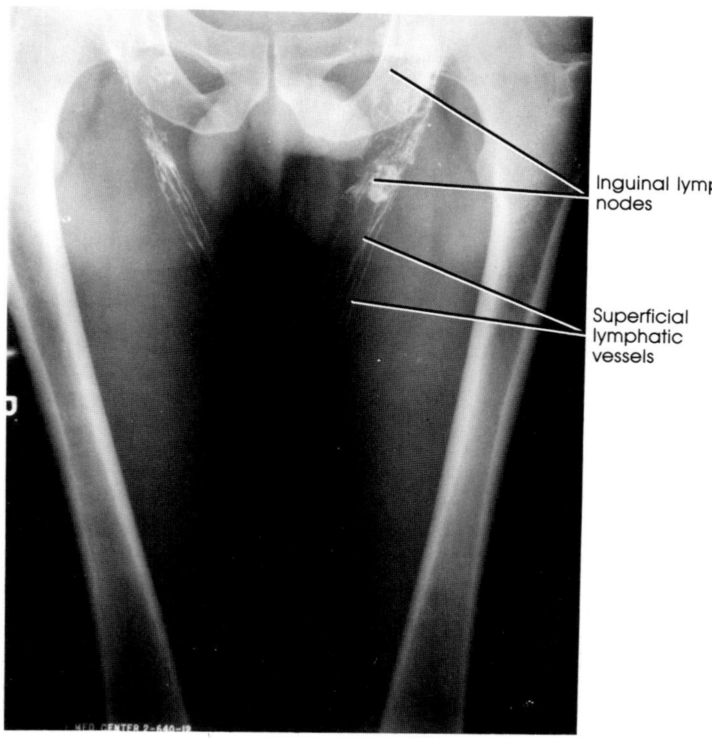

Fig. 30-94. Delayed radiograph of same patient as in Fig. 30-93. Superficial lymphatic vessels of thigh are opacified, and contrast medium is in superficial inguinal lymph node group.

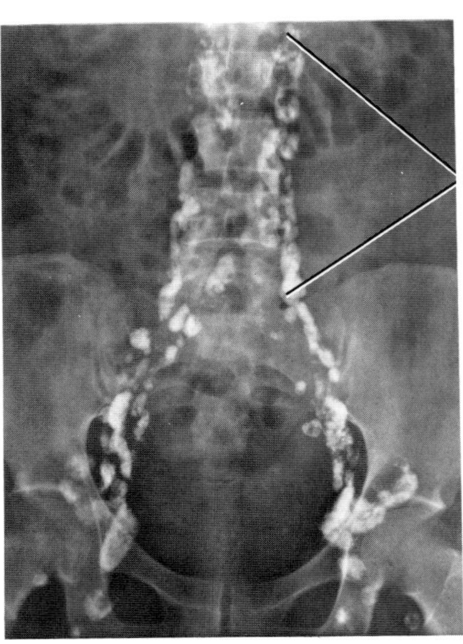

Fig. 30-95. Normal AP lymphangiogram.

ILIOPELVIC-ABDOMINOAORTIC REGION

Three radiographs, AP and 30-degree right and left AP oblique images, are taken for each of the two iliopelvic-abdominoaortic studies. The "lymphangiograms" are taken within the first hour after injection of the contrast medium (Figs. 30-95 and 30-96). These radiographs show the contrast medium within the lymph vessels that run concurrently with the femoral and iliac arteries, veins, and nerves, as well as the lymph vessels in the paraspinal areas. After the contrast medium has concentrated in the lymph nodes 24 hours later, "lymphadenograms" are taken (Fig. 30-97).

All radiographs are recorded on 14 × 17 inch (35 × 43 cm) films positioned to include the lower border of the ischium. The central ray is directed vertically and centered at the level of the iliac crests.

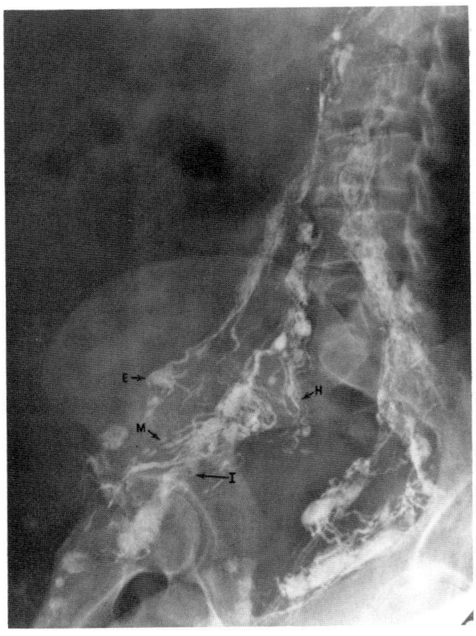

Fig. 30-96. Lymphangiogram of iliopelvic-aortic region. Right AP oblique position showing external chain, *E,* middle chain, *M,* and internal chain, *I,* of external and common iliac groups. *H,* Internal iliac group.

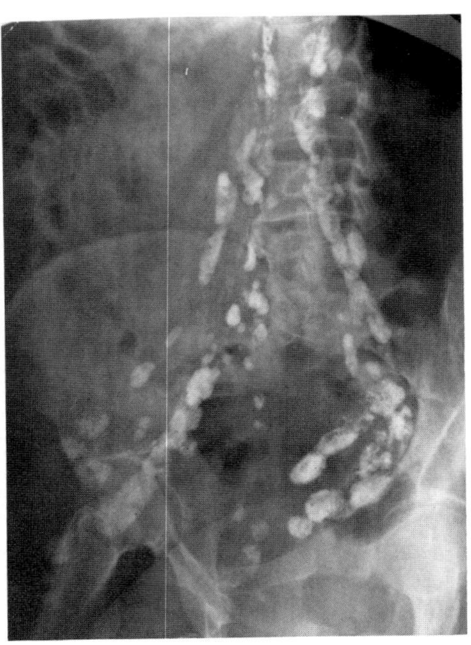

Fig. 30-97. Lymphadenogram 24 hours later of same patient as in Figs. 30-95 and 30-96.

THORACIC DUCT

Two radiographs, AP and left lateral images, are made for each of two serial studies of the thoracic duct. The contrast medium remains in the thoracic duct for less than an hour after completion of the injection; thus the studies must be timed accordingly (Fig. 30-98).

The exposures are made on 14 × 17 inch (35 × 43 cm) films that are adjusted to place the upper margin of the film 2 inches (5 cm) above the supraclavicular region. The central ray is directed perpendicularly to the midpoint of the film.

LOWER LIMB

Three AP projections, centered respectively at the level of the midtibias, the level of midfemora, and for the groin at the level of the symphysis pubis, may be taken for the demonstration of the lymphatic vessels. Radiographs are taken for the demonstration of the lymph nodes of the lower limbs 24 hours later.

The exposures are made on 14 × 17 inch (35 × 43 cm) films, and the central ray is directed vertically (Figs. 30-99 and 30-100).

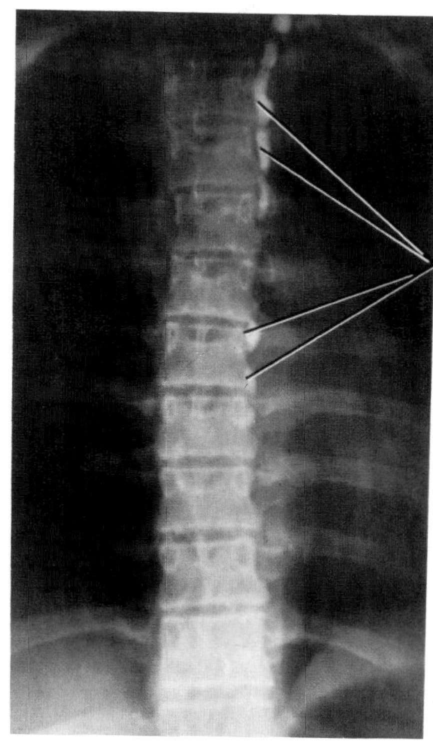

Fig. 30-98. AP projection showing opacification of superior portion of thoracic duct. Segmented appearance is caused by valves in lymph vessels.

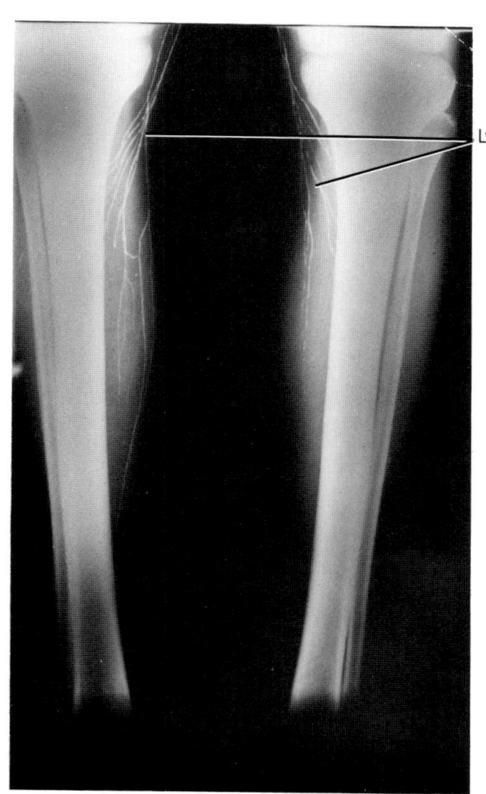

Fig. 30-99. Lymphangiogram of legs 10 minutes after injection.

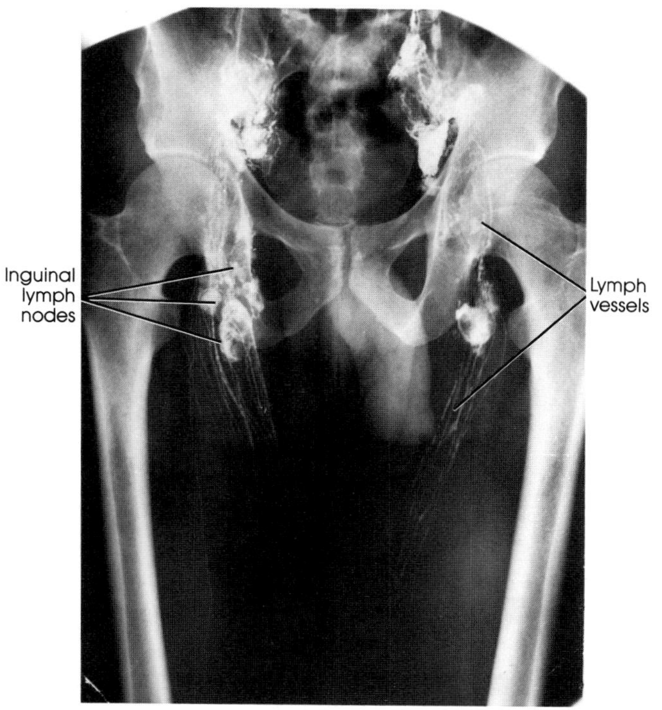

Fig. 30-100. Lymphangiogram of inguinal region and upper thighs.

Lymphatic Injection of Hand

The general procedure for lymphatic injection of the hand is the same as for the feet. Blue dye is injected into the dorsal surface of the first and second interdigital web spaces. A longitudinal skin incision is made on the dorsum of the hand, parallel to and on the ulnar side of the tendon of the musculus extensor pollicis longus over the base of the first or second metacarpal. A 30-gauge needle is used for cannulation. Four milliliters of the contrast medium is injected. This quantity is sufficient to visualize the lymphatics of the upper extremity and the lymph nodes of the axilla.

UPPER LIMB

AP and lateral images are taken on 14 × 17 inch (35 × 43 cm) films for the lymphangiograms and the later lymphadenograms of the arm and forearm. The films are placed diagonally to include the greatest length of the limb. The central ray is directed vertically and is centered to the elbow (Fig. 30-101).

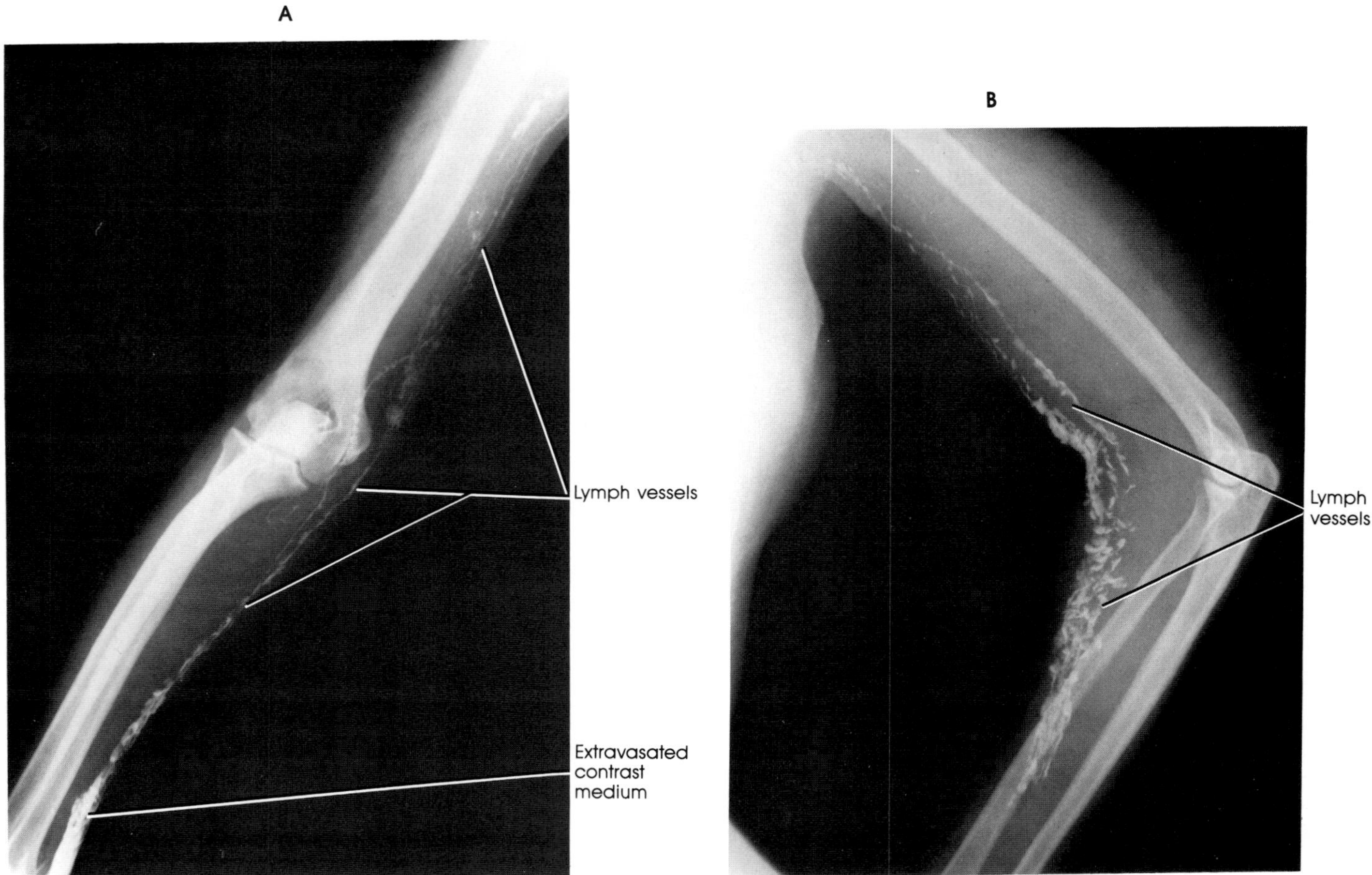

Fig. 30-101. A, AP and, **B,** lateral lymphangiograms of upper limb, showing fluting of vessels and extravasation of contrast medium.

AXILLA

AP and 45-degree AP oblique images are taken for each series of studies of the axilla. These studies may be made on 11 × 14 inch (30 × 35 cm) films that are adjusted to include the supraclavicular region. The central ray is directed vertically and is centered to the region of the coracoid process (Fig. 30-102).

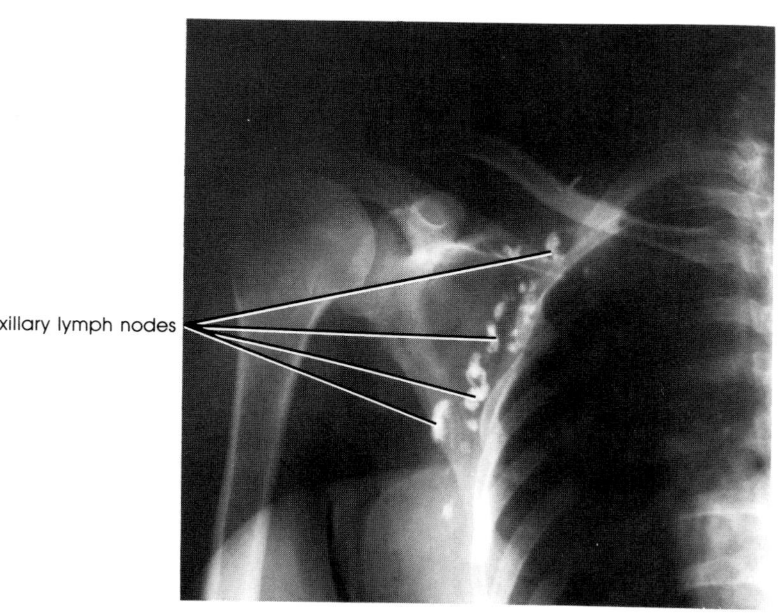

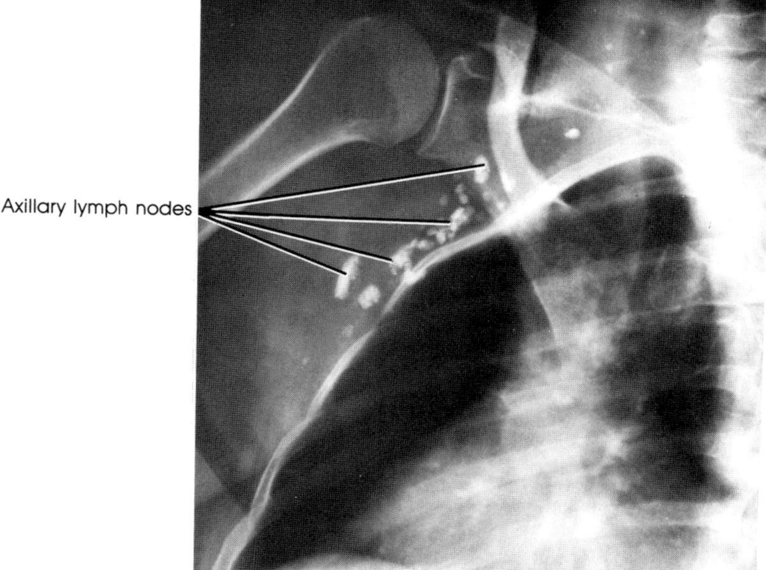

Fig. 30-102. A, Frontal and, **B,** oblique lymphadenograms of axilla.

Photographic subtraction, introduced by Ziedses des Plantes,[1] is a technique by which bone structure images are subtracted, or canceled out, from a film of the bones plus opacified vessels, leaving an unobscured image of the vessels. The technique can be applied in all forms of angiography, wherever the vessels are superimposed in bone structures.

With the increasing popularity of digital subtraction angiography (see Chapter 36), the use of photographic subtraction has decreased in many institutions. However, photographic subtraction remains relatively widely used and, in some cases, is increasing in popularity. One such area of increasing frequency occurs in evaluation of joint replacements (see discussion of contrast arthrography, Volume 1, Chapter 12 of this atlas).

[1]Ziedses des Plantes BG: Subtraktion: eine roentgenographische Methode zur separaten Abbildung bestimmter Tiele des Objekts, Fortschr Roentgenstr 52:69-79, 1935.

The purpose of subtraction in angiography and other specialized procedures is to fully define all vessels containing contrast material and at the same time eliminate the confusing overlying bone images. Following are a few terms that pertain to the subtraction technique:

registration Matching of one image over another so that bony landmarks are *precisely* superimposed. When so arranged, films are taped together to prevent slippage. Composites discussed herein may involve two or more films.

reversal film (also called a **positive mask** or **diapositive**) Reverse-tone duplicate of x-ray image, showing black changed to white and white to black. This positive transparency is obtained by exposing single-emulsion film through traditional x-ray film.

zero, or base, film (also called the **control film**) This film must show bone structures only, and there must be *no patient motion* whatever between it and subsequent contrast studies. For these reasons, zero film is exposed just before contrast medium is injected into vessels.

EQUIPMENT AND MATERIALS

Items needed for subtraction include the following:

1. A contact printer similar to the one illustrated in Fig. 30-103. Several units are available that can also be used to duplicate radiographs.
2. Radiographic processing facilities.
3. A horizontally oriented illuminator for registration of images.
4. Films:
   a. Subtraction *mask* film for making the reversal masks.
   b. Subtraction *print* film for making photographic prints of the final subtracted image.

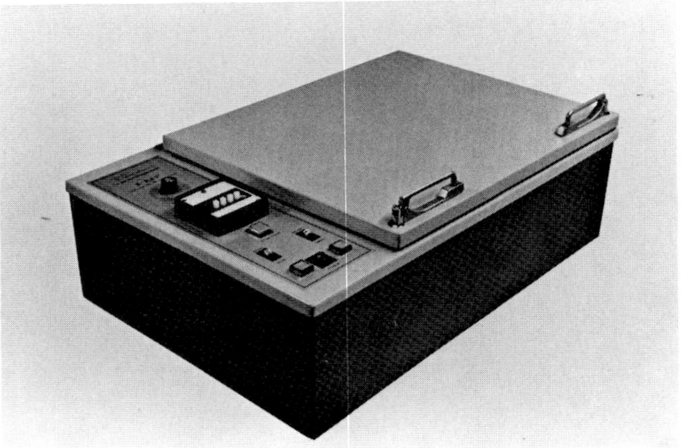

Fig. 30-103. Contact printer such as that used during exposure steps in producing subtraction prints.

First-Order Subtraction

The simplest method of photographic subtraction is called *first-order subtraction* (Fig. 30-104) and consists of obtaining a positive mask, or reversal, of the first film (zero film) of the angiographic series (the one that does not contain contrast material). When the reversal mask is superimposed over a film in the series that contains contrast material, the positive and negative images of the bones tend to cancel each other out, and only the vessels can be seen. The vessels are not canceled out because they were present on only one film—the one containing the contrast material. A contact printer makes a print of this combination of films.

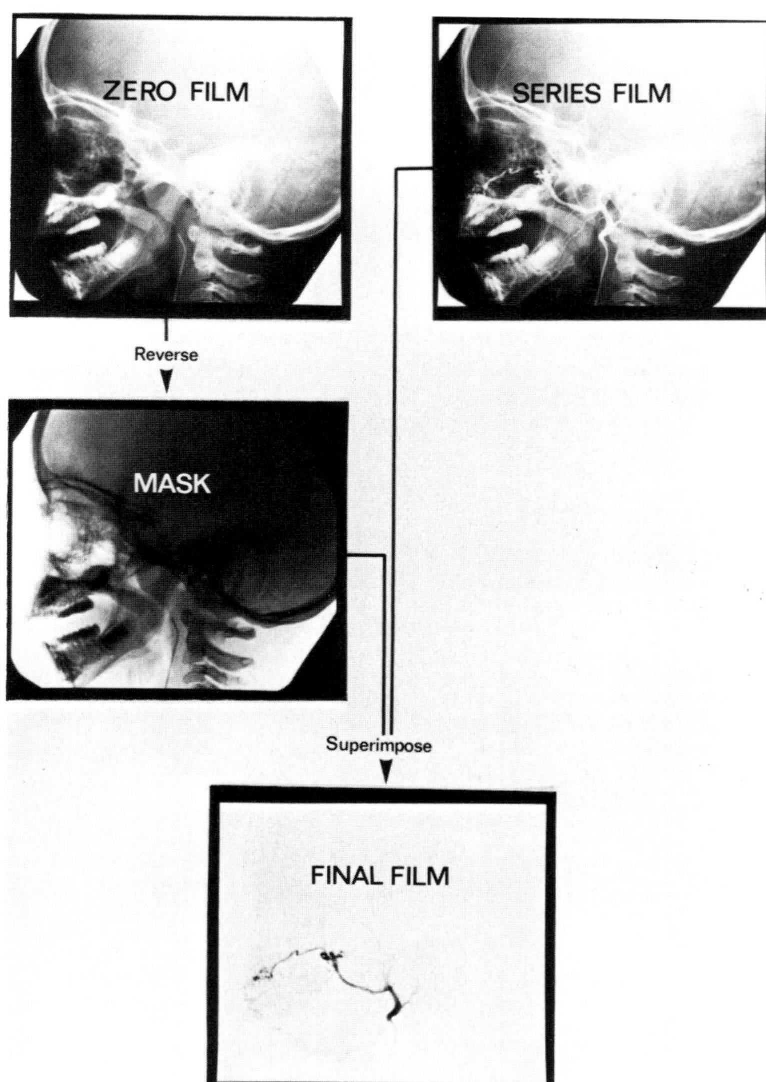

Fig. 30-104. First-order subtraction process.

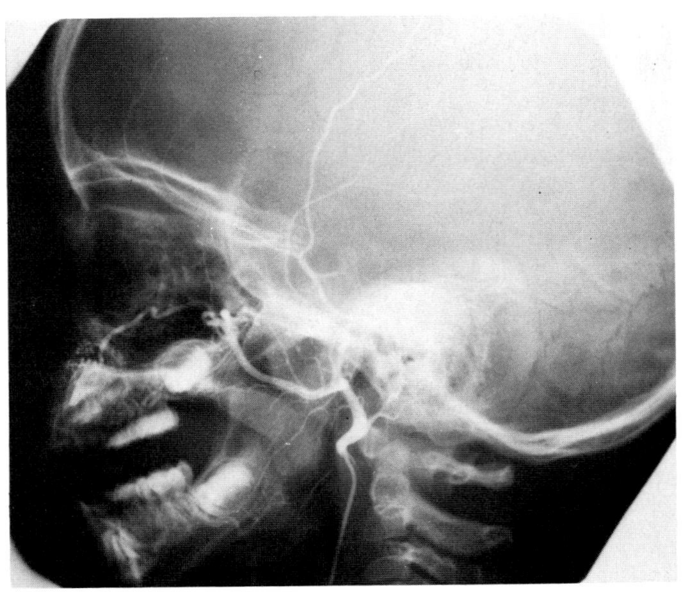

Fig. 30-105. Angiographic series radiograph.

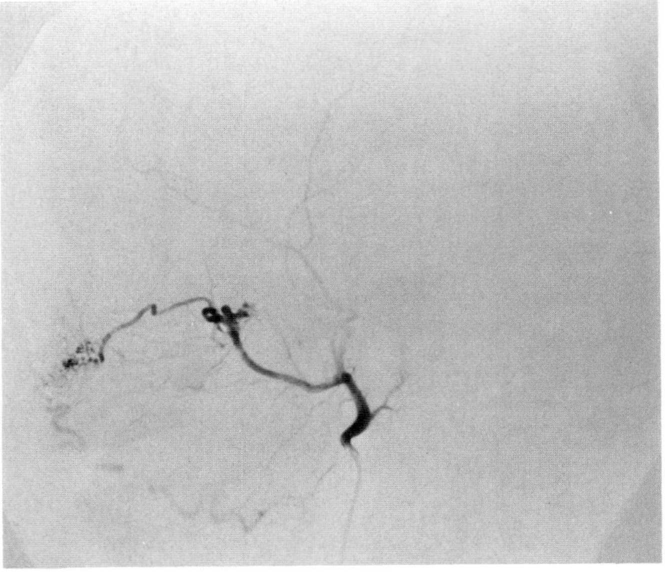

Fig. 30-106. First-order subtraction print.

FIRST-ORDER SUBTRACTION PROCEDURE

Step 1

In a darkroom the nonemulsion side of the sheet of subtraction mask film is placed in contact with the *zero film* and is exposed for approximately 5 seconds* to light. When processed, this becomes the *mask*.

Step 2

On a light box, the *mask* is carefully registered over the selected *series film* (Fig. 30-105). The two are taped securely together.

Step 3

In the darkroom the *mask-series film* combination is placed in contact with the emulsion side of a sheet of subtraction print film, which is then exposed for approximately 5 seconds* to light. This produces the final subtraction image (Fig. 30-106).

*Time will vary according to equipment and material used.

Second-Order Subtraction

The reversal of the zero film obtained in the first-order subtraction is usually not the exact reversal of the density of the selected angiographic film; thus the subtraction result is imperfect. The imperfection can be corrected with what is called *second-order subtraction*. This process involves producing another film, called a *secondary* or *correction mask*, which compensates for the slight differences. Hanafee and Shinno[1] led the way toward this improved subtraction method. Their method of second-order subtraction consists of superimposing the zero film on its own reversal mask. The additional print that results from the transmission of light through the two films, which in theory would be the exact opposite of each other, produces a faint radiographic image that corrects for the small "photographic mistake" between the first two. The reversal of the zero film, the correction film, and the film containing contrast material are carefully registered; this combination is then exposed to obtain the final subtraction print.

A further advancement toward the goal of complete subtraction was published by Sucher and Strand in 1974.[2] This second-order subtraction modification is called *composite-mask subtraction* or *white-over-white* technique. When correctly applied, this technique approaches almost total elimination of both bony structure and soft tissue, leaving a display of the vessels in high-contrast reproduction (Fig. 30-107).

[1]Hanafee W and Shinno JM: Second-order subtraction with simultaneous bilateral carotid, internal carotid injections, Radiology 86:334-341, 1966.
[2]Sucher DL and Strand RD: Composite mask subtraction, white over white technique, Radiology 113:470-472, 1974.

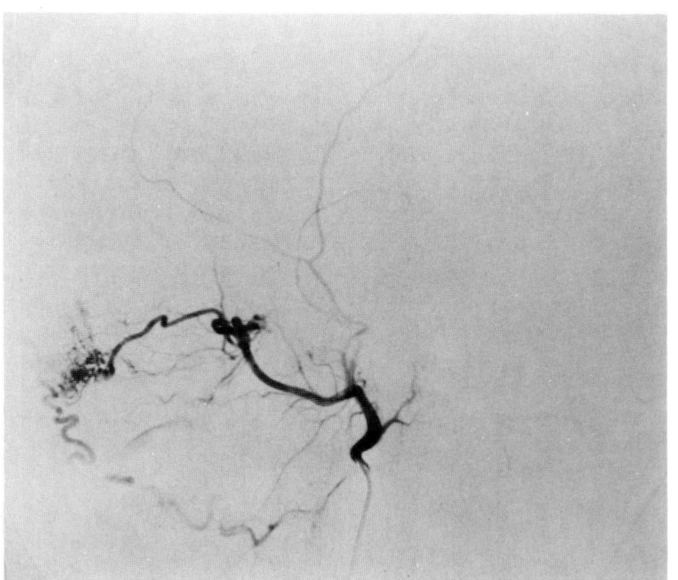

Fig. 30-107. Composite-mask, white-over-white technique. Bone has been completely removed, allowing improved visualization of vessels.

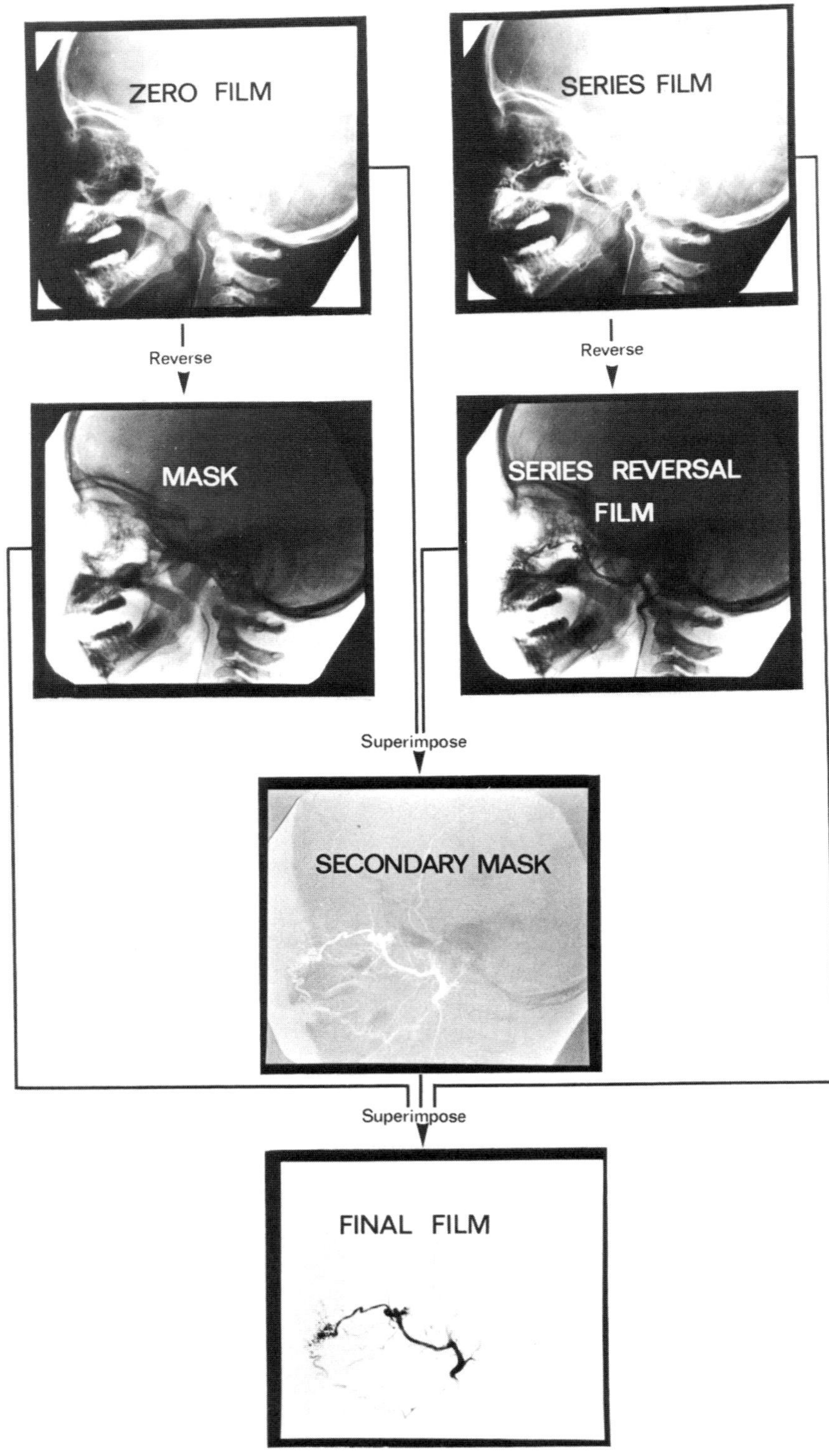

Fig. 30-108. Composite-mask subtraction process.

COMPOSITE-MASK SUBTRACTION PROCEDURE

The following steps may be followed by referring to Fig. 30-108.

Step 1

In a darkroom the nonemulsion side of a sheet of subtraction mask film is placed in contact with the *zero film* and is exposed for approximately 5 seconds* to light. When processed this becomes the *mask*.

Step 2

In a darkroom the emulsion side of a sheet of subtraction mask film is placed in contact with the selected angiographic *series film,* which is then exposed to light. This process produces the series reversal film.

Step 3

On a light box the *series reversal film* is carefully registered with the *zero film,* and the two are securely taped together.

Step 4

In a darkroom the *zero–series reversal film* combination is placed in contact with the emulsion side of a sheet of subtraction mask film and is exposed for approximately 20 seconds* to light. This process produces the *secondary mask*.

Step 5

On a light box the *series film* and the *mask* are carefully registered and taped securely. To this composite the *secondary mask* is carefully registered and taped.

*Time will vary according to equipment and material used.

Step 6

In a darkroom the *series film–mask–secondary mask* combination is placed in contact with the emulsion side of a sheet of subtraction print film and is exposed for approximately 35 seconds* to light. The final subtraction image is thus produced.

A comparison of second-order subtraction with composite-mask subtraction shows the steps to be almost identical. The only procedural difference is that in second-order subtraction the secondary mask is made by registering the zero film and the *zero reversal mask*. In composite-mask subtraction, the zero film and the angiographic *series reversal film* are superimposed to produce the secondary mask. Although the procedures are similar, the composite-mask subtraction technique is recommended when increased resolution is required.

In recent years marked advancement has been made by the production of films specifically designed for subtraction. In addition to the advantage of 90-second processing, these films often allow subtractions of adequate or even excellent quality to be made with the single-order subtraction technique. Composite-mask subtraction is recommended only when small structures require increased definition for visualization or when illustrations of high quality are needed for publications.

*Time will vary according to equipment and material used.

Definition of Terms

anastomose Join.

aneurysm A sac formed by local enlargement of a weakened artery wall.

angiography The radiographic study of vessels.

anomaly A variation from the normal pattern.

aortic dissection Tear in the inner lining of the aortic wall that allows blood to enter and track along the muscular coat.

arteriography The radiologic examination of arteries after the injection of a radiopaque contrast medium.

arteriovenous malformation An abnormal anastomosis or communication between an artery and a vein.

atherosclerosis Fibrous and fatty deposits on the luminal wall of an artery that may cause obstruction of the vessel.

bifurcation The place where an artery divides into two branches.

biplane Two x-ray exposure planes 90 degrees from another; usually frontal and lateral.

brachiocephalic Of the arms and head.

cerebrovascular Pertaining to the blood vessels of the brain.

cinefluorography Same as cineradiography; the making of a motion picture record of successive images on a fluoroscopic screen.

claudication Cramping of the leg muscles after physical exertion because of a chronically inadequate blood supply.

embolus Thrombus that detaches and moves freely in the bloodstream.

extravasation The escape of fluid from a vessel into the surrounding tissue.

film changer Device that transports films into and out of the exposure field for serial imaging.

hematoma A local swelling filled with effused blood.

hemostasis Stopping of blood flow or hemorrhage.

hydronephrosis Distention of the pelvis and calices of the kidney with urine caused by ureteral obstruction.

lesion An injury or other damaging change to an organ or tissue.

lymphadenography Radiographic study of the lymph nodes.

lymphangiography Radiographic study of the lymph vessels.

lymphography Radiographic evaluation of the lymphatic channels and lymph nodes.

meninges The three membranes that envelop the brain and spinal cord.

nephrectomy Surgical removal of the kidney.

nephrostomy Surgical opening into the kidney's collecting system.

nonocclusive Being not completely closed or shut; allowing blood flow.

percutaneous Effected or introduced through the skin.

percutaneous nephrolithotomy A uroradiologic procedure performed to extract stones from within the kidney or proximal ureter.

percutaneous transluminal angioplasty Surgical correction of a vessel from within the vessel using catheter technology.

stenosis Constriction or narrowing of a passage or an orifice.

thrombogenesis The formation of a blood clot.

thrombosis Formation or existence of a blood clot.

thrombus A blood clot obstructing a blood vessel or cavity of the heart.

uroradiology The radiologic and interventional study of the urinary tract.

venography The radiologic study of veins after the injection of radiopaque contrast medium.

SELECTED BIBLIOGRAPHY

Abrams HL: Abrams angiography: vascular and interventional radiology, ed 3, Boston, 1983, Little, Brown & Co.

Abrams HL: Angiography, ed 3, Boston, 1983, Little, Brown & Co.

Athanasoulis CA et al: Interventional radiology, Philadelphia, 1982, WB Saunders Co.

Bierman HR et al: Intra-arterial catheterization of viscera in man, Am J Roentgenol Radium Ther Nucl Med 66:555-568, 1951.

Bull JWD: History of neuroradiology, the presidential address delivered at the British Institute of Radiology, Oct 20, 1960, Br J Radiol 34:69-84, 1961.

Chase NE and Kricheff II: Cerebral angiography in the evaluation of patients with cerebrovascular disease, Radiol Clin North Am 4:131-144, 1966.

Chopp M et al: Clinical dosimetry during cerebral arteriography, Neuroradiology 20(2):79-81, 1980.

Clouse ME and Wallace S: Lymphatic imaging—lymphography, computed tomography and scintigraphy, ed 2, Baltimore, 1985, Williams & Wilkins.

Cromwell LD, Kerber CW, and Vermeere WR: A wedge filter for craniocervical angiography, AJR 129(6):1125-1127, 1977.

Doi K et al: X-ray imaging of blood vessels to the brain by use of magnification stereoscopic technique, Adv Neurol 30:175-189, 1981.

Dotter CT and Judkins MP: Transluminal treatment of arteriosclerotic obstruction: description of a new technique and preliminary report of its application, Circulation 30:654-70, 1964.

Ferrucci JT et al: Interventional radiology of the abdomen, ed 2, Baltimore, 1985, Williams & Wilkins.

Fisher HW: Viscosity, solubility, and toxicity in the choice of an angiographic contrast medium, Angiography 16:759-766, 1965.

Fitz CR and Harwood-Nash DC: Neonatal radiology; special procedure techniques in infants, Radiol Clin North Am 13:(2):181-198, 1975.

Fu WR: Angiography of trauma, Springfield, Ill, 1972, Charles C Thomas, Publisher.

Greitz T: A radiologic study of the brain circulation by rapid serial angiography of the carotid artery, Acta Radiol, suppl 140, 1956.

Gruntzig A and Hopff H: Perkutane rekanalisation chronischer arterieller Verschlusse mit einem neuen dilatationskatheter; modifikation der Dotter-Technik, Deutsch Med Wochenschr 99:2502-2511, 1974.

Hacker H: Detail angiography—direct x-ray enlargement in serial angiography, Electromedica 38:346-349, 1970.

Hinck VC and Dotter CT: Appraisal of current techniques for cerebral angiography, Am J Roentgenol Radium Ther Nucl Med 107:626-630, 1969.

Hoppe JO and Archer S: X-ray contrast media for cardiovascular angiography, Angiology 11:244-254, 1960.

Johnsrude IS et al: A practical approach to angiography, ed 2, Boston, 1987, Little, Brown & Co.

Judkins MP et al: Lumen following safety J-guide for catheterization of tortuous vessels, Radiology 88:1127-1130, 1967.

Kadir S: Diagnostic angiography, Philadelphia, 1986, WB Saunders Co.

Katzen BT: Interventional diagnostic and therapeutic procedures, New York, 1980, Springer-Verlag New York, Inc.

Kerber C et al: Selective cerebral angiography through the axillary artery, Neuroradiology 10(3):131-135, 1975.

Lammer J and Karnel F: Percutaneous transluminal laser angioplasty with contact probes, Radiology 168(3):733-737, 1988.

Lang EK: Transcatheter embolization of pelvic vessels for control of intractable hemorrhage, Radiology 140:331-339, 1981.

Langes EK et al: Catheter atherectomy: functional results in peripheral arterial disease, Angiology 40(9):830-834, 1989.

Lin JP: Techniques of cerebral angiography, Radiol Clin North Am 12(2):223-240, 1974.

Mani RL: A new double-curve catheter for selective femoro-cerebral angiography, Radiology 94:607-611, 1980.

Mani RL and Gross RC: Keyhole cone device for lateral magnification cerebral angiography, Am J Radiol 129(1):165-166, 1977.

Mills CS and Van Aman ME: Modified technique for percutaneous transfemoral pulmonary angiography, Cardiovasc Interven Radiol 9:52-53, 1986.

Molnar W and Stockum AE: Transhepatic dilatation of choledochoenterostomy strictures, Radiology 129:59, 1978.

Morris JL and Wylie I: Cerebral angiotomography, Radiology 120(1):105-109, 1976.

Newman GE et al: Peripheral artery atherectomy: description of technique and report of initial results, Radiology 169(3):677-680, 1988.

Newton TH: The axillary artery approach to arteriography of the aorta and its branches, Am J Roentgenol Radium Ther Nucl Med 89:275-283, 1963.

Newton TH and Potts DG: Radiology of the skull and brain—angiography, vol 2, book 1, Great Neck, 1986, Medibooks.

Numaguchi Y, Hoffman JC Jr, and Sones PJ Jr: Femoral percutaneous catheterization in infants and small children for cerebral angiography, Radiology 116(2):451, 1975.

Osborn AG: Introduction to cerebral angiography, New York, 1980, Harper & Row, Publishers Inc.

Rakofsky M: Quantified analysis of a carotid angiogram, Neuroradiology 20(2):53-71, 1980.

Ramsey RG: Neuroradiology, ed 2, Philadelphia, 1987, WB Saunders Co.

Reuter SR et al: Gastrointestinal angiography, ed 3, Philadelphia, 1986, WB Saunders Co.

Ring EJ and McLean GK: Interventional radiology: principals and techniques, Boston, 1981, Little, Brown & Co.

Roehm JOF et al: The bird's nest inferior vena cava filter: progress report, Radiology 168:745-749, 1988.

Rose BS, Simon DC, Hess ML, and Van Aman ME: Percutaneous transfemoral placement of the Kimray-Greenfield vena cava filter, Radiology 165:373-376, 1987.

Seldinger SI: Catheter replacement of the needle in percutaneous arteriography, Acta Radiol 39:368-376, 1953.

Shimizu H, Satô O, and Kobayashi M: A new method of autotomography with cerebral angiography (angioautotomography), Neuroradiology 9(4):203-208, 1975.

Smith DC and Tidwell J: Adjustable sliding aluminum wedge filter: device for angiographic enhancement, Radiol Technol 49(4):459-471, 1978.

Smith GA et al: Experimental evaluation of cerebral angiography, J Neurosurg 8:556-563, 1951.

Smith GR and Loop JW: A simple method of femorocerebral catheterization, Radiology 118(3):733-734, 1976.

Snopek AM: Fundamentals of special radiographic procedures, Philadelphia, 1984, WB Saunders Co.

Staton R: Lymphography, Radiol Technol 55:233-238, 1984.

Takahashi M: Magnification factor, position, and true size of an object in stereoscopic magnification radiography, Radiology 142(1):215-217, 1982.

Takahashi M and Ozawa Y: Stereoscopic magnification angiography using a twin focal-spot x-ray tube, Radiology 142(3):791-792, 1982.

Takahashi M et al: Serial cerebral angiography in stereoscopic magnification, AJR 126(6):1211-1216, 1976.

Thorn A and Voight K: Rotational cerebral angiography: procedure and value, Am J Neuroradiol 4(3):289-291, 1983.

Tortorici MR: Fundamentals of angiography, St Louis, 1982, The CV Mosby Co.

Von Sonnenberg E and Mueller PR: Practical interventional radiology, Philadelphia, 1989, WB Saunders Co.

Whitley JE and Whitley NO: Angiography: techniques and procedures, St Louis, 1971, Warren H Green, Inc.

Wilkens RA and Viamonte M, editors: Interventional radiology, Boston, 1982, Blackwell Scientific Publications, Inc.

Wood EH, Taveras JM, and Tenner MS: The brain and eye—an atlas of tumor radiology, Chicago, 1975, Year Book Medical Publishers, Inc.

Chapter 31

CARDIAC CATHETERIZATION

RONALD D. WEINSTEIN

Cardiac catheterization is a comprehensive term used to describe a minor surgical procedure that involves the introduction of a catheter into the heart and surrounding vasculature for the purpose of diagnostic evaluation or therapy associated with a variety of cardiovascular-related disorders in both children and adults.*

Cardiac catheterization can be classified as either a diagnostic study or an interventional procedure. The primary purpose for conducting diagnostic studies is to collect information or data necessary to evaluate the patient's condition. Interventional procedures involve applying therapeutic measures such as injecting certain cardiovascular medications (pharmacologic therapy) or inserting specially designed catheters (manipulative therapy) used to treat or improve certain disorders.

*For a description of the anatomy of the heart see Chapter 30.

□ All photographic illustrations provided courtesy of St. Luke Episcopal Hospital, Texas Children's Hospital, Texas Heart Institute of Houston, Texas.

□ Thanks are extended to J. Michael Chudik, B.S., R.T., Director of Cardiovascular Services, Grant Medical Center in Columbus, Ohio for his work in revising and expanding this chapter.

Historical Development

As early as 1844, experimentation in placement of catheters into the hearts of animals led to the successful catheterization of both the right and left ventricles of a horse by French physiologist Claude Bernard. The first human cardiac catheterization was reported in 1929 by Werner Forssman, a 25-year-old surgical resident, who placed a catheter into his own heart, then walked to the radiology department where a chest radiograph was made to document this medical achievement.

Catheterization of the heart soon became a valuable tool used primarily for diagnostic purposes. Through the 1940s the basic catheterization study remained relatively uncomplicated in nature and easy for the competent physician to perform; however, the risk to the patient was significant.

Physician-operated catheterization methods and techniques increased in number and complexity and were refined in the years that followed. These refinements included the development of the Seldinger and transseptal left heart catheter introduction approaches and techniques for selective catheterization of the coronary artery by Sones and Judkins during the 1950s.

During the 1960s and through the 1970s, tremendous advances in radiologic and cardiovascular medicine and technology occurred. Radiographic imaging and recording, physiologic monitoring, and cardiovascular pharmaceuticals, supplies, and equipment became increasingly reliable. From the 1970s to the present a major emphasis in the field of cardiac catheterization has been the increased dependency, applicability, and diversity of interventional techniques. Application of computers in the catheterization laboratory has also facilitated the development of this rapidly growing and extremely specialized subspecialty of the cardiovascular medical and surgical sciences. These advances and trends have enabled cardiac catheterization to evolve from a basically simple but hazardous diagnostic investigation to its current state as a sophisticated and low-risk diagnostic study or interventional procedure.

Indications, Contraindications, and Risks

There are general indications, contraindications, and risks associated with diagnostic and interventional cardiac catheterizations; these must be considered by the physician when attempting to determine the appropriateness of conducting any type of catheterization. Examples of these follow.

GENERAL INDICATIONS

Cardiac catheterization is performed to identify the anatomic and physiologic condition of the heart. Coronary angiography is currently the most definitive procedure for visualizing the coronary anatomy. The anatomic information evaluated from this procedure may include the presence and extent of obstructive atherosclerotic coronary artery disease, thrombus formation, coronary artery collateral flow, coronary anomalies, coronary artery size, aneurysms, and other coronary obstructions such as spasms.

The most common disorder necessitating catheterization of the adult heart is advanced coronary artery disease (nearly 80% of all cases). This disease is primarily caused by the accumulation of soft intracoronary fatty *(atheromatous)** material leading to *stenosis* or *occlusion* of the arteries. Coronary artery disease is symptomatically characterized by severe chest pain *(angina pectoris)* or by a heart attack *(myocardial infarction)*. Treatment of coronary artery disease includes both medical and surgical interventions.

One general indication for conducting diagnostic cardiac catheterization of the adult related to coronary artery disease is to assess the appropriateness and feasibility of various therapeutic interventions. For example, catheterization is performed before open heart surgery to provide essential information such as *hemodynamic* and angiographic data necessary to document the presence of disease and its anatomic and physiologic severity. In selected circumstances, postoperative catheterization is performed to assess the results of surgery. For relief of *arteriosclerotic* coronary artery stenosis, a manipulative interventional procedure called *percutaneous transluminal coronary angioplasty* (PTCA) may be indicated.

*All italicized terms are defined at the end of this chapter.

Diagnostic studies of the adult heart also aid in evaluating the patient who has confusing or obscure symptoms (such as chest pain of undetermined cause) and to evaluate nonsurgical diseases of the heart (for example, certain *cardiomyopathies*). National statistics have revealed that the typical adult heart catheterization patient is a male over the age of 45 years.

In children, diagnostic heart catheterization is employed in the evaluation of congenital and valvular diseases, disorders of the cardiac conduction system, and certain cardiomyopathies. Interventional techniques are also used in children primarily to alleviate the pathophysiology associated with certain congenital heart defects.

A special report, "Guidelines for Coronary Angiography," published in the *Journal of The American College of Cardiology** contains a thorough discussion of the indications for this procedure. These indications include patients with the following disease states:

1. Known or suspected coronary heart disease, both symptomatic and asymptomatic
2. Atypical chest pain of uncertain origin
3. Acute myocardial infarction (evolving, completed, and convalescent)
4. Valvular heart disease
5. Known or suspected congenital heart disease
6. Other conditions (such as diseases affecting the aorta and the presence of dilated cardiomyopathy)

These guidelines also consider the risks, benefits, and utilization of this procedure by listing each of the above disease categories into three classifications:

1. Class 1: conditions for which there is general agreement that coronary angiography is justified
2. Class 2: conditions for which coronary angiography is frequently performed but there is a divergence of opinion with respect to its justification in terms of value and appropriateness
3. Class 3: conditions for which there is general agreement that coronary angiography ordinarily is not justified

*J Am Coll Cardiol 4:935-950, Oct 1987.

CONTRAINDICATIONS AND ASSOCIATED RISKS

Cardiac catheterization, like other surgically related procedures, has associated inherent risk factors. According to Grossman* however, the only absolute contraindication for heart catheterization is refusal by a mentally competent patient.

Contraindications to perform coronary angiography are relatively few when the appropriateness of the procedure is based on the condition of the patient. Relative contraindications may include:

- Active gastrointestinal bleeding
- Renal insufficiency
- Recent stroke
- Fever from infection or presence of an active infection
- Severe electrolyte imbalance
- Severe anemia
- Short life expectancy because of other illness
- Digitalis intoxication
- Patient refusal of therapeutic treatment such as percutaneous transluminal coronary angioplasty (PTCA) or bypass surgery

Some of these conditions could be temporary or treated and reversed before a cardiac catheterization is attempted.

The risk of cardiac catheterization varies according to the type of procedure as well as the individual patient. Variables include the anatomy to be studied, the type of catheter and approach used, history of drug allergy, the basic cardiovascular disease and noncardiac disease or diseases present (such as asthma and diabetes), hemodynamic status, age, and other patient characteristics.

*See the bibliography at the end of this chapter.

The Society for Cardiac Angiography reviewed the catheterizations for 53,581 patients performed in 66 member laboratories from October 1979 to December 1980 and found the overall mortality to be 0.14%. Mortality varied from 1.75% in children less than 1 year of age to 0.25% in patients over 60 years of age; the vast majority of patients between these extremes (1 to 60 years) had a mortality of only 0.07%. The major complication rate reported for the entire group was 1.82%. Major complications included acute myocardial infarction, cardiac arrest, emergency surgery, and death.

The risks associated with cardiac catheterization have decreased dramatically in recent years. It should be noted, however, that as the severity of the patient's disease increases, so does the risk associated with the procedure. Therefore the benefits expected to be derived from cardiac catheterization data must be weighed against the associated risk.

Specialized Equipment

Cardiac catheterization has developed into a highly complex, sophisticated procedure requiring equipment and supplies with similar characteristics. Unlike earlier radiographic examinations of the intracardiac structures, modern cardiac catheterization requires more than a simple fluoroscope and perhaps some sort of recording modality such as overhead radiography.

Equipment required for cardiac catheterization can be categorized in three groups: cardiovascular, fluorographic imaging and recording, and ancillary. The following are selected examples of equipment typically contained in each group.

CARDIOVASCULAR EQUIPMENT

Catheters placed into the human vasculature are available in variations of length, shape, diameter, and number of exit holes. The selection of which available catheter to use in a particular circumstance is made by the physician. Most cardiac catheters are radiopaque and presterilized, and many are preshaped and disposable.

The catheter or catheters placed into the patient's vasculature either can function as a fluid column for recording pressure data or can serve as a conduit for fluid or drug infusion. Blood samples can be drawn directly from selected cardiac chambers for the purpose of *oximetry* or other laboratory analysis. Conversely, medications, radiographic contrast media, and other fluids may be rapidly administered through the catheter. To accomplish these and other tasks, a system of valves (stopcocks) are combined to form a manifold, which can be attached to the proximal end of the intracardiac catheter or catheters. Using a manifold does not require disconnecting the intracardiac catheter or catheters to perform such functions as drawing blood samples, administering medications, recording blood pressures, and heparin flushing. A typical disposable manifold is illustrated in Fig. 31-1.

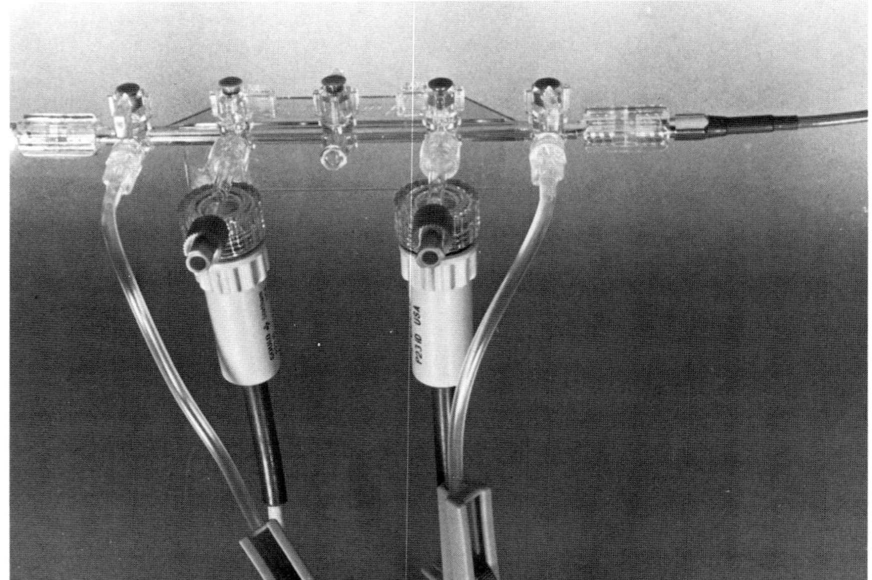

Fig. 31-1. Fifteen cm length disposable manifold setup for adult heart catheterization with two transducers connected below and one catheter attached on the right.

A major piece of equipment integral to cardiac catheterization procedures is a physiologic recorder (Fig. 31-2), which is used to monitor and record vital patient functions including the electrical activity within the heart and certain hemodynamic parameters such as the pressures within various intracardiac chambers. Patients are monitored during the entire catheterization (regardless of the type of procedure performed) with periodic electrocardiographic and pressure recordings.

To collect hemodynamic data during the catheterization, it is necessary to connect the physiologic recorder (requiring information in electrical form) to the catheter (carrying information in the form of physical fluid pressure) that is placed in the patient's vasculature. For cardiac catheterization, physiologic recorders usually have six, twelve, or sixteen channel capacity. A channel (or module) is an electrical component of the physiologic recorder capable of measuring an individual parameter such as a specific type of electrocardiogram or intravascular pressure. The number of channels required for a particular catheterization will increase as the amount of detailed required information increases.

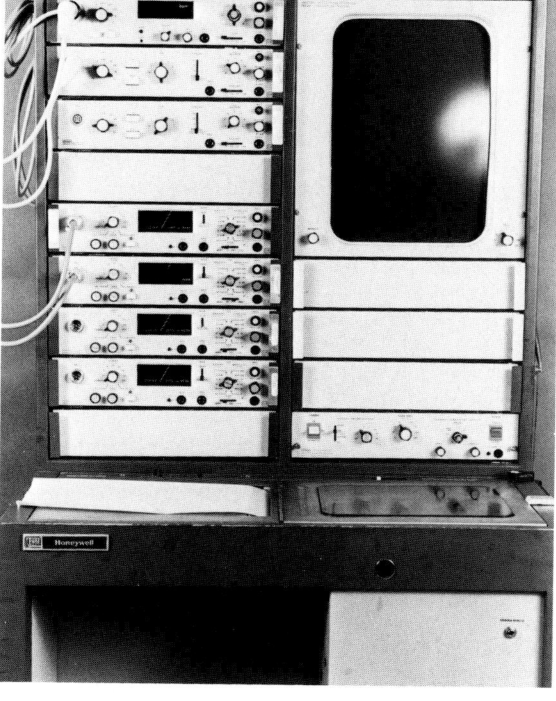

Fig. 31-2. Twelve channel capacity physiologic recorder used to monitor certain patient data during a heart catheterization. The unit illustrated has three electrocardiogram *(upper left)* and four blood pressure *(lower left)* operational channels available.

Devices called *transducers* (seen in Fig. 31-1) are interfaced between the manifold and the physiologic recorder to convert fluid (blood) pressure into an electrical signal.

Special needles, guide wires, and dilators used for cardiac catheterization are similar to those employed in other forms of special radiologic procedures. The constant flow, high-pressure injector (Fig. 31-3) for administration of radiographic contrast media during catheterization is also used in general angiography as described in Chapter 30. Administration of contrast media into the coronary arteries and certain other adult and pediatric vessels generally does not require the use of a high-pressure injector. The high-pressure injector is used extensively during cineangiography of intracardiac chambers, the aortic root, and pulmonary vessels. Most high-pressure injector manufacturers offer some optional equipment that may be of some use in the cardiac catheterization laboratory. One such feature is electrocardiogram (ECG) gating of the injection. This feature enables single or multiple injections to occur at a predetermined point during the heartbeat. This allows for injections that are synchronized with the movement of the heart and may minimize the incidence of premature ventricular contractions during the ventriculogram. Oximeters (Fig. 31-4) are used to determine the blood oxygen saturations of samples obtained during adult and pediatric catheterizations.

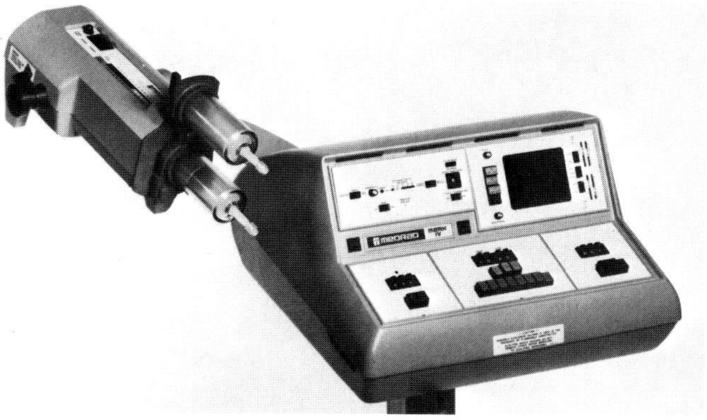

Fig. 31-3. High pressure injector for radiographic contrast media.

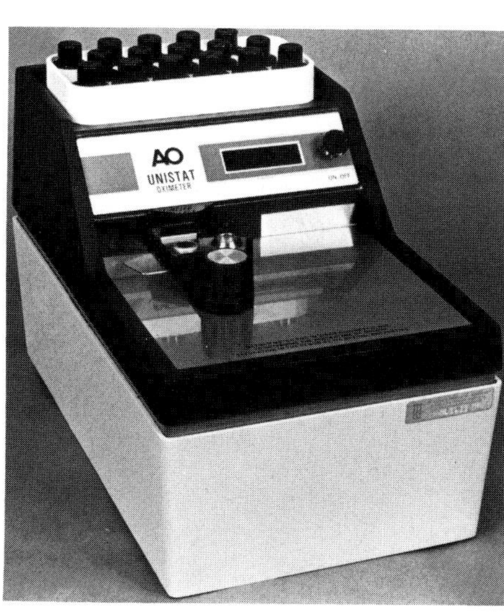

Fig. 31-4. Oximeter used to measure oxygen saturations in blood.

FLUOROGRAPHIC IMAGING AND RECORDING

The fluorographic imaging and recording equipment found in cardiac catheterization laboratories is essentially the same as that found in vascular angiography suites. The ultimate goal is to have an electro-optical system that is capable of producing and recording fluorographic images with the greatest amount of detail available. This is especially important in cardiac catheterization because of the relatively small anatomic detail associated with the pediatric heart, adult coronary arteries, and the smaller diameter catheters and guide wires used for certain interventional procedures.

Operation of a high-resolution imaging and recording system requires the inclusion of some essential pieces of equipment. One such piece of equipment is the image intensification tube. The image intensification tube should produce maximum detail necessary for cardiac catheterization and have the capability for one or two magnification stages to allow for enhanced visualization of small anatomic structures or catheters.

A television camera is coupled with the output phosphor of the image intensifier, and its signal is fed to television monitors placed so that images can be readily observed during the procedure. Videotape and/or videodisc systems record these images and allow for playback during the catheterization. Maximum available resolution from this optical system is crucial.

Permanent recording of the fluoroscopic image is typically made on 35 mm film and is termed *cinefluorography*. To accomplish this, a motion picture camera is attached to the image intensifier housing that records the fluorographic exposure images at 30 or 60 frames per second. Cinefluorography occurs simultaneously with television monitoring and image recording by a videotape and/or videodisc unit.

In addition to cinefluorography and video recording, some laboratories also employ single or biplane rapid film changers to produce serial, rapid sequence radiographic films that are advantageous in certain situations. The addition of rapid film changers, magnification, digital subtraction, and digital vascular imaging (fluoroscopic and angiographic) equipment can increase the effective use of the catheterization laboratory.

Digital subtraction and digital vascular imaging equipment is gaining more widespread acceptance in the catheterization laboratory. Although these systems have been used in the angiographic area for some time, they are now sufficiently developed to be acceptable when imaging the heart. The resolution of the earlier images has been the drawback to using them in the catheterization laboratory. The obvious solution to this problem, higher matrix sizes, allows for acceptable resolution but also creates another problem in the acquisition and storage of such large volumes of information. Another factor that compounds this problem is that the motion of the heart still requires acquisition rates of 30 frames per second. Digital image processing allows enhanced visualization of the information that is acquired by these systems (a very important fact to be aware of is that less contrast medium is needed because of this). Postprocessing analysis software gives the clinician the capability of doing automatic quantitation of vessel size, measurement of ejection fractions, and coronary flow studies. It is almost certain that digital imaging systems will at some time in the future replace cine film as the standard for cardiac catheterization laboratory imaging.

Fluorographic tubes must be capable of producing ionizing radiation for the long periods of time associated with fluoroscopy and must therefore be designed to withstand greater heat loading. For most catheterization imaging, multifocal spot, high-speed rotating fluorographic tubes are desirable. Extremely short exposure times are required to accommodate the rapid exposure sequencing of the various recording systems.

Procedures such as selective coronary arteriography and certain pediatric catheterizations require that the patient be carefully positioned to reduce the superimposition created by the cardiac vasculature. Moving the patient is not desirable during the catheterization, particularly when catheters have been carefully positioned to demonstrate specific anatomic structures or to record certain data. To obtain optimal projections, it becomes necessary to rotate the examination table or preferably the fluorographic equipment (image intensifier and fluorographic tube).

Normal and pathologic variations in the adult coronary anatomy and pediatric heart exist; therefore positioning of the patient cannot be specified for each type of catheterization procedure. Each patient's anatomy must be fluoroscopically evaluated to ascertain the optimal degree of rotation and cranial or caudal angulation necessary to visualize the structure or structures of interest.

Some catheterization laboratories employ a motor-driven cradle-top apparatus that is mounted to the top of the examination table. When it becomes necessary to place the patient into an oblique position, the cradle is simply rotated until the desired degree of angulation is reached. In many modern catheterization laboratories, the image intensifier and fluorographic tube are mechanically suspended in a C arm configuration to allow for equipment rotation around the patient and to provide cephalic/caudal angulations as well. In some interventional procedures, the use of biplane C arms (Fig. 31-5) is advantageous and allows for simultaneous imaging of cardiac structures in two different planes.

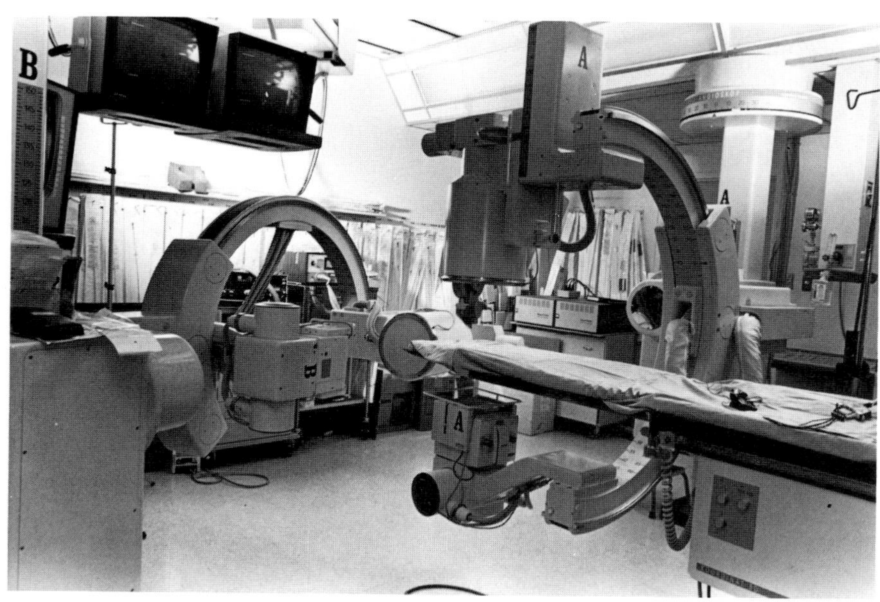

Fig. 31-5. Biplane C arm fluorographic and image intensifier arrangement.

ANCILLARY EQUIPMENT AND SUPPLIES

Because of the nature of the patient's condition and the inherent risk associated with cardiac catheterization, each catheterization room requires a fully equipped emergency cart. The cart typically contains emergency medications, cardiopulmonary resuscitation equipment, defibrillator, intubation equipment, and other related supplies. Oxygen and suction must also be readily available.

Several iodinated radiographic contrast media are approved for intravascular, intracardiac, and intracoronary use in both adults and children. Transient (temporary) electrocardiographic changes during and immediately following contrast media injection are common. Administration of nonionic contrast media or ionic low-osmolar contrast media is being used in many cardiac catheterization laboratories and has gained acceptance because of the properties associated with these media. Unfortunately, the newer contrast media are considerably more expensive than the earlier types. These agents have some definite advantages over ionic high-osmolar contrast media. They display a reduced incidence of cardiovascular reactions and side effects as a result of their lower osmotic pressure. Many catheterization laboratories are now using these newer contrast agents for all of their procedures that require the administration of contrast media. Other laboratories utilize the nonionic and/or low-osmolality contrast agents for pediatric and high-risk patients. These laboratories still use the ionic high-osmolar contrast media for low-risk patients.

Catheterization Methods and Techniques

Different cardiac catheterizations require various combinations of methods and techniques necessary to allow for precise data acquisition or the application of therapeutic interventions. Some of the methods and techniques common to most cardiac catheterizations are presented.

PRECATHETERIZATION CARE

Patient history, physical examination, chest radiograph, basic blood work, and an electrocardiogram (and other noninvasive cardiology procedures) are usually performed before cardiac catheterization. Various premedications are frequently administered for sedation and to control nausea.

Patients brought to the catheterization laboratory are typically not allowed anything to eat or drink for 4 to 6 hours before the procedure. During all catheterizations, a protocol or detailed record of the procedure including fluoroscopy time, medications administered, and supplies used should be maintained.

CATHETER INTRODUCTION

After the patient has been transported to the catheterization laboratory, electrocardiographic monitoring is initiated. The appropriate site for catheter introduction must be prepared using aseptic technique to minimize the risk of subsequent infection. Although specific sites for catheter introduction are numerous and vary according to patient age, habitus, physician preference, and procedure attempted, catheter introduction is accomplished by the cut-down or percutaneous approach.

The cut-down approach requires that a small incision be made in the skin to allow for the direct visualization of the artery and/or vein the physician wants to catheterize. The skin is aseptically prepared, infiltrated with local anesthetic, and the vessel or vessels bluntly dissected and exposed. After an opening is created in the desired vessel (*arteriotomy* and/or *venotomy*), the catheter is introduced and advanced toward the heart. Cut-downs are frequently performed in the right antecubital fossa to access the basilic or other large medial arm vein and/or the brachial artery.

For catheterization of the femoral artery and/or vein, often desirable in pediatric studies, a percutaneous approach is employed (see Seldinger technique as detailed in Chapter 30). In the Seldinger technique, the skin is aseptically prepared and infiltrated with local anesthetic. A special angiography needle is used to puncture the skin and placed into the desired vessel. A guide wire is then advanced through the needle and the needle removed, leaving the guide wire in the vessel. A dilator may be used to prepare the vessel for the larger diameter catheter. The catheter is next placed over the guide wire and the catheter advanced toward the heart. The guide wire may be removed or temporarily left in place to facilitate further placement of the catheter. It should be noted that both types of catheter introduction approaches have specific indications, precautions, advantages, and disadvantages.

DATA COLLECTION

The acquisition of certain data is essential regardless of the type of catheterization performed or the nature of the patient's illness. Physiologic data typically collected include hemodynamic parameters and electrocardiogram and oximetry readings. Selective cineangiography is also used to record anatomic information.

Hemodynamic parameters include blood pressure and *cardiac output*. The monitoring and recording of intracavitary (within the heart) as well as extracardiac vascular pressures require the catheter-manifold-transducer-physiologic apparatus system described earlier in this chapter. Cardiac output, an important indicator of the heart's overall ability to pump blood, can be measured in the catheterization laboratory. There are several methods that are used to obtain estimates of a patient's cardiac output. The electrocardiogram is continuously monitored during catheterizations and can be simultaneously recorded with intracavitary or extracardiac pressures (Fig. 31-6). Blood oxygen saturations are determined in various locations.

Selective angiocardiography requires cinefluorography of the vasculature during the injection of iodinated contrast media. The total fluoroscopy time for an average adult diagnostic catheterization is about 10 minutes, and the time the catheter or catheters actually remain in the vessels is about 35 minutes.

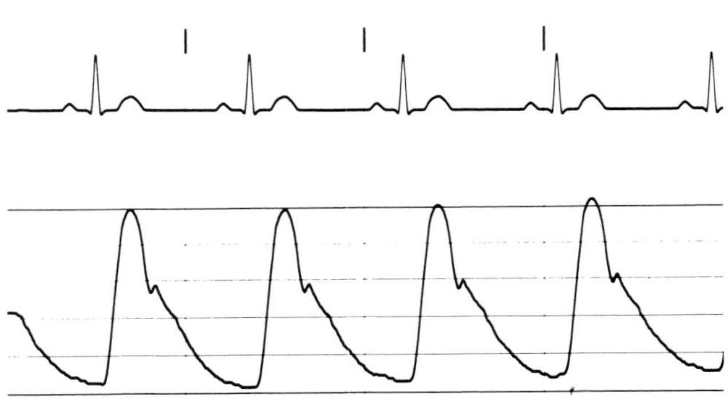

Fig. 31-6. Simulated normal electrocardiogram *(top)* and simultaneous aortic pressures *(bottom)*.

Catheterization Studies and Procedures

The primary purpose of a diagnostic cardiac catheterization is data collection, and the primary purpose of the interventional procedure is for therapy. The following section briefly describes some of the more commonly performed diagnostic and interventional heart catheterizations.

BASIC DIAGNOSTIC STUDIES: ADULT

Catheterization of the left side of the heart is a widely performed, basic, diagnostic, cardiac catheterization study. The catheter may be introduced through the brachial or femoral artery, advanced to the ascending aorta, and passed through the aortic valve into the left ventricle. Arterial oximetry is performed, and pressures are taken in the left ventricle; these measurements are repeated as the catheter is withdrawn across the aortic valve. Selective angiography of the right (Fig. 31-7) and left (Fig. 31-8) coronary arteries is performed, using different projections to allow for the evaluation of the extent of intracoronary stenosis. Coronary arteriograms are obtained in nearly 80% of all catheterizations of the left side of the heart.

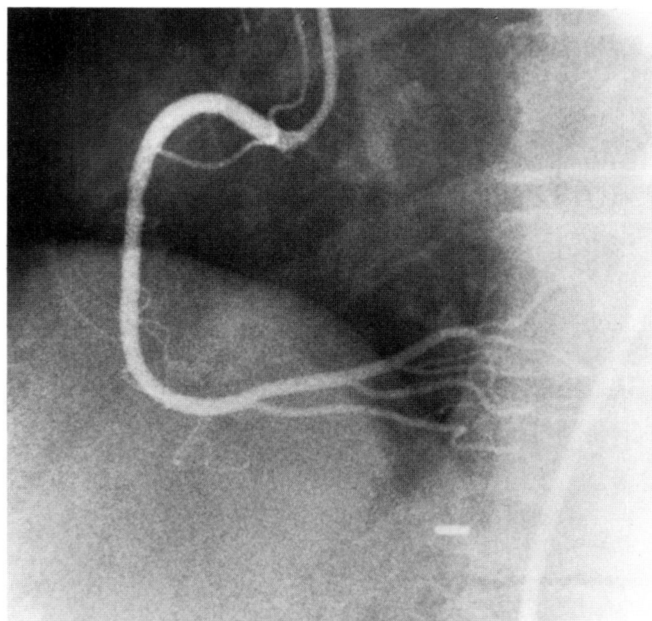
Fig. 31-7. Normal right coronary arteries.

Selective angiography of the left ventricle (Fig. 31-9) is performed in approximately 94% of catheterization studies of the left side of the heart. Left ventriculography provides information related to wall motion that can be used to estimate the *ejection fraction*.

Catheterization of the right side of the heart is another commonly performed study. A venous catheter is inserted in the groin or antecubital fossa and advanced to the vena cava, into the right atrium, across the tricuspid valve, to the right ventricle, and through the pulmonary valve to the pulmonary artery; it is advanced until wedged distally in the pulmonary artery. Oximetery is performed, and pressures recorded in various locations. Selective cineangiography is performed as appropriate.

It frequently becomes necessary to perform simultaneous catheterization of both the right and left sides of the heart. The same extremity can be used for catheterization of both sides of the heart. The right-sided pulmonary wedge pressure can then be superimposed on the left ventricular pressure, and oximetery performed on both sides of the heart.

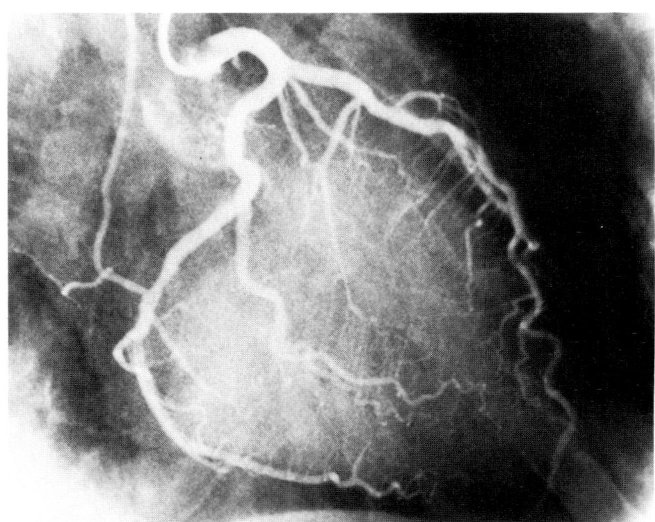
Fig. 31-8. Normal left coronary arteries.

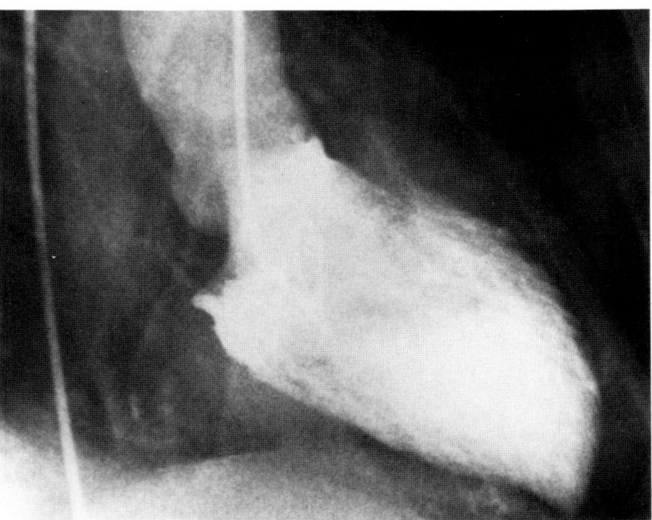
Fig. 31-9. Normal left ventriculogram (during diastole).

BASIC DIAGNOSTIC STUDIES: PEDIATRIC

A primary indication for diagnostic catheterization studies in children is the evaluation and documentation of specific anatomy, hemodynamic data, and selected aspects of cardiac function associated with congenital heart defects. Methods and techniques used for catheterization of the pediatric heart vary depending on the patient's age, heart size, type and extent of defect, and other coincident pathophysiologic conditions.

Pediatric cardiac catheters are often introduced percutaneously into the femoral vein and sometimes in older children into the femoral artery. In very young patients, it may be possible to pass a catheter from the right atrium to the left atrium (thereby allowing access to the left side of the heart) through either a *patent foramen ovale* or a preexisting atrial septal defect. Should the atrial septum be intact, temporary access to the left atrium may be obtained by using a transseptal catheter system.

ADVANCED DIAGNOSTIC STUDIES

Exercise hemodynamics are sometimes required in the evaluation of valvular heart disease, especially mitral stenosis. In such cases a simultaneous catheterization of both sides of the heart is performed including right and left pressures taken at rest, after the legs are raised, and during and after exercise. Exercise often consists of pedaling a stationary bicycle ergometer that is placed on top of the examination table.

Electrophysiology studies, performed on either adult or pediatric patients, involve the collection of sophisticated data that will subsequently allow a detailed mapping of the electrical impulse routes within the heart itself (used in determining the origin and site of heart rhythms and blocks). This technique is principally employed to define and localize disorders of the conduction system of the heart that produce *dysrhythmias*. After characterization of the precise defect from these data, an appropriate course of therapy can be undertaken.

Vasospastic or *variant angina* is an acute *paroxysm* of coronary artery spasm occurring for relatively short periods of time. Diagnosis of this disorder is typically made by routine electrocardiography during an episode of pain. Patients suspected of having coronary artery spasm but who lack confirmation as evidenced by an electrocardiogram may be candidates for an ergonovine study. Ergonovine maleate is a potent coronary *vasoconstrictor* to which variant angina patients are uniquely sensitive.

Very small amounts of ergonovine maleate may be administered intravenously after routine simultaneous catheterization of both sides of the heart and baseline selective coronary arteriography, which allows for assessment of the disease before, during, and after the patient is medicated. A positive response generally includes chest pain, electrocardiographic changes, slowing of the heart rate, and severe coronary artery spasm. At times the coronary artery spasm (demonstrable by coronary arteriography) may become intense enough to necessitate intracoronary administration of nitroglycerin (a *vasodilator*).

INTERVENTIONAL PHARMACOLOGIC PROCEDURES: ADULT

Interventional pharmacologic procedures in the adult consist of the intravascular administration of a medication during the heart catheterization for therapeutic purposes. An example is the administration of thrombolytic agents such as streptokinase (often through intracoronary infusion) in the catheterization laboratory during the early hours of an acute myocardial infarction in an effort to modify its course. It is estimated that thrombotic coronary artery occlusion is present in 75% to 85% of patients with acute myocardial infarction. When reperfusion of the *ischemic* myocardium is effective, the scarring is reduced. Reperfusion in the early stages of myocardial infarction offers higher potential for myocardial salvage. Another *thrombolytic* agent used in this type of procedure is a relatively new medication called tissue-type plasminogen activator (t-PA). The research and results associated with this medication have indicated a decreased morbidity and mortality for those receiving the agent during the first 2 hours after the onset of acute myocardial infarction symptoms. Because of this, administration of the medication occurs before the patient is brought to the catheterization laboratory.

INTERVENTIONAL MANIPULATIVE PROCEDURES: ADULT

Interventional manipulative cardiac catheterization techniques requiring special purpose catheters have expanded greatly since the late 1970s. One such technique, percutaneous transluminal coronary angioplasty (PTCA), employs balloon dilation of a discrete coronary artery stenosis. The first successful PTCA was performed in 1977 by Andreas Greuntzig, a Swiss cardiologist.

Following catheterization of the left side of the heart (Fig. 31-10) a specially designed guiding catheter is placed into the orifice of the stenosed coronary artery. Next, a special balloon-tip catheter (Fig. 31-11) is advanced through the guiding catheter until the balloon section is centered within the stenotic area.

In some cases an over-the-wire balloon system is used. If this type of system is utilized, the wire is first advanced through the balloon catheter and across the stenotic area. The balloon catheter is then advanced over the wire across the stenotic area and then inflated. A fixed-wire system only allows a specific amount of wire movement through the lumen of the balloon catheter. The over-the-wire system will allow the wire to cross the lesion first and continue to advance until the balloon portion of the catheter is centered in the stenotic area. Some new systems employ a balloon attached only to a hollow-core wire. Each of these systems has advantages when used in the proper situation and within the proper vessel. Once the proper balloon is across the stenotic area, slow precise inflation of the balloon portion of the catheter with contrast media fractures or compresses the fatty deposits in the muscular wall of the artery. The catheter is then deflated to allow for the rapid return of perfusing blood to the distal heart muscle. The inflation procedure, followed by arteriography, may be repeated several times until a satisfactory degree of patency is observed (Fig. 31-12). More than one lesion may be dilated during the same procedure.

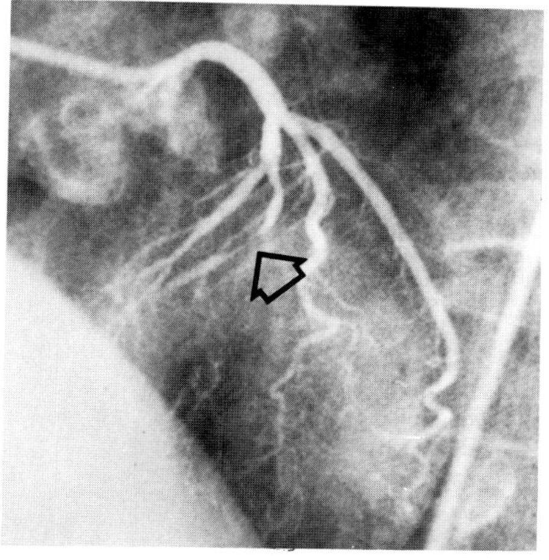

Fig. 31-10. Pre-PTCA stenotic coronary artery lesion (arrow indicates the stenotic area estimated at 100%, with no blood flow distal to the lesion).

It should be noted that PTCA is not appropriate for all patients with arteriosclerotic coronary artery disease. Of those angina patients with advanced coronary artery disease requiring coronary artery bypass surgery, about 10% are estimated to be suitable candidates for PTCA.

Approximately 70% to 80% of the single-lesion vessels dilated with the PTCA technique remain patent for 1 year after the initial procedure was performed. In the early 1980s, PTCA was combined with streptokinase infusion for the management of acute myocardial infarction. Because of the inherent risks associated with coronary artery dilation, open heart surgical facilities must be immediately available. Coronary occlusion is an example of a major complication associated with emergency surgery for the PTCA patient.

Another manipulative interventional procedure being performed with greater frequency in cardiac catheterization laboratories, rather than in operating rooms, is permanent pacemaker implantation (insertion). The procedure can be successfully performed on selected adult and pediatric patients without general anesthesia. Permanent pacemakers are typically used to treat patients with cardiac conduction disorders that are not responsive to medications.

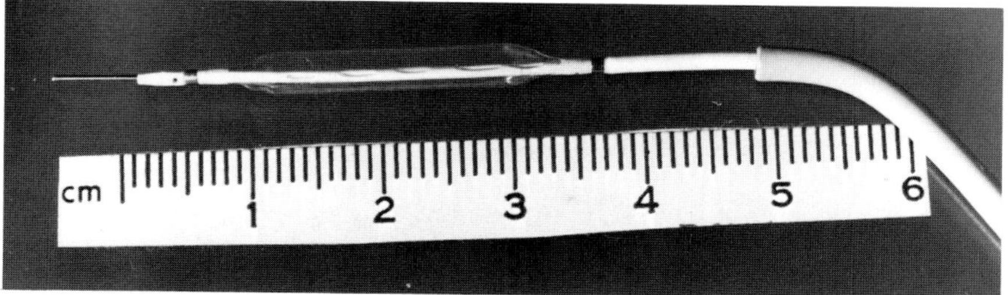

Fig. 31-11. Catheter tip system for transluminal coronary angioplasty. The three sections of this system are the outer guiding catheter *(right)*, central balloon catheter *(middle)*, and internal steerable guide wire *(left)*.

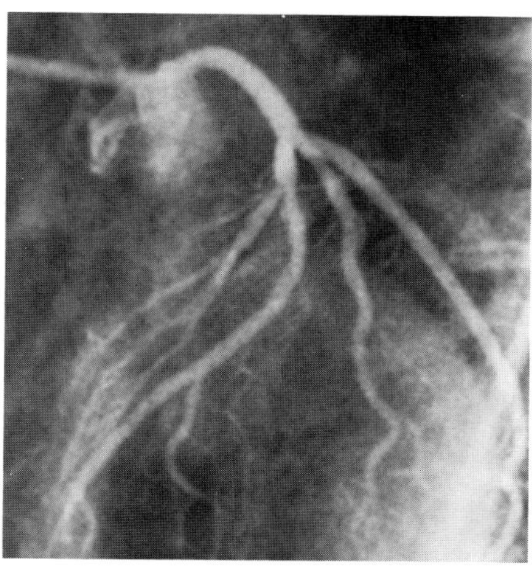

Fig. 31-12. Post-PTCA dilated coronary artery lesion (blood flow distal to the area dilated estimated to be 100%, indicating a successful procedure). Same patient as in Fig. 31-10.

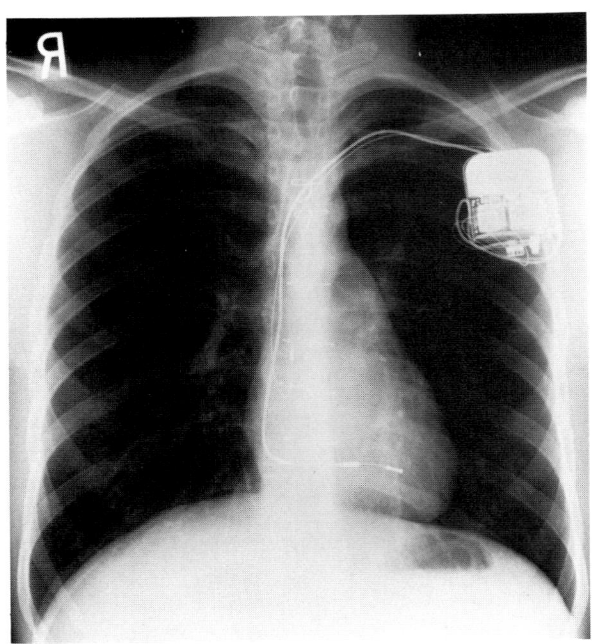

Fig. 31-13. Chest radiograph of a patient with a permanent pacemaker (note pacemaker location in the superior and anterior chest wall with distal leads located in both the right ventricle and the right atrium of the heart).

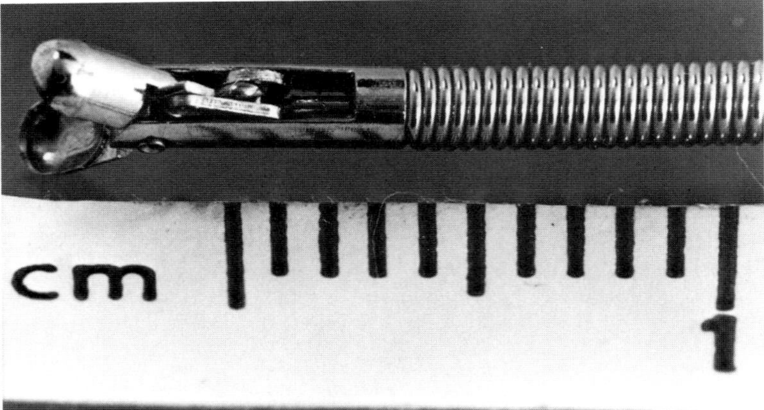

Fig. 31-14. Bioptome catheter tip used for endomyocardial biopsy (open tip closes to obtain small tissue sample).

The installation of a permanent pacemaker usually involves puncture of the subclavian vein and the introduction of pacemaker leads that are insulated electrical wires with distal electrodes. The leads are manipulated so that the tip is in direct contact with either the right ventricular or right atrial endocardium, or both. The proximal ends of the pacemaker leads are then attached to a battery pack that is implanted in a subcutaneous pocket created in the anterior chest wall (Fig. 31-13). Modern lithium-type batteries can last from 5 to 10 years.

Endomyocardial biopsy provides tissue for direct pathologic evaluation of cardiac muscle. A special biopsy catheter with a bioptome tip (Fig. 31-14) is advanced through a guiding catheter to the right ventricle under fluoroscopy. The instrument is then used to obtain myocardial tissue samples from the septal wall that are submitted for pathologic evaluation. Endomyocardial biopsy is frequently used to monitor cardiac transplantation patients for early signs of tissue rejection.

INTERVENTIONAL PROCEDURES: PEDIATRIC

A number of congenital cardiac defects in children are amenable to interventional procedures that can be performed in the catheterization laboratory. As with PTCA procedures, cardiovascular surgical support services must be readily available.

Certain pediatric interventional procedures, when successful, negate the need for surgical correction of the defect or defects. Some procedures, however, are performed for palliative purposes to allow the child to grow to a size and weight when subsequent open heart surgery is feasible.

One such technique, balloon atrial septostomy, may be used to enlarge a patent foramen ovalae or preexisting atrial septal defect. Enlargement of the opening enhances the mixing of right and left atrial blood, resulting in an improvement of the level of systemic arterial oxygenation. *Transposition of the great arteries* is an example of a condition for which atrial septostomy is performed.

Balloon septostomy requires a catheter similar to the type used in PTCA. The balloon is passed through the atrial septal opening into the left atrium, inflated with contrast media, then snapped back through the septal orifice, causing the septum to tear. It is often necessary to repeat this technique until the septal opening is sufficiently enlarged to allow for the desired level of blood mixing, as documented by oximetry, intracardiac pressures, and angiography.

In cases where the atrial septum does not contain a preexisting opening, an artificial defect can be created. A special catheter containing an internal folding knifelike blade (Fig. 31-15) is advanced into the left atrium employing a transseptal system approach. Once inside the left atrium, the blade is advanced out of its protective outer housing and pulled back to the right atrium, creating an incision in the septal wall. This blading technique may be repeated. A balloon septostomy is then performed to widen the new opening, and monitored by oximetry, pressures, and angiography.

Another condition that may be evident in the newborn is a patent ductus arteriosus. In utero the pulmonary artery shunts its blood flow into the aorta via the ductus arteriosus, which normally closes following birth. When this channel fails to spontaneously close it is referred to as a patent ductus arteriosus. In some instances, delayed closure can be induced with medication. When this is unsuccessful and the residual shunt is deemed significant, surgical closure (ligation) of the vessel is appropriate.

For some patients, occlusion of the patent ductus arteriosus can be accomplished in the catheterization laboratory. A catheter containing an occlusion device (such as an umbrella) is advanced to the ductus. After confirmation of proper positioning in the lesion by angiography, the occluder is released. Subsequent clotting and fibrous infiltration permanently stop the flow and subsequent mixing of blood.

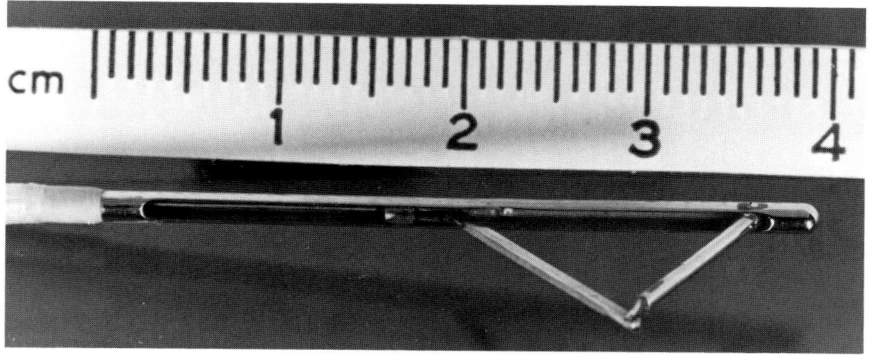

Fig. 31-15. Blading catheter tip used to incise septal walls in pediatric interventional procedures.

Postcatheterization Care

On completion of the catheterization procedure, all catheters are removed and arteriostomies and/or venostomies repaired as appropriate. If a cut-down was performed, skin incisions are also repaired. Wound sites are cleansed and dressed to minimize risk of infection. Elastic dressings are often used to encourage *hematostasis*.

Postcatheterization medications are prescribed by the physician. The puncture site must be observed for hemorrhage, and the status of the distal pulse is recorded on the protocol before the patient leaves the catheterization laboratory. Vital signs should be monitored on a regular schedule until at least 24 hours after the catheterization. Oral fluids should be encouraged, and pain medication may be indicated. Cardiac catheterization may also be performed on an outpatient or day-treatment basis. In these cases the patient is monitored from 4 to 8 hours in a recovery area and then allowed to go home. Instructions for home care recovery procedures are usually given to the patient or a family member before the patient leaves the recovery area.

Cardiac Catheterization on the Horizon

Techniques and methods for cardiac catheterization will continue to advance at an increasing rate. Fluorographic imaging and recording equipment will become even more sophisticated, yielding greater resolution and detail. Application of digital vascular imaging and other improved computerized image enhancements will allow for more precise catheter manipulation. It is likely that as diagnostic catheterization techniques improve, more specific data will be made available.

Many experts feel that the greatest area for growth in the field of cardiac catheterization is interventional procedures. Many procedures classified as experimental or investigational in the early 1980s are currently being performed with regular frequency. Application of laser technology combined with fiber optic direct visualization of intraluminal pathologic conditions is evolving as a new therapeutic modality for coronary artery disease patients. For example, laser angioplasty of the coronary anatomy is already being performed. In addition, atherectomy devices have also been applied to coronary artery disease. These devices actually cut the plaque out of the lumen of the artery. Balloon valvuloplasty is a therapeutic technique used to break open the leaflets of calcified valves by using a large balloon catheter. It is anticipated that many existing and new interventional procedures will provide some patients with viable, relatively low risk, and financially reasonable alternatives to open heart surgery. Current trends indicate that the number and variety of outpatient cardiac catheterizations will continue to increase.

It is expected that the types of equipment and procedures performed in cardiac catheterization laboratories of the future will be significantly different from those associated with existing facilities. However, despite changes in cardiovascular technology and medical techniques, cardiac catheterization laboratories will continue to provide essential patient care services necessary for the diagnosis and treatment of a vast number of cardiovascular-related diseases.

Definition of Terms

angina pectoris A severe form of chest pain and constriction near the heart usually caused by a decrease in the blood supply to the cardiac tissue. This decrease is most often associated with stenosis of a coronary artery as a result of atherosclerotic accumulations or spasm. Incidence of pain generally lasts for a few minutes and is more likely to occur after stress, exercise, or other activity resulting in an increased heart rate.

arteriosclerotic General pathologic condition characterized by thickening and hardening of arterial walls leading to a general loss of elasticity.

arteriotomy Surgical opening of an artery.

atheromatous Degenerative changes in the inner lining of arteries caused by deposition of fatty tissue and subsequent thickening of arterial walls occurring in atherosclerosis.

cardiac output The amount of blood pumped from the heart per given unit of time. The cardiac output can be calculated by multiplying the stroke volume (amount of blood in milliliters ejected from the left ventricle each heart beat) by the heart rate (number of heart beats per minute). A normal, resting adult with a stroke volume of 70 ml and a heart rate of 72 beats per minute would therefore have a cardiac output of approximately 5.0 liters per minute.

cardiomyopathies A relatively serious group of heart diseases typically characterized by enlargement of the myocardial layer of the left ventricle, resulting in decreased cardiac output. Hypertrophic cardiomyopathy is a condition often studied in the catheterization laboratory.

cinefluorography High-speed, 35 mm motion picture film recording of a fluoroscopic image. Recording of fluoroscopic images while structures contain radiographic contrast media is correctly termed "cineangiography."

dysrhythmia An abnormal heart rhythm as seen in an electrocardiogram (also referred to as an "arrhythmia").

ejection fraction Measurement of ventricular contractility expressed as the percentage of blood pumped out of the left ventricle during contraction. The ejection fraction can be estimated by evaluation of the left ventriculogram. The normal ejection fraction range is between 57% and 73% with an average of 65%. A low ejection fraction indicates failure of the left ventricle to pump effectively.

hematostasis The arrest of blood flow in a hemorrhage.

hemodynamics The study of those factors involved in the circulation of blood. Hemodynamic data typically collected during heart catheterization are cardiac output and intracardiac pressures.

ischemic A local decrease of blood supply to myocardial tissue associated with temporary obstruction of a coronary vessel, typically as a result of a thrombus (blood clot).

myocardial infarction An acute ischemic episode resulting in myocardial damage and pain (commonly referred to as a "heart attack").

occlusion Obstruction or closure of a vessel, such as a coronary vessel, as a result of thrombus or spasm.

oximetry The measurement of oxygen saturation in the blood.

paroxysm Sudden, periodic onset of a disease symptom, such as spasm.

patent foramen ovale An opening between the right atria and left atria that normally exists in fetal life to allow for the essential mixing of blood. The opening normally closes shortly before or after birth.

percutaneous transluminal coronary angioplasty (PTCA) Manipulative interventional procedure involving the placement and inflation of a balloon catheter in the lumen of a stenosed coronary artery for the purpose of compressing/fracturing the diseased material, thereby allowing for subsequent increased distal blood flow to the myocardium.

stenosis The narrowing or constriction of a vessel, orifice, or other type of passageway.

thrombolytic An agent such as a drug that causes the breakup of a thrombus.

transducer A device used to convert one form of energy into a different form of energy. Transducers used in cardiac catheterization convert fluid (blood) pressure into an electrical signal that is fed into the physiologic recorder.

transposition of the great arteries A congenital heart defect in which the aorta arises from the right side of the heart and the pulmonary artery arises from the left side of the heart. This condition requires interventional therapy.

variant angina Rare type of angina pectoris that occurs during rest and that may be a result of coronary artery spasm. Also called "Printzmetal's angina."

vasoconstrictor A drug or other agent that causes the blood vessels to narrow their internal openings (lumens).

vasodilator A drug or other agent that causes the blood vessels to widen their lumens.

vasospastic Characterized by spasm of a blood vessel.

venotomy Surgical opening of a vein.

SELECTED BIBLIOGRAPHY

Berne R and Levy M: Cardiovascular physiology, ed 4, St Louis, 1981, The CV Mosby Co.

Braunwald E: Heart disease: a textbook of cardiovascular medicine, vols 1 and 2, Philadelphia, 1980, WB Saunders Co.

Daily E and Schroeder J: Hemodynamic waveforms—exercises in identification and analysis, St Louis, 1983, The CV Mosby Co.

Ford RD: Cardiovascular disorders, ed 4, Philadelphia, 1984, Springhouse Corp.

Grossman W: Cardiac catheterization and angiography, ed 2, Philadelphia, 1980, Lea & Febiger.

Hurst JW: The heart, ed 5, vols I and II, New York, 1976, McGraw-Hill Book Co.

Verel D and Grainger RG: Cardiac catheterization and angiography, ed 3, New York, 1978, Churchill Livingstone, Inc.

White R: Fundamentals of vascular radiology, Philadelphia, 1976, Lea & Febiger.

Zimmerman HA: Intravascular catheterization, ed 2, Springfield, 1972, Charles C Thomas, Publisher.

Chapter 32

SECTIONAL ANATOMY FOR RADIOGRAPHERS

TERRI BRUCKNER

An understanding of the relationships between organ and skeletal structures is essential for the identification and localization of specific anatomic structures when using computed imaging modalities. The trend in the development of new imaging methods is most definitely toward sectional reconstruction, whether using x-ray, magnetic resonance, or diagnostic ultrasound imaging. The purpose of this chapter is to provide the radiographer who possesses a background in general anatomy with an orientation to sectional anatomy and to correlate such with structures demonstrated on images from the various radiology modalities.

The cadaver sections were selected as being representative of major organ structures for each of the body regions and are depicted from the inferior surface. The major anatomic structures normally seen when using current imaging modalities have been labeled. For each cadaver section presented, representative images have been included to provide an orientation to anatomic structures normally seen using the available imaging modalities. When axial images are viewed, it is useful to imagine that one is standing at the patient's feet and looking toward the head. With this orientation, the patient's right side will be to the viewer's left and vice versa. The anterior aspect of the patient is usually at the top of the image, and the posterior is at the bottom. All relational terms in the following discussion refer to the body in normal anatomic position.

Cranial Region

The computed tomography (CT) localizer, or scout, image (Fig. 32-1) represents a lateral image of the cranium. CT imaging for the cranium is generally performed with the gantry angled 15 to 20 degrees to the orbitomeatal line (OML). Magnetic resonance (MR) imaging of the cranium generally results in images parallel to the orbitomeatal or infraorbitomeatal plane. For further details on patient positioning, see the chapters describing computed tomography (Chapter 34) and magnetic resonance imaging (Chapter 37). Three identifying lines represent the approximate levels for each of the labeled cadaver sections and images for this region. The cranial cadaver section seen in Fig. 32-2 is sectioned through the frontal and parietal bones. The outer layer of gray matter (cortex) is clearly differentiated from the deeper white matter (myelinated fibers). The numerous convolutions (gyri) and fissures (sulci) are demonstrated. The cerebral hemispheres are separated by the longitudinal fissure. Invaginated in this fissure is a fold of dura mater, the falx cerebri. The superior sagittal sinus is a venous drainage system that runs through the superior margin of the falx and is closely related to the contour of the superior skull margin. In cross section, the anterior and posterior aspects of this sinus can be seen in the midline deep to the bony plates. Two of the five cerebral lobes are seen (frontal and parietal). The division between these lobes is the central sulcus. The corona radiata is a tract of white matter that connects all parts of the cerebral hemisphere to the basal ganglia.

The corresponding CT image (Fig. 32-3) demonstrates the structures discussed above. The superior sagittal sinus appears white because of the introduction of contrast medium.

The axial section through the midcranial region (Fig. 32-4) demonstrates the primary structures of the cerebral hemispheres. The falx cerebri is shown within the longitudinal fissure with the superior sagittal sinus in the anterior and posterior margins. The hemispheres are joined by a tract of white fibers known as the corpus callosum. The anterior portion of the corpus callosum is the genu, and the posterior portion is the splenium. In this section, the frontal, temporal, and occipital lobes are visualized along with the fifth lobe (insula or island of Reil), which is deep to the temporal lobe at the lateral fissure of Sylvius. At this level, the anterior and posterior horns (cornu) of the lateral ventricles are seen. The membranous layer between the anterior horns is the septum pellucidum. Within each posterior horn is the choroid plexus, a capillary network for the formation of cerebrospinal fluid. Deep to the cortex, much of the cerebrum is composed of tracts of white matter. Several areas of gray mat-

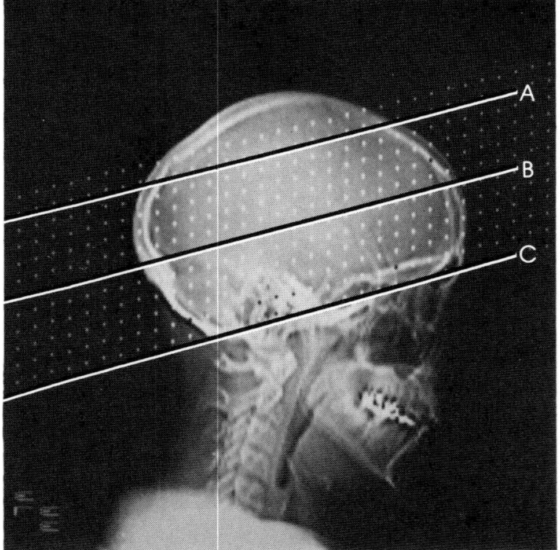

Fig. 32-1. CT localizer or scout image of skull.

ter are found deep within the white matter. These areas of gray matter relay information and are known collectively as the basal ganglia or cerebral nuclei. The major components of the basal ganglia are the caudate nucleus, the lentiform nucleus (composed of the putamen and the globus pallidus), and the amygdaloid nucleus. (Some texts include the claustrum with the basal ganglia.) The lentiform nucleus is separated from the caudate nucleus and the thalamus by a tract of white matter known as the internal capsule. The caudate nucleus is located lateral to each anterior horn of the lateral ventricles. The midline third ventricle is visualized at this level. The thalamus, which serves as a central relay station for sensory impulses to the cerebral cortex, is located surrounding the third ventricle. Between the third ventricle and the splenium of the corpus callosum is the pineal body. This is an important anatomic landmark because of its tendency to calcify in adults. Branches of the anterior cerebral arteries are found in the longitudinal fissure, just anterior to the genu of the corpus callosum. Branches of the middle cerebral arteries are found in the lateral fissures.

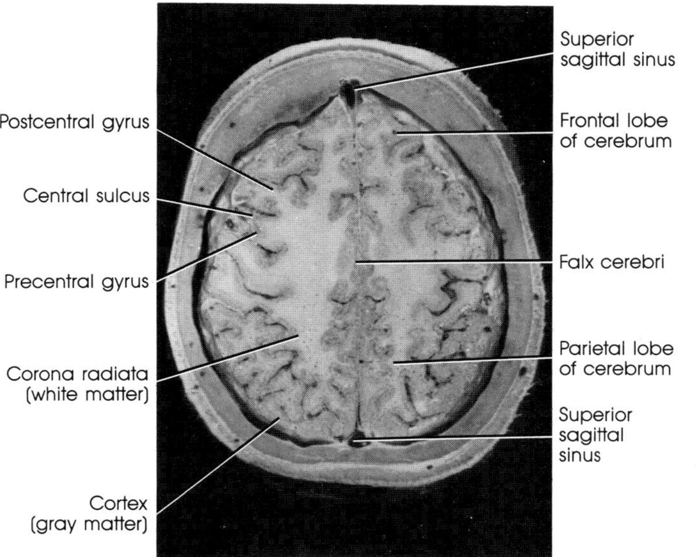

Fig. 32-2. Cadaver section corresponding to level A in Fig. 32-1.

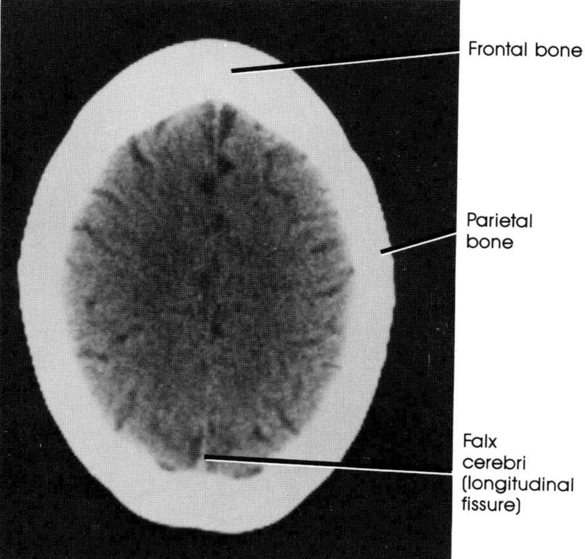

Fig. 32-3. Computed tomography (CT) image representing the anatomic structures located at level A in Fig. 32-1.

(Courtesy Theresa Spotts, R.T.)

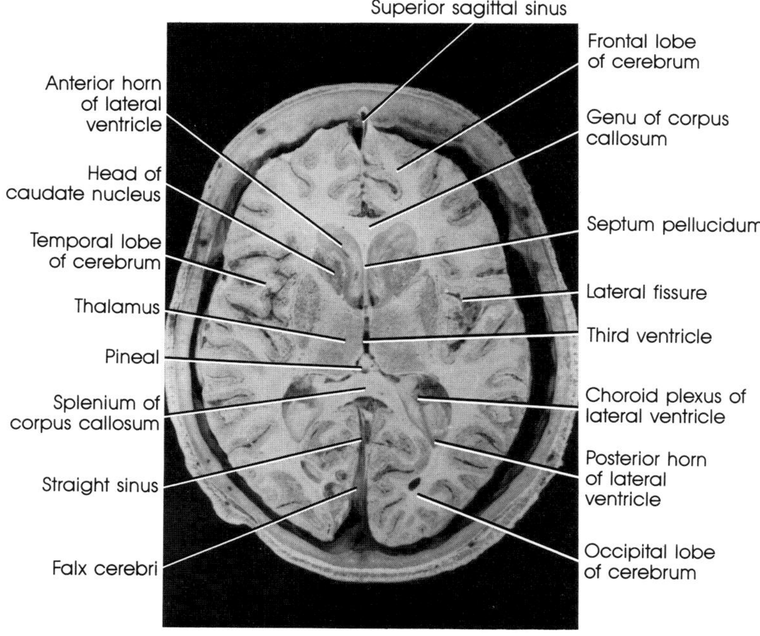

Fig. 32-4. Cadaver section corresponding to level B in Fig. 32-1.

Cranial region

Fig. 32-5 is a magnetic resonance (MR) image that corresponds to the cadaver section discussed previously. In this T1-weighted image, bone cortex appears black because of a lack of signal return. The high content of fat in the marrow cavity will appear white on these images. Cerebrospinal fluid within the ventricle appears dark. Note the differentiation between gray and white matter structures.

The cross section through the base of the cranium (Fig. 32-6) demonstrates the inferior portions of the cerebrum, the brainstem, the cerebellum, and the associated major skeletal structures. The temporal lobes are found in the middle cranial fossa between the lesser wings of the sphenoid and the pars petrosa. The hypophysis cerebri (pituitary gland) is located in the sella turcica, formed by the body of the sphenoid bone. Posterior to the sphenoid bone is the pons, a portion of the brain that relays impulses between the medulla oblongata and the cerebrum. The basilar artery lies in the midline directly anterior to the pons. The major portion of the posterior fossa is occupied by the cerebellum.

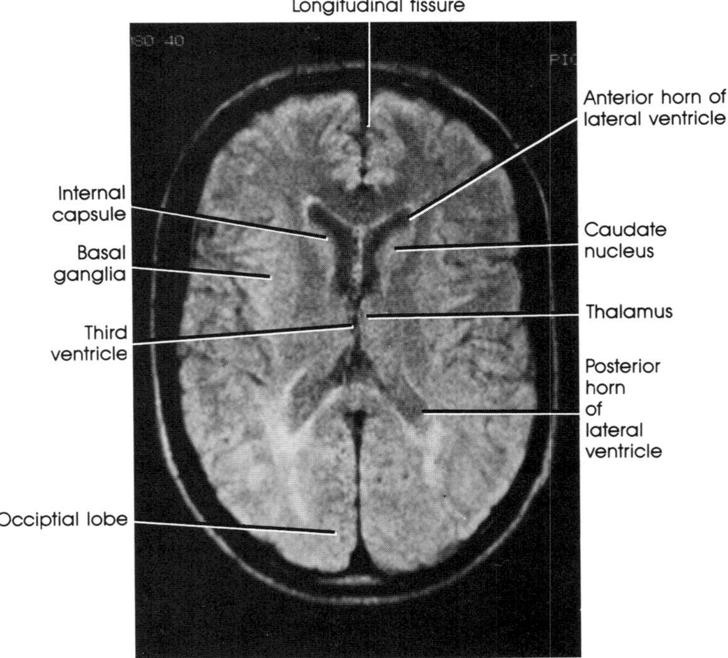

Fig. 32-5. Magnetic resonance (MR) image representing the structures located at level B in Fig. 32-1.

(Courtesy Picker International.)

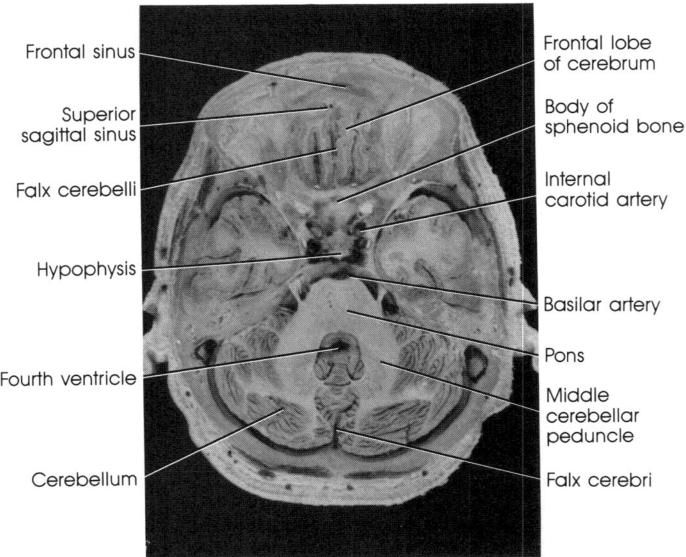

Fig. 32-6. Cadaver section corresponding to level C in Fig. 32-1.

The cerebellum functions as a reflex center for coordinating skeletal muscle movements. The cerebellum is divided into two hemispheres that are joined by the midline vermis. A fold of dura mater, the falx cerebelli, is found between the cerebellar hemispheres. The fourth ventricle is seen between the pons and the cerebellum. Posterior to the cerebellum the transverse dural venous sinuses are seen passing laterally in the margin of the tentorium cerebelli.

Fig. 32-7 is a magnetic resonance image through the orbits and posterior fossa. (Note the difference in orientation to the orbitomeatal plane between this MR image and the preceding cadaver and CT images.) The optic nerves can be seen extending posteriorly from the eyeballs toward the optic chiasm. The ethmoid air cells and sphenoid sinuses are both visualized at this level. Posterior and lateral to the sphenoid sinuses are the internal carotid arteries in the carotid canal.

The cadaver section labeled Fig. 32-8 is through the third cervical vertebra. At this level the hyoid bone (which serves as an attachment for the muscles of the tongue) is visualized. The submandibular (salivary) gland is found lateral to the hyoid at this level. Immediately posterior to the submandibular glands are the internal and external carotid arteries. These arteries are enclosed in the carotid sheath along with the internal jugular vein and vagus nerve. The vertebral arteries can be seen in the neck within the transverse foramina of the cervical vertebrae. The sternocleidomastoid muscles, which attach to the mastoid processes and the sternum and clavicle, are visualized lateral to the internal jugular veins.

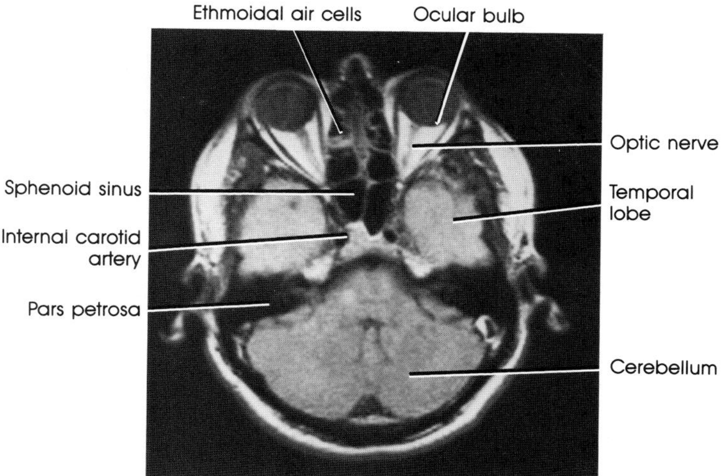

Fig. 32-7. MR image representing the anatomic structures located at level C in Fig. 32-1.

(Courtesy Picker International.)

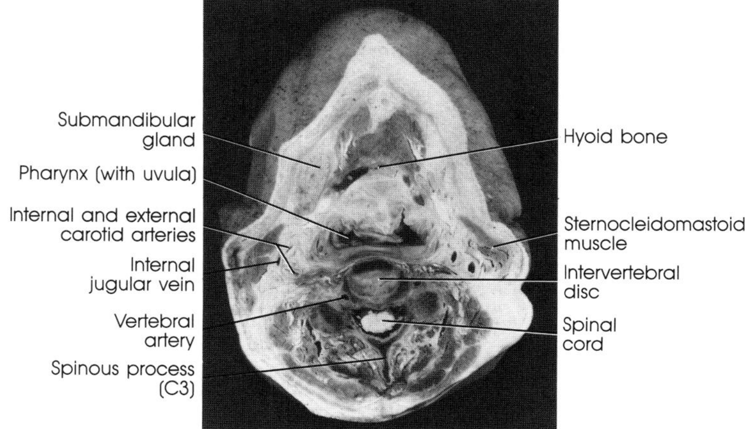

Fig. 32-8. Axial cadaver section through the third cervical vertebra.

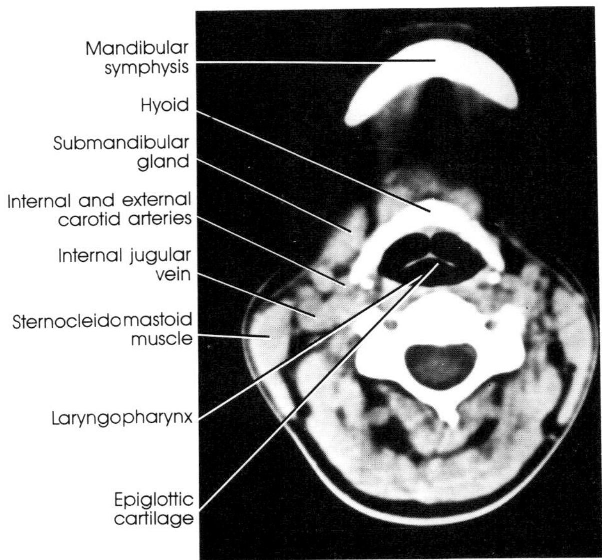

Fig. 32-9. CT image through the third cervical vertebra corresponding to Fig. 32-8.

(Courtesy Lyn VanDervort, R.T.)

Fig. 32-9 is a CT image through the hyoid bone. This image demonstrates the symphysis of the mandible anterior to the hyoid (with the suprahyoid muscles between). Deep to the hyoid bone is the epiglottic cartilage. The internal jugular vein and internal and external carotid arteries can be located but are not optimally visualized because of the lack of contrast media enhancement for this particular scan. Cadaver image (Fig. 32-10) and CT scan (Fig. 32-11) correspond to the body of the sixth cervical vertebra. The thyroid cartilage (Adam's apple) is seen surrounding the larynx and vocal

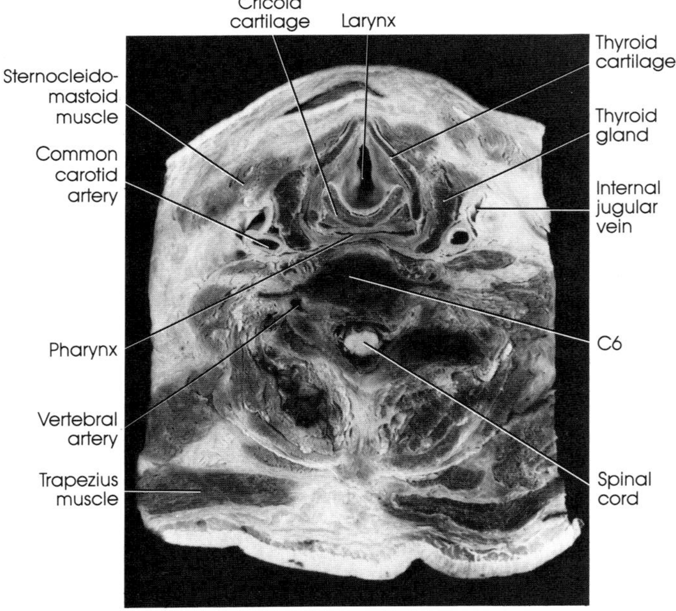

Fig. 32-10. Cadaver section through the sixth cervical vertebra.

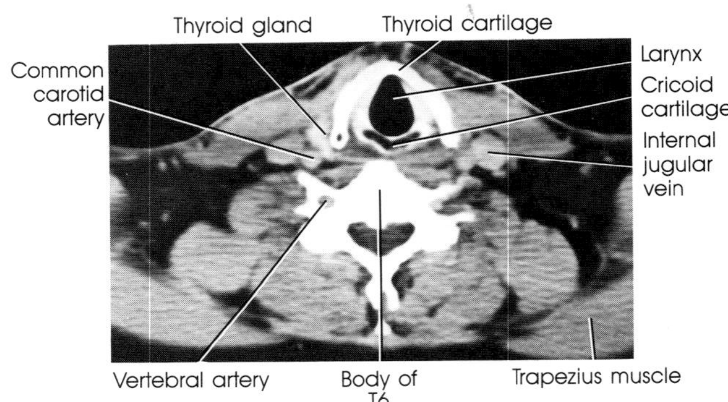

Fig. 32-11. CT image through the sixth cervical vertebra corresponding to Fig. 32-10.

(Courtesy Angelique Jacopin, R.T.)

cords. The cricoid cartilage (the lower edge of which signals the end of the pharynx) is seen posterior to the vocal cords. The thyroid gland has an H-shaped configuration with two lateral lobes connected by a horizontal portion (isthmus). The lobes of the thyroid gland are found on the posterolateral aspects of the thyroid cartilage (and in lower sections lateral to the trachea) and appear highlighted on CT scans because of normal iodine content. At this level the common carotid artery, internal jugular vein, and vagus nerve are seen on each side of the pharynx enclosed within the carotid sheath. The vertebral arteries are noted again within the transverse foramina of C6.

It is increasingly common to find images in the sagittal and coronal planes. CT scanners have the capability to image in the axial plane and reconstruct the information in these alternate planes. MR, on the other hand, is capable of direct axial, sagittal, and coronal imaging. Representative images have been selected in the sagittal and coronal planes to help interpret the anatomy demonstrated.

Fig. 32-12 is a midline sagittal MR image of the cranium. The relationship between the cerebral hemisphere, cerebellum, and brainstem is demonstrated. In this image the frontal, parietal, and occipital lobes of the cerebrum are seen and correspond to the cranial bones. The corpus callosum is a white matter tract that connects the hemispheres and is found at the inferior aspect of the parietal lobe. Cerebrospinal fluid appears dark on this T1-weighted image, making it relatively easy to trace the ventricular system. The anterior horn of the lateral ventricle is inferior to the genu of the corpus callosum. The midline third ventricle receives cerebrospinal fluid by way of the foramen of Monro and is not optimally visualized in this image. Cerebrospinal fluid drains from the third ventricle via the cerebral aqueduct of Sylvius, which can be found within the midbrain (between the corpora quadrigemina and the cerebral peduncles). The fourth ventricle is also a midline structure and is situated between the pons and the cerebellum. The large air-filled sphenoid sinus is located anterior to the pons. Superior to this, the pituitary gland (hypophysis cerebri) rests within the sella turcica. Directly superior to the pituitary is the optic chiasm. Several vascular structures are well demonstrated in this image. The basilar artery appears between the clivus and the pons. The great cerebral vein of Galen is posterior to the splenium of the corpus callosum. Between the cerebrum and the cerebellum, the straight sinus (one of the dural venous sinuses) is noted within the tentorium cerebelli.

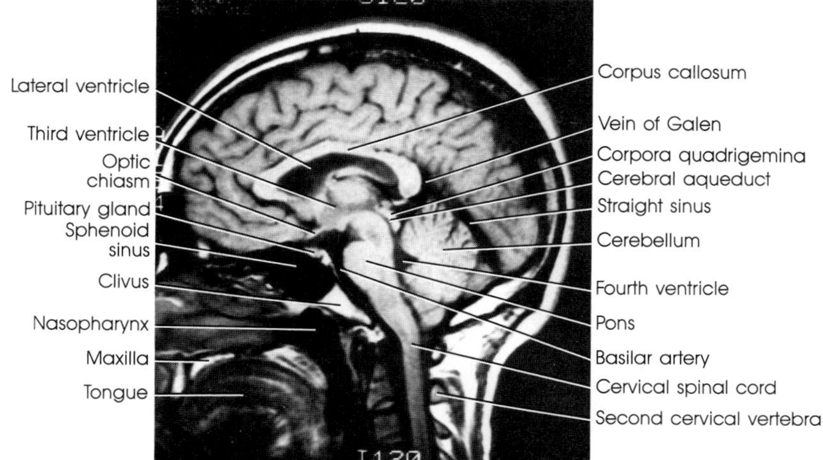

Fig. 32-12. Sagittal MR image through the midsagittal plane.

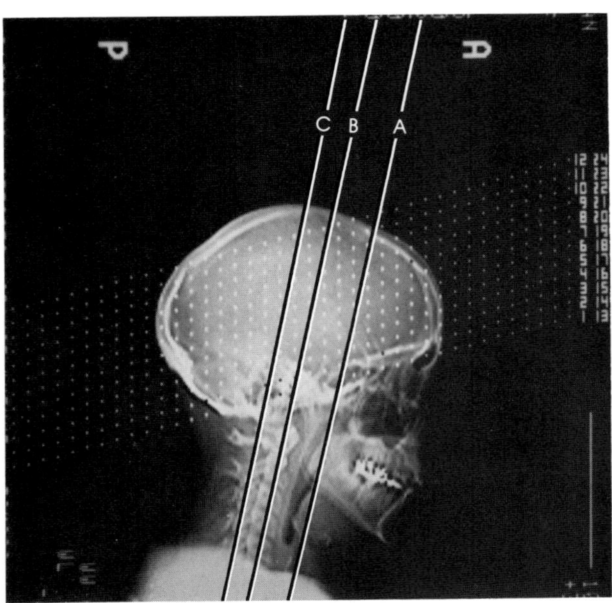

Fig. 32-13. CT localizer or scout image of the skull.

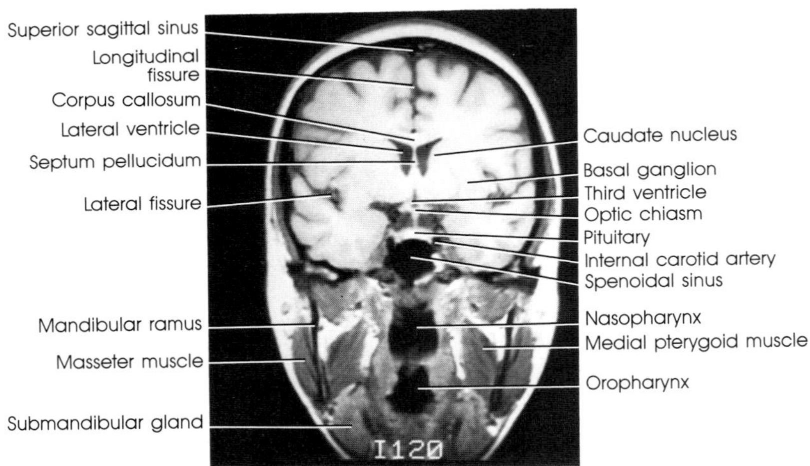

Fig. 32-14. Coronal MR image corresponding to level A in Fig. 32-13.

A CT localizer (Fig. 32-13) is included for reference in the next three coronal images. Fig. 32-14 is a coronal MR image through the anterior horns of the lateral ventricles and the pharyngeal structures. The anterior portions of the cerebral hemispheres are joined by the corpus callosum, which is immediately superior to the lateral ventricles. The membrane between the anterior horns (of the lateral ventricles) is the septum pellucidum. On the lateral aspect of each cerebral hemisphere is the lateral fissure of Sylvius, which divides the frontal lobe from the temporal lobe. The insula lies deep to this fissure. Structures of the basal ganglion can again be identified. The caudate nucleus is seen lateral to the anterior horns. Inferolateral to the caudate nucleus are the putamen and globus pallidus (labelled basal ganglion). The anterior portion of the third ventricle is found in the midline inferior to the lateral ventricles. Inferior to the third ventricle are the optic chiasm and the pituitary gland. The superior and inferior sagittal sinuses occupy the margins of the falx cerebri in the longitudinal fissure between the hemispheres of the cerebrum. The internal carotid arteries occupy the cavernous sinus along with several cranial nerves and are found lateral to the pituitary and sella turcica. Branches of the middle cerebral arteries occupy the lateral fissures of the cerebrum. Several air-filled structures are seen on this image and they are (from superior to inferior) the sphenoid sinus, nasopharynx, and oropharynx. This image also demonstrates the rami of the mandible along with the masseter and pterygoid muscles. The submandibular (salivary) glands are found deep to the gonion (angle) of the mandible.

Fig. 32-15 is a coronal MR image through the bodies of the lateral ventricles, the brainstem, and the anterior cervical vertebrae. The third ventricle is well demonstrated and bordered laterally by the thalamus. The cartilaginous structures of the external ear surround the external auditory meatus and canal. The dark region (low signal return) medial to the external ear canal corresponds to the petrous portion of the temporal bone. Within this region the seventh and eighth (facial and vestibulocochlear) cranial nerves are found in the internal auditory canal. The first three cervical vertebrae are detailed in this section with the dens (odontoid process) of the axis (C2) seen between the lateral masses of the atlas (C1). The vertebral arteries are demonstrated within the transverse foramina, lateral to the bodies of cervical vertebrae. The internal carotid arteries are found more laterally in the neck between the sternocleidomastoid muscles and the cervical spine. The large whitish masses inferior to the external auditory canals are the parotid (salivary) glands.

Fig. 32-16 shows a coronal MR image through the lateral ventricles, brainstem, and spinal cord. The splenium of the corpus callosum is found between the lateral ventricles. Inferior to the splenium is the midline pineal gland. The cerebral aqueduct of Sylvius is also a midline structure found within the midbrain. On either side of the cerebral aqueduct are the superior and inferior colliculi (corpora quadrigemina), which are associated with visual and auditory reflexes. Two large white matter tracts are seen extending laterally, inferior to the colliculi. These are the middle cerebellar peduncles, which serve as pathways connecting the cerebrum and cerebellum. Portions of the cerebellum are visualized superior and inferior to the middle cerebellar peduncles. The medulla oblongata is the most inferior segment of the brainstem and is continuous with the spinal cord as it passes through the foramen magnum. The large dark area (signal void) corresponds to the bony mastoid portion of the temporal bone.

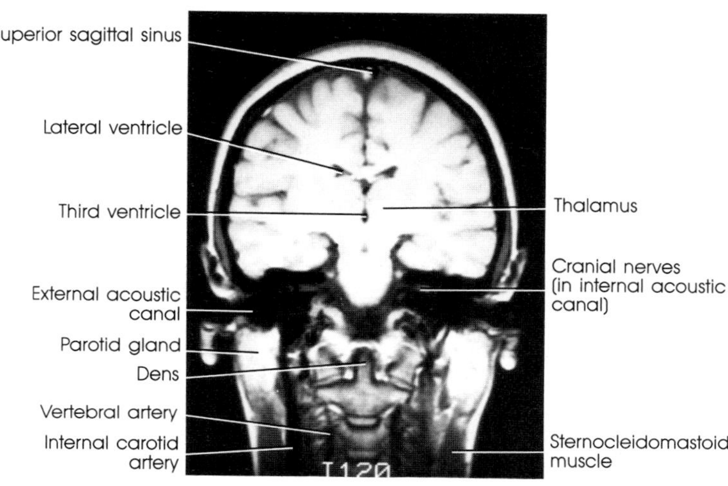

Fig. 32-15. Coronal MR image corresponding to level B in Fig. 32-13.

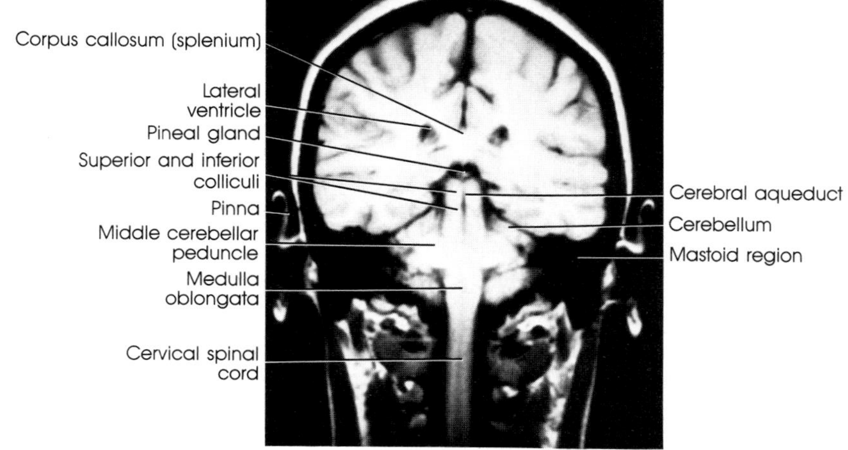

Fig. 32-16. Coronal MR image corresponding to level C in Fig. 32-13.

Cranial region

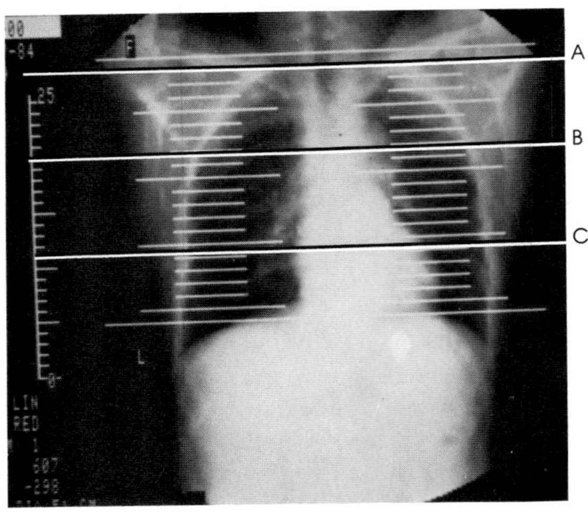

Fig. 32-17. CT localizer or scout image of thorax.

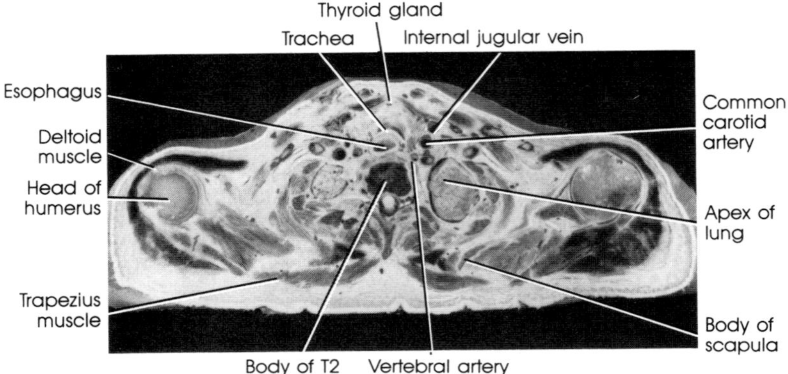

Fig. 32-18. Cadaver section corresponding to level A of Fig. 32-17 at the second thoracic vertebra.

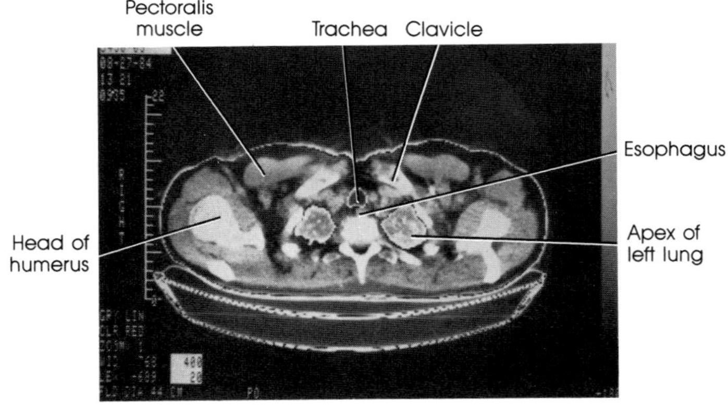

Fig. 32-19. CT image corresponding to Fig. 32-18.

(Courtesy Theresa Spotts, R.T.)

Thoracic Region

The CT localizer, or scout image, represents an AP projection of the thoracic region with three identifying lines (Fig. 32-17). These lines demonstrate the approximate three levels for each of the labeled cadaver sections for this region.

The cross section and CT images (Figs. 32-18 and 32-19) at the level of T2 demonstrate the relationship between the vertebral column, esophagus, and trachea. The inferior portion of the thyroid gland, which extends from C6 to T1, is positioned lateral to the trachea. The vertebral arteries are positioned lateral to the vertebral column, and the common carotid arteries are found lateral to the trachea. At this level the internal jugular veins are anterior to the carotid arteries. The apices of the lungs are visualized along with the first two ribs, the glenohumeral joint, and the sternal extremity of the clavicle. The trapezius, pectoral, and deltoid muscles are clearly seen. The muscles of the rotator cuff (supraspinatus, infraspinatus, subscapularis, and teres minor) stabilize the glenohumeral joint. At this level the supraspinatus, which lies superior to the scapular spine, is visualized.

The cross section and CT scan (Figs. 32-20 and 32-21) at the level of T5 demonstrate the great vessels superior to the heart. (The heart is normally positioned between T7 and T11, with the majority of the organ lying to the left of the midline.) The ascending aorta is found anteriorly in the midline; the descending aorta is related to the left anterior surface of the vertebral bodies. (This relationship between descending aorta and vertebral column is continuous through the thorax and abdomen.) The superior vena cava is located to the right of the ascending aorta, and the pulmonary trunk is located to the left of the ascending aorta at this level. The pulmonary trunk originates from the right ventricle of the heart and divides into the right and left pulmonary arteries, which carry deoxygenated blood to the lungs. In these figures the right and left pulmonary arteries are seen at the hilus of each lung. The azygos vein, which serves as a vessel for collateral blood flow (anastomosis) for obstruction of the inferior vena cava (IVC) or portal vein, is positioned anterior and to the right of the vertebral column from its origination near the diaphragm until it empties into the superior vena cava at the level of T4 or T5. At the T5 vertebral level the trachea divides into the left and right primary bronchi. The thoracic duct, one of the major channels for lymphatic drainage, generally originates at the twelfth thoracic vertebra and ascends the thorax in the posterior mediastinum between the aorta and the azygos vein. The duct ultimately empties into the venous blood system at the junction of the left subclavian and internal jugular veins.

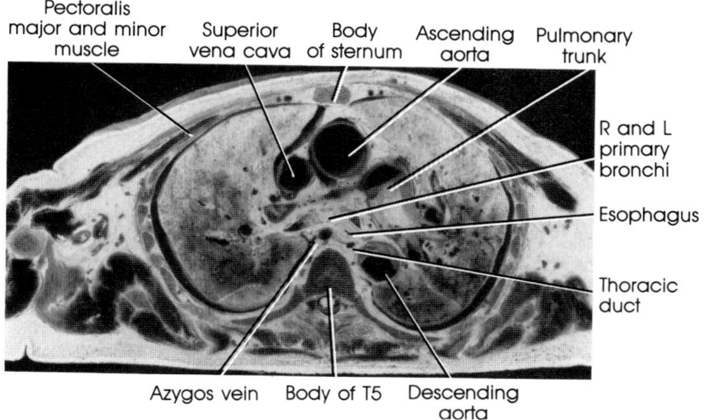

Fig. 32-20. Cadaver section corresponding to level B of Fig. 32-17 at the fifth thoracic vertebra.

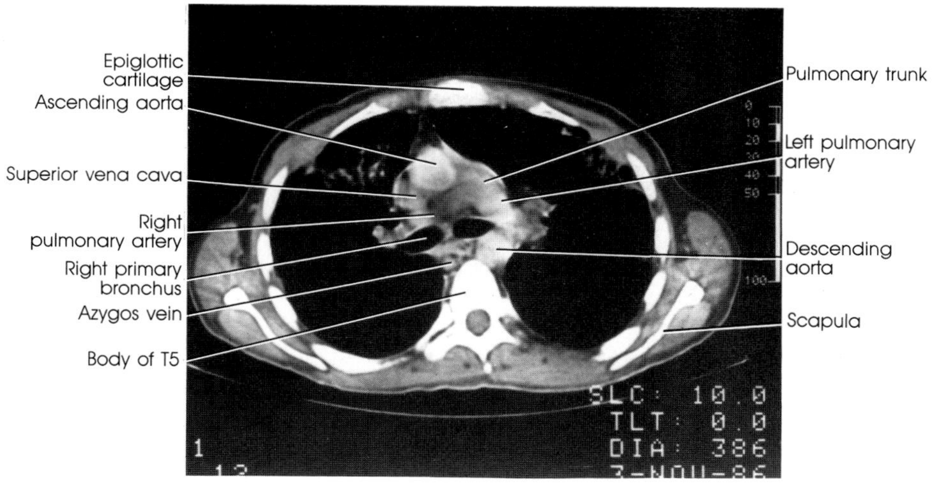

Fig. 32-21. CT image corresponding to Fig. 32-20.

Thoracic region

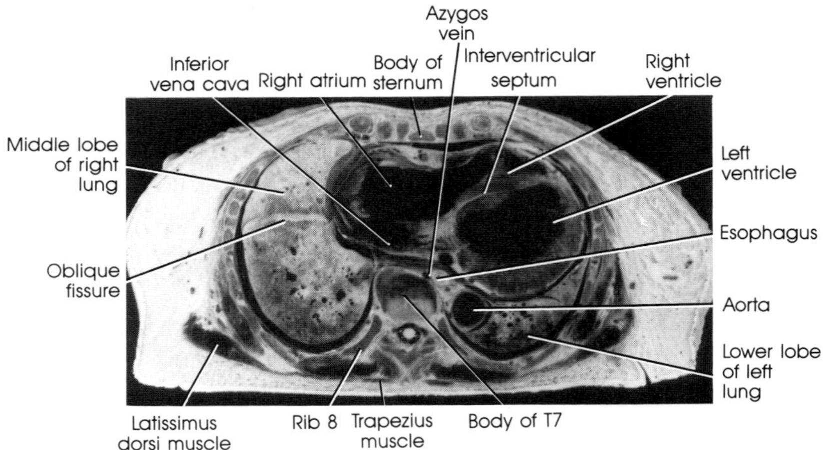

Fig. 32-22. Cadaver section corresponding to level C in Fig. 32-17 at the seventh thoracic vertebra.

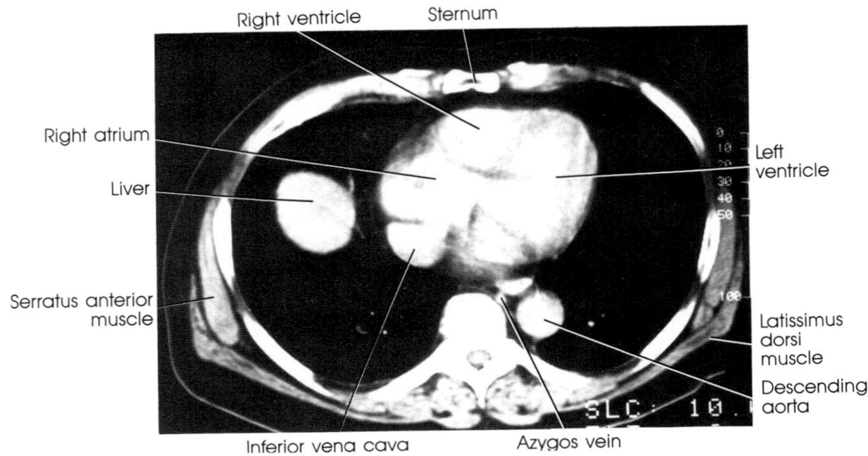

Fig. 32-23. CT image corresponding to Fig. 32-22.

The cross section and CT image at T7 (Figs. 32-22 and 32-23) demonstrate the lungs and the midsection of the heart. Generally, when the heart is imaged in cross section, the left atrium will be the most superior structure encountered, and the pulmonary veins will be seen emptying into it. The right atrium will be seen lying the farthest toward the right side of the body anterior and somewhat inferior to the left atrium. The inferior vena cava may be seen at this level as it enters the right atrium. (The superior vena cava may be seen emptying into the right atrium in more superior images.) The right ventricle lies to the left of the right atrium and anterior to the more muscular left ventricle. The interventricular septum can be seen between the ventricles. The right lung is divided into three lobes: superior, middle, and inferior. The superior lobe is superior and anterior, the middle lobe is inferior and anterior, the inferior lobe is inferior and posterior. The left lung is divided into two lobes: superior and inferior. (The superior lobe of the left lung corresponds to the superior and middle lobes of the right lung.) The inferior lobes are separated from the other lobes by the oblique fissures.

Fig. 32-24 presents a sagittal image through the midline structures of the neck and upper thorax. The air-filled pharynx and trachea are easily identified. The cartilaginous flap within the laryngeal portion of the pharynx is the epiglottis. Spinal structures are well seen in this image, and the relationship between the intervertebral disks and the spinal cord is clearly depicted. The major blood vessels of the superior thorax are seen posterior to the manubrium. The most anterior of these vessels is the left brachiocephalic vein, which ultimately unites with the right brachiocephalic vein to form the superior vena cava. Posterior to the brachiocephalic vein one sees a portion of the aortic arch with the origin of the left common carotid artery. Inferior to the arch is the left main pulmonary artery.

The MR coronal image in Fig. 32-25 is slightly posterior to the midcoronal plane and also demonstrates structures of the neck and superior thorax. The inferior cervical and superior thoracic vertebrae can be identified. On the patient's left side, note the humeral head, clavicle, acromion process, and acromioclavicular joint. The tracheal bifurcation is seen on this image. The aortic arch and pulmonary trunk are found in close proximity to the left mainstem bronchus. From the superior aspect of the arch extends the left subclavian artery. The heart and lungs are not ideally imaged in this scan because of motion artifacts. (See Chapter 37 on magnetic resonance imaging for methods to overcome this problem.)

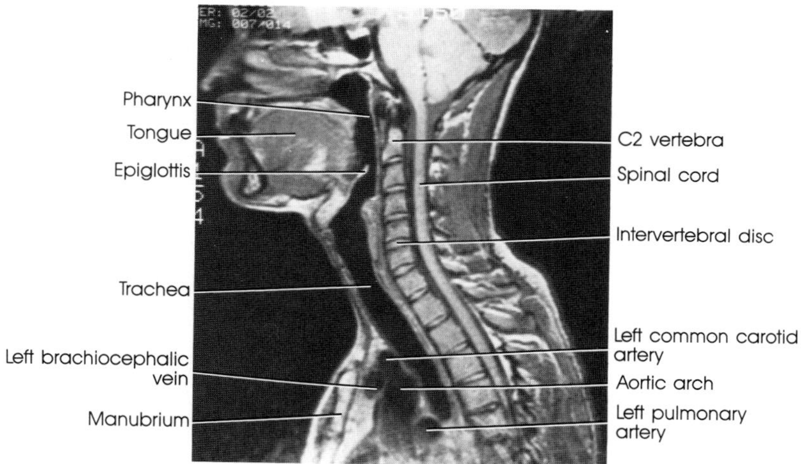

Fig. 32-24. Midline sagittal MR image through the neck and upper thorax.

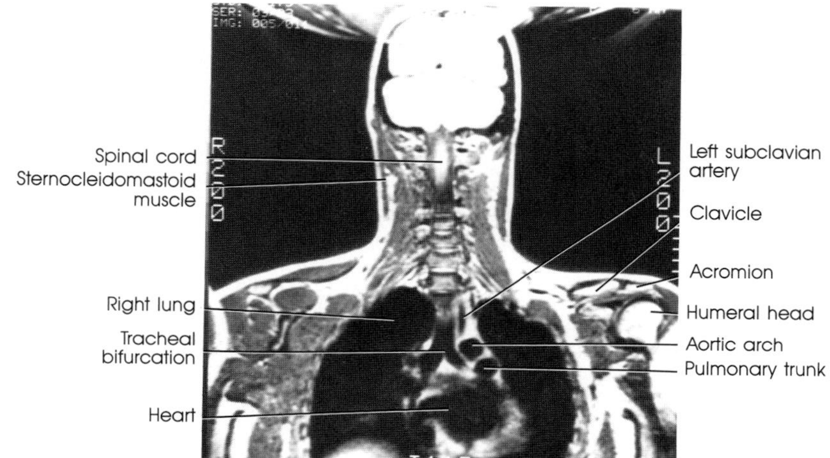

Fig. 32-25. Magnetic resonance image of the neck and thorax through the midcoronal plane.

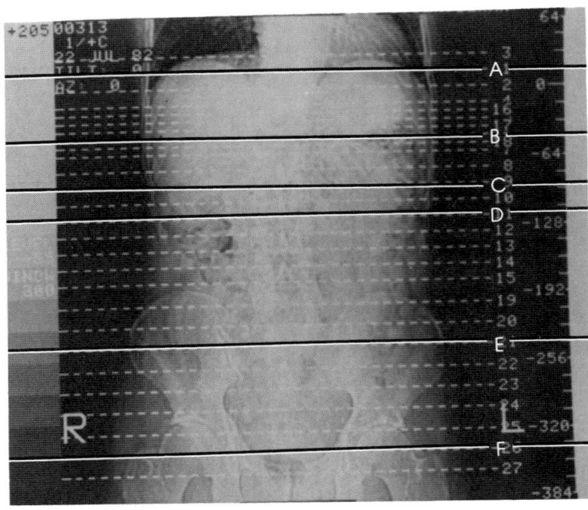

Fig. 32-26. CT localizer or scout image of the abdominopelvic region.

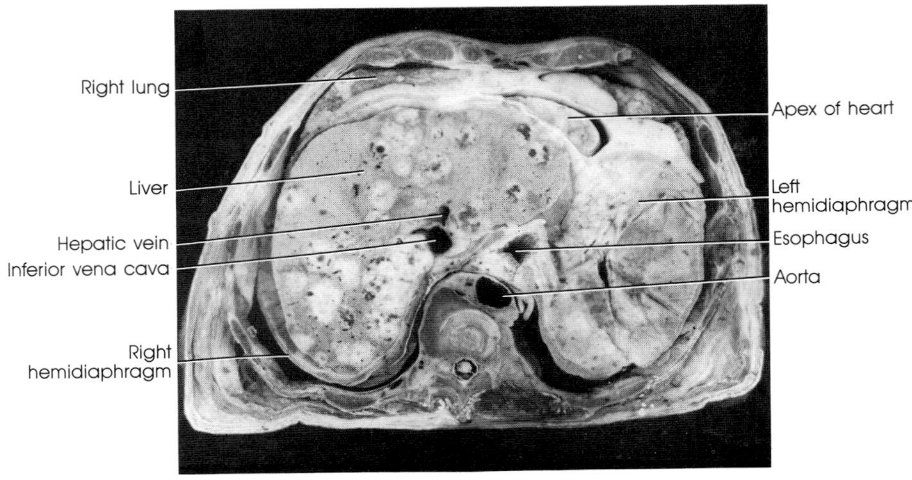

Fig. 32-27. Cadaver section corresponding to level A in Fig. 32-26 at the tenth thoracic vertebra.

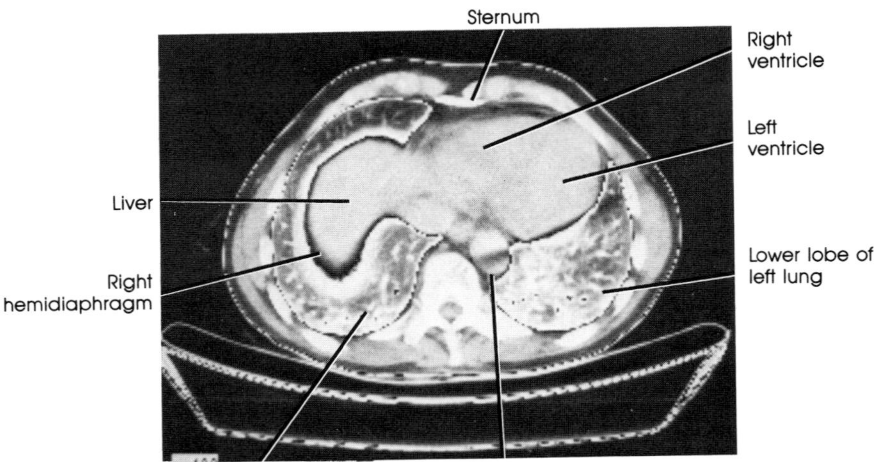

Fig. 32-28. CT image corresponding to Fig. 32-27.

Abdominopelvic Region

The CT localizer, or scout image (Fig. 32-26), representing an AP projection of the abdominopelvic region has six identifying lines demonstrating the levels for each of the labeled cadaver sections and images for this region.

Fig. 32-27 and 32-28 represent structures seen at the T10-11 levels (corresponding to level A in the localizer, Fig. 32-26). The cadaver section (Fig. 32-27) demonstrates the right hemidiaphragm surrounding the superior portion of the liver, and the left hemidiaphragm in its entirety. The apex of the heart is seen to the left of the liver. The esophagus, posterior to the liver, has migrated toward the patient's left as it nears its entrance into the stomach. The aorta is in its normal position, anterior and slightly left of the vertebral body. The inferior vena cava (IVC) appears embedded within the liver. Hepatic veins are draining into the IVC at this level. The CT scan (Fig. 32-28) is at a slightly more superior level. The lower lobes of both lungs are seen. The right hemidiaphragm is seen surrounding the superior portion of the liver. The inferior portion of the heart details the right and left ventricles.

The cross section and CT scan at the level of T12 (Figs. 32-29 and 32-30) demonstrate the relationship between the liver, stomach, and spleen. The stomach is located between the levels of T11 and L2, in the anterior aspect of the left upper quadrant. The spleen, located between the levels of T12 and L1, is in the posterolateral aspect of the left upper quadrant posterior to the fundus of the stomach. The liver is generally found between T11 and L3 and occupies the entire right upper quadrant. The right lobe of the liver has two small subdivisions, the caudate and quadrate lobes, which are bounded by the gallbladder, the ligamentum teres, and the inferior vena cava. The left lobe of liver stretches across the midline and into the left upper quadrant. The suprarenal (adrenal) glands are normally located superior to the kidney. The right adrenal gland is found at this level between the liver and the right diaphragmatic crus. The abdominal aorta is positioned anterior and to the left of the vertebral column with the celiac trunk projecting anteriorly. The three branches of the celiac trunk (hepatic, splenic, left gastric arteries) supply the liver, spleen, and stomach with oxygen-rich blood. The splenic artery runs a very tortuous course and normally cannot be visualized in its entirety in axial sections. The IVC can be seen in its normal position anterior and to the right of the vertebral column. The muscles of the abdomen are located between the lower rib cage and the iliac crest of the pelvis. This group of muscles includes the external oblique, internal oblique, and transverse abdominal muscles. The two rectus abdominis muscles are located on the anterior aspect of the abdomen on either side of the midline and extend from the symphysis pubis to the xiphoid process. The psoas muscles originate from the body of the twelfth thoracic vertebra and the transverse processes of the lumbar vertebrae and descend the abdomen lateral to the vertebral bodies. The quadratus lumborum muscles are located posterolateral to the psoas muscles through the abdomen.

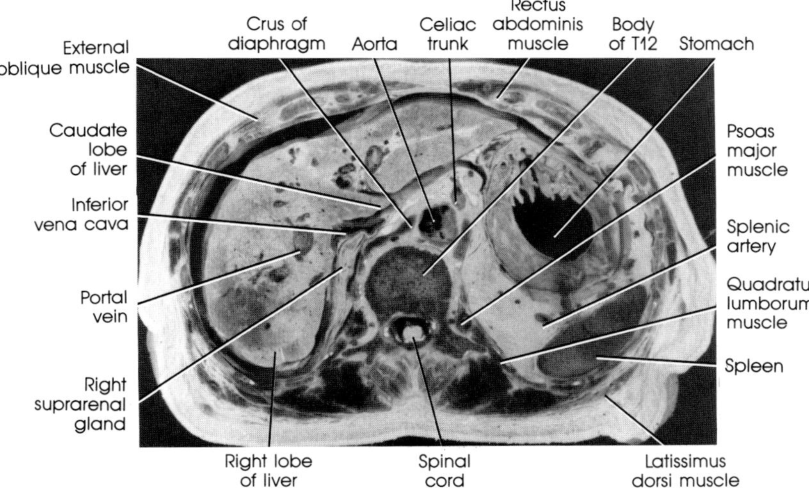

Fig. 32-29. Cadaver section corresponding to level B of Fig. 32-26 at the twelfth thoracic vertebra.

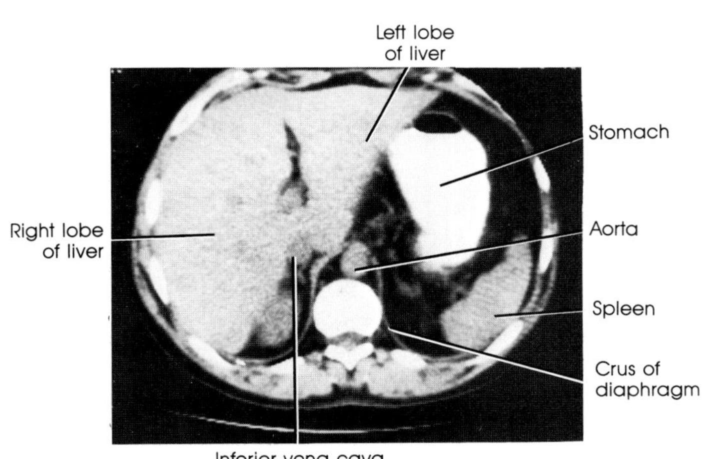

Fig. 32-30. CT image corresponding to Fig. 32-29.

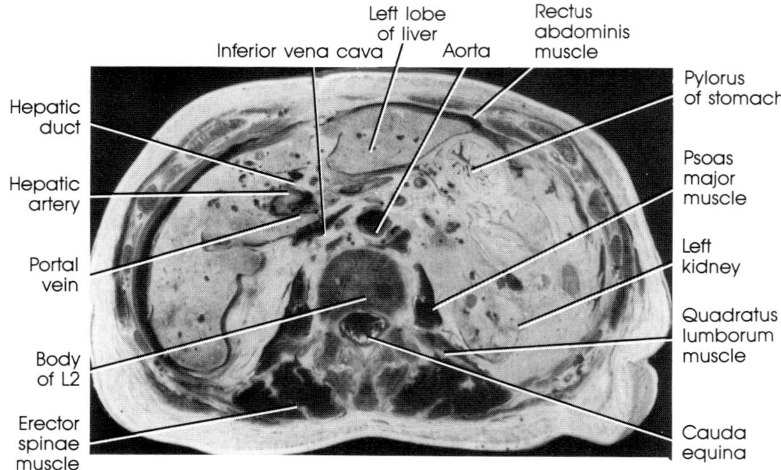

Fig. 32-31. Cadaver section corresponding to level C of Fig. 32-26 at the second lumbar vertebra.

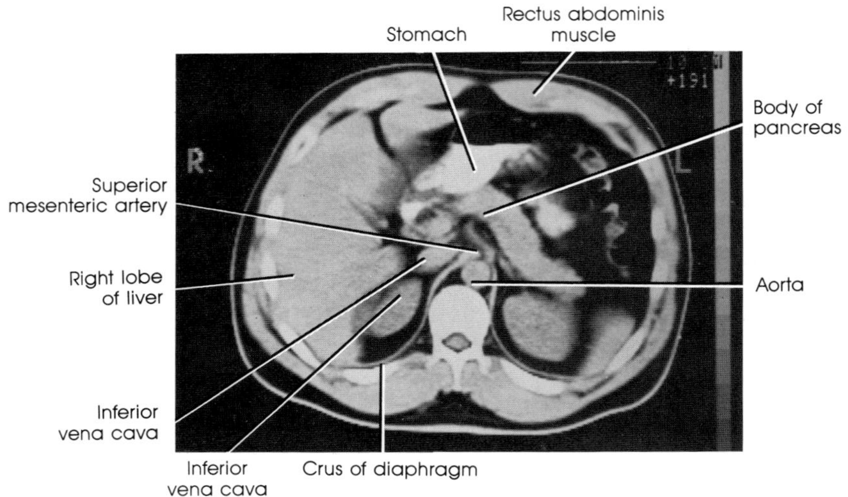

Fig. 32-32. CT image corresponding to Fig. 32-31. Note the crus (tendinous origin) of the diaphragm surrounding the aorta.

The cross section and CT scan at the level of the second lumbar vertebra (Figs. 32-31 and 32-32) demonstrate the inferior aspect of the liver with the porta hepatis. At the porta hepatis the vasculature of the liver can be seen in its normal configuration with the hepatic duct lying anterior to the hepatic artery and the portal vein lying posterior to the hepatic artery. The superior pole of the left kidney is visualized along with the pylorus of the stomach. The pancreas lies essentially in a horizontal plane posterior to the stomach and liver. The head of the pancreas is near the liver and surrounded by the duodenum (C-loop). The tail of the pancreas is slightly superior to the head and is located near the hilus of the spleen. Posterior to the left lobe of the liver and the neck of the pancreas, the junction of the splenic vein and the superior mesenteric vein is visualized. This junction is the origin for the portal vein. The superior mesenteric artery lies anterior and to the left of the aorta and can be seen originating from the aorta in the CT scan. The IVC is seen as the left renal vein empties into it. Lateral to the vertebral body are the psoas muscles. The quadratus lumborum muscles are seen between the psoas muscles and the transverse processes of the lumbar vertebrae. The spinal cord normally terminates at the level of the first lumbar vertebra. Inferior to L1, the spinal nerves (cauda equina) are seen within the spinal canal.

Fig. 32-33 and 32-34 represent the level of the intervertebral disk between L2 and L3. At this level the gallbladder is seen lying against the inferior aspect of the liver. The pylorus of the stomach and the first, or horizontal, portion (bulb) of the duodenum is anterior in the abdomen. The descending colon is seen in the left posterior and lateral aspect of the abdomen. The ascending colon is seen in Fig. 32-33 lateral to the right kidney as it makes its anterior turn toward the transverse colon (hepatic flexure). This level demonstrates the hilus of each kidney and the head, neck, and body of the pancreas (across the midline). The inferior vena cava is seen behind the head of the pancreas with the right renal vein emptying into it. The superior mesenteric vessels and aorta are located posterior to the body of the pancreas.

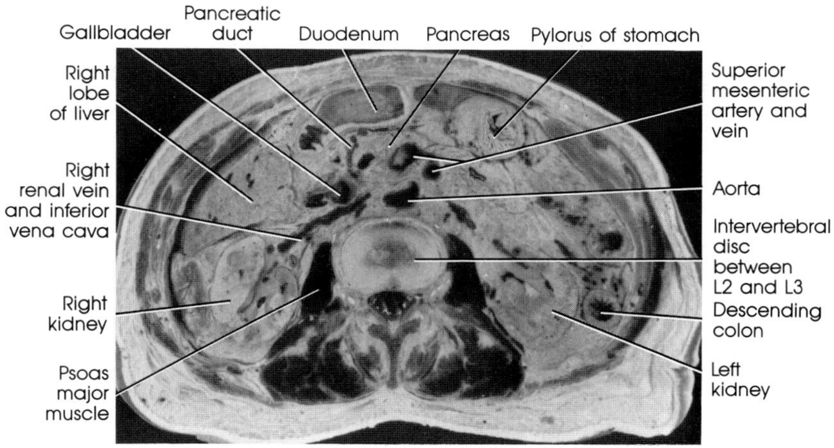

Fig. 32-33. Cadaver section corresponding to level D of Fig. 32-26 at the interspace between the second and third lumbar vertebrae.

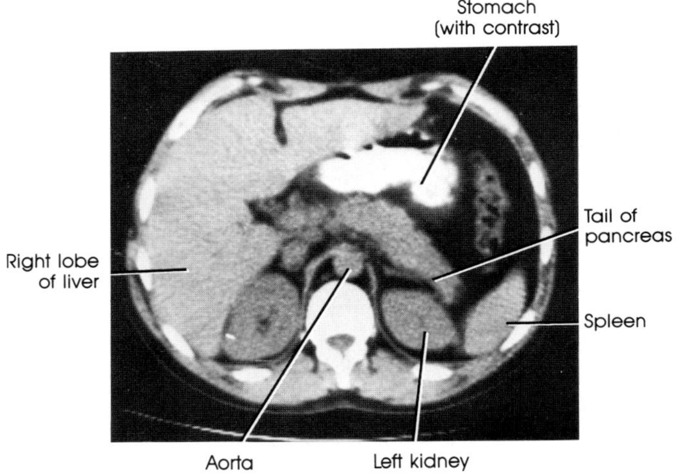

Fig. 32-34. CT image corresponding to Fig. 32-33.

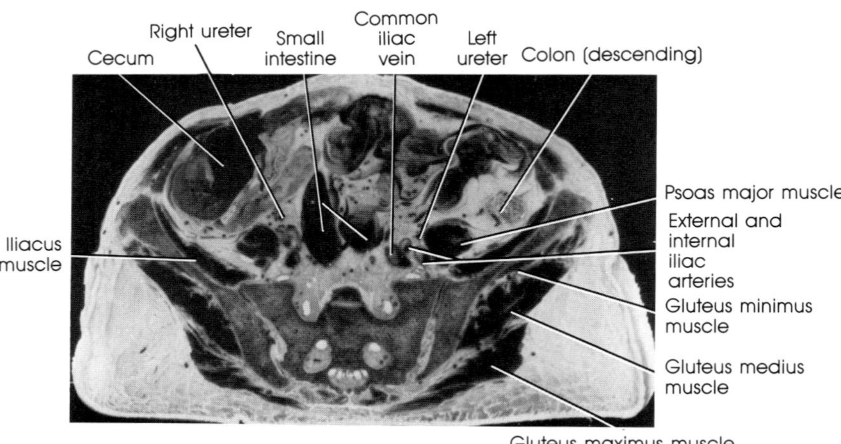

Fig. 32-35. Cadaver section corresponding to level E of Fig. 32-26 at the anterior superior iliac spine (ASIS).

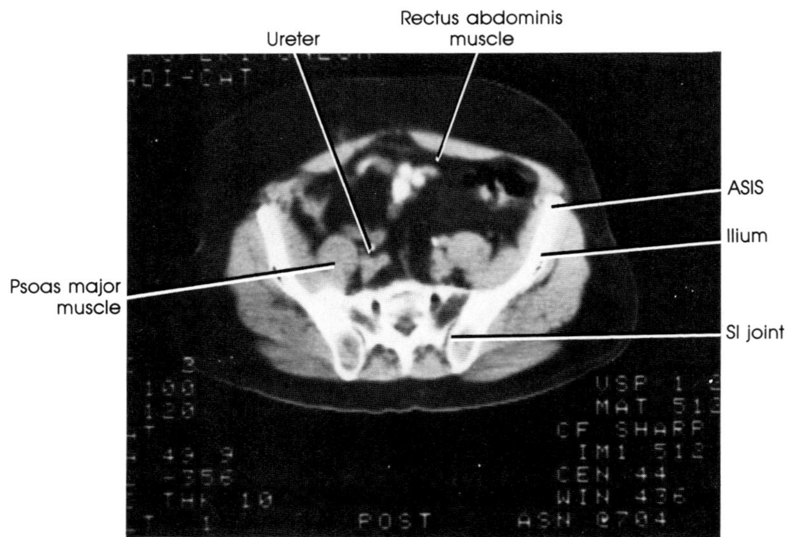

Fig. 32-36. CT image corresponding to Fig. 32-35.

(Courtesy Tom Meridith, R.T.)

The cross section and CT scan seen in Fig. 32-35 and 32-36 are at the midsacral level and demonstrate the wing (ala) of the ilium, the anterior superior iliac spine (ASIS), and the sacroiliac (SI) joints. At the posterolateral aspect of the ilium the three gluteal muscles are visualized. The iliacus muscle is seen lining the internal aspect of the iliac wings near the psoas muscles. The cecum is found at the right anterior aspect of the pelvic cavity and the descending colon at the left lateral aspect. Multiple loops of small intestine are found throughout this level in the images. The abdominal aorta bifurcates at the fourth lumbar vertebra into the common iliac arteries. Each common iliac artery divides at the level of the ASIS into internal and external iliac arteries. The internal iliac arteries tend to be located in the posterior pelvis and branch to feed the pelvic structures. The external iliac vessels will be found progressively anterior in succeeding inferior sections to become the femoral vessels at the superior aspect of the thigh. The internal and external iliac veins unite inferior to the ASIS to form the common iliac veins, and the IVC is formed anterior to the fifth lumbar vertebra by the junction of the common iliac veins. The common iliac veins are positioned at the anterior aspects of the sacrum with the internal and external iliac arteries lateral to the veins in these images. Through the abdomen and at this level the ureters are located along the anterior aspect of the psoas muscles and can be seen filled with contrast in the CT image (Fig. 32-36). In the female pelvis, the ovaries are normally located laterally in the pelvis near the anterior superior iliac spines.

The cross section and CT scan seen in Fig. 32-37 and 32-38 are at a level just superior to the pubic symphysis. The ischial spines, acetabula, femoral heads, and greater trochanters are visualized. The relationship between the rectum, vagina, wall of the bladder, and superior aperture of the urethra is demonstrated from posterior to anterior in the pelvic region. The external iliac vessels are now known as the femoral vessels, with the name change occurring at the inguinal ligament, which is found between the pubic symphysis and the ASIS. The iliopsoas muscles (formed by the junction of the psoas and iliacus muscles) are found anterior to the femoral heads; the internal obturator muscle, with its characteristic right-angle bend, is found medial to the acetabulum.

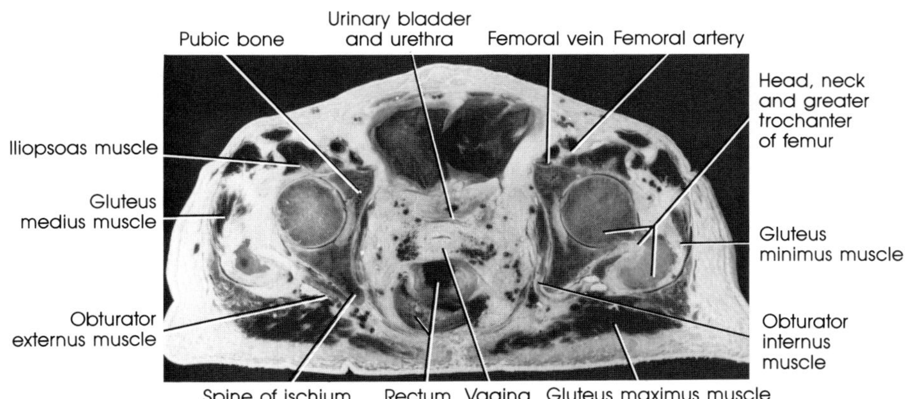

Fig. 32-37. Cadaver section corresponding to level F of Fig. 32-26 at the coccyx (female).

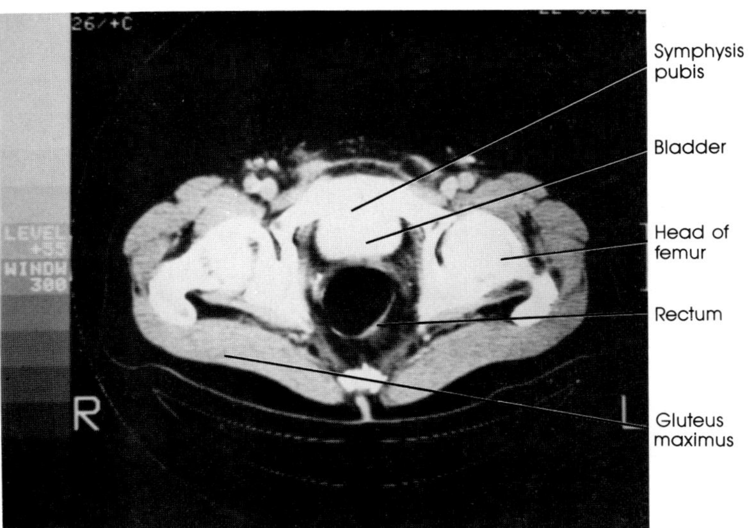

Fig. 32-38. CT image corresponding to Fig. 32-37.

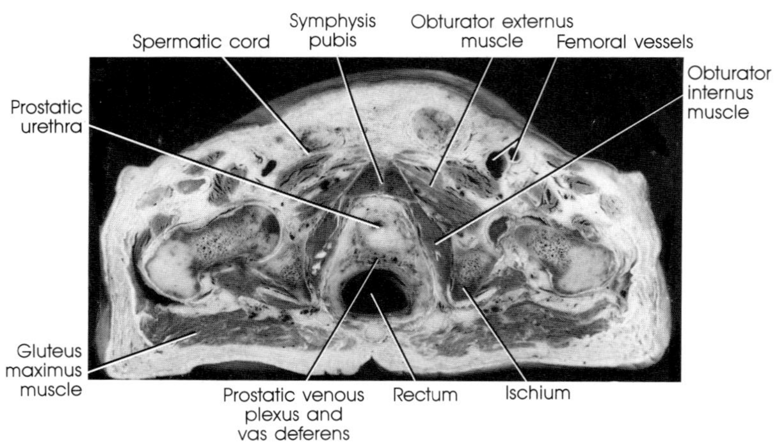

Fig. 32-39. Cadaver section corresponding to level F of Fig. 32-26 at the coccyx (male).

Figs. 32-39 and 32-40 are of a male pelvic cadaver section and a corresponding MR image. These figures highlight structures of the male reproductive system. At this level the relationship between the rectum, prostate gland, and symphysis pubis is noted. The prostatic portion of the urethra is seen within the prostate. Posterior to the prostate are the prostatic venous plexus and the vas deferens. The spermatic cord contains the ductus deferens and the testicular vessels and it is found superficial and lateral to the pubic symphysis.

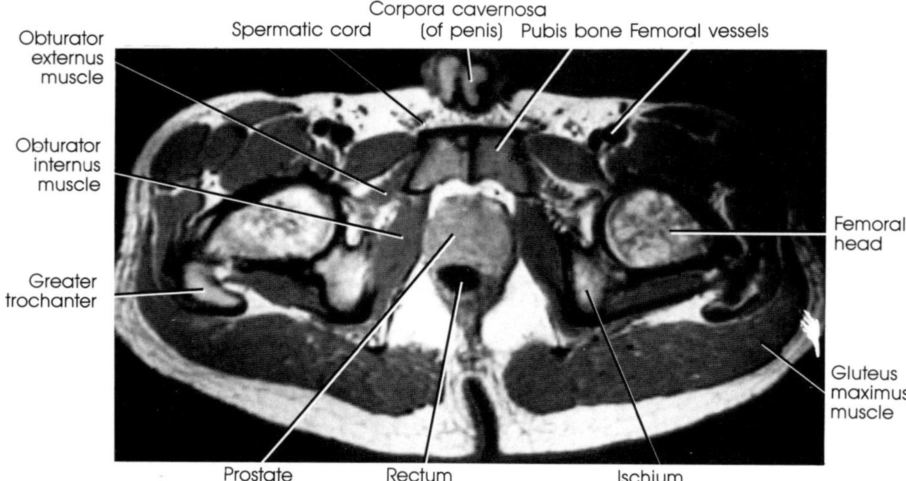

Fig. 32-40. MR image corresponding to Fig. 32-39.

Fig. 32-41 is a sagittal MR image of the structures of the abdomen and pelvis near the midline. The third, fourth, and fifth lumbar vertebrae, sacrum, and coccyx are visualized. The cauda equina is seen descending the spinal canal. Anterior to the vertebral bodies is the distal portion of the abdominal aorta. At the level of the fourth lumbar vertebra, the aorta bifurcates to form the right and left common iliac arteries. The large areas of signal void anterior to the sacrum represent the rectum. The bladder is anterior to the rectum and superior to the prostate. The urethra appears faintly traversing the prostate. The corpus spongiosum and corpora cavernosa of the penis are inferior and anterior to the symphysis pubis. The right and left testes are seen inferior to the penile structures. The rectus abdominis muscle extends superiorly from the pubis in the anterior abdominal wall.

A coronal MR image through the femoral heads and greater trochanter is found in Fig. 32-42. The femoral heads are demonstrated within the acetabula. The crests of the ilia are visualized with their associated musculature. The internal surface of the iliac bone is lined by the iliacus muscle. In this image the psoas muscles are seen joining the iliacus muscles to form the iliopsoas muscles. Gluteus medius and minimus muscles are found external to the iliac bones. The bladder and prostate are seen within the pelvic cavity. Superior to the bladder is a portion of the sigmoid colon. The right ductus deferens is found lateral to the neck of the bladder. Between the rami of the pubic bones are the corpus spongiosum and the corpora cavernosa. The scrotum is seen inferior to the penis and between the gracilis muscles of the thighs.

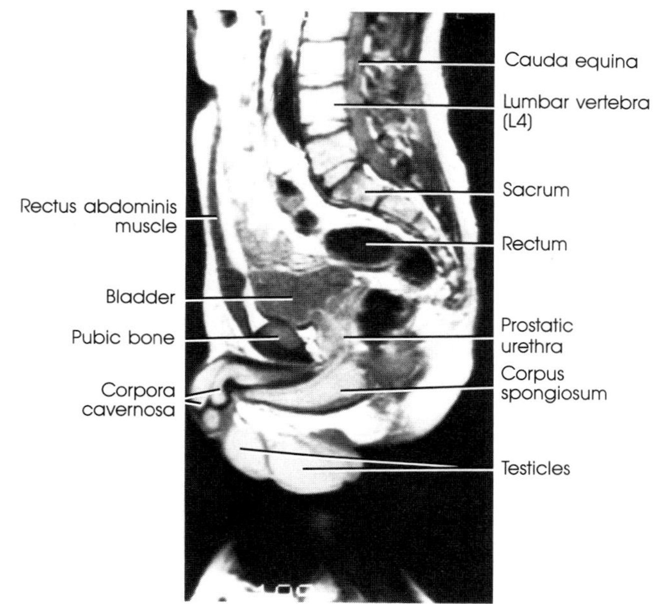

Fig. 32-41. MR image of the abdominopelvic region at the midsagittal plane.

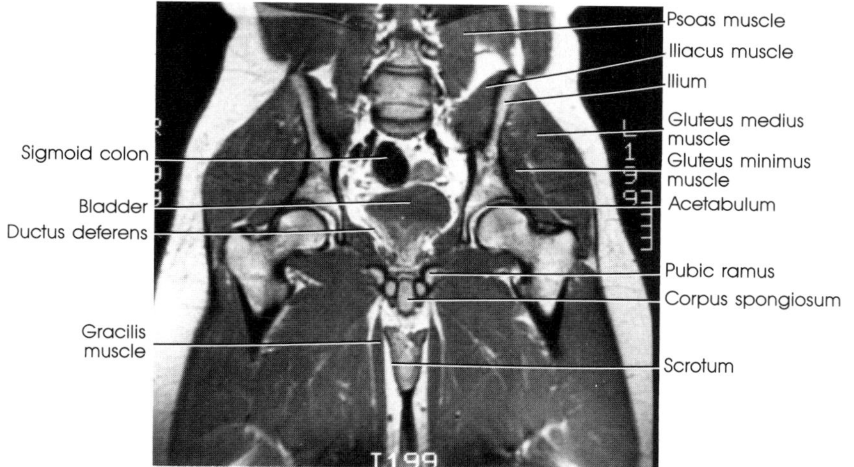

Fig. 32-42. MR image of the abdominopelvic region at the midcoronal plane.

SELECTED BIBLIOGRAPHY

Bo WJ, et al: Basic atlas of cross-sectional anatomy, ed 2, Philadelphia, 1990, WB Saunders Co.

Cahill DR: Atlas of human cross-sectional anatomy, Philadelphia, 1984, Lea & Febiger.

Carter BL, et al: Cross-sectional anatomy: computed tomography and ultrasound correlation, Englewood Cliffs, NJ, 1977, Appleton-Century-Crofts.

Chiu L, Lipcamon J and Yiu-Chiu V: Clinical computed tomography, Rockville, Md, 1986, Aspen Publishers, Inc.

Christoforidis A: Atlas of axial, sagittal, and coronal anatomy, Philadelphia, 1988, WB Saunders Co.

Elster A, Goldman A and Handel S: Magnetic resonance imaging, Philadelphia, 1987, JB Lippincott Co.

Hagen-Ansert S: The anatomy workbook, Philadelphia, 1986, JB Lippincott Co.

Keiffer S and Heitzman E: An atlas of cross-sectional anatomy, Hagerstown, Md, 1979, Harper & Row.

Koritke J and Sick H: Atlas of sectional human anatomy, Germany, 1988, Urban & Schwarzenberg, Inc.

Ledley RS, Huang HK and Mazziotta JC: Cross-sectional anatomy: an atlas for computerized tomography, Baltimore, 1977, Williams & Wilkins.

Metrewelli C: Practical abdominal ultrasound, Chicago, 1978, Year Book Medical Publishers Inc.

Novelline R and Squire L: Living anatomy: a working atlas using computed tomography, magnetic resonance and angiography images, St Louis, 1986, The CV Mosby Co.

Peterson R: A cross-sectional approach to anatomy, Chicago, 1978, Year Book Medical Publishers Inc.

Taylor K: Atlas of gray scale ultrasonography, New York, 1978, Churchill Livingstone, Inc.

Wagner M and Lawson TL: Segmental anatomy, New York, 1982, Macmillan Publishing Co.

Wicke L: Atlas of radiologic anatomy, ed 4, Baltimore, 1987, Urban & Schwarzenberg, Inc.

Chapter 33

COMPUTER FUNDAMENTALS AND APPLICATIONS IN RADIOLOGY

JANE A. VAN VALKENBURG

The progressive and evolutionary growth in medicine would not be possible without the aid of computers. As a result of the applications of the computer in the storage, analysis, and manipulation of data, pathologic conditions can be diagnosed more accurately and earlier in the disease process, resulting in an increased patient cure rate. The increasing use of computers in medical science clearly demonstrates the need for qualified personnel who can understand and operate computerized equipment. This chapter is designed to introduce the fundamental concepts and principles of computer technology and to briefly discuss the application of the computer in diagnostic imaging, management utilization, and education.

Definition

The computer is a fast, computational, electronic machine that receives input data, processes the data by performing arithmetic or logical operations using a program stored in its memory, and then generates output data that are displayed on the appropriate equipment. As a machine, the computer is limited to performing arithmetic or logical operations and cannot make rational, diagnostic judgments. However, the development of medical artificial intelligence–based expert computer systems, such as ICON, provides the capability to compare the observations of the radiologist to clinical information and compare this information to similar cases, allowing the radiologist and/or physician to make more informed judgments.

Artificial intelligence may be defined as comparing computer function with human judgment. In medicine, artificial intelligence has been concentrated on developing computer systems that contain detailed data about specific medical subjects. In contrast, the expert computer systems contain vast amounts of data used for making decisions about a specific problem. Expert systems are designed to duplicate the human reasoning process, thereby providing a differential diagnosis or critique of the diagnosis. When the artificial intelligence system and the expert system are integrated, the information generated aids in analytical reasoning and decision making. The artificial intelligence–based expert system used in radiology is known as the IMAGE/ICON system.

Historical Development

The Oriental abacus is known as the first digital calculator; it was used as early as the 6th century B.C. The abacus is a device with beads strung on parallel wires that are attached to a frame.

In 1642 a young Frenchman, Blaise Pascal, built a small mechanical adding device to aid him in his work as an accountant. The device consisted of cogwheels in a box; each cogwheel had ten teeth, and each tooth on the cogwheel represented one digit from 0 through 9. As one of the wheels passed from the position of 9 to 0, a small sprocket on the wheel would interdigitate with the next wheel and provide an automatic carryover. This was the first mechanical adding machine and was known as the "arithmetic machine." The concept is used today in the mechanical paper-tape adding machines and was the forerunner of the clock industry.

In 1694 Gottfried Wilhelm von Leibnitz, using Pascal's "arithmetic machine" concept, developed a mechanism that used step-cylinders instead of cogwheels. The machine could add, multiply, and divide and was known as a "calculating machine." The machines developed by Pascal and Leibnitz, improved by further developments, are the predecessors of the modern keyboard adding machines.

A French inventor, Joseph Jacquard, displayed an automatic weaving loom at the Paris Industrial Exhibition in 1801. The sequence of the loom's operations was based on coded information punched into thick paper cards. The pattern of the tapestry woven on this loom was produced by the holes in the punched cards. The positioning of the threads was determined by the presence and position of the holes on the card. To produce a single tapestry, approximately 24,000 punched cards were used.

In 1822 Charles Babbage, considered the originator of the modern computer, presented an outline for a machine that could calculate celestial tables used to aid in the navigation of ships. Errors in calculating these tables had caused ships to go off course and often resulted in shipwrecks. The machine's calculations were based on the constant variation, or difference, in a series of multiplications, additions, divisions, or squares and could tabulate up to 20 decimals with seven differences. Because this "difference machine," as it was called, required accurate precision in the positioning of the cogs, wheels, shafts, and sprockets, the engineering technology was not available to accurately construct it, although the design was sound (Fig. 33-1). Although he spent 20 years attempting to build this machine, Babbage was never able to complete it.

Meanwhile, Babbage had been presented with one of Jacquard's tapestries and was intrigued by Jacquard's idea of a punched card and its application to constructing a machine to do calculations. In 1834, Babbage presented the principle of what he called an "analytic engine," from which today's computer was developed. Babbage divided the construction of this machine into two main components: the "store," which is comparable to the *memory*,* and the "mill," which is similar to the *central processing unit* in modern computers. The mill performed the calculations and was controlled by a punched card. The store held the numbers for use as the calculation proceeded. Babbage devoted years of his life to the development of this analytic engine, but unfortunately it was never finished. After his death, the analytic machine was constructed using his complete and detailed drawings.

*All italicized terms are defined at the end of the chapter.

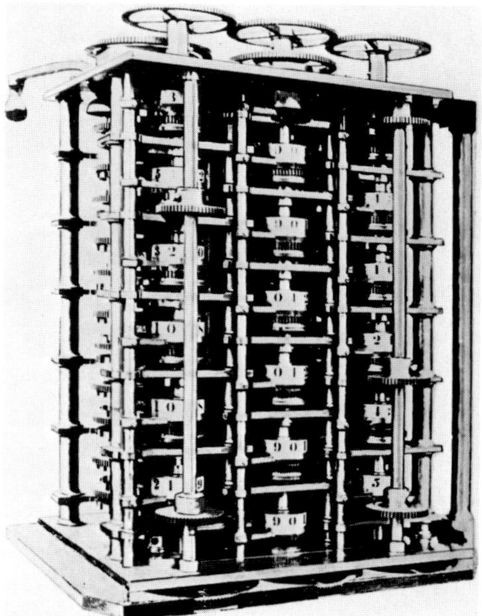

Fig. 33-1. The idea for a "difference machine" that would compute mathematical tables, such as logarithms, was first conceived by Babbage in 1812. After 20 years of labor, financial diffculties compelled him to stop work and the machine was never completed.

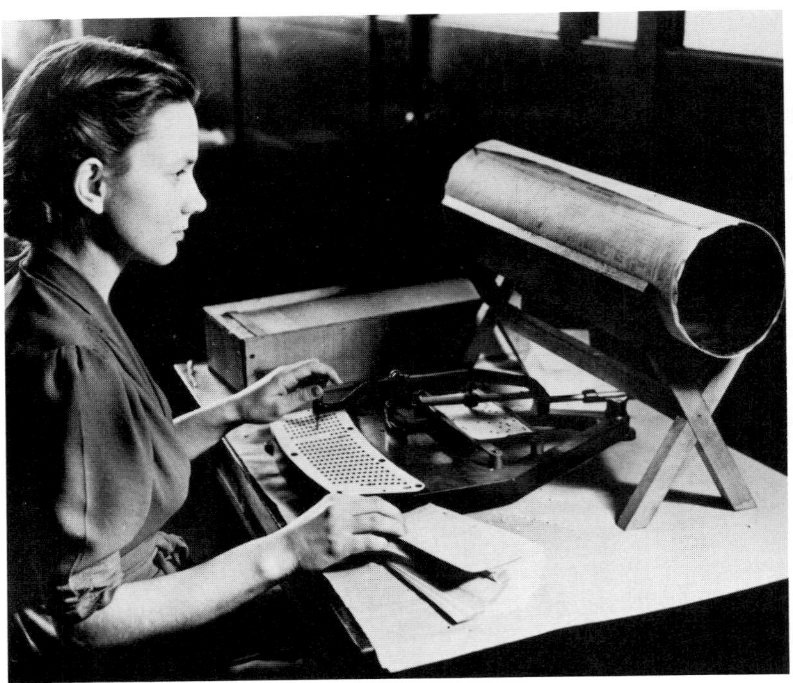

Fig. 33-2. Device used by Hollerith to punch programs, single and manually, in cards.

(Courtesy IBM Corp.)

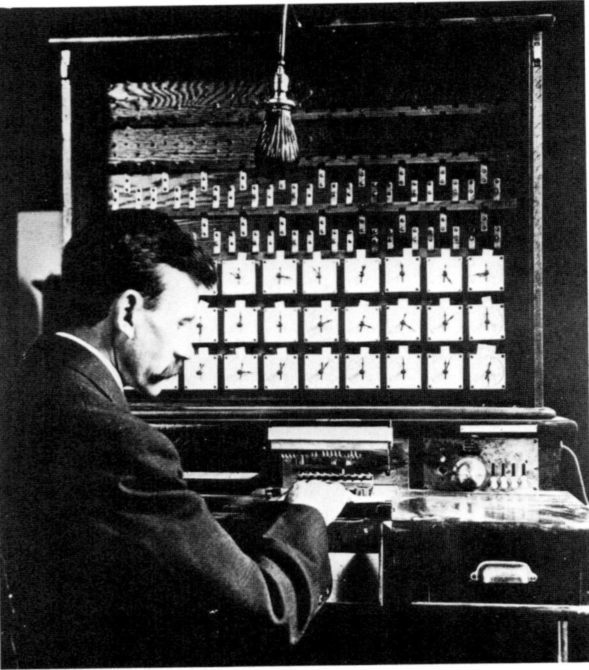

Fig. 33-3. The dial cabinet used by Hollerith to count the holes in the punched cards. The properly punched cards were then filed for future use.

(Courtesv IBM Corp.)

Table 33-1. Important events in computer development

Date	Developer	Event
1937-1944	Howard Aiken, Harvard University	Using Babbage's mechanical design, IBM joined Aiken in the development of Mark 1, an electromechanical, automatic, sequenced-controlled calculator; program sequencing was done with paper tape.
1943-1946	John Mauchley and J. Presper Eckert, University of Pennsylvania	A high-speed electronic calculator, the Electronic Numeric Integrator and Calculator (ENIAC); first machine to use vacuum tubes, which allowed faster switching functions.
1946-1952	John Von Neumann, University of Pennsylvania	Designed a machine with a stored memory, Electronic Discrete Variable Automatic Computer (EDVAC); capable of reading instructions from memory and executing them in proper sequence that allowed programming.
1951	Eckert-Mauchley	The first commercially available computer, Universal Automatic Computer I (UNIVAC), using a stored memory; used by the U.S. Census Bureau; company later bought by Sperry-Rand Corporation.
1954	Bell Telephone Laboratories	First computer to use solid-state transistors and diodes, Transistor Digital Computer (TRADIC); allowed development of much smaller machines.
1963-1964	Numerous researchers	Integrated circuits and semiconductors; development based on principles presented by Wilhelm Schottky.
1973	Numerous researchers	Miniaturization of electronic circuits or microchips; marketing of the minicomputer to general public.

During the 1880s, Herman Hollerith and James Powers, who worked with the U.S. Bureau of Census, were concerned about tabulating the census for the growing American population and decided that an automatic process for counting the census must be developed (Fig. 33-2). Working independently, they each constructed versions of punched-card tabulating machines, and the 1890 census was tabulated using these machines. Hollerith obtained a patent on his machine and founded a company to further develop his ideas (Fig. 33-3). In 1911, this company merged with two other companies to form the Computer Tabulating Recording Company; and in 1924 this company became the International Business Machine Corporation, IBM, a leader in the development of computer technology.

After 1920 computer development progressed at a rapid rate. For a summary of the important events in the advancement of computer development see Table 33-1.

The significant changes in the development of computers are referred to as *generations*. The notable changes that signify the evolution of computer development are listed in Table 33-2.

Table 33-2. Evolution of computer development

Generation	Development	Date
First	Vacuum tubes	1943-1946
Second	Solid-state transistors	1954
Third	Integrated circuits and semiconductors	1963-1964
Fourth	Silicon chips or microchips	1973

Types of Computers

There are three categories of computers: the microcomputer, the minicomputer, and the mainframe computer. The smallest computer, the microcomputer, usually contains the circuitry or *central processing unit (CPU)* on a single integrated-circuit chip. The main limitation of this system is that it is typically a one-person or one-function system.

Minicomputers usually have faster responding CPUs and more memory and storage. Unlike most microcomputers, minicomputers are multiuser or multitasking systems; several people (2 to 30) may use the system at one time. They are capable of more tasks and can use various programs because they contain several chips or one or more printed circuit boards filled with many integrated circuits.

Mainframe computers are used when there is an increased need for data storage, processing speed, and memory requirements and when the number of users increases. The distinction between the mainframe computer and the minicomputer is becoming less distinct as a result of innovative technology and miniaturization of computer components. Tasks that were once performed only by mainframe computers are now being handled by the minicomputers. The advantage of the large mainframe system is its ability to process large amounts of data efficiently (Fig. 33-4). Mainframe computers are used by the U.S. Census Bureau, Internal Revenue Service, large corporations, research libraries, universities, and other organizations requiring the processing, acquisition, and storage of large amounts of information.

The supercomputer is a type of mainframe computer developed to process mathematically intense operations, such as rapid processing of deep-space images for NASA, astronomical projections, and real-time national weather forecasting; this type of computer is currently used by the U.S. Census Bureau. These supercomputers, or maxicomputers, claim to have computing speeds approaching ten billion floating point operations per second, one billion bytes of memory, and can switch from one transmission state to another in one-thousandth of a billionth second, or one picosecond. The supercomputer will become the fifth generation of computers and incorporate artificial intelligence. The next decade promises revolutionary changes in the development of computer circuitry, resulting in future minicomputers that have the capabilities of maxicomputers and making obsolete the supercomputers presently being used.

The computers used in radiology departments are usually microcomputers and minicomputers. Applications of these computers are divided into two categories: *control* and *data management*. Microcomputers are typically used to control operations in radiographic/fluoroscopic rooms, automatic processing regulation, and rapid film changers. Minicomputers are found in computed tomography units or in any equipment where image reconstruction is performed. Both microcomputers and minicomputers are used for word processing, billing systems, and inventory management. *Real-time* imaging, which is used in ultrasound and digital radiography where immediate data manipulation is important, requires special purpose *hardware* interfaced with a minicomputer.

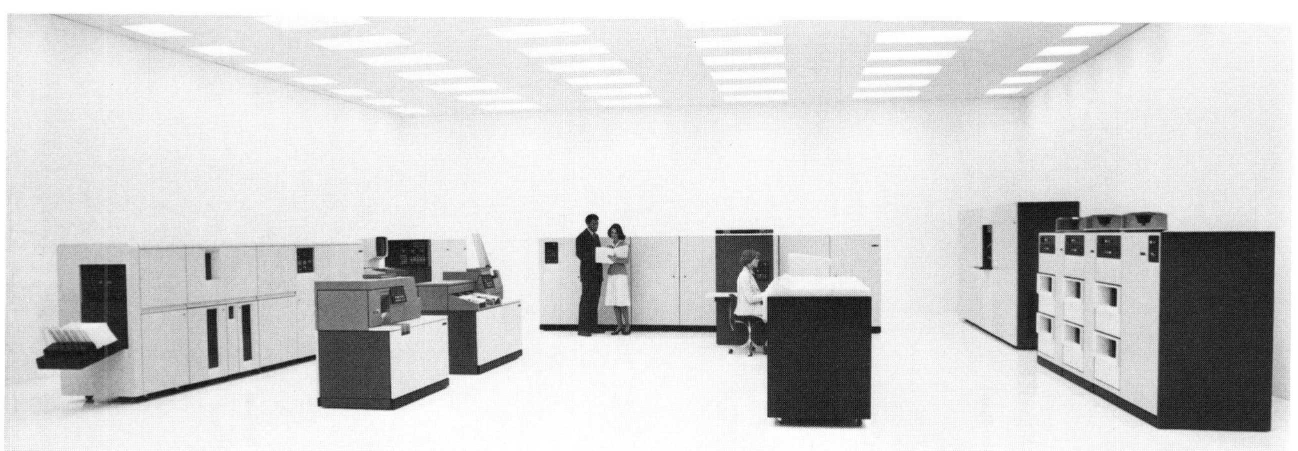

Fig. 33-4. Mainframe computer system with disk drives and magnetic tape memory systems.

(Courtesy IBM Corp.)

Functional Components of a Computer

The term *hardware* is used to describe the functional equipment components of a computer and is everything concerning the computer that is visible. *Software* designates the parts of the computer system that are invisible, such as the *machine language* and the programs. A computer *program* is a clearly defined set of instructions that gives the computer specific tasks to perform. Programs are written in high-level languages that are intelligible to the user and translated into machine languages that are then intelligible to the computer.

The computer hardware consists of four functionally independent components (Fig. 33-5): (1) the *input* devices; (2) the CPU, which houses (a) the *control unit,* and (b) the *arithmetic/logic unit (ALU);* (3) the *primary memory* unit; and (4) the *output* devices.

INPUT DEVICES

Input devices are the units that "read" the instructions represented on the input medium (such as punched cards), transform this information into *binary* digits, and then feed this information to the CPU for processing.

Common input media are punched cards and punched paper tape. Keyboards (similar to a typewriter) and video *terminals* are devices that may also be used to give instructions to the CPU. The input device reads the coded instructions represented by the holes punched in the cards or paper tape, typed on a keyboard, or drawn directly on a video terminal by means of a light pen attachment. The coded instructions enable the input device to translate the external data into binary representations that can then be handled by the CPU.

Other forms of input devices are magnetic ink readers, *optical scanners,* and magnetic *disks* or tapes. Magnetic ink, made from iron oxide particles, is used to provide direct instructions to the input device. Optical scanners are frequently used by testing agencies to score examinations by using a light or lens system to scan a sheet of paper for information that is then converted to digital information by the input device. Magnetic disks and tapes may contain information or data to be screened and changed to binary representations by the input device (Fig. 33-6).

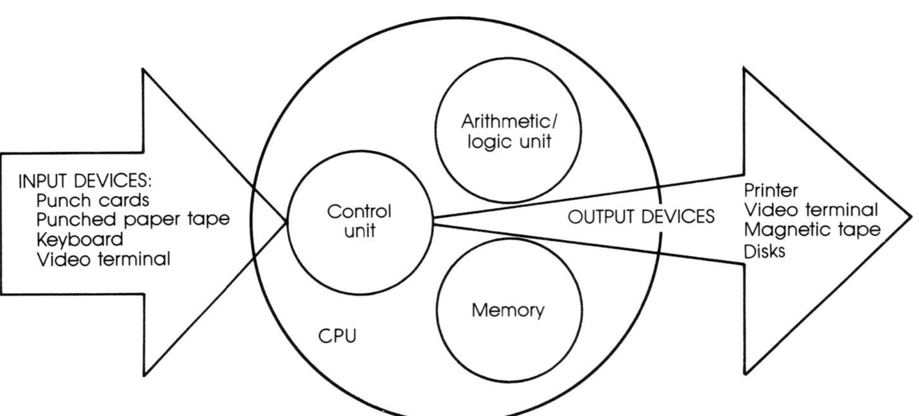

Fig. 33-5. Fundamentals of a computer. Central processing unit (CPU) or operating system.

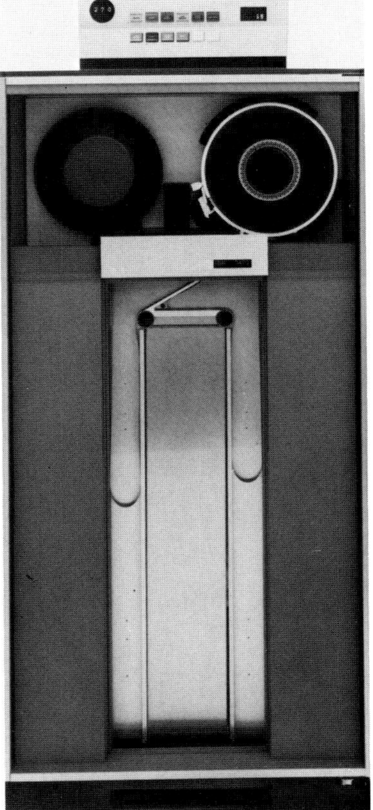

Fig. 33-6. Magnetic tape memory system. The tape loops, in the lower center area, and is suspended in vacuum compartment to facilitate the tape passage at high speeds.

(Courtesy IBM Corp.)

CONTROL UNIT

The sequence of events or tasks performed by the computer is regulated and coordinated by the control unit housed within the CPU. The control unit retrieves information from the memory and sends it to the arithmetic/logic unit to be processed; after this processing, the control unit then sends that data back to the memory for storage or to the appropriate output device. The function of the control unit is similar to a policeman stationed at a busy intersection and preventing mass confusion by directing traffic into the proper lanes in an orderly fashion.

On initiation of a specified program by the operator, the control unit retrieves the information from the memory and sends it to the ALU for processing. On completion of the tasks by the ALU, the control unit transmits the processed information or data back to the memory or to an output device, as instructed by the operator. The time frame for these functions to occur happens in microseconds, milliseconds, and nanoseconds, depending on the circuitry of the machine, which determines the speed of the functions.

ARITHMETIC/LOGIC UNIT

The arithmetic/logic unit (ALU) does all of the computations, comparisons, and logical operations using binary numbers for additions, subtractions, multiplications, and/or divisions. The control unit determines the numbers to be acted on and what the operation will be. Following the calculations, the information can be displayed immediately or placed in the memory for future use.

The calculations take place within the ALU in areas known as *registers* or "accumulators." To combine two numbers, for instance, the numbers would be called from the memory by the control unit and placed in two separate registers. The control unit passes control to the ALU to perform the computation. When completed, the result is displayed on an output device or sent back to the memory for future use.

MEMORY

There are two types of memory storage: primary and secondary. The primary memory is an integral part of the circuitry and can store data for immediate retrieval when needed. Data contained in the primary memory can be transferred back and forth to the CPU for further calculations. The primary memory is described according to the storage capacity and is quantified by the letter *K*. The letter K is derived from the metric system and denotes the quantity of 1000. However, because 1024 rather than an even 1000 is a mathematical integral power of 2, the letter K stands for 1024 when applied to computer technology. For example, a 256K memory means that approximately 256,000 locations exist within the primary memory for data storage, however, the more accurate figure is 262,144 locations. The memory is divided into small sections called "locations," with each location having a storage *address*. The address is usually represented by a number or numbers that the CPU uses to find the information for further processing or display.

Within the primary memory of a computer, there are two types of addressable memory: the *random access memory (RAM)* and the *read only memory (ROM)*. One may read, change, delete, and store on the RAM memory with immediate access to data; but if the voltage to the computer should suddenly drop or fluctuate, the information is lost unless it has been stored in secondary or auxiliary storage areas, such as magnetic tapes or disks. Therefore to correct this deficiency in the primary memory and to prevent the loss of important instructions that are needed to operate the computer without reprogramming for each usage, the ROM memory was developed; its contents are generally imprinted at the factory. Instructions and information within the ROM memory are nonvolatile; and whether the computer is on or off, it is not affected. Although the CPU can retrieve the information on the ROM, the information or instructions cannot be changed or deleted or new instructions stored. The ROM memory is used primarily to secure programs that are used frequently and need to be accessible as soon as the power is turned on.

In computers with a smaller capacity, the ROM may be removed by the operator and changed; for example, the cartridges used for video games. The computers used in a radiology department have a ROM as an integral part of the circuitry that is "burned in" at the factory. When performing diagnostic imaging studies, a very fast transmission of data must occur between the CPU and the ROM; therefore in these computers, the ROM is often located within the CPU. The ROM is a program and it is usually considered as software. In the types of computers where the ROM is part of the circuitry and is purchased as an integral part of the computer and not separately, it is then referred to as firmware. The ROM memory can be changed in these special types of computers, but a person skilled in computer circuitry is needed to do the task.

The primary memory, consisting of the RAM and the ROM, are limited in storage capacity; and it is relatively expensive to add circuitry for storage purposes. Use of less expensive and mass capacity storage areas is necessary to keep records for long periods of time. The secondary memory storage areas, such as magnetic tapes, disks, and magnetic drums, fill this need. These secondary or auxiliary storage mediums can be removed from the computer and be stored separately. When needed, they can then be inserted into a device that is interfaced with the computer and information retrieved from them by use of the storage address.

OPERATING SYSTEM

An operating system is a set of programs to help other programs use the computer and its peripheral devices; for example, printers and video terminals. These sets of programs serve four basic functions: (1) they request programs and cause the computer to execute the instructions in the program; (2) they manage the input and output and use of peripheral devices; (3) they manage the information within the files and the priority of processing; and (4) they manage the information stored in the RAM memory.

The control unit within the CPU directs the functions of the operating system and sees that the correct programs are performed. The CPU responds to the request for a program, locates the program in the operating system, copies it into a workspace in the primary memory, and begins execution of the program's instructions. An operating system eliminates the need to write instructions into every program the operator wishes to perform.

Contained within each operating system are three management systems for instructions, sometimes called "managers." The input/output (I/O) manager coordinates all transfers of information between devices connected to the computer. This manager also knows which peripheral device is connected to what other devices in the computer. This permits each peripheral device to send and receive information in different ways from different locations. The file manager handles all the information that is to be stored in auxiliary storage areas by packing the information into indexed groups. The file manager also keeps track of where individual files are located in order to retrieve the information when it is needed by recording the file name and location with the indexed information groups. When a storage disk or magnetic tape is inserted into the computer, the file manager reads where the file is stored, locates it, and loads (copies) it into a waiting area called a *buffer*. The third manager handles all of the computer's immediate records stored in the RAM memory.

In an operating system, when a program is requested from an input device such as a video terminal, the CPU monitors the terminal, interprets the request for a program, and then requests the file manager to retrieve the data from the files, unless it is stored in the RAM memory where it can be immediately found.

The file manager searches its directory for the file needed and loads the file onto a buffer. The file manager reports the file's status to the CPU. If the file is not found, the file manager reports that the file is "not found." If the file is found, the manager informs the CPU that the file is in the buffer.

The CPU then requests that the memory manager reserve a portion of the primary memory for the program. The program moves from the buffer to the designated space and the CPU starts operation of the program.

If the program should need additional memory, or to use a peripheral device, a request is transmitted to the CPU, which then refers this request to the memory manager, I/O manager, or file manager. When the program is completed, the CPU gains control of the system and waits for additional commands.

OUTPUT DEVICES

Output devices display the results of the computations or tasks the computer has been instructed to complete. The most common devices are the video terminal and/or *cathode ray tube (CRT),* the high-speed printer, and magnetic tapes or disk drives. Other types are the card punch and paper-tape punch. These output devices will only respond when directed by the control unit of the CPU.

The copies made by high-speed printers and the information recorded on magnetic tapes or disks provide permanent records of the tasks completed. The printers are usually used when visual data are required, whereas magnetic tape drives and disk drives are used when data need to be stored for records or possible further computations and usage (Fig. 33-7). The data stored on magnetic tapes or disks can be retrieved and displayed on a video screen (CRT) when desired and further data added or deleted.

Mass information is usually stored on magnetic tapes, which are inexpensive and can store millions of pieces of information. The reel-to-reel magnetic tape drives are rather large and the initial cost is quite expensive; therefore this output device is used when large amounts of information are to be stored.

Magnetic disk drives are the most popular output devices and are called either a "hard" disk drive or a "floppy" disk drive. The hard disks are rigid, larger, can store megabytes (M-bytes) of information, and are about the size of a long-playing phonograph record. In 1972, when IBM introduced these "hard" disks, they were called "30-30" disks, or *Winchester disk* drives, because each disk would hold 30 M-bytes of information.

Floppy disk drives range in size from 3½ to 8 inches in diameter and are made of a flexible plastic material. These disks or diskettes are lightweight and relatively inexpensive. They are used primarily in microcomputers and minicomputers; however, they have a slower access time and lower storage capacity than other recording media.

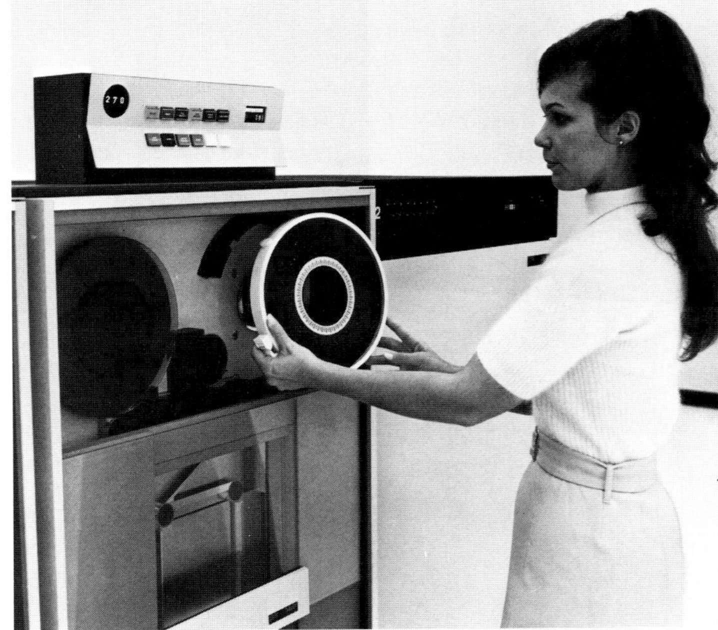

Fig. 33-7. Magnetic tapes may be removed for storage and then retrieved for use at a future date.

(Courtesy IBM Corp.)

Computer Operations

ANALOG COMPUTERS

Unaltered electricity, demonstrated in the form of a continuous sine wave, can be used to run a computer. A computer designed to operate directly from unaltered or continuous electricity is called an *analog computer*. The tasks performed by this type of computer depend on the ability to measure distinctions in the various voltages and the precision of the circuitry. Because the electricity is in an unbroken or continuous sine wave, discrete values are difficult to measure, and if a new or different function needs to be performed, the circuit would have to be rewired.

DIGITAL COMPUTERS

To overcome the inherent problems with analog computers, *digital computers* were developed. Digital computers break up the electricity sine wave into distinct, measurable values (Fig. 33-8). A familiar example of this would be the digital electronic timing system used in sporting events that breaks the time or sine wave into hundredths of a second. A computer is capable of breaking the sine wave into millionths of a second. With this finer digitization, the sine wave would almost approach a smooth-looking curve.

Because digital computers are faster and more accurate, most modern computers are digital. Much of the information from examinations performed in a radiology department is initially in the form of raw or unaltered electricity; therefore to obtain more uniform and consistent results, the computers contain an *analog-to-digital converter (ADC)* that changes the sine wave into digital form and discrete values.

BINARY SYSTEM

A digital computer operates on a binary system that is similar to the Morse code, but instead of dots and dashes, two digits are used—the 1 and the 0. The American Standard Code for Information Interchange (ASCII) established a standard code consisting of a string of eight zeros and ones and referred to as a *byte*. Each individual digit is called a *bit* or *binary digit*. The coded instructions contained in the first four bits tell the computer if the information is a number, letter, or symbol. For example, a prefix of 1011 signifies a number, and 1100 or 1101 a letter, depending on its placement within the alphabet. A different set of instructions represents a method of encoding four bits of memory into a binary representation of one decimal digit or number and is known as a binary coded decimal or BCD. An example of a binary coded decimal method is: 0 = 0000; 1 = 0001; 2 = 0010; 3 = 0011; 4 = 0100; 5 = 0101; 6 = 0110; 7 = 0111; 8 = 1000; 9 = 1001.

The binary system forms the basis for digital electronics by allowing only two voltage levels. Information is stored by activating electronic switches or "logic gates" to an "off" position, represented by 0, and to the "on" position, represented by 1. By stringing these zeros and ones together, coded instructions are received by the computer as to which function or task to perform.

Integrated, microscopic circuits are etched onto wafer-thin layers of silicon. Each of these silicon layers or chips contains a circuit that has a carefully and specifically designed maze of logic gates or switches. These integrated circuits, or transistors, on each of the silicon chips are then assembled into a larger circuit on a board with the output of one circuit, or transistor, interfacing with the input of another. The circuit boards are designed to enable the computer to perform specialized functions.

Although the complexity of a computer can become enormous as a result of the number of circuit boards involved, the basic circuitry or electronics using the binary system and logic gates remains the same.

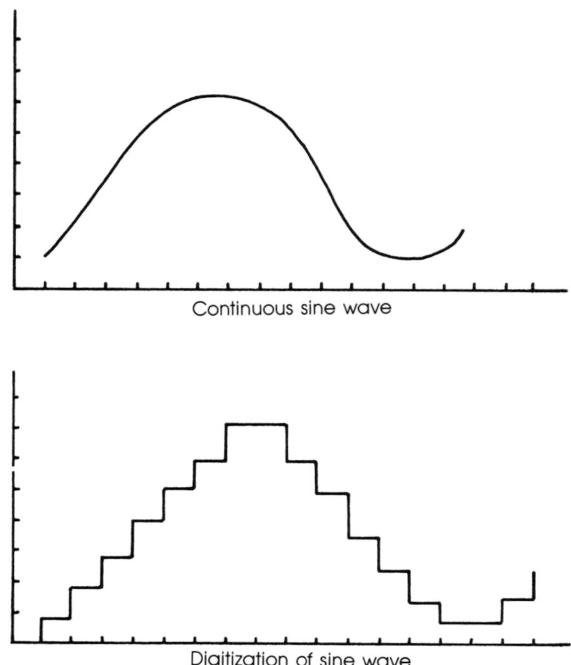

Fig. 33-8. A continuous sine wave is used in analog computers. Digital computers use a sine wave broken into distinct time increments.

PROGRAMMING

A computer program is a series of simple arithmetic steps in the binary system that occurs in a millionth of a second in the circuitry of the computer. The construction of the transistors and circuit boards within a computer determines the *machine language* that must be used to operate a specific computer; therefore a certain type or brand of computer will only operate on the machine language designed for it.

Computer programs stored within the primary memory or inserted in the secondary memory are known as computer *software*. When coded instructions are received by the control unit, data are retrieved from the memory and transferred to the ALU in the order of their memory location for computations.

Since the development of computer programs is time-consuming, tedious, and prone to programming errors that can become costly, the computer industry devised what are known as "high-level *languages*." These high-level languages can be translated into a specific machine language by special programs called *compilers* or interpreters. Some of the high-level languages developed to perform specific types of tasks that are relevant to a certain field or discipline are listed in Table 33-3.

The use of high-level languages, such as FORTRAN (which is used in imaging processing), has allowed the formation of sophisticated computer systems that can process the large amounts of data generated by the equipment used in a radiology department. The explosive growth of digital imaging modalities has resulted in the development of an integrated medical image management system known as "picture archiving and communication system" or PACS. The PACS system is a group of computer programs that allows a radiology department to electronically acquire images on a terminal or CRT, transport them to various places, store the images, and catalog them on magnetic tapes or optical disks.

Table 33-3. High-level computer languages

BASIC	Beginner's all-purpose symbolic instruction code; the standard language provided with most personal computers.
COBOL	Common business-oriented language; used for financial applications; sometimes used for medical information systems.
ALGOL or PASCAL	Algorithmic language; languages used by mathematicians.
FORTRAN	Formula translation; language for scientific programs that performs calculations based on complex formulas.
PL/1	Programming language, version 1; developed by IBM to replace COBOL, FORTRAN, and ALGOL; used as a literary searcher and filer.
MUMPS	Massachusetts General Hospital utility multiprogramming system; originally developed for medical information–processing applications; most radiology information management systems have been developed from this language.

Applications in Radiology

Although the CPU of a computer system defines the processing of data, the interface with the *peripheral* input/output devices is important in radiology. The various imaging modalities depend on specific peripheral imaging devices that interface with a computer; therefore when purchasing a computer system, an important consideration is the ability to upgrade the system to accommodate the newer peripherals.

BASICS OF INTERFACING PERIPHERAL DEVICES

The transfer of data between the CPU, memory, and input/output devices must occur rapidly when performing an examination in a radiology department. To enable computers to process this rapid influx of data, a "bus" structure was developed to provide standardization and flexibility in the operating system. The bus consists of parallel conductors on a circuit board, known as a "mother" board. The circuit boards that contain the CPU, memory, and the interface to the peripheral input/output devices are plugged into the mother board, allowing communication with each other by way of the bus.

The parallel conductors on the bus serve three definite functions: (1) address lines, which select a memory location or a specific input/output interface; (2) data lines, which carry a specified number of data bits; and (3) control lines, which carry the timing, status, and initiation of signals from one device to another. Because the bus communicates the data to and from the CPU by means of these parallel circuits instead of a string of serial bits, the processing is many times faster (Fig. 33-9).

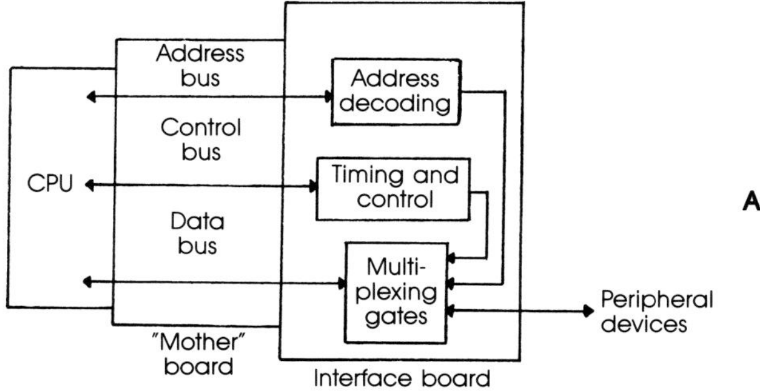

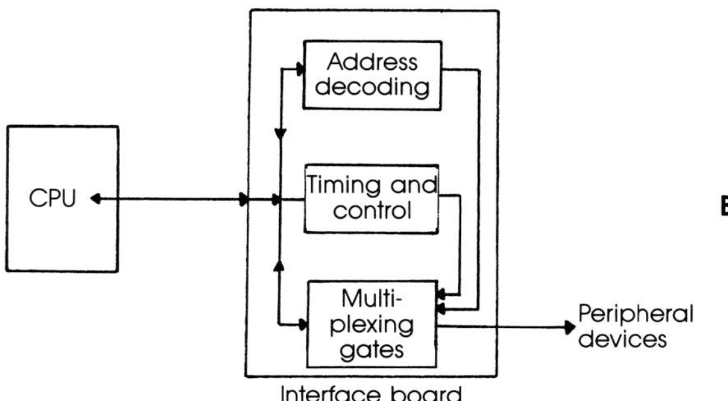

Fig. 33-9. A, Simplified diagram of bus system. Allows rapid data transfer, up to 32 bits at a time. **B,** Data transferred to CPU in a serial or single string of bits; takes much longer for transmission.

ANALOG-TO-DIGITAL CONVERTERS AND VIDEO IMAGE PROCESSORS

Devices that produce images of real objects, such as patients, produce an analog rather than a digital signal. The electrical signal being emitted from the output phosphor of an image intensifier on a fluoroscopic unit, the scintillation crystal of a nuclear medicine detector, the ionization chamber or scintillation detector of a computed tomography (CT) unit, or the piezoelectric crystal of an ultrasound machine, is in analog form with a variance in voltage. For these signals to be read as data by the computer, they must be digitized and converted into the binary number system. The peripheral device that performs this task is the analog-to-digital converter, which transforms the sine wave into discrete increments with binary numbers assigned to each increment. The assignment of the binary numbers depends on output voltage, which in turn represents the degree of attenuation of the various tissue densities within the patient.

The basic component of an analog-to-digital converter (ADC) is the "comparator" that outputs a "1" when the voltage equals or exceeds a precise analog voltage, and a "0" if the voltage does not equal or exceed this predetermined level. The most significant parameters of an ADC are: (1) *digitization depth* (the number of bits in the resultant binary number); (2) *dynamic range* (the range of voltage or input signals that result in a digital output); and (3) *digitization rate* (the rate that digitization takes place). Achieving the optimal digitization depth is necessary for resolution quality and flexibility in image manipulation. Digitization depth and dynamic range are analogous to producing optimal contrast and latitude in a radiograph.

To produce a video image, the field size of the image is divided into many cubes or a matrix, with each cube assigned a binary number proportional to the degree of the attenuation of the x-ray beam or intensity of the incoming signal. The individual three-dimensional cubes with length, width, and depth are called "voxels" (volume element), with the degree of attenuation or intensity of the incoming voltage determining their composition and thickness (Fig. 33-10). For ex-

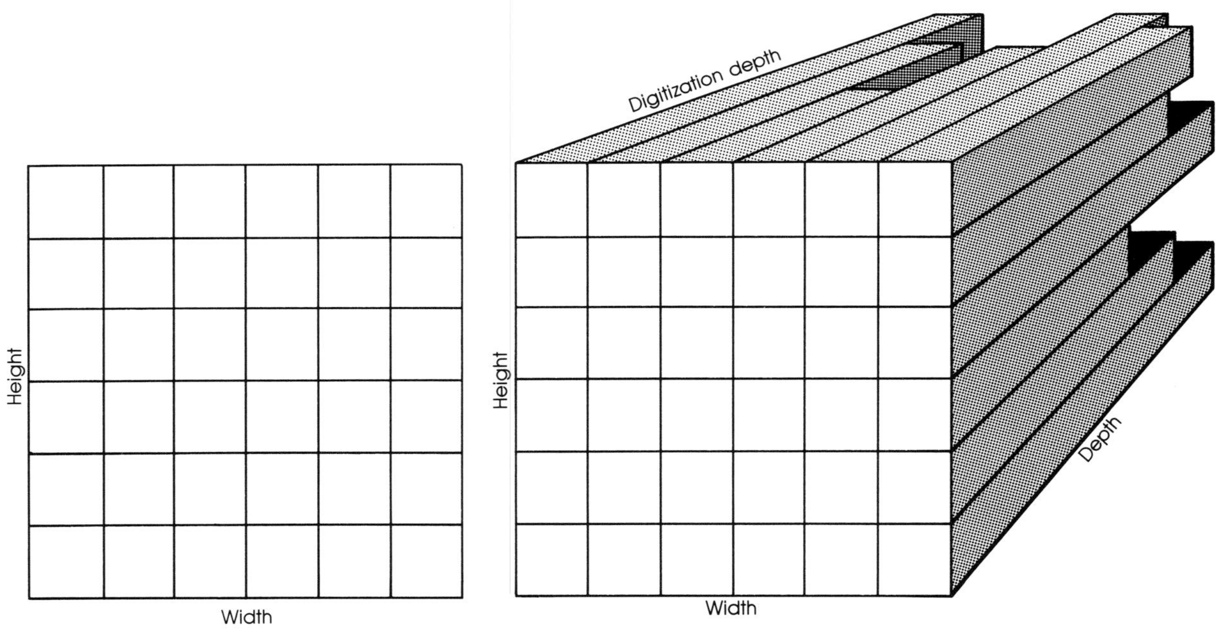

Fig. 33-10. Comparison between pixel (left) and voxel (right).

ample, the contrast media used in a CT or digital fluoroscopy examination would produce voxels with less digitization depth than the surrounding tissues, as a result of the attenuation of the x-ray beam. Digitization depth allows flexibility in the manipulation of the image.

Because the technology for displaying three-dimensional objects has not been fully developed, a two-dimensional square or "pixel" (picture element) represents the voxel on the television display monitor or cathode ray tube. The matrix is an array of pixels arranged in two dimensions, length and width, or in rows and columns. The more pixels contained in an image, the larger the matrix becomes with the resolution quality of the image improving. For instance, a matrix containing 256 × 256 pixels equals a total of 65,536 pixels or pieces of data; whereas a matrix of 512 × 512 pixels contains 262,144 pieces of data. One should not confuse field size with matrix size. You can have a small field size and a large matrix size, or vice versa, depending on the equipment. The larger matrix also allows for more manipulation of the data or the image displayed on the television monitor and is very beneficial and useful in the imaging modalities, such as digital subtraction fluoroscopy, CT, nuclear medicine, and ultrasound.

After the image has been produced on the video display unit, hard copies are then made on single-emulsion film, using a multiformat camera, or a laser camera that directs a laser beam onto a single-emulsion film. The laser camera also permits the images to be reproduced on paper. The images may also be stored on magnetic tape or on a disk for future reference. A computer system that has one or more peripherals included in the system, like the one described above, is called *multiprogramming* (Fig. 33-11).

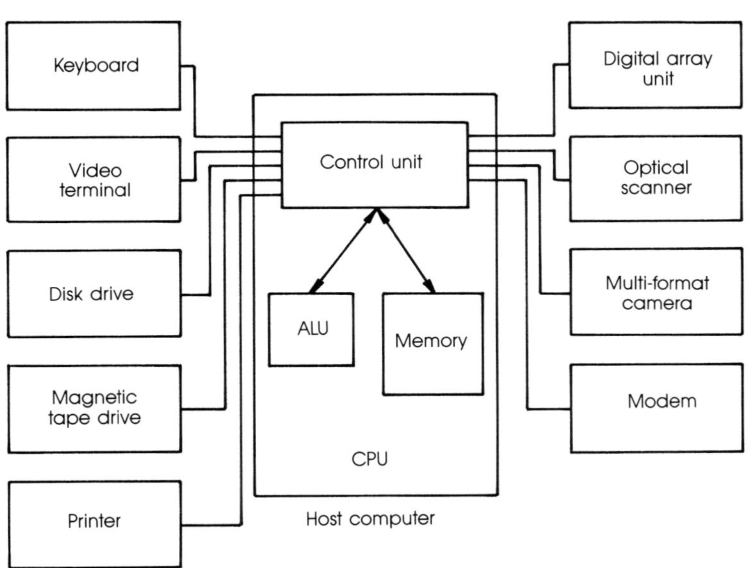

Fig. 33-11. Host computer with various input/output devices.

Applications in radiology

ARRAY PROCESSORS AND OTHER SPECIAL PURPOSE PROCESSORS

To acquire a 512 × 512 pixel matrix at 30 television frames per second, an analog-to-digital converter must be able to process 10^7 digitizations per second, with each pixel being eight to ten digits deep to allow for satisfactory image manipulation. The hardware developed to handle this mass amount of data is the "array processor" or "special purpose processor." The array processor was initially designed to calculate arithmetic operations at speeds ten to 1000 times faster than the CPU and has since progressed to the point that it has become a specialized small computer but is still considered peripheral to the host computer. Its function is to speed the processing of the matrices and other array of numbers by means of highly repetitive arithmetic operations.

The arithmetic operations performed within the array processor are aided by fast Fourier transforms that reduce the amplitude and increase the frequency of the sine wave through mathematic manipulation to allow faster processing. Because sine waves are not of equal intensity, Fourier transformation is a complex mathematical summation and/or multiplication of the sine waves that depict a spatial location within the body to provide a more accurate analysis and manipulation of the data. Other methods that speed up the processing are matrix multiplication, inversion, and convolution. Mathematic operations achieve speeds of up to 14 *m*illion *fl*oating-point *o*perations *p*er *s*econd (megaflops); because of the special design of the array processor, many of the different operations are performed simultaneously. One definition given of an array processor is:

> It has at least one adder and one multiplier that can run simultaneously and do floating-point arithmetic; it can be programmed; and it achieves high performance through parallel processing or "pipelining."

The alternatives to the array processor for arithmetic operations are the dedicated "single component" microprocessor and the "bit-slice" microprocessor. These two special processors are less expensive, but have considerably slower *response time* than the array processor.

Array processors are designed to handle massive amounts of data. Therefore they are justified for use where vast amounts of photons or signals are being emitted, such as the case in several radiologic procedures (e.g., from the output phosphor of an image intensifier, an ionization chamber, scintillation detector of a CT unit, or the antenna of a magnetic resonance imaging device). All of these units require an array processor to "crunch the numbers" so that they may be handled by the host computer (Fig. 33-12). For a 512 × 512 matrix image, the reconstruction process, without the use of an array processor, can take several minutes; whereas, with an array processor, the task can be completed in less than 5 seconds (some less than 1 second) with each rotation of an image requiring at least 5 million operations.

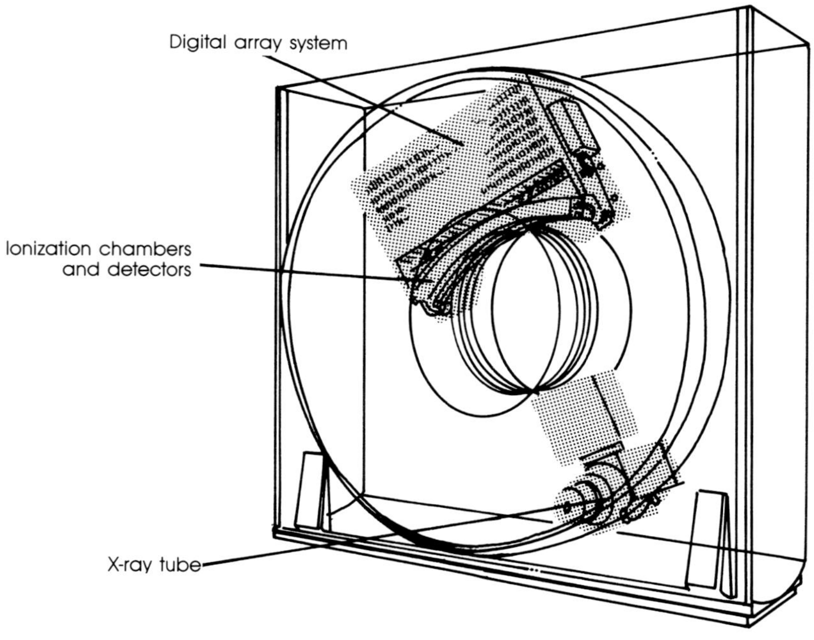

Fig. 33-12. Gantry of a third-generation CT unit. The digital array system contains the ionization chambers and detectors, an analog-to-digital converter, and a digital array unit. The attenuated x-rays are converted to an electrical signal, digitized, and transmitted to the array processor for image reconstruction.

GRAPHIC DISPLAY DEVICES

Although many graphic display systems are available, they have not been used extensively in the medical imaging field. True graphic display is used extensively in the designing-type industries, for example, automobiles and architecture. Gray level mapping is used in computed tomography, MRI, sonography, and nuclear medicine and is referred to as graphs. However, radiation therapy departments have used graphic display devices to demonstrate two-dimensional representations of tumors or even three-dimensional representations of tumors, with shading within the graphic.

A graphic display system houses a display processing unit (DPU) and a dedicated computer with its own set of commands, data formats, and memory. The display processing unit creates an image on a display monitor and then regenerates this image 30 to 60 times a second to avoid a flicker in the image. For image display and regeneration of the image, the "raster-scan" or television-type system is used, dividing the picture into horizontal lines. The regeneration of the image takes place one line at a time.

A display list processor, which is housed in the host computer, transmits instructions to the display processing unit to create a graphic picture. The DPU then executes these instructions from 30 to 60 times per second to maintain the image on the television screen.

Many graphic display systems use the "frame buffer" display technology, where the digitization depth of each voxel is written into the display processing unit's memory. There is less flexibility in the manipulation of the image with this system, but it allows for "selective erasure" of background intensity levels or anatomic structures. Another advantage of this system is that the host computer can perform contrast stretching, windowing, and other functions without disturbing the image data stored in the display processing unit's memory.

Gray level mapping may be thought of as a graph of the gray levels within an image, and it is sometimes referred to as histogram stretching, windowing, or contrast enhancement. A histogram of the image is produced by using gray level mapping and represents a bar chart of the number of pixels versus gray levels (Fig. 33-13). The capability of producing a gray scale histogram or graph is made possible by having a scan conversion memory tube within the computer system that uses a logarithmic transformation of the image into relative exposure values. The histogram is then easily changed into a graph representing the gray levels within an image. A low-contrast histogram (Fig. 33-13, *A*) representing an image has a narrow histogram or a steep slope, whereas a high-contrast histogram (Fig. 33-13, *B*) has a wider histogram or a wider slope.

In medical imaging equipment, the term *window width* refers to the width of the steep part of the curve, or the contrast within the image; *window level* refers to the location of the steep part of the curve within the gray levels and is analogous to image brightness or darkness (Fig. 33-14). The gray level map or graph can be thought of as analogous to the density scale of a radiographic film, an H & D, or a characteristic curve. A windowing operation is the selection of a certain range of the gray scale displayed as an image and the use of the full brightness scale of the television equipment to display only a specific preselected range of gray levels. The remainder of the gray scale outside of the window is subtracted from the gray scale map, leaving only the desired portion of the image displayed as illustrated in Fig. 33-14.

Machine language is coded in binary numbers (0 and 1; "on" or "off") and the shortest possible word is a *bit*. Each voxel depicts an individual depth level of grayness and is represented by a bit, or two characters, a 0 and 1. The number of shades of gray in an image, representing depth, that can be present is determined by a formula, 2 raised to the power of the number of bits, or 2^n. A gray scale with discrete values is assigned to the bits of voxel depth; for example, 2^2 equals 4 gray levels; 2^8 equals 256 gray levels; 2^{10} equals 1024 gray levels; and 2^{16} equals 65,536 gray levels. Bytes, or longer words, are necessary in digital imaging for faster processing. An 8-bit word is known as a *byte;* however, by convention, the computer system is referred to as an 8-bit system, or a 10-bit system or a 16-bit system. Gray levels are conceptualized as being parallel to contrast latitude: the more levels or shades of gray, the more contrast latitude. Discrete values assigned to the "brightness" of the levels of gray are known as Hounsfield units in computed tomography; however, this concept is used by computer systems in digital radiography, nuclear medicine, magnetic resonance imaging, and sonography.

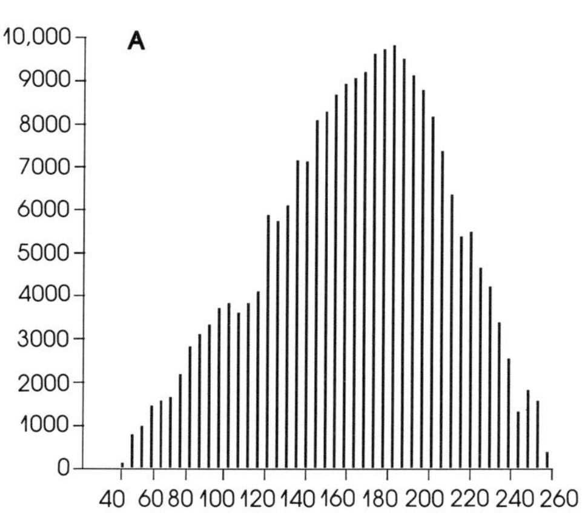

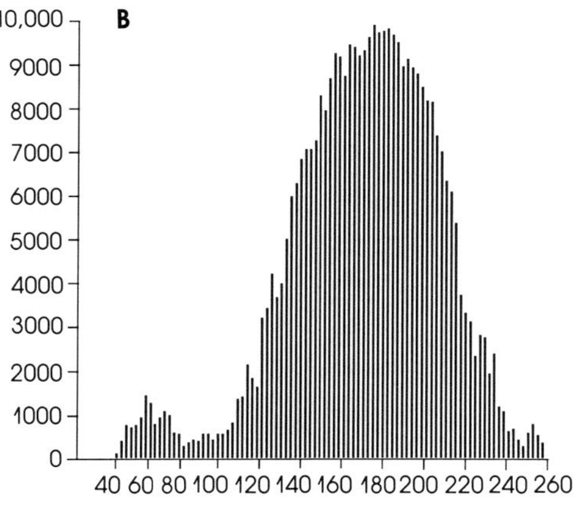

Fig. 33-13. A, Histogram demonstrating low (long scale) contrast in an image, and **B,** histogram demonstrating high (short scale) contrast in an image.

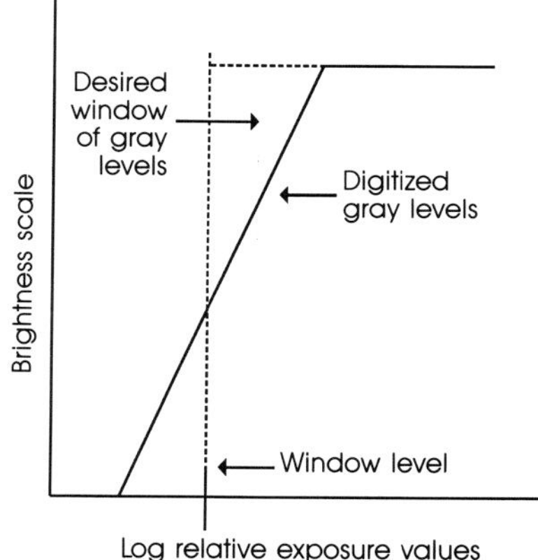

Fig. 33-14. Gray level windowing.

Applications in radiology

Digital Imaging Processing

Within the computer system, digital images are represented as groups of numbers. Therefore these numbers can be changed through applying mathematic operations, and as a result the image is altered. This important concept has provided extraordinary control in contrast enhancement, image enhancement, subtraction techniques, and magnification without losing the original image data.

CONTRAST ENHANCEMENT

Contrast enhancement is accomplished by windowing, which has been explained in the previous section of this chapter (see graphic display devices). Window width encompasses the range of densities within an image. A narrow window is comparable to the use of a high-contrast radiographic film. As a result, image contrast is increased. Increasing the width of the window allows more of the gray scale to be visualized, or more latitude in the densities of the image visualized (Fig. 33-15). A narrow window is valuable when subtle differences in subject density need to be visualized better. However, the use of a narrow window increases image noise, and the densities outside of the narrow window are not visualized.

A

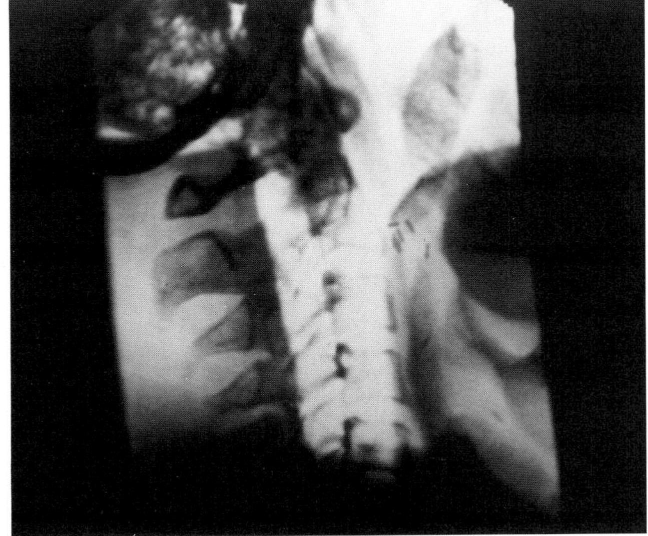

B

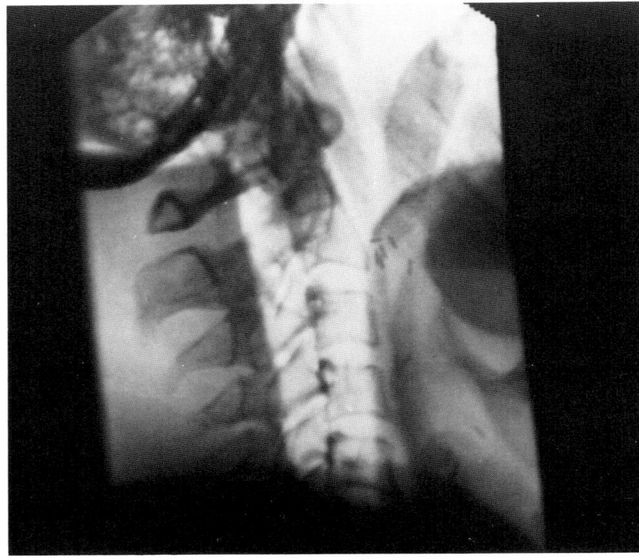

C

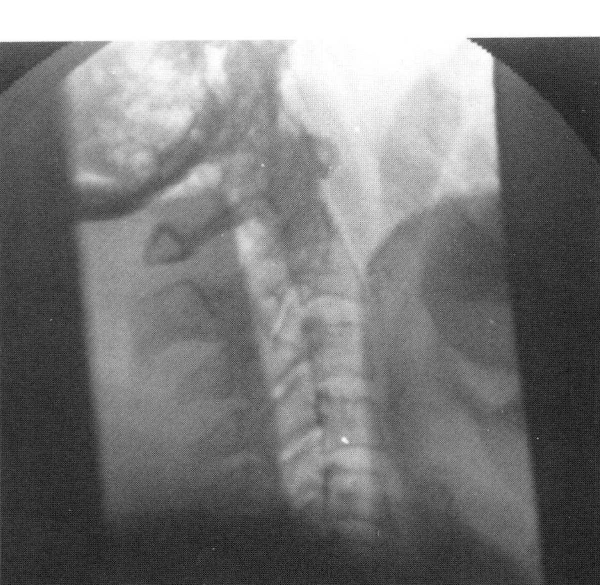

Fig. 33-15. Lateral cervical spine image using different window settings. Window levels of: **A,** 381; **B,** 658; and **C,** 2544. Notice as the window level increases in numeric value, the scale of contrast increases (more long scale).

IMAGE ENHANCEMENT OR RECONSTRUCTION

A method of image enhancement or reconstruction is accomplished by the use of digital processing or filtering, which can be defined as accenting or attenuating selected frequencies in the image. The filtration methods used in medical imaging are classified as: (1) convolution, (2) low-pass filtering, or smoothing; (3) band-pass filtering; and (4) high-pass filtering, or edge enhancement. The background intensities within a medical image consist mainly of low spatial frequencies, whereas an edge, typifying a sudden change in intensities, is composed of mainly high spatial frequencies; for example, the bone to air interface on the skull when using computed tomography. Spatial noise originating from within the computer system is usually high spatial frequencies. Filtration reduces the amount of high spatial frequencies inherent in the object. The percentage of transmission versus spatial frequency, if plotted on a graph, is called modulation transfer function (MTF). One effort of continual research in medical imaging is to develop systems with higher modulation transfer function.

Convolution is accomplished automatically with computer systems that are equipped with fast Fourier transforms. In the systems that do have fast Fourier transforms, the convolution process is implemented by placing a filter mask array, or matrix, over the image array, or matrix, in the memory. A filter mask is a square array or section with numbers, usually consisting of an area of 3 × 3 elements. The size of the filter mask is determined by the manufacturer of the equipment, although larger masks are not often used because they take longer to process. The convolution filtering process can be conceptualized as placing the filter mask over an area of the image matrix, and then multiplying each element value of the filter mask by the image value directly beneath it, obtaining a sum of these values, and then placing that sum within the output image in the exact location as it was in the original image (Fig. 33-16). Convolution filtering is performed primarily to attenuate the higher frequencies within the image. The result of the convolution process is a blurring of the higher frequencies or intensities within the image.

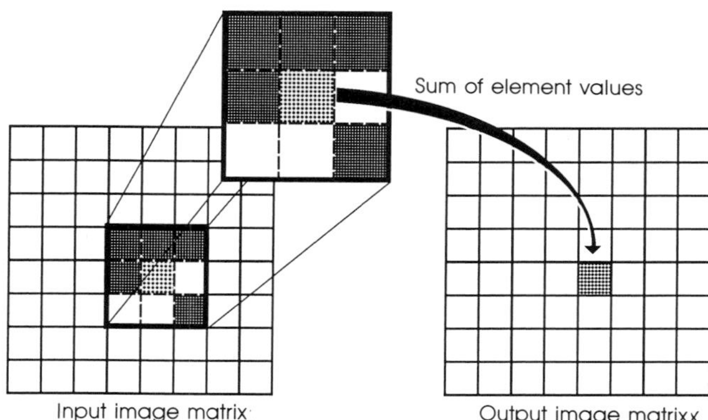

Fig. 33-16. Convolution filtering.

9	8	7	9
7	6	3	7
8	9	9	8
9	6	7	6

9	8	7	9
7	7.3	7.3	7
8	7.1	6.7	8
9	6	7	6

Fig. 33-17. Smoothing, or low-pass, filtering.

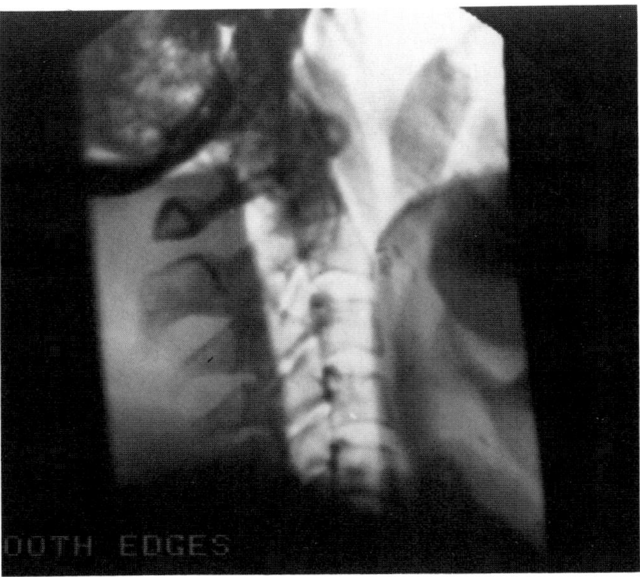

Fig. 33-18. Smoothing technique.

Smoothing, or low-pass filtering, can also be used to remove the high-frequency noise within an image. Smoothing is accomplished by replacing the individual pixel values in the output image by gaining an average of the pixel values around each pixel. To clarify the concept, each pixel's value in the output image is replaced by gaining the simple average of it and eight neighboring pixels (Fig. 33-17). The averaging of the pixels is completed for each pixel within the matrix. The smoothing process smooths or attenuates the sudden differences in intensities or densities in the image by attenuating the higher frequencies within the image matrix (Fig. 33-18).

Band-pass filtration removes or attenuates all frequencies or intensities within the image except those in a preselected range. Band-pass filtering corresponds to the windowing process previously discussed.

High-pass filtration or edge enhancement uses a special edge filter to produce an edge sharpening effect. If a standard high-pass filter were to be used in medical imaging, a remarkably high-contrast image would be produced. An edge filter provides a more diagnostic image by averaging the gray levels similar to the convolution process and then establishing a threshold within the gray level scale. Thresholding allows saturation to black of all the gray levels below the threshold value, and saturation to white of all the levels above the threshold. The thresholding process generates a higher contrast image of the anatomic area of interest and is particularly useful in demonstrating small structures. Research is being conducted with mammography equipment using high-pass filtration to accentuate the structural fine details within the breast and to minimize the background of the breast tissue. Digital subtraction angiography is well known for using high-pass filtration or edge enhancement to accentuate smaller vessels filled with contrast media (Fig. 33-19).

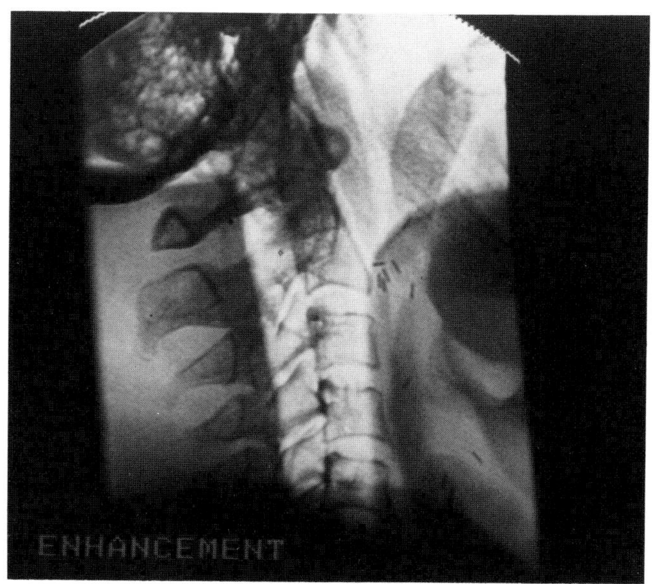

Fig. 33-19. Edge enhancement.

SUBTRACTION TECHNIQUES

The advantages of using digital subtraction include the ability to visualize small anatomic structures and to perform the examination via venous injection of contrast media. The most common digital subtraction techniques are temporal subtraction and dual energy subtraction. Hybrid subtraction is a combination of these two methods.

Temporal subtraction may be defined as a digital imaging process based on time intervals or limited by time, and in its simplest form it is produced by obtaining a mask (similar to a scout radiograph) and subtracting the pixel values of the mask from the pixel values of a postinjection image (see Volume 3, Chapter 30, photographic subtraction). There should be no change in the images except for the contrast media–filled vasculature, and the subtracted image should primarily demonstrate the opacified blood vessels. However, a serious problem with this technique is the probability of patient motion between exposures. To correct the motion problem, a time interval difference (TID) mode is used for the digital processing. The TID technique involves obtaining a series of mask images and storing the images in adjacent memory locations. When the contrast medium is injected, a series of exposures is made at very rapid rate; for example, 15 images per second for 4 seconds. The postinjection images are identified as frame numbers and stored in adjacent memory locations. The frames, or postinjection data, are then subtracted from the masks, or original data, by allowing the computer to follow a set, programmed procedure. Examples of this set procedure may be: subtracting mask #1 from frame #2; mask #2 from frame #4; and so on.

Dual energy subtraction does not require the acquisition of images before the injection of contrast media. After an iodinated contrast medium is injected, a series of rapid exposures is made at a high kVp setting above the K-edge of iodine, 35 keV; and another series of exposures is made at a low kVp setting, below the 35 keV attenuation coefficient of iodine. The high kVp setting will diminish the bone contrast in the image, whereas the low kVp setting will enhance the less dense anatomic structures (i.e., the small vessels). A subtraction process of the two sets of images is then performed, with the outcome being increased contrast of the opacified vessels. To digitally perform the dual subtraction technique after the images have been acquired, the densities of the straight line portion of the film's H & D curve are correlated to the desired window level to produce the image. Advantages of dual subtraction are (1) patient motion is not as much of a problem as in the temporal subtraction method; and (2) the high kVp and low kVp images allow the display of bone only or soft tissue only, or a combination of the tissues.

Hybrid subtraction is a combination of the temporal subtraction, TID, and the dual energy subtraction methods. When using the hybrid subtraction method, a set of masks is obtained for the high kVp setting and for the low kVp setting. Therefore, two sets of masks and two sets of frames with iodinated contrast media are acquired. The low kVp masks are subtracted from the frames with contrast media, and the high kVp masks are subtracted from the high kVp frames. The hybrid subtraction procedure eliminates bone, leaving only the contrast-filled vessels.

Mask registration is a procedure that is useful when patient motion occurs between the time of the mask exposures and the time of the contrast media frames. To correct the motion problem, the absolute density value of each pixel within the matrix of each mask and each frame is calculated and portrayed as a reregistration of the image. The calculation of the absolute values of the pixels is similar to the smoothing filtration method described previously.

MAGNIFICATION

Magnification, sometimes called zooming, is a process of selecting an area of interest and copying each pixel within the area an integer number of times. Large magnifications may give the image an appearance of being constructed of blocks. To provide a more diagnostic image, a smoothing or low-pass filter operation can be done to smooth out the distinct intensities between the blocks.

THREE-DIMENSIONAL IMAGING

When three-dimensional imaging was first introduced, the images were less than optimal because of the resolution being too low to adequately visualize anatomic structures deeper within the body. The images often only adequately displayed the more dense structures closer to the body surface, or surface boundaries, which appeared blocky and jagged; therefore the data depicting the soft tissue or less dense structures were not visualized. By using fast Fourier transforms (3DFT), new algorithms for mathematic calculations, and the development of computers with faster processing time, the quality of three-dimensional images has become smooth, sharply focused, and realistically shaded to demonstrate soft tissue. The terminology used to describe the ability to demonstrate soft tissue in three-dimensional imaging is referred to as a volumetric rendering technique.

Volumetric rendering is a computer program whereby "stacks" of sequential images are processed as a volume with the gray scale intensity information in each pixel being interpolated in the z axis (perpendicular to the x and y axes). Interpolation is necessary because the field of view of the scan (the x and y axes) is not the same as the z axis because of interscan spacing. Following this computer process, new data are generated by interpolation, resulting in each new voxel having all the same dimensions. The volumetric rendering technique enables definition of the object's thickness, a crucial factor in three-dimensional imaging and in visualizing subtle densities.

Generation of three-dimensional imaging typically requires a "stack" of 50 scans with a resolution of 256 × 256, for a total of 6 megabytes of information and the processing capability of 5 million instructions per second. An average examination takes approximately 25 to 40 minutes of scan time to complete. The entire examination, from the time the patient enters until he or she exits from the department, would more than likely be over an hour.

OPTICAL STORAGE AND RETRIEVAL SYSTEMS

Because of the storage and retrieval problems within a radiology department, there is currently a trend to develop optical storage technology. Optical storage technology embraces the concept of using some form of optical device to record and retrieve information from a light-sensitive medium. The optical devices currently being used are either gas or diode lasers. The media being used for recording are rectangular plates or disks resembling a long-playing phonograph record.

Manufacturers of optical disk systems use minute holes made in the disk by the laser beam for the recording of information. The pits, made in the media surface, range in size from 1 to 2 micromillimeters in size, with the spacing between the rows 1.5 to 2 micromillimeters. This permits the ability for storage of 40,000 to 50,000 images on a single side of an optical disk.

Digital computer imaging systems using the binary system can send instructions to the optical laser system to encode the disk. The length of the pits and the distance between them made by the laser beam on the disk represent a digital coding scheme that can be retrieved. The advantages of this system are that, unlike radiographs, a disk does not deteriorate and requires very little storage space.

To retrieve the information on the disk, a reading laser produces a light source on the surface of the disk. If no information is on the portion of the disk where the laser is focused, the light is reflected back. When the reading laser is focused on an area that has been encoded, or where there is a pit, the light is partially refracted, according to the length and depth of the pit. The refraction of the light is then transmitted to the surface where a photodetector is excited, produces a lower voltage, and is processed through digitization of the sine wave.

Digital optical systems can be used throughout the radiology department for the processing, storage, and retrieval of data; they can be used not only in the area of image processing but also for management services. As the technology develops, the costs of obtaining this system will be reduced. The radiology department of the future may not use radiographic films. A radiologist will be able to correlate, integrate, and evaluate images with the medical records of a single patient by use of a digital optical system.

Another form of image processing that was developed primarily by NASA and that will have an impact on the practice of radiology is the use of a digitizing camera for the analysis of data. A radiograph exposed and processed using current methods can be digitized by placing the film or a microdensitometer on a lightbox in front of a digitizing camera that operates in a similar fashion to that of the optical laser devices. The image is then digitized and processed by the computer system, which allows for the manipulation of the image. Such a system would obviate repeat radiographs in a radiology department.

An innovative application of the digitizing camera and special image processors is being used. This application is called "teleradiography," and it uses the digitizing camera to digitize the radiographic images of examinations on patients in rural areas for transmission by means of a *modem* over conventional telephone lines to a remote medical center. The images are then processed by a special image processor and displayed on video terminals for diagnosis by physicians in prominent medical centers. This system would enable small, rural hospitals to provide improved medical care without the great expense of obtaining sophisticated computer equipment. It is predicted that networks will be established among large medical research centers and smaller hospitals and clinics through the use of teleradiography, for the purpose of providing more accurate diagnosis in pathologic conditions and trauma situations.

INFORMATION AND MANAGEMENT SYSTEMS

Most of the information and management computer systems used in radiology have been developed from the MUMPS programming languages. The modules contained in the majority of information management systems are registration, scheduling, process control, film file management, and reporting. The use of these modules also contributes to the quality control of the department.

The function of the registration module is to record the information typically found typed on a card file in the department—the dates and types of examinations a patient has had. Use of computer files provides more accurate recording of information and much faster retrieval of the file.

Combined with the registration program is the scheduling module that makes the patient's appointment. This program aids in smoothing out the department's workload, thus providing better use of equipment and personnel. Another function of this program is to check the patient's file for previous examinations and to sequence the examinations in the proper order. This module can also check to see what rooms are available for this study, calculate the average time it takes to complete the examination, print workloads for the entire department or a particular room, and produce schedules for the nursing stations, outpatient clinics, and physicians.

The process module tracks the process of performing and interpreting the examination. This process starts with the arrival of the patient in the department and includes the examinations performed, the rooms used, the technologist who performed the examination, the number of radiographs per examination, if retakes were done and the reason for the retakes, and if any medications or contrast media were used. Before the patient leaves, a computer check is done to determine if the patient needs any pending examinations and whether all examinations have been completed. The program will also record the time that the report was dictated, transcribed, and signed by the radiologist. Use of this module or program can provide a very detailed repeat analysis that can be used to justify repair of equipment, new equipment purchases, or the need for inservice education or further education of the technologists.

Computer management of the film file provides a library system that records the files within the department and their location, or individual radiographs loaned to outside departments, doctors, clinics, and other medical facilities. The system can provide lists of files or radiographs that are overdue, which helps in the recovery of these medical records before they are lost. Used with a scheduling module, a list of patients and the previous examinations completed on each patient can be produced so that they may be retrieved from the file archives the day before the scheduled examinations. Lastly, this program will also print adhesive labels that can be attached to the file jacket to record the date and type of examination performed.

A reporting program assists in the preparation and interpretation of the examinations. This module usually includes a word processing program used by the transcriptionist. Using CRTs in transcription and proofreading can save clerical time and improve the accuracy of the reports. Some systems even allow the radiologist to electronically sign the reports. A teaching file can also be developed with this system by having the radiologist dictate a code to be included with the transcription. The code enables the computer to identify the more interesting cases to be used for educational purposes.

All of these modules can be used on a *time-sharing* basis. Time sharing is a computer system in which each person using the system is given, for a small fraction of time, the total use or resources of the larger, multiprogram computer. The use of the large computer is rotated among the users under the direction of the operating programs and is determined by priorities. A time-sharing computer system makes a computerized information management system cost effective, even for small hospitals and clinics.

The other modules that can be included in an information management system contain administrative and financial programs. The most common of these is the billing system that can provide very accurate and detailed itemized lists of expenses.

An overall benefit from all of these modules and the data or information generated is the potential to enhance quality control throughout the entire department and hospital. Management decisions, based on the statistics provided by such a system, will promote efficiency and improve operations within a department or hospital, thereby providing quality patient care.

APPLICATIONS IN EDUCATION

Computers have been used to facilitate learning for the past 20 years. The development of miniaturized transistors and semiconductors allowed the mass distribution of microcomputers and minicomputers that has resulted in the adoption of computer-assisted instruction at all educational levels.

One must distinguish between computer-assisted instruction (CAI) and computer-managed instruction (CMI). CAI programs involve the learning of new information and actually assist in the teaching process. Methods incorporated in CAI are the presentation of new material, reinforcement through immediate feedback, questioning, and graphics. To ensure that learning has occurred, the students can be tested for knowledge and repeat the training if necessary. CMI uses testing procedures and then directs the student to reference material for further information or help with no initial instruction being performed by the computer. Many CMI programs often serve as nothing more than electronic bookkeepers, because their function is to grade the tests, provide test scores, and provide statistical data on these tests.

Instruction using a CAI system is concentrated on the presentation and learning of concepts, principles, and rules, or what is known as the "cognitive domain" of learning. Its effectiveness is limited in the teaching of psychomotor skills, such as radiographic positioning, and in the "affective domain," the learning of professional attitudes and empathy. Learning in these latter two domains may be enhanced by adding a video disk system to the computer system.

Although CAI has a high potential for the enhancement of learning, it will not replace the instructor in the classroom or in the clinical setting, just as the computer will not replace human judgment in making a diagnosis. A distinct advantage of CAI is that students exposed to this method of instruction will have the opportunity to become familiar with computers and their operation, and therefore will more readily adapt to the computerized equipment in the clinical setting.

Summary

Radiology departments in the future will become more reliant on the computer for imaging, therapeutic purposes, file management, billing, quality assurance, patient monitoring, education, and research. Radiologists will find their time absorbed and divided among the various imaging and therapeutic procedures. As this occurs, technologists will gain additional responsibility and be required to possess the knowledge and skills necessary to understand and operate the computerized equipment and systems. Therefore it is essential that technologists know how to operate a computer just as they must know how radiation is produced.

Definition of Terms

address The label, name, or number identifying a register, location, or unit where data are stored; in most cases, address refers to the location in the computer memory.

algorithm A defined set of instructions that will lead to the logical conclusion of a task.

analog computer Computer that performs operations on continuous signals.

analog-to-digital converter An input device for changing continuous (analog) signals into digital form (i.e., discrete numbers).

arithmetic/logic unit (ALU) That part of the computer that performs computations, comparisons, and logical operations.

assembler A computer program used to assemble machine code from symbolic code.

assembly language A computer programming language that is machine-oriented and can be translated directly into machine instructions.

baud rate The rate at which information is transmitted serially from a computer; expressed in bits per second.

binary A numbering system based on twos rather than tens (decimals); the individual element can have a value of 0 or 1, and in computer memory is known as a bit.

bit Constructed from the words *BI*nary digi*T*. The term refers to a single digit of a binary number. For example, the binary number of 101 is composed of three bits.

boot The process of initializing a computer operating system; also referred to as "booting up."

buffer An auxiliary storage area for data input in order to match the speed differences between machines.

bug A common term used to describe an error in operation or in a program.

byte A term used to define a group of bits, usually eight, and being treated as a unit by the computer.

cathode ray tube (CRT) An electronic tube (like the familiar television tube) that makes the computer output visible; sometimes called a VDU (visual display unit).

central processing unit (CPU) The brain of the computer; it is the circuitry that actually processes the information and controls the storage, movement, and manipulation of the data.

character Any letter, digit, or punctuation mark; characters are usually represented by a binary code composed of eight bits, or one byte.

command A portion of code that represents an instruction for the computer.

compiler A set of programs that compiles or converts a program into the machine language instructions for a particular computer.

console Usually the front panel of the CPU by which the operator supervises and controls the machine.

control unit That part of the CPU that directs the sequence of operations, such as which instruction is to be executed next.

cursor A character, usually an underline or a graphics block, that indicates position on a display screen.

data acquisition unit A peripheral device that acquires signals from equipment and transmits them to the computer.

data base A large file of organized information that is produced, updated, and manipulated by one or more programs.

data management system A group of commands that create, update, and reference a data base.

digital computer A computer in which discrete numbers are used to express data and instructions.

digitization depth The dimension of depth within a matrix, represented by a number of pixels, which, in turn, signifies the levels or shades of gray available within an image.

digitization rate The amount of time needed to change data from analog form to digital form.

direct access Access to data independent of the previously obtained data; it may also be called "random access."

disk A circular plate coated with magnetic material and used to store data.

diskdrive A device used to read data from and to write data onto disks.

downtime The time a computer system is out of operation, usually for repairs and/or maintenance; often expressed as a percentage of the normal operating hours.

dynamic range The range of voltage or input signals that result in a digital output.

file A collection of related data or information kept as a unit.

generation A group of computers produced within the same period, based on the model of an earlier product.

hard copy Any readable output from a computer; it is usually on paper, but in radiology the output of images is usually on radiographic film.

hardware The physical devices and/or equipment of a computer system.

high-level language A computer language in which each user instruction corresponds to multiple instructions when converted to machine code; examples: FORTRAN, FOCAL, COBOL, and ALGOL.

hybrid computer A computer with both analog and digital computing capability.

input The information the computer receives via media; for example, magnetic tape, disks, punched cards, or keyboard.

input/output terminal (I/O terminal) A machine or device capable of both feeding information into and retrieving it from the computer.

instruction A program step that tells the computer exactly what to do for a single operation in a program.

interface A device that serves as a common boundary between two other devices; a connection between two pieces of computer hardware.

interrupt A temporary suspension of processing by the computer; caused by input from another part of the computer or by an auxiliary device or machine.

K A symbol for 1000; in computer language, it means 2^{10} or 1024 and denotes the number of units a computer can store in its memory; example: $32 \times 1024 = 32{,}768$ or 32K.

language A defined set of characters that, when used alone or in combinations, form a meaningful set of words and symbols; used to write instructions for a computer; examples: ALGOL, COBOL, BASIC, and FORTRAN.

machine language A programming language consisting only of numbers or symbols that the computer can understand without translation.

magnetic memory Any memory device using magnetic fields as a means of storing data; for example, magnetic tape or disks.

memory The storage of information and data by the computer.

modem (*MO*dulator/*DEM*odulator) A device that allows data to be transmitted long distances, usually over telephone lines, by impressing digital pulses onto an analog carrier wave.

multiprogramming The ability of a computer system to permit execution of more than one separate task at a time; is used in timesharing and/or multiuser systems.

multitasking A computer system or a single machine that can process several programs.

off-line Portions of the computer that are not under the direct control of the CPU or the operator.

on-line Portions of the computer that are directly under the control of the CPU and the operator.

optical scanner A device that scans the light either reflected or transmitted through a surface and then converts the signal into a machine-readable input.

output The results generated when the computer has performed the requested combinations of tasks.

peripheral A device that is separate but connected to the computer for the purpose of supplying input and/or output capability.

primary memory A portion of a computer that is used to store information, either data or programs; the size of a computer may be referred to by the amount of user memory; usually measured in kilobytes.

random access The ability to access locations of data without regard to sequential data; access may be accomplished by going directly to the location.

random access memory (RAM) Pertaining to a storage device in which access time is effectively independent of the location of the data.

read only memory (ROM) A memory that is similar to the RAM except that data cannot be written into it, but is capable of being read.

real time Computer operations that occur fast enough to be analyzed and used immediately for decision making.

register A device in the CPU that stores information for future use.

response time The time between the input of information into a computer and the response or output.

serial processing Digital computer processing in which programs are run sequentially, rather than simultaneously or together.

software A general term that applies to any program or set of instructions that can be loaded into a computer.

storage capacity The amount of data that can be stored in the computer memory, usually expressed in terms of kilobytes.

terminal An input/output device, usually consisting of a keyboard and display screen.

time sharing The process of accomplishing two or more tasks at (apparently) the same time; the computer will process one task at a time, but only a small portion, before switching to the next; because the computer can process a large amount of data in a short period of time, the switching between tasks is not noticed by human observation.

Winchester disk drive A smaller, less-expensive, hard disk drive capable of transferring data at an increased rate with sophisticated error detection and correction procedures.

word The number of bits processed as a single unit in an arithmetic operation.

word length The number of bits composing a word.

write To record data on a memory device.

x-y digitizer An input device that allows the motion of the cursor or pen to be transduced and fed into the computer as a series of x-y coordinates.

SELECTED BIBLIOGRAPHY

Bushong SC: Radiologic science for technologists—physics, biology, and protection, ed 4, St Louis, 1988, The CV Mosby Co.

Chandler, R: PACS: applications in the modern radiology department, Admin Radiol, June, 1987.

Convey HD, et al: Computers in the practice of medicine, introduction to computer concepts, vol I, 1980, Reading, Mass, Addison-Wesley Publishing Co, Inc.

Cook LT, et al: Image processing: shape analysis, texture analysis, and three-dimensional display, Appl Radiol 13(3):123-134, 1984.

Curry T, et al: Christensen's introduction to the physics of diagnostic radiology, ed 3, Philadelphia, 1984, Lea & Febiger.

Edwards M, et al: Computers in radiology—interfacing with peripheral devices, Appl Radiol 2:37-46, March/April 1984.

Enlander D: Computers in medicine—an introduction, St Louis, 1980, The CV Mosby Co.

Fishman EK, et al: Volumetric rendering techniques: applications for three-dimensional imaging of the hip, Radiology 163:737-738, 1987.

Gonzoley R, et al: Digital image processing, Reading, Mass, 1977, Addison-Wesley Publishing Co, Inc.

Gould RG: Digital hardware in radiography and fluoroscopy, Appl Radiol 13(3):137-140, 1984.

Greenfield GB and Hubbard LB: Computers in radiology, New York, 1984, Churchill Livingstone.

Hunter TB: The computer in radiology, Rockville, Md, 1986, Aspen Publications.

Kuni CC: Introduction to computers and digital processing in medical imaging, Chicago, 1988, Year Book Medical Publishers.

Lehr JL: Computer languages and the operating systems, Appl Radiol 13(1):35-41, 1984.

Lehr JL, editor: Planning guide for radiologic installations: fascicle 9: computer information systems, Chicago, 1977, American College of Radiology.

Lehr JL: Software: basics and applications in radiology, Semin Ultrasound 4(4):260-269, December 1983.

Lieberman DE: Computer methods, the fundamentals of digital nuclear medicine, St Louis, 1977, The CV Mosby Co.

Ney D, et al: Interactive real-time multiplanar CT imaging, Radiology 170:275-276, 1989.

Novick G: Introduction to computer hardware and internal representation, Appl Radiol 12(6):51-62, 1983.

Powis RL, et al: A thinker's guide to ultrasonic imaging, Baltimore, 1984, Urban & Schwarzenberg, Inc.

Robb WL: Future advances and directions in imaging research, Am J Radiol 150:39-42, 1988.

Rowberg AH: Digital hardware in CT and NMR, Appl Radiol 13(4):71-74, 1984.

Seeram E: Computed tomography technology, Philadelphia, 1982, WB Saunders Co.

Simborg DW: Local area networks: why? what? what if?, MD Computing, Computers in Medical Practice 1(4):10-20, 1984.

Strong HM and Cerva JR: Image storage and transmission technology, Semin Ultrasound 4(1):270-279, 1983.

Swett HA and Miller PL: ICON: a computer-based approach to differential diagnosis in radiology, Radiology 163:555-558, 1987.

Swett HA, et al: Expert system-controlled image display, Radiology 172:487-493, 1989.

Trux PG: The current state of operating systems: 1983 and 1984, MD Computing, Computers in Medical Practice 1(4):58-63, 1984.

Ubaldi S, et al: The use of microcomputers in radiologic technology training programs: focus on education, Radiol Technol 53(3):271-273, 1981.

Chapter 34

COMPUTED TOMOGRAPHY

KENNETH C. JOHNSON
ALAN H. ROWBERG

This chapter presents the fundamental concepts of *computed tomography (CT),** compares it with conventional radiography, and describes some typical applications. Many of the factors that affect the resulting diagnostic image are also discussed.

As seen in Fig. 34-1, CT is the process of creating a cross-sectional tomographic plane *(slice)* of any part of the body. The image then is reconstructed by a computer using x-ray absorption measurements collected at multiple points about the periphery of the part being *scanned*.

Today, CT is a well-accepted imaging modality for neurologic and body procedures, with a growing emphasis on body applications because of magnetic resonance imaging's (MRI's) maturation and acceptance in neurologic diagnosis. The reasons for this shift include the reduced scan times and improved low contrast resolution of today's CT scanners.

Many benefits are realized from the capability of CT to present a cross-sectional image of the body and its ability to distinguish more minute differences among various tissues than with conventional radiography. In addition, the CT image can be altered at the viewing console to optimize the presentation of the diagnostic information.

*All italicized terms are defined at the end of this chapter.

Comparison with Conventional Radiography

Reviewing conventional radiography helps explain the uniqueness of CT diagnostic information. When a conventional x-ray exposure is made (Fig. 34-2), the transmitted radiation passes through the patient and is detected by x-ray film or an image-intensifier phosphor. First, for each exposure to radiation, one diagnostic image with a fixed density and contrast is produced. Second, three-dimensional body structures are superimposed as a two-dimensional image on the cathode ray tube and on the x-ray film. Thus the highlighting of certain anatomy requires exact positioning of the patient, often the use of contrast agents, and frequently more than one exposure.

Compare the conventional radiograph to the CT image shown in Fig. 34-3. In a typical CT study, from 10 to 20 or more individual slices are required for a single CT examination.

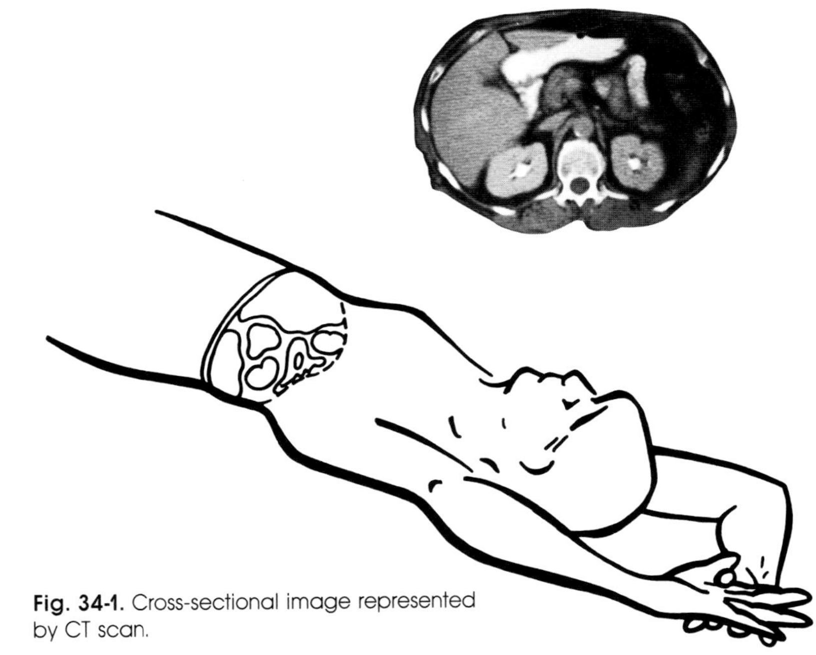

Fig. 34-1. Cross-sectional image represented by CT scan.

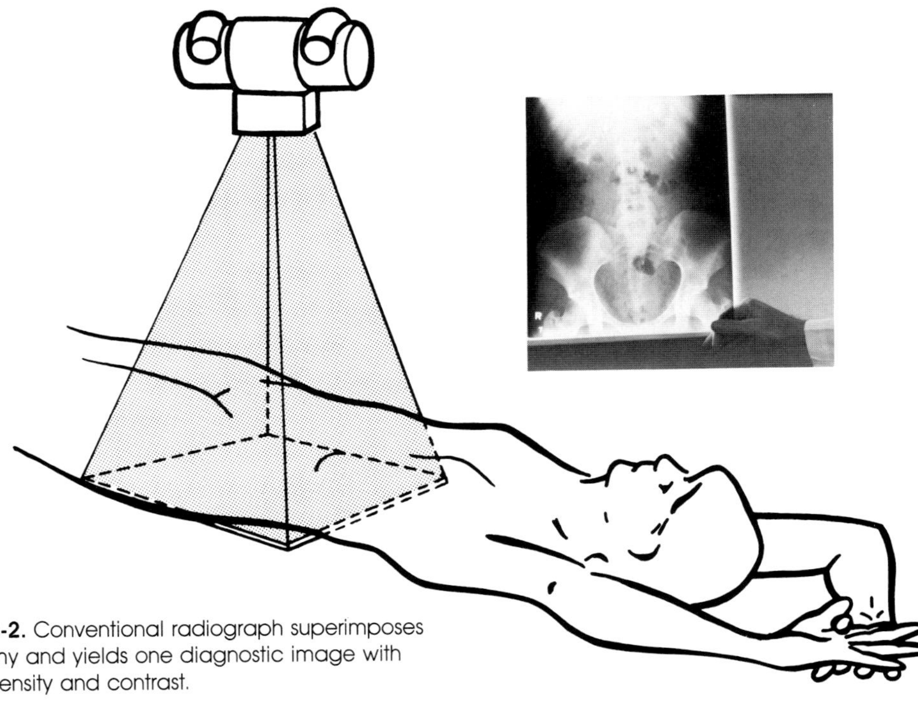

Fig. 34-2. Conventional radiograph superimposes anatomy and yields one diagnostic image with fixed density and contrast.

Low tissue density that would normally be obscured by higher-density anatomy on a conventional radiograph can be clearly visualized with CT. For this reason CT is valuable in neurologic work in which the brain is surrounded by the skull. Likewise, in many body examinations, low tissue density that would otherwise be hidden or blend with surrounding anatomy can be clearly visualized.

Although it seems obvious, it should also be noted that the CT image displays the entire cross section of the slice of anatomy that was scanned. Thus the size and location of any pathologic condition can be determined with extreme accuracy within a given CT slice. With conventional radiography, multiple exposures and contrast media are often required to estimate the size and location of the diseased area. Further, the series of CT scans identifies the location of the pathologic finding in three dimensions when each slice is analyzed and may be viewed in three dimensions with three-dimensional software packages.

Contrast. CT measures and can reveal significantly more minute differences in x-ray attenuation than can be recorded by conventional radiography. For example, conventional radiography requires a minimum difference in tissue of 2% to 5% to radiographically separate the structures. CT can resolve differences in tissue density as low as 0.3%. In Fig. 34-4 the gray and the white matter in the brain can be distinguished easily. The x-ray detectors used in CT have a wider dynamic range than film, so greater contrast sensitivity is possible in an imaging environment that contains the large density range from air or lungs to soft tissue to bone.

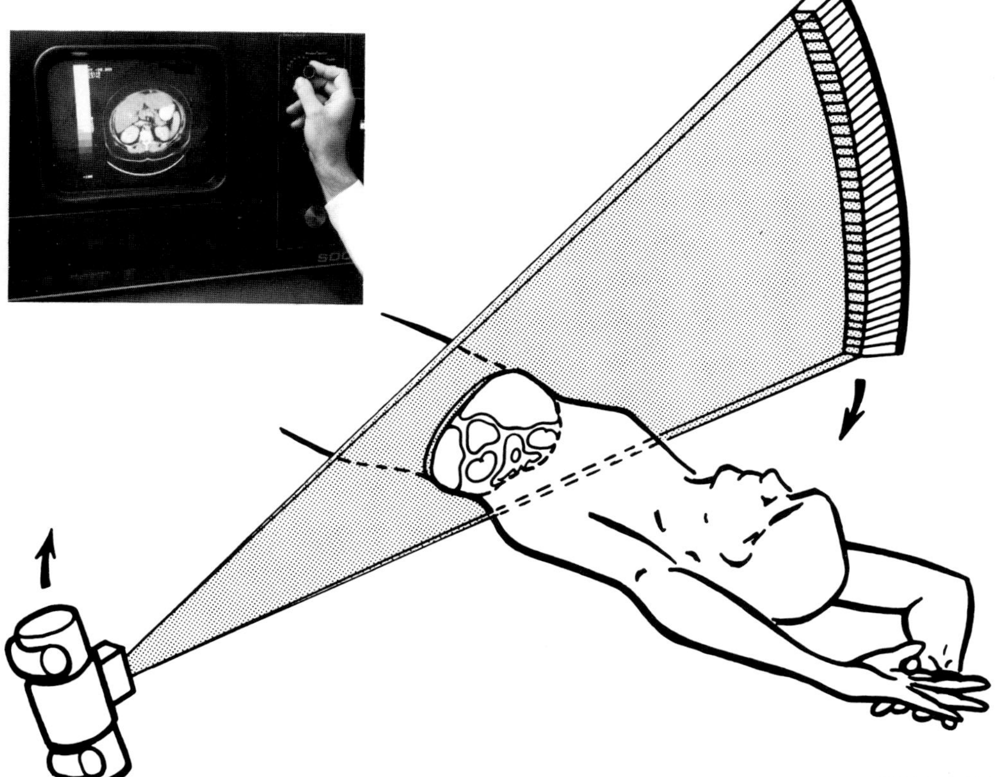

Fig. 34-3. CT scan provides cross-sectional image that can be altered at viewing console.

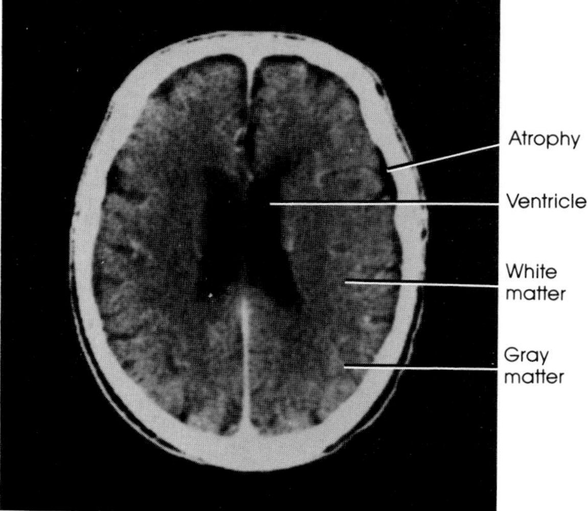

Fig. 34-4. CT brain scan differentiates between gray and white brain matter.

IMAGE MANIPULATION

In conventional radiography, only a single radiograph with a fixed contrast and density is obtained for each patient exposure to radiation. Once the film has been processed, the patient must be exposed to radiation again to produce another image. The CT image, on the other hand, is the result of complex mathematical calculations that the computer performs to reconstruct an image that is stored in the computer's memory. The CT image is displayed on a *cathode ray tube (CRT)* and can be altered in many ways.

When viewing the image on the CRT, the operator can adjust the brightness and contrast of the image as desired. The image can also be magnified, and the computer will calculate statistical values for various regions as specified by the operator. The manner in which the image obtained from a CT slice can be manipulated is demonstrated in Fig. 34-5. Both soft tissue and very dense anatomy can be examined within a single slice. Table 34-1 shows typical settings of window width and window levels used to view CT images.

Table 34-1. Typical window width and window level settings (in Hounsfield units)

CT examination	Window width	Window level
Brain	250	30
Spinal cord	350	50
Skull, vertebrae, or other bone	2000	500
Lungs	2000	−700
Mediastinum	450	40
Abdomen	150	50

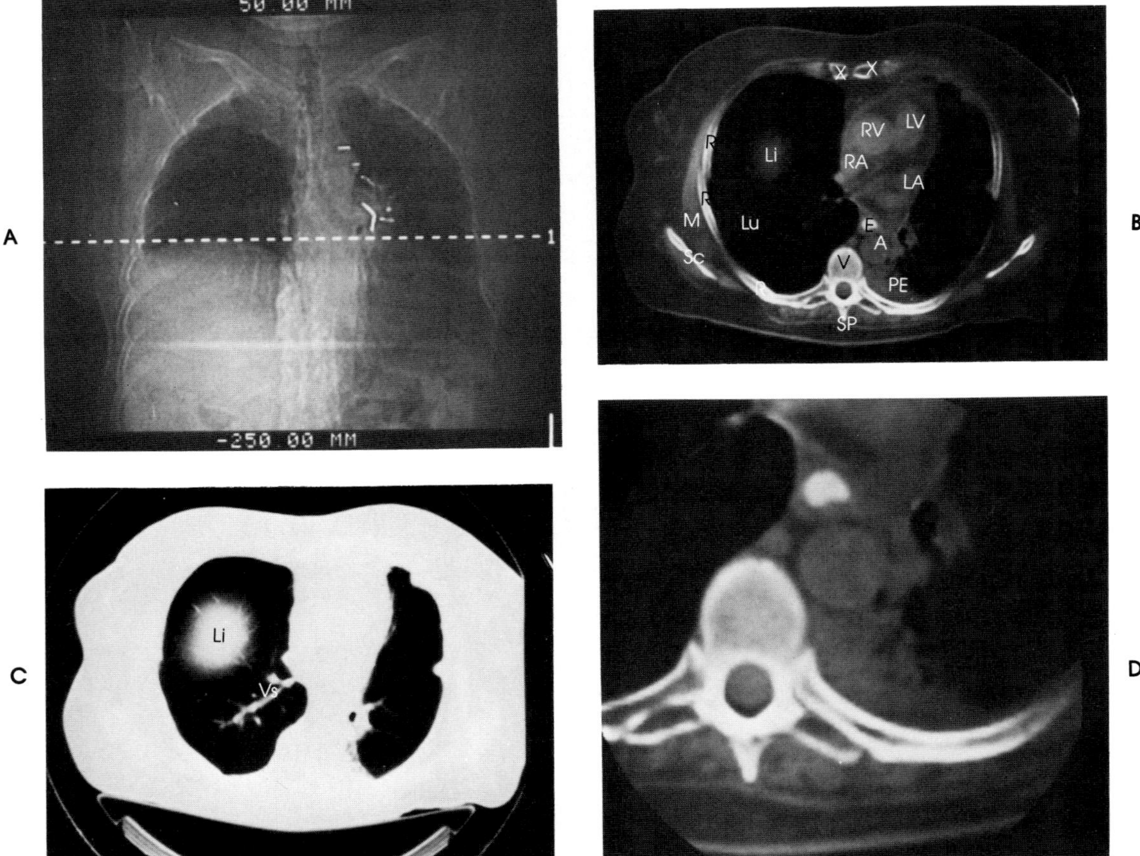

Fig. 34-5. Manipulation of CT image. **A,** AP localizer image locating CT slice *(dashed line)*. **B,** CT image adjusted for viewing wide range of body tissues. *A,* Aorta; *E,* esophagus with contrast medium; *LA,* left atrium; *Li,* apex of liver; *Lu,* lung; *LV,* left ventricle; *M,* muscle; *PE,* pleural effusion; *R,* rib; *RA,* right atrium; *RV,* right ventricle; *Sc,* scapula; *SP,* spinous process; *V,* vertebral body; *X,* xiphoid. **C,** CT slice adjusted to study low-density tissue. *Li,* Apex of liver; *Vs,* lung vessels. **D,** Magnified view of specific area.

In addition to these capabilities, others are available such as the ability to create sagittal or coronal images from the cross-sectional projection. Fig. 34-6 demonstrates sagittal and coronal images of the neck and upper thorax that were obtained by having the computer reconstruct the data it obtained from the various transverse slices. These sagittal and coronal images were produced with no additional radiation exposure to the patient.

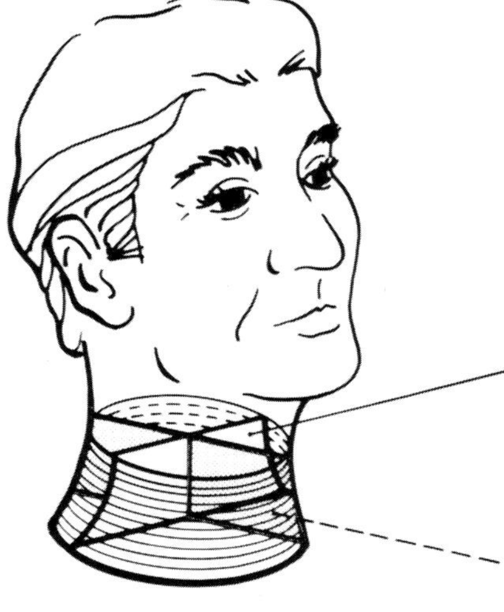

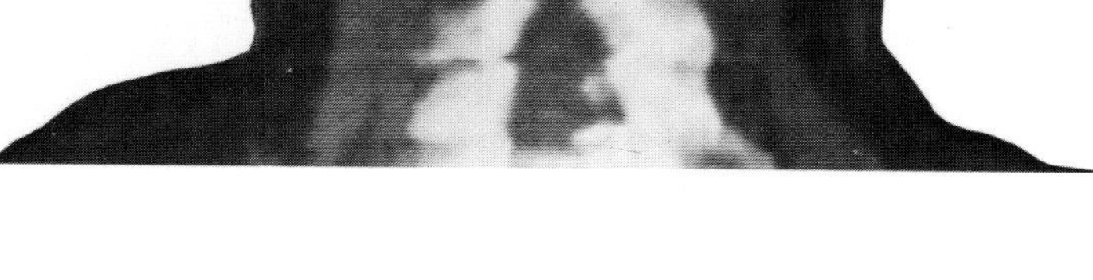

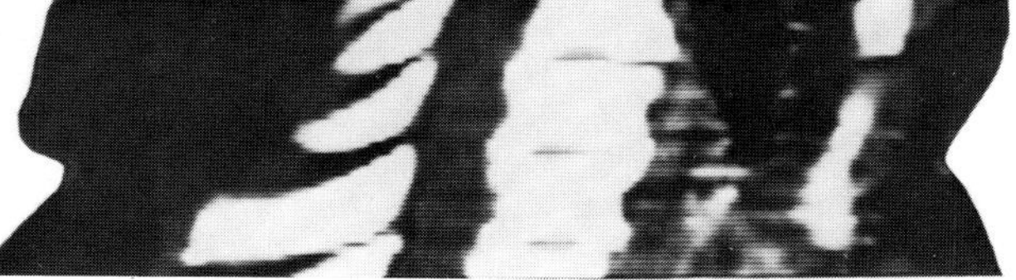

Fig. 34-6. Coronal and sagittal reconstructions of neck and upper thorax generated from axial CT slices.

LIMITATIONS

Although CT has many advantages, it also has limitations. Among these limitations is the time it takes to perform a single examination. Completion of most examinations requires 15 to 30 minutes or longer. Thus most scanners are limited to performing a maximum of 15 to 20 examinations during a typical 8-hour day.

Another limitation of CT is its use in dynamic studies. The time required to scan each slice is 1 second or more. The table is then moved and the next slice taken. Thus, to image a large anatomic area, a considerable amount of time is involved. Various approaches are being developed to maximize the number of slices that can be visualized in a short period for dynamic studies. Dynamic scanning may also be used to scan repeatedly at the same location, without moving the table between slices, thus visualizing the flow of contrast in and out of a location, and to estimate the flow dynamics in a region. A number of design factors as well as x-ray tube cooling may limit the overall rate at which dynamic scanning may be done.

Another current limitation of CT as compared with conventional radiography is in its ability to resolve small structures. Conventional radiography has a resolving power down to approximately 0.1 mm, whereas CT can currently only resolve pathologic features larger than 1 mm. Thus conventional radiography can resolve smaller anatomic detail as long as sufficient contrast is available.

Historical Development

The first successful clinical demonstration of CT was conducted in 1967 by Godfrey Hounsfield from the Central Research Laboratory of EMI, Ltd., in England. In 1971 the first full-scale unit for head scanning was installed at Atkinson Morley's Hospital, Wimbledon, England. Its value for providing neurologic information enabled it to gain rapid acceptance.

The first CT units in the United States were installed in 1973 at the Mayo Clinic and Massachusetts General Hospital. In 1974 Dr. Robert Ledley at Georgetown University Medical Center developed the first scanner capable of visualizing any section of the body.

The early generations of scanners, such as the one in Fig. 34-7, were designed so that the x-ray tube and detector or detectors were required to go through a complex series of motions to collect the absorption data for reconstructing an image. As a result, these systems required 15 seconds to 5 minutes to gather sufficient data for reconstructing an image. Because of this inherently slow scanning speed as well as other limitations, these early systems were used almost exclusively for neurologic work, for which they provided unique, useful diagnostic information. The scanning geometry made scanning time proportional to the field of view since the x-ray source had to be moved mechanically across the entire scan field diameter for each scan. The scan time of the early systems was so long that it limited usefulness in the body, where natural motions such as patient breathing and intestinal peristalsis blurred the images. Thus these scanners were often referred to as head scanners.

The majority of scanners being produced today employ a fan beam of radiation that rotates in a continuous, 360-degree motion around the patient. The time for collecting the required data to reconstruct an image typically ranges from 1 to 10 seconds, depending on the particular system being used and the examination being conducted. These fast scan times have greatly reduced or eliminated *artifacts* that were caused by peristalsis, vascular pulsations, or respiratory artifacts on slower scanners. As a result, systems such as the one shown in Fig. 34-8 have many applications for scanning any portion of the anatomy; thus the term "whole-body scanners."

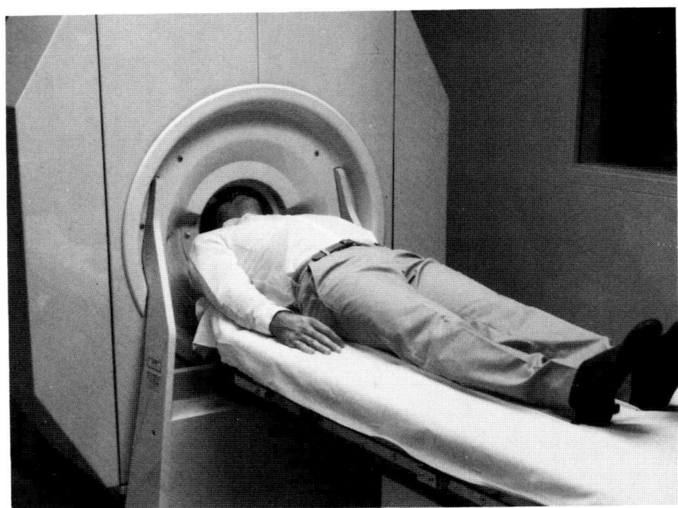

Fig. 34-7. Early CT scanner capable of examining head only.

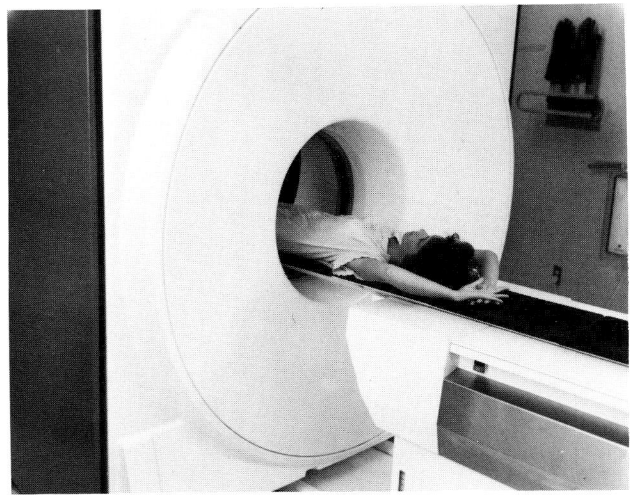

Fig. 34-8. Whole-body scanner capable of examining cross section of any part of body.

Two basic designs of radiation detectors are used in today's CT scanners. In some systems the detectors rotate in conjunction with the tube (Fig. 34-9). In other systems the tube rotates within a stationary array of detectors (Fig. 34-10).

Another significant design difference is in the design of the x-ray tube system. Some systems utilize cables that limit the rotation of the system, whereas others utilize a slip ring technology that enables continuous rotation of the tube.

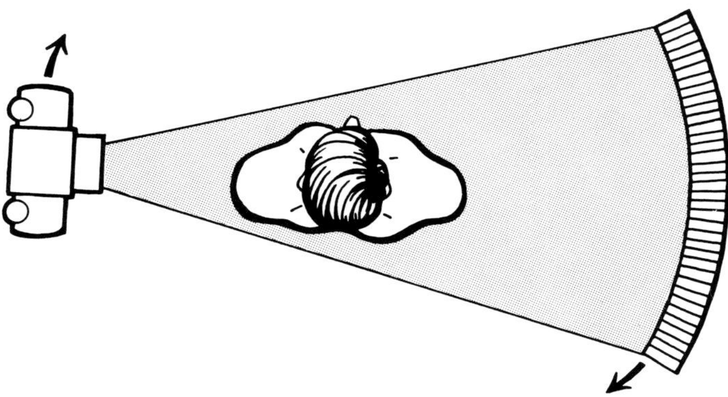

Fig. 34-9. CT system with rotating tube and detector array.

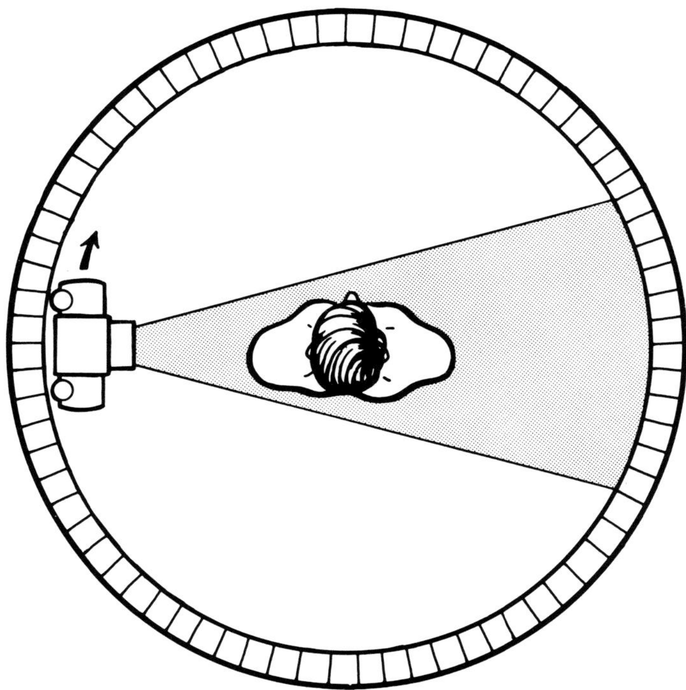

Fig. 34-10. CT system with rotating tube and stationary detectors around perimeter.

Equipment and Methodology

As illustrated in Fig. 34-11, the major areas and equipment required for generating a CT scan include the patient examination area, the operator's console, the computer room, and the diagnostic viewing console.

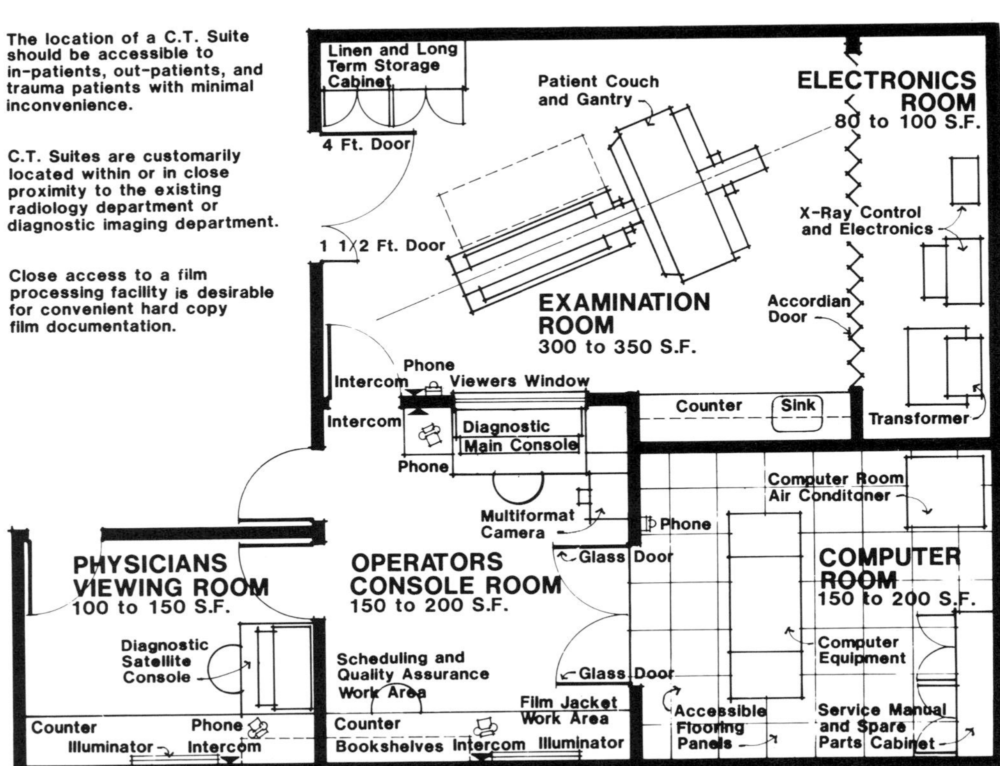

Fig. 34-11. Typical CT scanning suite.

(Courtesy Hospital Technology Series Guideline Report, published by the American Hospital Association, Chicago, copyright 1983.)

Computed tomography

EXAMINATION ROOM

The major components in the patient area are the patient table and *gantry* as seen in Fig. 34-12. This table and the gantry should be positioned so that the operator can see into the gantry to observe the patient when the technologist is seated at the operator's console. It is often advisable to add mirrors or a television system to help observe the patient who is on the far side of the gantry from the operator's console.

The gantry houses the x-ray tube and detector system. The entire motion of the detector and x-ray tube rotation occurs within the housing of the gantry. To obtain other than perpendicular, cross-sectional projections with respect to the patient table, it is possible to tilt most gantries before acquiring the data.

The patient table is generally automated in the vertical and the horizontal directions so that the patient can be properly positioned within the gantry. Because of the very thin slices (as thin as 1.0 mm) that are often studied, maintenance of an extremely accurate and reliable linkage between the gantry and the indexing mechanism for the patient table is mandatory.

The patient is generally placed in the supine position. Most systems use external positioning lights that work as follows. Once the patient has been properly restrained, the tabletop is elevated and moved longitudinally until the desired external anatomic landmark is aligned with the positioning lights (Fig. 34-13.) A command is then fed into the computer to advance the tabletop into the gantry so that the desired body area will be in the correct location to be scanned.

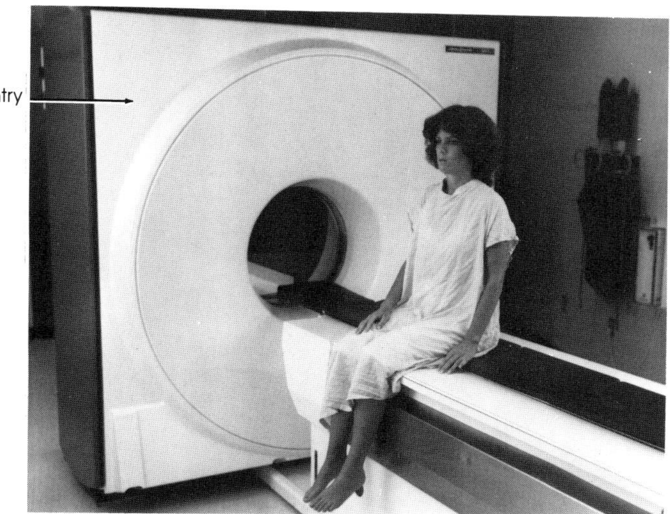

Fig. 34-12. Patient area with table and gantry.

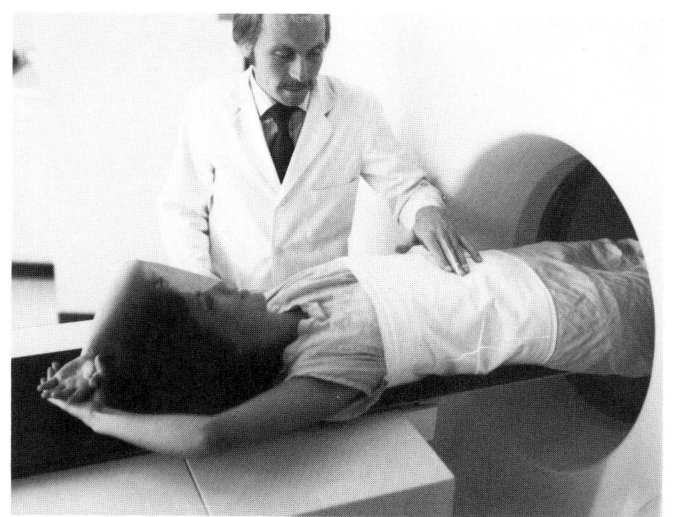

Fig. 34-13. Technologist using external landmarks and laser positioning lights to position patient.

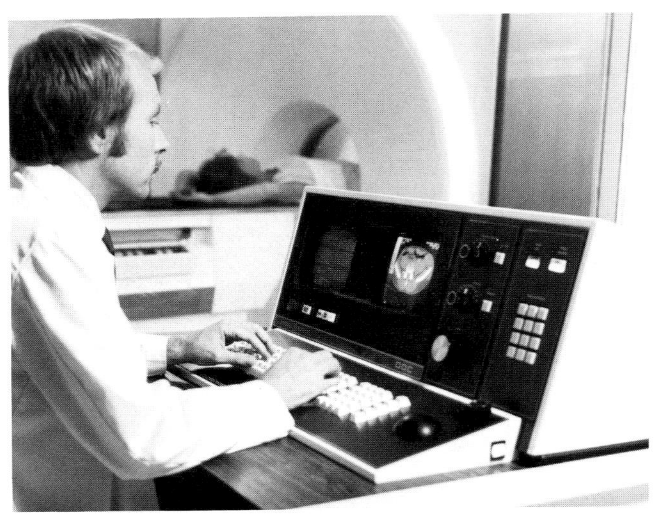

Fig. 34-14. Technologist generating CT scan at operator's control console.

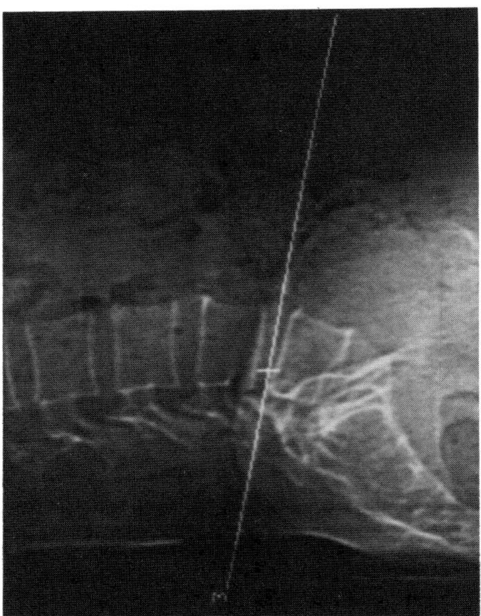

Fig. 34-15. Localizer image showing line positioned by operator to indicate where CT slice is to be taken.

OPERATOR'S CONSOLE ROOM

Once the patient has been positioned on the table and moved into the gantry, the technologist controls the CT system from the operator's console as shown in Fig. 34-14. Many improvements have been made to simplify the commands for the technologist so that an understanding of complex computer terminology is minimized. This simplification allows the technologist to focus most attention on the patient and the diagnostic results. Although the computer assists the technologist, the technologist has a significant role in controlling a number of variables (discussed in a later section) that have a direct impact on the diagnostic information obtained.

Before the technologist can begin the scan, patient data must be entered into the computer: the proper radiographic technique parameters must be selected, and the x-ray tube rotor must be initiated. After the exposure for an individual slice has been completed, the table is automatically indexed (moved) to the position for the next slice. Depending on heat storage capacity and tube cooling characteristics, the next scan is taken. It is possible to make fairly rapid exposures on some systems, whereas others may require a delay of a few minutes or more between scans.

Today, most CT systems include the capability that enables the technologist to generate a *localizer image* of the patient that is viewed at the operator's viewing console. The technologist marks the specific area that is to be scanned on the CRT, and the system describes exactly how to position the table and gantry to visualize this section. A typical localizer image is shown in Fig. 34-15. Not only does this localizer image capability enable improvement of productivity, but also it is useful during examinations such as of the spinal column.

COMPUTER ROOM

As a scan is produced, the *data acquisition system (DAS)* converts the x-ray *attenuation* measurements into digital signals that are sent to the computer. The computer performs a great number of complex calculations to reconstruct the cross-sectional image of the object. The actual technique and time required to reconstruct the image can vary considerably, depending on a number of factors such as the design of the equipment and the *software*.

Another significant factor that varies according to the equipment used is the amount of data (images) that can be stored in the computer. Some systems can store only a few dozen images, whereas others have the capacity to store hundreds. Once the computer's disk storage is filled, images must be erased before additional scans can be made. When the computer's disk is full, it is possible to transfer the information to floppy disks, magnetic tape, or optical disks for permanent storage, but interruptions in the normal scanning schedule should be prevented. Thus the large storage capacity is a desirable feature.

A typical computer system is shown in Fig. 34-16. To provide the most reliable service, most computers are installed in a room separated from the other functions. The reasons for this separation are that air-conditioning and power requirements for a computer are critical and must be optimized. In many cases, most of the radiographic electronics are also housed in this area. Caution should be taken, however, to ensure that these units do not have a negative effect on the computer's performance.

DIAGNOSTIC VIEWING CONSOLE

Although a separate console for diagnostically evaluating the CT image and formatting (transferring the image to special x-ray film) the film is generally desirable, some systems combine the operator's console and the diagnostic viewing console. This combined console generally leads to scheduling difficulties and limits the volume of work that can be performed. Fig. 34-17 shows an example of a typical viewing console that allows independent viewing of the diagnostic image while the technologist continues scanning. When viewing the image on the CRT, the technologist can produce a photographic copy at any time with a multiformat camera. For the best image quality, most CT units use a camera that exposes a multiformat single-emulsion film.

In addition to making a photographic copy of the image, it is also possible to permanently store the data on an optical disk, magnetic tape, or floppy disk so that the information can be reentered into the computer's memory at a later time to again view the image on the CRT. Once the data have been reentered, the image can be manipulated as before, enabling additional images to be made without any additional radiation exposure to the patient.

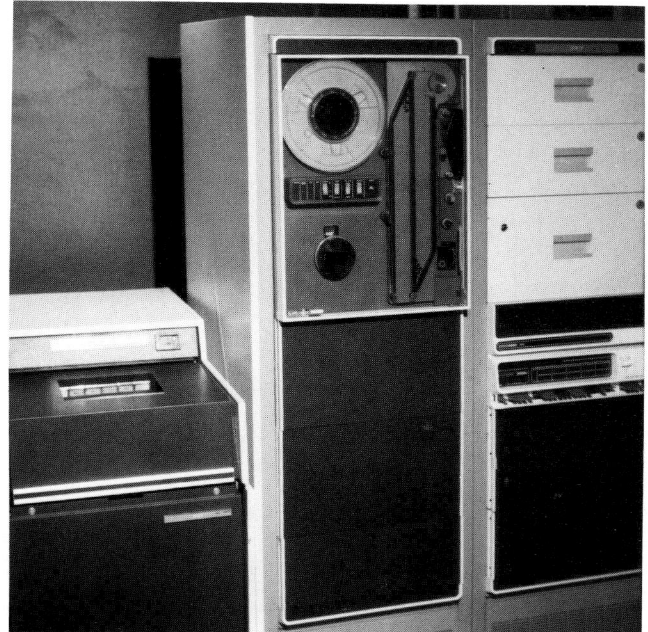

Fig. 34-16. Typical CT computer system.

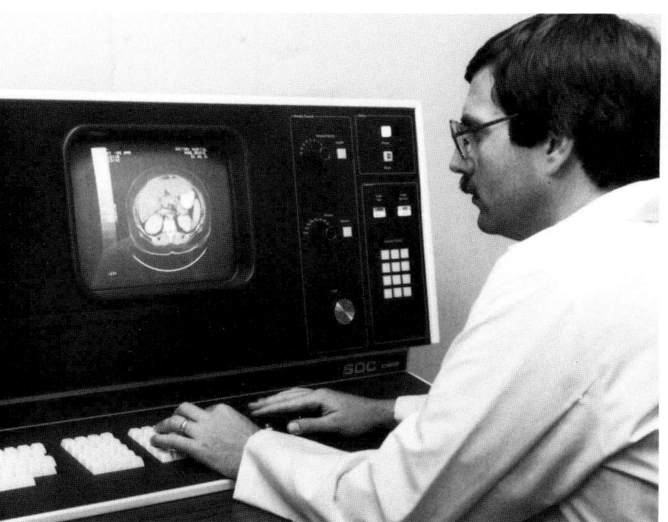

Fig. 34-17. Diagnostic viewing console.

Reconstructed Image Parameters

The CT image that is viewed on a CRT is actually made up of thousands of small *pixels* (*pi*cture *el*ements). As illustrated in Fig. 34-18, the *matrix* is defined as the number of pixels that are used to display the image on the CRT. Most CT systems use a 256 × 256, a 320 × 320, a 512 × 512, or a 1024 × 1024 matrix for displaying the images. Some systems use a coarser matrix for providing the technologist with a "quick look" at a reconstructed image. For the same field of view, a larger matrix size gives finer spatial resolution and generally better images. However, the images may take longer to acquire, increase the radiation exposure and take longer to reconstruct, require more disk space to be stored in the computer, and require more magnetic tape to be put into archives.

When viewing the image on the CRT, one should be aware that the pixel is associated with a volume of the patient. The *voxel* (*vo*lume *el*ement) is defined as the area of the pixel multiplied by the thickness of the slice. The slice thickness is generally determined by the examination being performed and may range from 1.0 to 10 mm in thickness. Although the thinner slice generally provides better resolution, a greater number of slices are required to examine a given area, and the radiation dose to the patient generally increases.

A *CT number* is defined as a relative comparison of the x-ray attenuation of each voxel of tissue with an equal volume of water. A number of factors affect actual CT numbers, and thus an absolute scale of CT numbers for various tissue is not possible. Water is given a CT number of zero. Tissues denser than water are given positive CT numbers, and less dense tissues are given negative values. Following is the formula for calculating the CT numbers:

$$\text{CT number} = k\,\frac{(\mu\text{tissue} - \mu\text{water})}{\mu\text{water}}$$

where: k = magnifying constant
μ = absorption coefficient

On all modern scanners, k = 1000 and the resultant scale of CT numbers is expressed in Hounsfield units (HU), where the units range from −1000 for air, to 0 for water, to 1000 or more for dense bone. Fat is generally around −50 HU, blood about 40 HU, and soft tissues in the range of 20 to 100 HU. Very old CT scanners used a magnifying constant (k) of 500.

Once a CT image has been reconstructed, the computer assigns a specific CT number to each pixel in the CRT display. When an image is then displayed on the CRT, the operator can adjust these numbers as desired to alter the gray scale of the display. The actual CT numbers being displayed are generally shown on the CRT adjacent to the image.

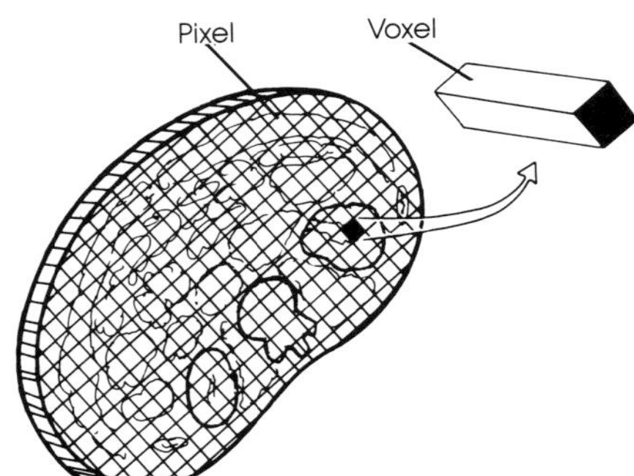

Fig. 34-18. CT image is composed of a matrix of pixels, each representing a volume of tissue (voxel).

Computed tomography

Examination Protocols

Many variables affect the diagnostic information that is obtained from a CT scan. A fairly common misconception is that, since a computer is involved, everything is automated. This section describes some of the factors that must be specified by the physician or technologist.

Four typical CT examinations are presented in Figs. 34-19 to 34-22. Since CT techniques are continually changing, these are intended as guidelines only. The actual protocol should be established by the professional staff in the medical facility.

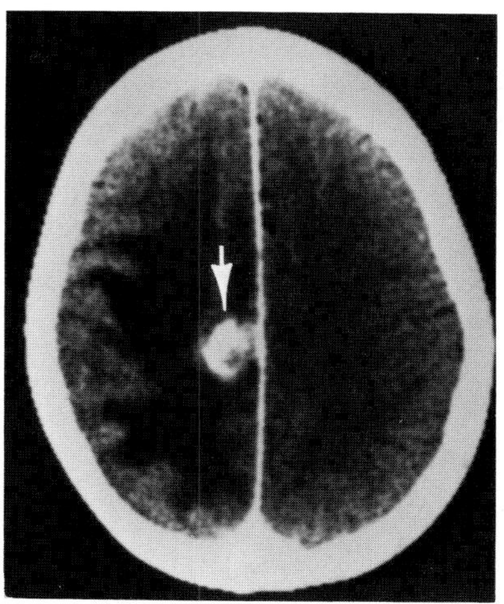

Fig. 34-19. CT brain scan showing metastatic brain tumor *(arrow)*; 1 cm thick slice with contrast medium enhancement.

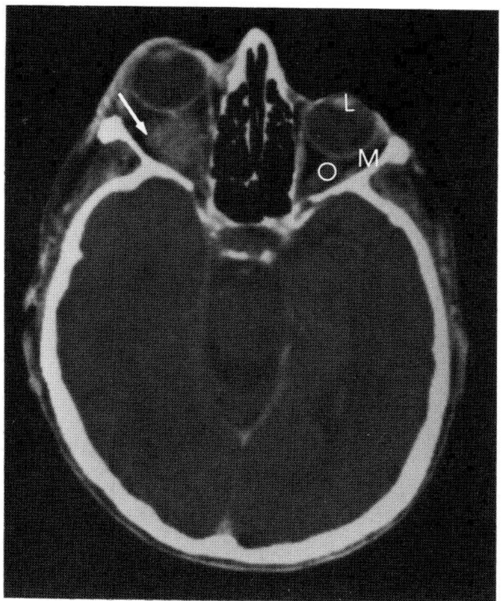

Fig. 34-20. CT scan of orbits showing pathologic condition *(arrow)*; 5 mm thick slice with contrast medium enhancement. *L*, Lens of eye; *M*, lateral rectus muscle; *O*, optic nerve.

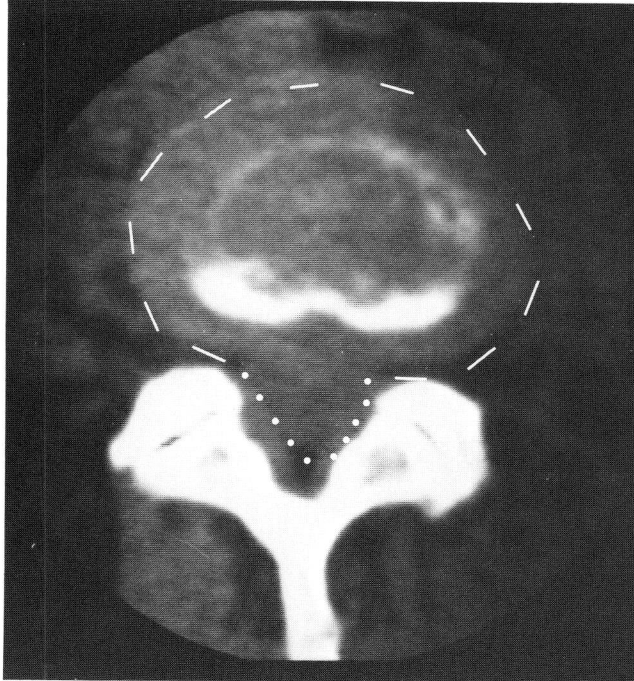

Fig. 34-21. CT scan of spine showing bulging intervertebral disk *(dashed line)* pressing against epidural sac *(dotted line)*; 1.5 mm thick slice, contrast medium not used.

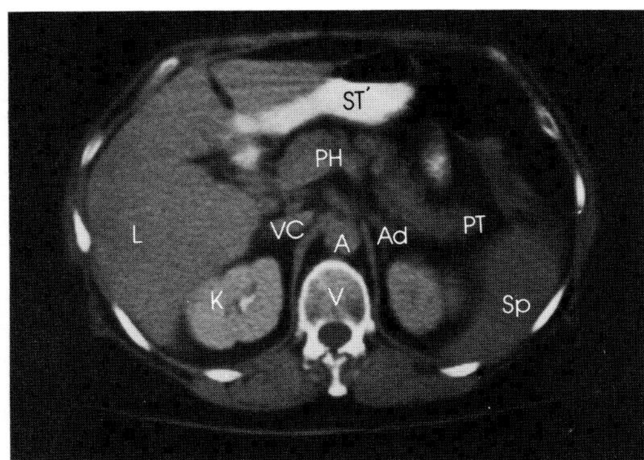

Fig. 34-22. CT scan of normal pancreas; 1 cm thick slice with contrast medium enhancement. *A*, Aorta; *Ad*, adrenal gland; *K*, kidney; *L*, liver; *PH*, head of pancreas; *PT*, tail of pancreas; *Sp*, spleen; *ST*, stomach with contrast medium; *V*, vertebral body; *VC*, inferior vena cava.

(Courtesy of Doctors Hospital, Columbus, Ohio.)

PATIENT PREPARATION AND USE OF CONTRAST AGENTS

The patient preparation for most CT examinations is minimal. In certain cases a contrast medium is used to enhance designated areas and to better differentiate disease processes. These factors contribute to the immense value of CT in diagnosing certain trauma cases, particularly neurologic trauma.

Although the specified preparation varies according to the institution and physician, the following are frequently used:

- Brain scans
  - Without contrast—no preparation
  - With contrast—nothing orally for 4 hours before examination
  - With and without contrast—nothing orally for 4 hours before examination
- Body scans
  - Abdomen and pelvis—Nothing orally after midnight; clear liquid breakfast permitted; standard bowel preparation for lower gastrointestinal study (the presence of any barium will generally cause significant artifacts)
  - Chest and extremities—no preparation

Contrast agents may be administered intravenously or orally. IV contrast medium is occasionally needed to enhance the contrast in CT scans of the brain, body, and extremities. The contrast medium used is the same as that employed for excretory urography. Oral contrast agents (barium or an iodinated contrast agent for gastrointestinal work) are used for enhancement in certain body examinations.

Position of patient

Patient positioning is determined by the desired plane of anatomy that is to be imaged, the ability of the patient to cooperate, the limitation of the gantry angulation, and the diameter of the opening for the patient into the gantry. In many cases the gantry is positioned perpendicularly to the patient table. However, it is often desirable to scan at other angles. Most brain scans are taken with the gantry placed at a caudal angle of approximately 15 to 20 degrees to the patient's orbitomeatal line. Most body scans are typically taken perpendicularly to the patient table. One exception is the CT examination of the spine for which slices through the disk space are obtained at various required angles. Up to 25 degrees of angulation may be required for imaging of the L5-S1 intervertebral disk space.

Positioning of the patient involves two major concerns: the accuracy with which the patient can be positioned (generally a specific position optimizes the diagnostic information) and the patient's comfort. Any movement during the examination is undesirable and can lead to a loss of diagnostic information. Therefore such actions as cushioning the head and placing pillows under the knees are recommended. Restraining straps should be used whenever possible to help immobilize the patient while not causing undue discomfort.

Slice thickness and locations

When operating a CT scanner, the technologist must specify the thickness and location of each slice.

Generally, thin slices (from 1.0 to 5 mm) are used for fine detail on examinations such as visualization of the optic nerve, the pituitary gland, and the posterior fossa. Another application requiring thin slices is production of sagittal and coronal reformatted images from the cross-sectional scans.

For routine brain scans and most body scans, a 1 cm slice thickness is generally acceptable. A common exception is scanning of the adrenal gland, for which thinner slices are typically taken.

If extremely fine detail is needed, the technologist may overlap the areas of each slice. For most examinations the slices are contiguous (adjacent or touching). In some studies, such as a generalized survey for lymphoma or metastases, 1 cm slices are generally taken every other centimeter.

The total number of slices depends on the size of the anatomic area to be examined and the preceding variables. As a general guideline, most brain scans take between 9 and 11 slices. A pancreas typically consists of 11 slices, the liver and spleen range is from 11 to 14 slices, and the kidney takes 14 to 16 slices. If unenhanced and contrast-enhanced images are desired, the number of slices taken doubles.

Quality assurance

The CT system is a complex system, and quality assurance is very important. A great deal of preventive maintenance is required to keep most systems properly calibrated. Although most of this work is generally performed by the vendor, the technologist should be routinely involved in scanning phantoms and performing other tests to ensure that the scanner is operating properly.

Definition of Terms

artifact Area of information on reconstructed image that does not exist in reality. It may be caused by operator motion, patient motion, or equipment peculiarities.

attenuation of x rays Process of energy absorption, described by percent of radiation absorbed while x rays pass through object.

cathode ray tube (CRT) Television screen used to display CT image and to communicate with computer.

computed tomography (CT) Process resulting in visualization of cross-sectional image of body part. Image is created by computer using multiple x-ray attenuation readings taken around periphery of object.

computerized axial tomography (CAT) Early term used to describe CT scanning. Since images produced are taken at various angles, "axial" has been deleted.

CT numbers Numbers used to define relative absorption coefficient for each pixel of tissue in image as compared with absorption coefficient of water.

data acquisition system (DAS) Radiation detection system that measures amount of radiation passing through patient.

gantry Framework that holds x-ray tube and radiation detection system.

localizer image Image used to localize specific body part.

matrix Two-dimensional array of numbers used to describe number of pixels in CT image display, e.g., 256 × 256, 320 × 320, 512 × 512, or 1024 × 1024.

pixel Picture element. CT image displayed on CRT is composed of many small squares (pixels), each of which represents specific volume of body. Each pixel is assigned CT number for image display purposes.

scan Motion of x-ray tube and radiation detector system required to collect data for reconstructing CT image.

slice Cross section of body part that is scanned for generating CT image.

software Computer programs that control CT system.

voxel Volume element—basic element that defines volume of tissue that each pixel represents in reconstructed image.

SELECTED BIBLIOGRAPHY

Boethius J et al: CT localization in stereotaxic surgery, Appl Neurophysiol 43:164-169, 1980.

Boethius J et al: Stereotaxic computerized tomography with a GE 8800 scanner, J Neurosurg 52:794-800, 1980.

Chiu LC, Lipcamon JD, and Yiu-Chiu VS: Clinical computed tomography: illustrated procedural guide, Rockville, Md, 1986, Aspen Systems.

Coulam CM et al, editors: The physical basis of medical imaging, New York, 1981, Appleton-Century-Crofts.

Curry TS et al: Christensen's introduction to the physics of diagnostic radiology, ed 3, Philadelphia, 1984, Lea & Febiger.

Federle FP et al: Computed tomography in the evaluation of trauma, Baltimore, 1982, Williams & Wilkins.

Genant HK, editor: Computer tomography of the lumbar spine, San Francisco, 1982, University of California.

Godwin JD, editor: Computed tomography of the chest, Philadelphia, 1984, JB Lippincott Co.

Haaga JR et al: Computed tomography of the whole body, ed 2, vols I and II, St Louis, 1988, The CV Mosby Co.

Hammerschlag SB et al: Computed tomography of the eye and orbit, Norwalk, Ct, 1983, Appleton-Century-Crofts.

Haughton V: Computed tomography of the spine, St Louis, 1982, The CV Mosby Co.

Hendee WR: The physical principles of computed tomography, Boston, 1983, Little, Brown, & Co, Inc.

Kubota K et al: Some devices for computer tomography radiotherapy treatment planning, J Comput Assist Tomogr 4:697-699, 1980.

Lee JKT, Sagel SS, and Stanley RJ, editors: Computed body tomography with MRI correlation, ed 2, New York, 1989, Raven Press.

Lee SH and Rao Krishna CVG, editors: Cranial computed tomography and MRI, ed 2, New York, 1987, McGraw-Hill.

Mancuso AA et al: Computed tomography and magnetic resonance of the head and neck, ed 2, Baltimore, 1985, Williams & Wilkins.

Moss AA et al: Computed tomography of the body, Philadelphia, 1983, WB Saunders Co.

Naidich DP et al: Computed tomography of the thorax, New York, 1984, Raven Press.

Naidich TP et al: Superimposition reformatted CT for preoperative lesion localization and surgical planning, J Comput Assist Tomogr 4:693-696, 1980.

Newton TH et al, editors: Radiology of the skull and brain, vol 5. Technical aspects of computed tomography, St Louis, 1981, The CV Mosby Co.

Newton TH et al, editors: Modern neuroradiology, vol 1. Computed tomography of the spine and spinal cord, San Anselmo, Calif, 1983, Clavadel Press.

Post MJD, editor: Radiographic evaluation of the spine, New York, 1980, Masson.

Stevens JM, Valentine AR, and Kendall BE: Computed cranial and spinal imaging: a practical introduction, Baltimore, 1988, Williams & Wilkins.

Van Maes PFGM et al: Direct coronal body computed tomography, J Comput Assist Tomogr 62:58-66, 1982.

Chapter 35

COMPUTED RADIOGRAPHY

MARCUS W. HEDGCOCK, JR.
RICHARD C. PASKIET, JR.

Since the days of Wilhelm Conrad Roentgen, radiography has been continuously improved and diversified. Even in the 1990s, the fluorescent x-ray film-screen combination remains the most widely used radiographic method. However, film-screen radiography limits image manipulation to "hot-lighting" or duplication.

Various methods for enhancing the diagnostic capability of x-ray images have been used over the years; for example, stereoscopic radiography. In stereoscopic radiography two images of the same anatomic structure are obtained, with the x-ray tube shifted 6 degrees after the first image is obtained. The two resulting x-ray images are then placed side by side on a light box and viewed by using a stereoscope. This three-dimensional viewing helps the radiologist to some degree, but the process is operationally cumbersome. More recent modalities, such as computed tomography (CT) and ultrasound, are *digital**; they provide cross-sectional images and allow the image to be manipulated. Conventional projection radiography (which accounts for nearly 70% of a radiology department's volume) has until recently, however, remained an *analog* modality.

*All italicized terms are defined at the end of this chapter.

Analog and Digital Information

Analog information is represented in a continuous fashion, whereas digital information is represented in discrete units. An analogy is the difference between oil paints and a box of crayons. The oil paints can be mixed to provide an infinite number of color shades, whereas the box of crayons can provide only the number of colors in the box. The advantage of digital information is that we know the location and nature of each digital level and can adjust each accordingly. All digital imaging systems, such as computed tomography, ultrasound, and computed radiography, acquire information by a process called *analog-to-digital conversion*. After the x-ray or ultrasound beam has passed through the patient, it is still an analog signal. This signal varies smoothly from zero (where all the radiation has been absorbed by some part of the patient) to the maximum intensity (where no radiation has been absorbed).

In a computed tomographic scanner (Chapter 34), the analog-to-digital conversion occurs when the x-ray beam strikes the detector located in the gantry. Each detector corresponds to an anatomic location that absorbed the radiation, and the detectors have a limited number of responses. The number of responses the detectors can make is called the gray level display of the system. If the system has 256 gray levels (0 being black, 256 being white), the computer assigns the gray level of these 256 shades that is closest to the intensity of the radiation striking the detector. The system then reproduces the image by combining the responses of all of the detectors. In a computed radiographic system, the analog-to-digital conversion occurs when the exposed image plate is scanned with a laser, and the emitted light pattern is then converted to digital information by the image reader, as explained below.

Computed and Analog Radiography

Computed radiography, often abbreviated CR, refers to conventional projection radiography, in which the image is acquired in digital format using an imaging plate rather than film. Conventional projection radiography includes all of the radiographic procedures that are now performed using a film-screen system. These include the familiar radiographic procedures that comprise the majority performed in an imaging facility: chest, abdomen, and orthopedic radiographs and contrast-enhanced radiographic studies, such as excretory urography and barium studies examining the gastrointestinal tract.

The major obstacle to developmental changes in the field of conventional projection radiography is that one specific medium, x-ray film, serves three distinct functions in the radiographic process; x-ray film is the sensor to acquire the diagnostic information, it is used to display the information, and it is used to store the information.

Historical Development

At the 1981 International Congress of Radiology (ICR) meeting in Brussels, Fuji Photo Film Co., Ltd. introduced the concept of computed radiography employing *photostimulable phosphor* plate technology. In 1983, the first clinical use of computed radiography was performed in Japan, and in early 1990 over 300 systems were in clinical use worldwide.

The operating principle of the phosphor plate, explained later in this chapter, has been shown to provide excellent image quality. Computed radiographic technology is digital and supports the development of a variety of computer-based diagnostic information processing systems. As such, computed radiography provides the missing link for the completely electronic radiographic imaging department and is now a practical imaging modality.

Converting conventional projection radiography into a digital format can be accomplished (1) by digitizing the standard radiographic film images, or (2) by acquiring a digital image directly by having the x rays strike an electronic sensor or an image intensifier, or by using an imaging plate that is then scanned with a laser and the emitted light read by an electronic sensor. The second technique described is currently the best option for computed radiography when a reusable imaging plate is used. In the remainder of this chapter, computed radiography refers to imaging performed using these imaging plates.

Unlike scanned projection radiography or intensifier-based systems that require that the images be acquired on dedicated equipment, the reusable photostimulable phosphor plate system can be used with any standard radiographic imaging equipment. The key to computed radiography's development is the separation of the functions of sensing, displaying, and storing information. Each function uses separate media and devices, and each function can be separately manipulated, yet central control of the final image is maintained through computer technology.

Operational Components: Separation of Image Acquisition, Display, and Storage Functions

IMAGE ACQUISITION FUNCTIONS

The image acquisition or "sensor" function served by the photostimulable phosphor imaging plate, like x-ray film, receives the portion of the x-ray beam that has passed through the patient. A CR imaging plate looks physically much like an intensifying screen (Fig. 35-1), and the plate is placed in a cassette similar to an x-ray film cassette. The computed radiography imaging plate cassette is made of lightweight aluminum with the tube side composed of honeycombed carbon fiber to produce a rigid, low x-ray attenuation surface. The imaging plate (IP) contains a layer of Europium-doped barium fluorohalide ($BaFX:Eu^{2+}$) crystals (the photostimulable phosphor). When x rays strike the crystals, BaFX is changed to a new semistable state. It is the distribution of these semistable molecules that forms the *latent image*. The $BaFX:Eu^{2+}$ phosphor is applied to a polyester support base and then coated with a clear acrylic protective layer (Fig. 35-2). Below the phosphor is a supporting layer that protects the phosphor layer from external shocks. The supporting layer also prevents reflection of the laser light. Next is a backing layer that protects the imaging plate from scratches during transfer and storage. Last is a bar code label that contains a number assigned to the imaging plate. This bar code provides a mechanism for associating each imaging plate with patient identification and related examination and positioning information.

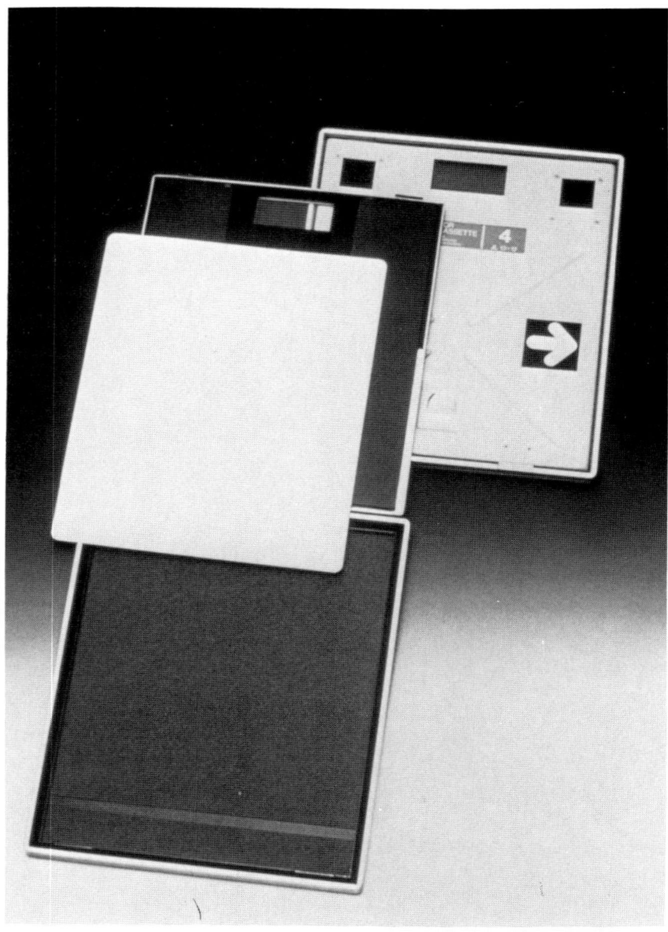

Fig. 35-1. Computed radiography photostimulable phosphor imaging plate (center left) shown lying on opened cassette. Back of closed cassette shown on upper right.

The imaging plate is flexible and less than 1 mm thick. A unique property of the phosphor material is its "memory" capability; it has the ability to maintain a latent image for a certain period of time after exposure to x rays. (Although some image degradation occurs as time lapses, a plate will retain a diagnostic image for up to 6 hours.)

A valuable characteristic of the imaging plate is its extreme dynamic range. The imaging plate demonstrates an excellent linear response to the intensity of exposure over a broad range. When the imaging plate response is compared with the characteristic, or H & D, curve of radiographic film (Fig. 35-3), the superior performance capability of the imaging plate is seen to provide far more information in the low and high exposure regions of the image.

The *image reader* (Fig. 35-4) is another important component of the image acquisition control in computed radiography. The image reader converts the continuous analog information (latent image) on the imaging plate to a digital format. As the imaging plate is scanned by the laser in the image reader, the portion of the plate struck by a laser emits light. This emitted light is directed by high-efficiency light guides to the photomultiplier tubes where the light is converted to digital electrical signals. The first reader systems became available in 1983 and were capable of processing only 40 plates per hour. Reader systems in 1990 are more compact and are capable of processing approximately 70 plates per hour. Several image readers can be interfaced to one recorder unit, and for high-volume applications, such as chest radiography, stand-alone systems with integrated image processors are available. In any of the reader systems, the imaging plate is transported internally through all the various stages of processing.

DISPLAY FUNCTIONS

The display of computed radiography data is basically the result of *spatial frequency response processing* and *gradation processing,* which are used to control the contrast and density of the displayed image. Spatial frequency response controls the sharpness of boundaries between two structures of different densities. Gradation processing controls the range of densities used to display structures on the image; gradation processing is similar to the window settings used in computed tomography for display. These two different characteristics, contrast and density, are optimized by the digital image processor for the specific anatomic region being studied.

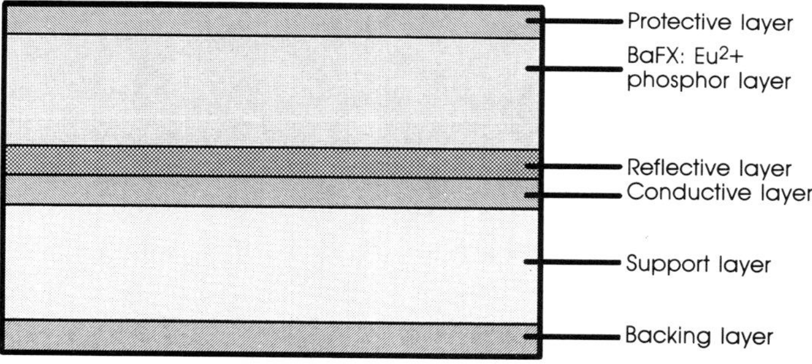

Fig. 35-2. Schematic diagram of layered composition of photostimulable imaging plate.

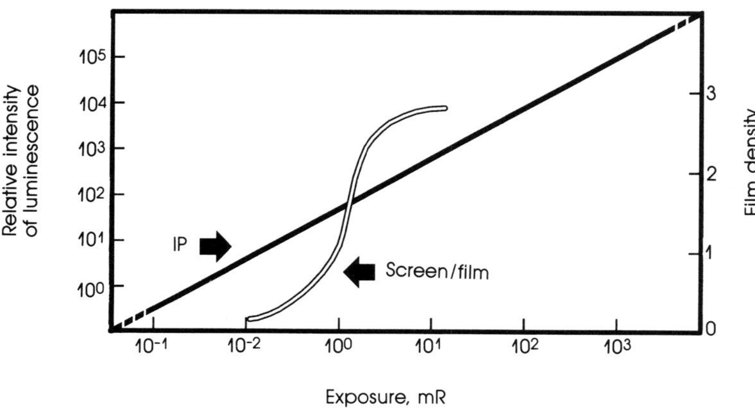

Fig. 35-3. Comparison of radiographic film H and D response curve to linear imaging plate response.

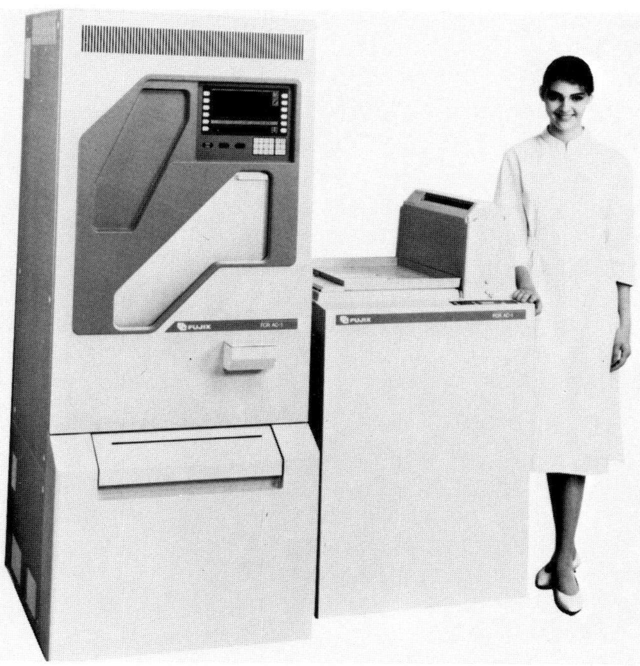

Fig. 35-4. Example of a computed radiographic system. The image reader device is on the far left. Film processor is seen to the right of the image reader.

To produce an image for viewing, the computed radiography computer system constructs (formats) the image from the raw data as read from the photostimulable plate. Because the computed radiographic image is in digital format, the raw image data can be manipulated to accentuate or suppress various features of the image; the image can be tailored to a specific clinical task. This is similar to the operation of other digital imaging modalities such as computed tomography, where the window and level setting of the image can be changed to visualize a specific structure such as the liver or lung.

If no special parameters are specified by the user, the image is reconstructed using the *default,* or preset, settings that the specific medical center has decided produces the best-quality images. If special image characteristics are desired to highlight specific structures, the reconstruction factors can be changed by the technologist or other user. The final image can be displayed on a monitor or produced as a hard-copy image on film or other medium. Unlike computed tomography, the computed radiography image is reconstructed each time from the raw data. If the image is displayed on a monitor, the image characteristics can be adjusted visually by the user to examine all features of the image to best advantage. To assist in the display process, various work stations with high-resolution *CRT* (cathode ray tube) monitors can be directly interfaced to the computed radiography unit.

There is little doubt that the electronic work station represents the alternator (viewbox) of the future. Work stations will be linked to a central image archive (an "electronic file room") and also to the text data in the radiology and hospital information systems, to provide a central clearing area for all information (images and text) needed by the imaging specialist. The functions for these work stations continue to be expanded (Table 35-1). These work station functions allow the user to alter the image display to best advantage for interpretation. The gradational enhancement (contrast) and spatial frequency (sharpness) enhancement can be varied on the work station, which is similar to formating the hard copy image. If, for example, two images have been taken sequentially, or taken using different energy characteristics (see dual energy subtraction discussed below), the images can be subtracted much like angiography with the use of radiographic film and digital subtraction systems. The image also can be "zoomed" or magnified. The density of a portion of the image can be estimated by selecting a region of interest (ROI). The image can also be rotated, flipped, or inverted. Statistical analyses can be performed on portions of the image, by calculating surface areas and estimated volumes, or by characterizing the change in density in a part of the image. Most important for daily operations, however, the work station contains a data base that enables the user to easily locate images and create lists of images for conferences, interpretation, or teaching files.

Table 35-1. Work station functions

Gradational enhancement	ROI display
Spatial frequency enhancement	Rotation/inversion
Subtraction/addition	Statistical analysis
Image magnification	Data base functions

The number of CRT monitors required for an interpretation work station is still under review. However, it is clear that at least two monitors, and probably more (four to six), will be needed. The monitor resolution factor remains a point of contention among experts in this field. Currently, 1K × 1K (kilobyte) *matrix* monitors are generally used. The resolution is adequate for most studies, and the cost is within reason. However, 2K × 2K monitors are expected to be the norm for primary review work stations. With 2K × 2K resolution, all studies can be appropriately displayed with little or no loss of diagnostic information. The main deterrent at this time to routine use of 2K × 2K monitors is cost, which should become lower as availability increases. Finally, there is discussion concerning the use of 4K × 4K monitors. These monitors cannot be used to full potential until the computed radiographic image resolution is increased from the current 2K × 2K, which would require major changes in the system scanning architecture to acquire data at the 4K × 4K ratio. Cost remains a major consideration for the use of these very high–resolution monitors.

Computed radiography also offers several options for film-based display. Fig. 35-5 shows a 2-on-1 format of an identical shoulder image. The image on the left demonstrates the shoulder with display factors similar to those of a conventional film-screen radiograph. An *edge enhanced* image is also automatically displayed as seen on the right image. Certain studies and pathologic conditions benefit from this enhanced image.

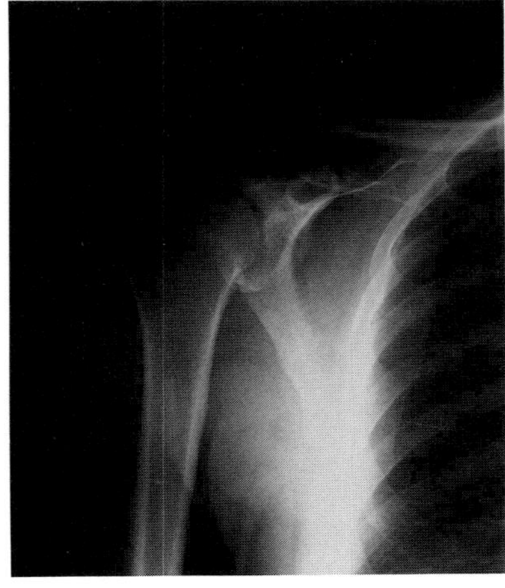
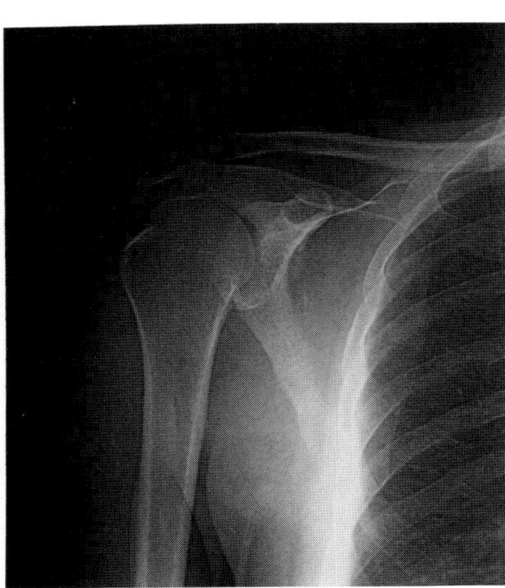

Fig. 35-5. Computed radiograph of a shoulder with conventional (left image) and edge-enhanced (right image) display parameters.

STORAGE FUNCTIONS

Computed radiography decreases image archive storage space requirements by reducing the size of films stored and by converting bulky film storage to electronic storage. Benefits include tremendous space savings, reduction in image retrieval time, and decreased film loss from nonreturns.

Several points must be considered regarding the design of electronic image archive devices. Flexibility is important. The device should interface with desired modalities and be expandable. The amount of storage on the electronic image archive should be adequate for the amount of data to be stored. Storage capacity of an electronic image archive depends on several variables, including the size of the basic storage unit (usually optical disk), the number of units on-line (jukebox size), and the ratio of data compression that is used.

An optical disk is currently the long-term storage medium of choice for computed radiography images. Computed radiography images contain more total data per individual image than any other digital modality, such as computed tomography or ultrasound (Table 35-2). Each computed radiography image contains about 6 *megabytes* of data. For example, a PA and a lateral chest image contain about 12 megabytes of data, which requires the same amount of electronic storage as the first four volumes of digital text found in the *Encyclopaedia Britannica*. One 12-inch dual-sided dual-density 2 *gigabyte* optical disk platter has the ability to store up to 800 computed radiography images with reversible 2:1 compression, or 7200 computed radiography images if 18:1 nonreversible compression is used. Such a factor alone projects the space savings benefit. By using an optical disk jukebox, approximately 200,000 radiographs can be stored in a space the size of a refrigerator.

With optical electronic storage, there is no deterioration of digital data. When such data are retrieved at a later date for image review and/or to make a copy on film, the reproduced image will be an exact duplicate of the initial image. In addition, any number of copies may be made using the original data, each being an original image. With these storage media, computed radiography image data can be searched for, retrieved, transmitted, or processed with tremendous ease.

Other large-capacity memory devices can be used for digital data storage. Magnetic tape, digital cassettes, streamer tape, or even verbatim cards can all serve these storage needs with various degrees of efficiency. Naturally, x-ray film can still be used to store visual analog patterns for image data filing purposes.

With a computed radiography system, flexibility can exist with the three primary options of (1) maintaining an active film file for display and storage purposes, (2) reviewing data on work stations and using long-term archiving devices for permanent electronic files, and (3) employing a combination of these methods to accommodate individual preferences.

Characteristics of a Computed Radiographic Image

Three factors are directly responsible for computed radiography image resolution: (1) the dimension of the crystals in the imaging plate, (2) the size of the laser beam in the image, and (3) the image-reading matrix. Computed radiography contrast resolution is currently greater than that of conventional film, but spatial resolution is slightly less than film. Computed radiography resolution averages from 2 to 5 lp/mm (line pairs per millimeter), whereas standard film can demonstrate 3 to 6 lp/mm. With further advances in imaging plate phosphor quality, a reduction in the microbeam laser size, and an increase in matrix dimension and image, spatial resolution will become inherently superior to that of conventional film-screen parameters. Present-day diagnoses are not hampered by the current resolution factors. However, chest imaging and mammography will further benefit from the increased spatial resolution that these examinations demand.

Table 35-2. Capacities of various electronic data storage media

Medium	Capacity
Magnetic tape (2400 feet reel)	166 Mbytes
Winchester magnetic disk	700-1400 Mbytes
Optical disk	
Single optical disk	
12 inch	2 Gbytes
18 inch	6.8 Gbytes
Multiple platter optical "jukebox"	200-1000 Gbytes
Optical tape (2400 feet reel)	200 Gbytes

1 gigabyte = 1000 megabytes.

Clinical Applications

In the clinical environment, the sequence of events in computed radiography imaging is shown in Fig. 35-6. The computed radiography process begins at the reception desk, where demographic information such as patient name, birthdate, sex, ID number, and examination ordered is entered into a reception terminal. Early systems used a magnetic card that accompanied the patient examination request and was presented to the technologist.

The technologist exposes the imaging plate in the same manner as a conventional film-screen cassette is used. The exposure may be made using either a tabletop, mobile, or table/wall bucky technique. The exposed imaging plate cassette is taken to the control terminal of the computed radiography reader unit. Here the patient ID number is selected from an examination terminal (or the ID card is "read" for patient and examination information) and the cassette is scanned with the bar code reader, linking each specific exposed imaging plate to the correct patient and image data. This replaces the typical ID camera step in film radiography.

The technologist inserts the exposed cassette into the cassette insertion area of the reader unit shown inside the box in Fig. 35-6 and the reader door is then closed. Once inside, the cassette is automatically opened, and the imaging plate is removed and replaced with an erased plate for rapid "cassette" turnaround. If an imaging plate changer magazine (which will retain 30 imaging plates for arteriographic or mass examination studies) is used instead of a single plate cassette, the magazine is inserted into its appropriate space and the plates are automatically removed one at a time for reading. The reading process on the original plate is then initiated.

The internal functions of a computed radiography system are illustrated in Fig. 35-7. Inside the system and not apparent to the technologist is the image plate reader assembly, which scans the imaging plate. The plate is transported through the system at right angles to a red *helium-neon laser* beam until the entire plate is sequentially scanned. When the barium fluorohalide crystals on the exposed photostimulable plate are exposed to the laser beam, the crystal layer emits the energy in the form of light, which was retained in its "memory" following x-ray exposure. The light intensity emitted is proportional to the amount of x rays that initially excited the crystal

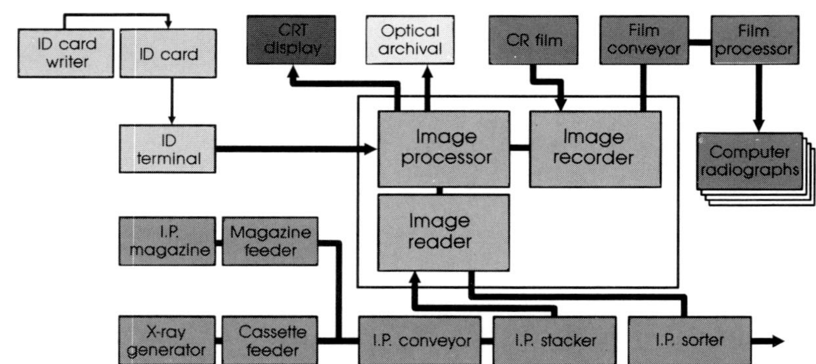

Fig. 35-6. Computed radiography sequence flow chart.

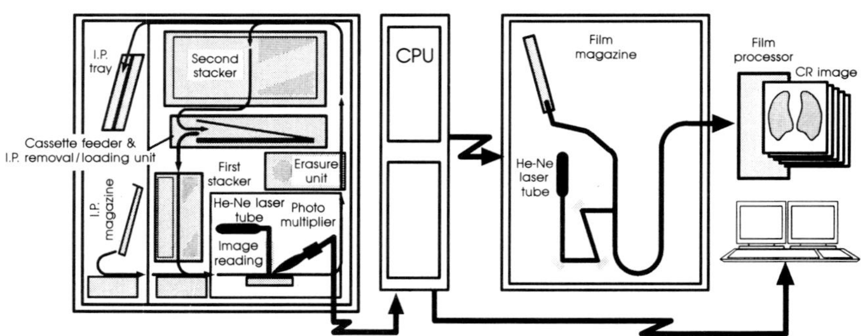

Fig. 35-7. Generalized internal functions and components of a computed radiography system.

layer. Tracking with the laser beam is a light guide, or photomultiplier pick-up tube, which collects the light emissions from all scanned areas and converts the light energy into electrical signals. Through an analog-to-digital converter, the electrical signal is converted into digital information, which is related spatially and is proportional in intensity to the original x-ray exposure in each segment of the imaging plate (Fig. 35-8).

The imaging plates offer wide exposure latitude. To make effective use of this latitude, the computed radiography system employs a sampling procedure for sensitivity adjustment during the plate reading stage. During the scanning process, a sample of the image data is acquired. These rough image data plus the entered anatomic data are examined to analyze the image characteristics and determine the best reading sensitivity and exposure latitude display parameters. By using this sampling capability, it is possible to normalize and digitize the entire luminescent area where the x-ray image exists. Errors in technical exposure factors are virtually eliminated. Exposure factors 500% greater than or 80% less than that which would normally be used to present the information aesthetically on a conventional film-screen system can be corrected by using the computed radiography system. These examples are obviously the extreme limits of correction and would rarely occur, but it must be realized that even gross technical errors are correctable when using the computed radiography system. Moreover, a general reduction in patient exposure can be realized when using computed radiography, compared with using the conventional 400-speed film-screen combination.

Technical corrections are achieved with computer-aided auto-ranging techniques. Optimized computed radiography display parameters are achieved through *histogram* analysis in proportion to the linear dynamic range of the imaging plates and tailoring the final image characteristics to an agreed upon subjective H & D curve for best display of the anatomic structure(s) of interest.

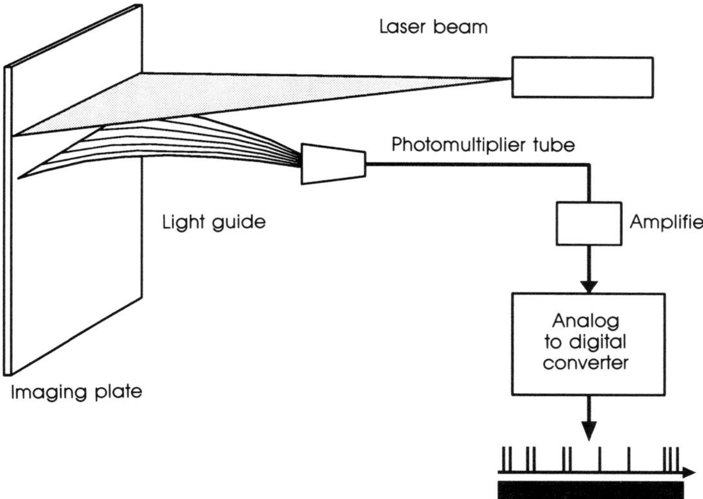

Fig. 35-8. Reading of computed radiographic imaging plate and conversion to digital information.

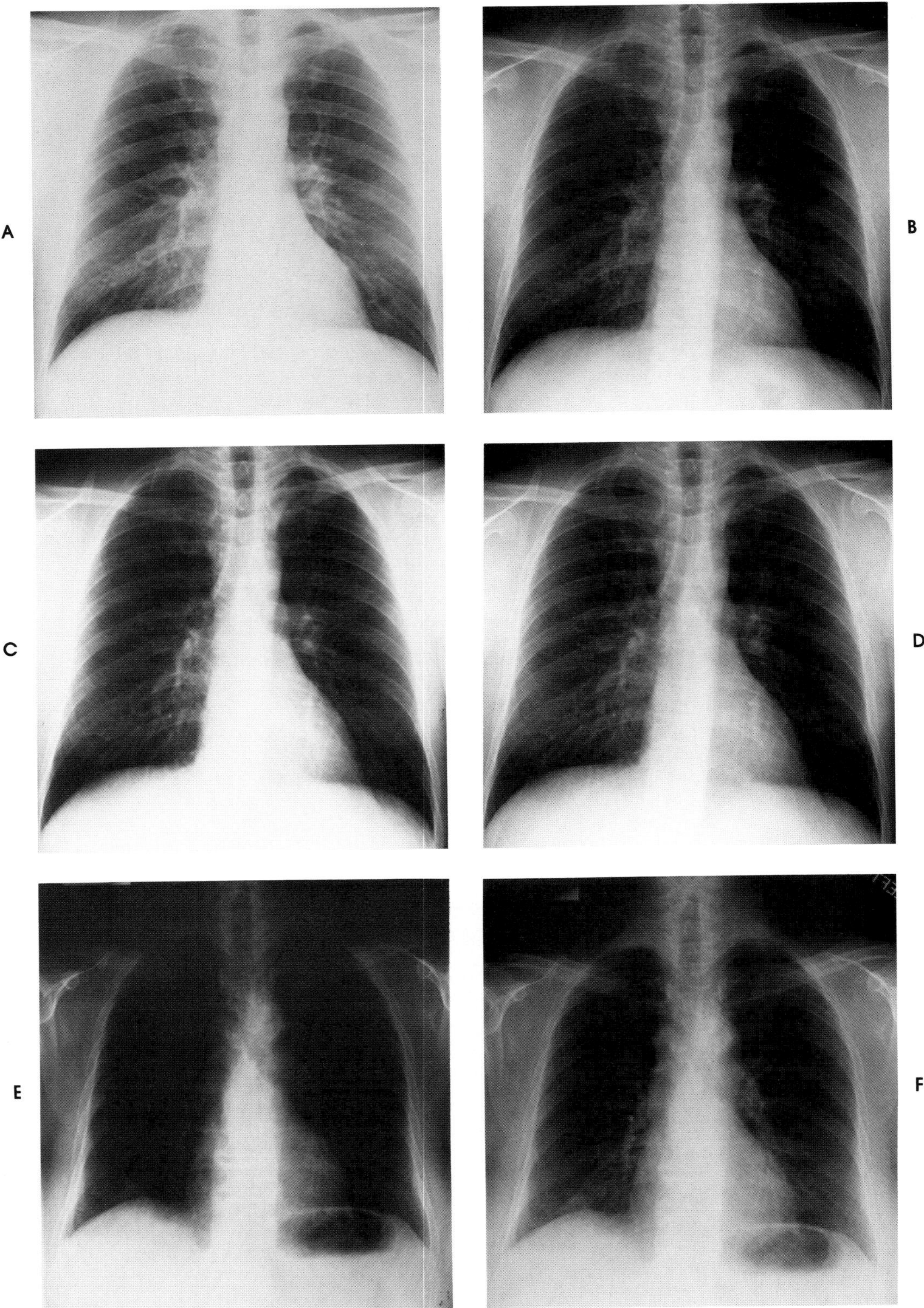

Fig. 35-9. Six images **(A** to **F)** showing pairs of analog (left images) and computed radiographs (right images) acquired simultaneously. Note that despite the widely differing exposure factors, the computed radiographic image does not vary in quality, although the analog radiographs are clearly suboptimal in quality. In the computed radiographic images, the left image has been formatted with display parameters like those of a conventional radiograph; the right image is edge-enhanced. **A,** Analog radiograph and, **B,** CR image, both using exposure factors of 125 kVp, 1 mAs. **C,** Analog radiograph and, **D,** CR image, both using 125 kVp, 2.5 mAs. **E,** Analog radiograph and, **F,** CR image, both using 125 kVp, 6.3 mAs.

To understand the effects of this process, consider the chest radiographs in Fig. 35-9, *A* through *F*. Analog and computed radiographic images were simultaneously obtained using a cassette containing both a radiographic film and an imaging plate. Despite technique factors that produced inadequate analog radiographs, all of the computed radiographic images are of consistent and appropriate penetration and quality. The "sampling" process normalized the image for the particular anatomic region being studied.

After the exposure of the imaging plate and its subsequent scanning by the helium neon laser, the image on the plate is erased. The energy remaining on the imaging plate after reading is completely eliminated by exposing the plate to a uniform, bright sodium-vapor light. The plates are reusable for thousands of times. In fact, the plate may well be mechanically destroyed or damaged before any degradation of the crystalline structure would ever be realized.

Other Techniques to Improve Diagnostic Efficacy

Several other techniques (besides manipulation of the images on the work station) are available to improve the diagnostic power of computed radiography. These include acquisition techniques, such as *dual energy* imaging, higher resolution plates, analysis of computed radiography imagery by computer, and networking for review centralization.

Image analysis by computer allows the user to extract more diagnostic information from the image. This is a relatively new technique, but promises to open new diagnostic horizons for diagnosis using computed radiography. Fig. 35-10 shows profiles of bone mineral in the hand of a patient with rheumatoid arthritis; this can be used to diagnose this condition and determine improvement following therapy.

Clinical Acceptance

Computed radiography is being used at an increasing number of medical centers in all applications where conventional projection radiography can be used, such as chest, bone, and mobile radiography, and contrast-enhanced examinations such as excretory urography and gastrointestinal radiography. Angiographic applications are primarily performed using digital radiography; angiographic applications are addressed in Chapter 36 in this Atlas.

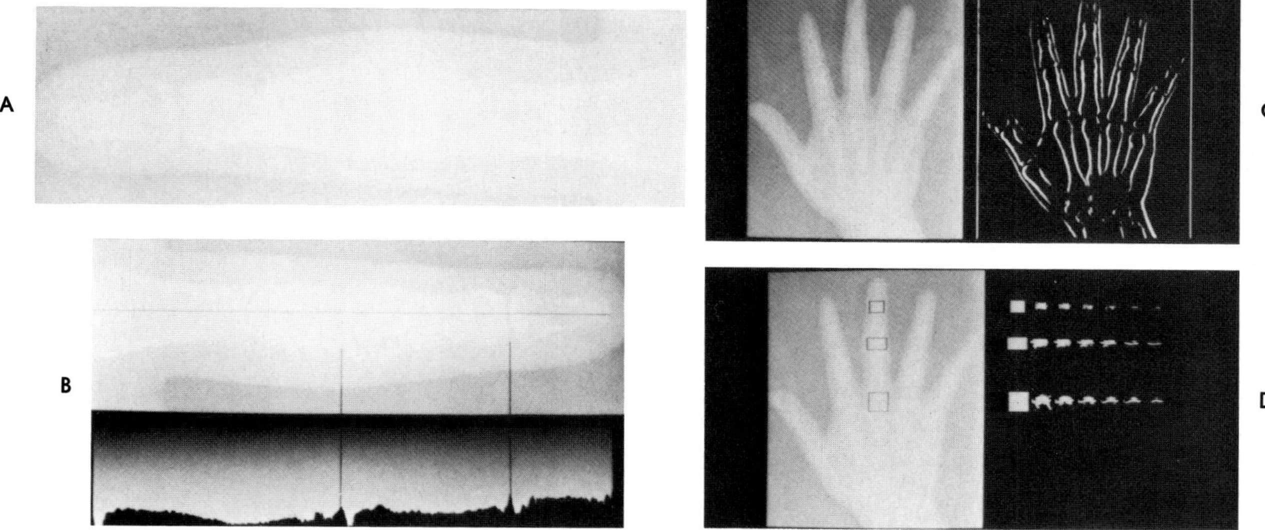

Fig. 35-10. Analytic techniques used on computed radiographic image of the hand to characterize the feature of the bones and detect abnormal variations. **A,** Computed radiographic image of third digit. **B,** Profile of density distribution of digit. **C,** Edge recognition algorithm. **D,** Transverse edge recognition at phalanx joints.

Quality Assurance Concerns

A positive design feature of a computed radiography system is its ability to minimize resultant image *artifacts,* whether induced from system irregularities or operator errors. Periodic failures in these safeguards, however, are inevitable and will affect image quality.

System noise, artifacts, and unevenness in an image are determined by the noise inherent in the imaging plate (structure noise) and reader system (quantum noise). Digital processing errors can create artifacts and density irregularities.

Several artifacts can be controlled by the operator. Dust on the imaging plate can be seen on the resulting image. It is, therefore, important to maintain a periodic schedule of cleaning the imaging plate surfaces for quality assurance, similar to the quality control maintenance used for radiographic intensifying screens. In addition, grids of a particular ratio and line factor are recommended for various examinations. If these recommendations are not followed, a *moiŕe* pattern of laser light scanning lines or data loss can occur. These errors cannot be controlled by the technologist and require system adjustments. It must be understood, however, that scatter radiation is detrimental to computed radiography image quality just as in conventional film-screen image quality. Grids must be used when the examination or the patient's body build warrants. Although computed radiography systems are able to correct for gross technical errors, there is a limit to the minimum dosage required for appropriate penetration and a diagnostic image. Each computed radiography operating institution must independently establish the radiation dose reduction limits. An inadequate dose will result in images demonstrating quantum mottle or areas devoid of data.

Pitfalls

In correctly produced computed radiography images the number of disadvantages is few and will not cause diagnostic problems, even with a relatively inexperienced computed radiography operator. The primary undesirable characteristics are edge enhancement artifacts. In certain circumstances, edge enhancement creates an appearance that may be confused with a pathologic disorder. On the edge-enhanced image, a dark band may appear at the interface between structures that differ widely in density. This effect is primarily seen in computed radiography images involving metal prostheses and barium contrast studies. The dark line of the edge-enhancement artifact is always perfectly symmetric around the dense object, which makes it relatively easy to distinguish from a lesion causing lucency. In computed radiographic images of the chest the pulmonary vasculature is very prominent on the edge-enhanced image, however, the "standard technique" image shows the vasculature to have an appearance identical to that of standard film radiographs.

Benefits of Computed Radiography

When using a computed radiography system certain benefits are readily apparent, including the following:

IMPROVED DIAGNOSTIC ACCURACY AND EXPANDED DIAGNOSTIC SCOPE

By storing laser-scanned x-ray images on high-sensitivity imaging plates, minute differences in x-ray absorption are detected, providing highly detailed and easily readable diagnostic information. The wide exposure latitude permits diagnosis on an entire area of interest, allowing imaging from bones to soft tissue with a single exposure. Computer analysis of images can provide increased diagnostic information to assist in the medical treatment of a patient.

X-RAY DOSAGE REDUCTION

The high-speed imaging plate coupled with the efficient information read-out of the high-precision laser spot scanning device allows the patient to be exposed to a lower x-ray dose than that using a conventional film-screen system. This is especially worthwhile for pediatric examinations. Reductions vary somewhat with the type of examination performed, as shown in Table 35-3.

Table 35-3. Radiation dose for diagnostic quality image by computed radiography compared with standard radiography

Procedure	Decrease in dose relative (%)
Chest radiography	14-20
Upper GI series	5
Excretory urography	50
Pelvis radiography phantom study	12

REPEAT RATE REDUCTION

Because of the computed radiography system's wide technique latitude, technical errors are easily corrected to provide prime diagnostic information. When a film-screen combination is used, technical errors in either direction can markedly degrade the image quality. Technical errors have much less effect on the final quality of a computed radiographic image. This benefit obviously increases *throughput* and reduces the patient's discomfort, because it lessens the need to repeat the examination. The technical latitude of computed radiography is a tremendous asset in the area of portable radiography.

TELERADIOGRAPHIC TRANSMISSION

Image plate reader devices can be linked via dedicated phone lines, microwave transmission, or other teleradiographic means to centralize the review of image data. This means of image sharing could obviously benefit affiliated hospitals or clinics that are separated by large geographic distances and share professional staff. Teleradiology could also provide immediate consultation with specialists, which benefits not only the patient but also the level of efficiency of the institution.

Many radiology departments have contemplated a PACS (Picture Archive and Communication System) for the immediate or near future. Hesitation to implement PACS by many has been caused not only by fears of multimodality/multivendor interfacing, but also by the requirement that conventional projection radiography (which represents approximately 70% of a radiology department's volume) be digital format compatible. Computed radiography is the link needed for PACS. With computed radiography, all imaging modalities can be integrated and share processing, display, and archiving ventures.

Department Efficiency

The computed radiography system eliminates all darkroom work. With this plus the previous benefits, departmental efficiency is ultimately increased.

Summary

Computed radiography will improve both the operational and diagnostic efficiency of radiology departments. By placing conventional projection radiography in digital format, computed radiography forms the keystone for PACS. Computed radiography improves the efficiency of conventional projection radiography by providing consistent image quality, decreasing the repeat exposure rate, minimizing patient radiation exposure, and decreasing lost images. By realizing such, many departments have already realized that computed radiography is proving to be a justifiable long-term investment.

Definition of Terms

analog Any information represented in continuous fashion rather than discrete units.

analog-to-digital conversion The process of converting a continuous (analog) signal to discrete (digital) units.

artifacts Observable, undesirable image features resulting from faulty image processing techniques.

bit Smallest piece of computer information.

byte 8 bits.

gigabyte (G-byte) 1000 megabytes.

megabyte (M-byte) 1000 bytes.

cathode ray tube (CRT) An electron tube (like a television tube) that makes the computer output visible; sometimes called a VDU (video display unit).

computed radiography (CR) Digital imaging process using a photostimulable chemical plate for the initial acquisition of image data; the display parameters of the image can be manipulated by a computer at a later time.

default The parameters by which the system operates; if no changes in instructions are made by the operator, the preset operating parameters or controls of the system prevail.

digital Any information represented in discrete units (see also analog).

dual energy imaging An x-ray imaging technique in which two x-ray exposures are taken of the same body part by using two different kilovoltages; the two images are processed in such a way as to remove image contrast resulting from either soft tissue or bone.

dynamic range The orders of magnitude over which the system can accurately portray information.

edge enhancement The technique of setting the spatial frequency response so that structures of a given type, usually the bones, stand out in bold relief.

gigabyte (G-byte) 1000 megabytes.

gradation processing The technique of setting the range of values over which an image is displayed, similar to the window setting in computed tomography; gradation processing allows one to select a wide range of values to display structures with widely differing densities, or a narrow range to display structures close together in density, for example a body part such as the mediastinum.

helium-neon laser An intense, coherent beam of light in the red wave-length.

histogram A graphic representation of the frequency distribution of gray levels, which represent the anatomy in a computed radiographic image (see Chapter 33, Fig. 33-14 for an example).

image plate reader The component of the computed radiography system that scans the image plate with a laser, converting the analog information on the image plate into an electrical signal; an analog-to-digital converter then changes the electrical signal to a digital signal.

latent image A nonobservable representation of a structure, such as the varied energy changes inherent in the crystalline structure of imaging plates.

matrix The grid-like pattern of an image, composed of a certain number of *pixels,* both in the horizontal and the vertical planes.

megabyte (M-byte) 1000 bytes.

moiré A fine network of wavy lines that have a watered appearance on the displayed image.

photostimulable phosphor A special luminescent material that stores x-ray energy and emits light proportional to the stored x-ray energy when stimulated by energy such as visible light from a laser.

pixels (*pi*cture *el*ements) The small squares that form the image; pixels have depth in bits usually 8, 12, 15, etc.; the greater the pixel depth, the larger the gray scale.

region of interest (ROI) An area on the image judged of primary clinical interest.

spatial frequency response The frequency response is the image sharpness and controls how prominently the "edges" are seen in one structure of one density compared with the "edges" in an adjacent structure of another density; the technique used in the computed radiography system is called "unsharp masking," in which an unsharp (blurred) image is used as the mask image to enhance the spatial frequency response.

spatial resolution Spatial resolution refers to how small an object can be detected by an imaging system, and how close together two similar objects can be and still be identified as separate objects; the measure usually used is line pairs per millimeter (lp/mm); for example, if the spatial resolution is 10 lp/mm, it means that 10 lines per millimeter can be distinguished as discrete lines, but if there are more than 10 lines per millimeter some lines will "run together" and appear to be a single line.

throughput The rate at which items can be processed through a system; originally a systems analysis term, the term is now commonly used in medicine; if a radiology department can perform a maximum of 60 chest radiographs per hour, this is the maximum throughput for chest radiographs.

SELECTED BIBLIOGRAPHY

Anasuma K: Technical trends of the CR system. In Tateno Y, Iinuma T and Takano M, editors: Computed radiography, Tokyo, 1988, Springer Verlag.

Barnes GT, Sones RA and Tesic MM: Digital chest radiography: performance evaluation of a prototype unit, Radiology 154:801-806, 1985.

Fraser RG, Breatnach E and Barnes GT: Digital radiography of the chest: clinical experience with a prototype unit, Radiology 148:1-5, 1983.

Hindel R: Review of optical storage technology for archiving digital medical images, Radiology 161:257-262, 1986.

Huebener KH: Scanned projection radiography of the chest versus standard film radiography: a comparison of 250 cases, Radiology 148:363-368, 1983.

Johnson GA and Ravin CE: A survey of digital chest radiography, Radiol Clin North Am 21(4):655-665, 1983.

Kuni CC: Introduction to computers and digital processing in medical imaging, Chicago, 1988, Year Book Medical Publishers Inc.

Long BW: Computed tomography: photo stimulable phosphor image plate technology, Radiol Technol 61(2):107-112, 1989.

Long BW: Image enhancement using computed radiography, Radiol Technol 61(4):276-280, 1990.

McAdams HP, et al: Histogram-directed processing of digital chest images, Invest Radiol 21:253-259, 1986.

Sakuma H, et al: Plain chest radiograph with computed radiography: improved sensitivity for the detection of coronary artery calcification, AJR 151:27-30, 1988.

Templeton AW, et al: A digital radiology imaging system: description and clinical evaluation, AJR 149:847-851, 1987.

Tateno Y: An introduction to clinical utilization of CR. In Tateno Y, Linuma T and Takeno M (editors): Computed radiography, Tokyo, 1987, Springer-Verlag.

Tesic MM, et al: Digital radiography of the chest: design features and considerations for a prototype unit, Radiology 148:259-264, 1983.

Chapter 36

DIGITAL SUBTRACTION ANGIOGRAPHY

WALTER W. PEPPLER

Digital electronic technology has increased the speed of image processing and decreased costs to the point where totally electronic radiographic image detection, storage, and display are beginning to replace film in a number of procedures. More importantly, radiographic images stored in a digital memory can be manipulated in ways that are impossible with film. Such manipulation enables the radiologist to isolate image information that is too low in image contrast to be recognized on a conventional radiograph. The ability to "see" what previously had been invisible has opened new areas for radiographic study. One area that has gained widespread acceptance is *digital subtraction angiography** (DSA).

*All italicized terms are defined at the end of this chapter.

□I wish to thank John C. McDermott, M.D., from the University of Wisconsin at Madison for his assistance in developing this chapter.

Historical Development

DSA was developed during the 1970s by groups at the University of Wisconsin, the University of Arizona, and the Kinderklinik at the University of Kiel. This work led to the development of commercial systems that were introduced in 1980. Within the next few years many manufacturers of x-ray equipment introduced DSA products. After several years of rapid change, the systems evolved to those available today. The primary changes since the introduction of DSA in 1980 include improved image quality, larger *pixel matrices* (up to 1024 × 1024), and fully *digital* systems. Image quality has improved for two reasons: (1) the component parts (e.g., the image intensifier, television camera) have been improved, and (2) the component parts have been more effectively integrated into the system, since the early systems were built using component parts selected "off the shelf," and they may or may not have been properly matched.

INTRAVENOUS VS. INTRAARTERIAL INJECTION

The most notable change in digital subtraction angiography was not in equipment design but in clinical practice. The initial success and promise of DSA was based on intravenous (IV) injection of contrast media. Intravenous procedures were less risky and less expensive than the intraarterial procedures used for conventional angiography and could be performed on an outpatient basis. This was quite an advantage, because conventional intraarterial film *angiography* usually required an overnight hospital stay. In addition IV DSA was less painful for the patient. However, IV DSA had serious limitations; image artifacts were caused by patient motion (e.g., cardiac motion, bowel peristalsis, diaphragmatic motion, swallowing, and coughing), less than optimal results were obtained in patients with reduced cardiac output, limitations were imposed by the larger volume of contrast medium required for IV injection, and problems occurred with superimposition of vessels (because all arteries are opacified with IV injections). Therefore, over the last several years the standard of practice has evolved so that the majority of DSA procedures are currently performed using intraarterial injection of contrast material. DSA now permits the use of a smaller volume of more dilute contrast medium and thus, the risks associated with the injection of contrast media have been reduced. *Nonionic contrast media* have also been introduced, and studies have shown the newer contrast agents to be safer than conventional, or *ionic contrast, media* and to be better accepted by patients. Improvements in catheter procedures have reduced the overnight hospital stay to several hours in the ambulatory surgery department for recovery. However, the main reason for the transition to intraarterial injection is because of the very significant increase in image quality. Intravenous injection of contrast media produces not only poorer image quality but also more variable results compared with that obtained routinely using intraarterial injections.

ECONOMICS AND DSA

The widespread acceptance of DSA has resulted in an economic benefit, because there are significant cost savings of intravenous and intraarterial DSA in comparison with film angiography. The DSA images are readily available without delay after the contrast medium is injected, resulting in decreased examination time for the patient. Also, because the technique is very sensitive to small amounts of contrast medium, smaller catheters are used in the intraarterial DSA method and this has allowed arteriography to be performed on an outpatient basis.

THE EXTINCTION OF FILM ANGIOGRAPHY?

With the widespread acceptance of DSA, and specifically intraarterial DSA, there are some proponents who believe that film arteriography may become a procedure of the past. Film arteriography still maintains an advantage in resolution with up to 10 lp/mm compared with about 2 lp/mm for DSA, and it is still mandatory in visceral arteriography. Because DSA is extremely sensitive to motion artifact, the presence of bowel peristalsis and respiratory motion within the abdomen results in significant image degradation. Therefore, in visceral angiographic work, film arteriography is still considered the gold standard. This is particularly important when arteriography is performed in a patient with gastrointestinal bleeding, because resolution is critical. Also, cut film arteriography of the visceral vessels is mandatory in patients with collagen vascular disease and in those with subarachnoid hemorrhage, cerebral vascular aneurysms, or cerebral vasculitis.

Equipment and Apparatus

An image intensifier–television system (fluoroscopy) can be used to form images with little electrical interference, provide moderate resolution, and yield diagnostic quality images when combined with a high-speed *image processor* in a DSA system as shown in Fig. 36-1.

The DSA procedure room is much like a standard angiographic suite. Both film and digital capabilities are usually present and the fluoroscopic equipment operates in the conventional way. However, a brief review will help explain the DSA system. The input surface of the *image intensifier* is coated with an x-ray–sensitive phosphor, typically cesium iodide (CsI). The image-intensifier phosphor is contained within a vacuum and enclosed in glass. X-rays that are absorbed by the CsI *input phosphor* emit visible light detected by electronics within the image intensifier. The detected light, proportional to the amount of radiation absorbed, is electronically amplified and accelerated across the image tube and is emitted at the *output phosphor* of the image intensifier by another light-emitting phosphor, approximately 1 inch in diameter. The resulting light intensity is brighter by a factor of 5000 to 10,000 times than if the CsI phosphor had been used alone.

The television camera (TV) is focused onto the image-intensifier output phosphor and converts the light intensity into an electrical signal. The television camera forms an image by electronically scanning a photosensitive *semiconductor* (called the target) on which the light has been focused. The presence of light on a small portion of the target changes the electrical properties in that target region. These changes are detected by the television camera.

The scanning of a narrow electron beam across the television target in 525 parallel lines at a rate of 525 lines per 1/30 second synthesizes an image line by line. With normal fluoroscopic operation, the video image is displayed on a television monitor. The scanning rate is so fast that the human eye does not notice the scanning process but sees a two-dimensional image on the television screen. The images are called *frames* and are presented at a rate of 30 per second.

In a DSA system, each of the television lines is further divided into segments called pixels (picture elements). The electronic video signal corresponding to each pixel is *digitized* and stored in a digital memory. Typically each line is divided into 512 or 1024 pixels, and the digitized value (gray level) assigned to each pixel is usually in the range of zero (representing black) to 1023 (white). The image in *memory,* which is made up of a total of 512 × 512, or 1024 × 1024, pixels (the number of lines times the number of pixels per line), is also stored on a digital disk for later review and analysis.

The image processor consists of a computer and image processing hardware. The computer controls the various components (e.g., memories, image processing hardware, and x-ray generator), and the image processing hardware gives the system the speed to do many image processing operations in *real time.* The computer and the operator communicate via a keyboard and special function keys to operate the DSA system.

The control room is usually separated from the procedure room and has a leaded glass window for observation. Typically there is a video monitor on the operator's console as well as one in the procedure room next to the fluoroscopic monitor. At the operator's console there is also a computer monitor for communicating with the computer. The video monitors display the subtraction images in real time as the images are obtained during the imaging sequence. At a later time, films *(hard copy)* are produced using a multiformat camera or laser imager (Fig. 36-2).

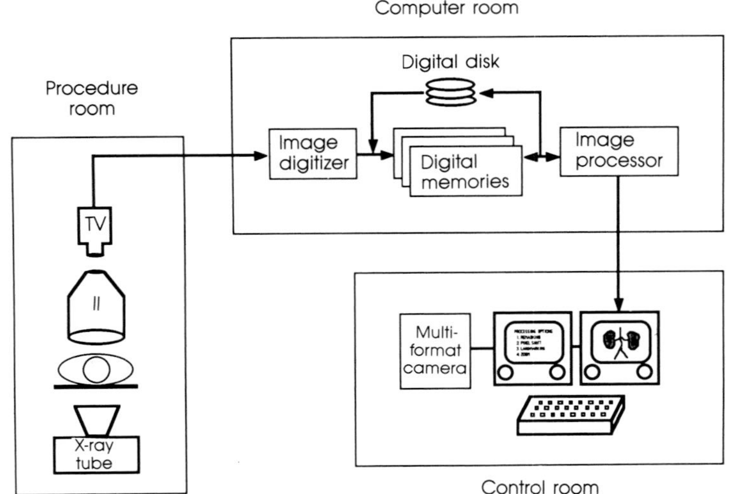

Fig. 36-1. Block diagram of a digital subtraction angiography (DSA) system.

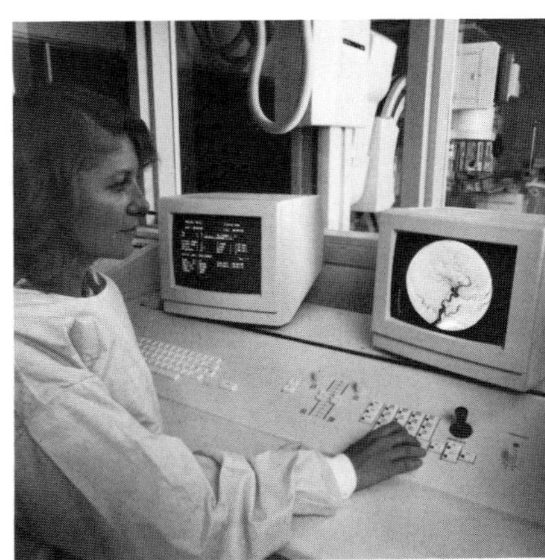

Fig. 36-2. The operator console of a digital subtraction angiography system with the procedure room in the background.

(Courtesy of Philips Medical Systems.)

Performing DSA Procedures

A DSA study begins by placing the catheter in the patient in the same manner used for conventional angiography. The injection techniques vary, but typically 40 to 50 ml of iodinated contrast medium is injected at a rate of 20 ml/sec for intravenous procedures, and 15 to 20 ml at a rate of 10 ml/sec for intraarterial procedures. An automatic pressure injector is used to ensure consistency of injection and to facilitate computer control of injection timing and image acquisition.

The intravascular catheter is positioned using conventional fluoroscopic apparatus and technique, and a suitable imaging position is selected. At this point an image that does not have a large dynamic range should be established; no part of the image should be significantly brighter than the rest of the image. This can be accomplished by proper positioning, but it often requires the use of compensating filters or bolus materials. The compensating filter can be either water bags or thin pieces of metal inserted in the imaging field to reduce the intensity of bright regions. Metal filters are usually affixed to the collimator, and water or saline bags are placed directly on or adjacent to the patient. If proper bolus placement is not performed, significant reduction of image quality will result. The reason for this is that the DSA video camera operates most effectively with video signals that are at a fixed level. Automatic controls in the DSA system adjust the exposure factors so the brightest part of the image is at that level. An unusually bright spot will satisfy the automatic controls and cause the rest of the image to lie at significantly reduced levels where the camera performance is worse. An alternative to proper bolus or filter placement is to adjust the automatic sensing region, which can be displayed on the image, to exclude the bright region. This solution is less desirable than using compensating filters, and for some positions of the bright spot it is not always possible.

Misregistration is a major problem in DSA; it occurs when the *mask* and the images displaying the vessels filled with contrast medium do not exactly coincide. Misregistration is sometimes caused by voluntary movements of the patient, but it is also caused by involuntary movements, such as bowel peristalsis or the contraction of the heart. Preparing the patient by describing the sensations associated with contrast-medium injection and the importance of holding still and, of course, having the patient suspend respiration during the procedure can help eliminate voluntary movements. Compression bands, glucagon, and cardiac gating can be effective in reducing misregistration caused by involuntary movement. Misregistration is less of a problem in intraarterial DSA than in intravenous DSA, because there is an inherently larger signal in intraarterial DSA so the misregistration signals are less significant and also because the time is reduced between the mask and the postinjection (contrast-filled) image. In addition, because a smaller volume of contrast medium is required with intraarterial injection, the patient's discomfort and the likelihood of coughing or swallowing are reduced, so misregistration problems are also less likely.

As the imaging sequence begins, a mask image is digitized and stored in the digital memory. This mask image and those that follow are produced when the x-ray tube is energized and the x rays are produced, usually one exposure per second at 65 to 95 kVp, and between 5 to 150 mAs. The radiation dose received by the patient for each image is approximately the same as that used for serial film angiography. Each of these digitized images is electronically *subtracted* from the mask, and the subtraction image is amplified (contrast enhanced) and displayed in real time so that the subtraction images appear essentially instantaneously during the imaging procedure. The images are simultaneously stored on a *digital disk* or *video tape recorder*. Video tape recorders are often used when images are acquired at a rate of 30 per second, because most digital disks cannot operate at high imaging rates. Real-time digital disks capable of recording images at a rate of 30 per second are quite expensive and are usually restricted to cardiac applications where high imaging rates are more common.

During the imaging procedure, the subtraction images appear on the display monitor. In many cases a preliminary diagnosis can be made at this point or as the images are reviewed immediately following each exposure sequence. However, a formal reading session, typically performed from hard copy film, occurs at a later time, at which time the final diagnosis is made.

Some *post-processing* (described below) is performed after each exposure sequence to improve the visualization of the anatomy of interest or to correct for misregistration. More involved post-processing, including quantitative analysis, is performed after the patient study has been completed, and then radiographs are produced using a *laser printer* or *multiformat camera*. In either case, several images appear on each film. The films are used during the formal reading session and are also kept for archival purposes.

Image Post-Processing

After the images have been obtained and stored on a disk, there are several ways of manipulating, or post-processing, the images. The most common is to adjust the contrast and brightness to produce an optimum display of the image. The contrast and brightness adjustments are equivalent to the window and level adjustments performed on CT or MRI images. The terms "contrast" and "brightness" are often used for DSA because of the similarity to adjusting the contrast and brightness on a television set.

REMASKING

Another common post-processing task is to correct misregistered images. The most effective way to fix misregistration is simply to *remask* the image. To remask, another mask image is chosen that is properly registered with the image of interest; the procedure is usually simple. The most efficient way to remask images is as follows. Rather than choosing new masks one at a time (which may or may not work), the image containing the maximum iodine signal should be selected as the "mask." Then a "live" (in this case without iodine) image that subtracts from the "mask" without misregistration is sought. The reversal of the role of the images reverses the polarity of the subtraction image (i.e., from white contrast to black contrast). However, the original polarity can be restored by pressing the contrast inversion button. This procedure usually produces an acceptable image with the least effort (Fig. 36-3).

PIXEL SHIFTING

In some cases an acceptable mask cannot be found. One way to salvage such runs is by *pixel shifting*. In this technique one of the images is shifted with respect to the other to compensate for the movement of the patient between the two images. Shifts of a fraction of a pixel are necessary in many cases to obtain proper registration. Most processors allow at least horizontal and vertical translation and some permit rotation as well. Pixel shifting can be a tedious procedure that requires a great deal of patience. In addition to many possible pixel shifts, several combinations of mask and live images may have to be tried. Unfortunately, in many cases it is more expedient to simply repeat the run. A reliable automatic pixel registration routine is much more likely to be used.

EDGE ENHANCEMENT

Using *edge enhancement,* also called unsharp masking, the edges of vessels can be accentuated (or enhanced) so that small details can be made more obvious. The procedure involves defining a *convolution matrix* that operates on the image. Predefined matrices are usually available so that an understanding of the underlying operations is not usually necessary. A real-time edge enhancement operation is available on some processors so that by simply turning a knob, various amounts of edge enhancement can be obtained.

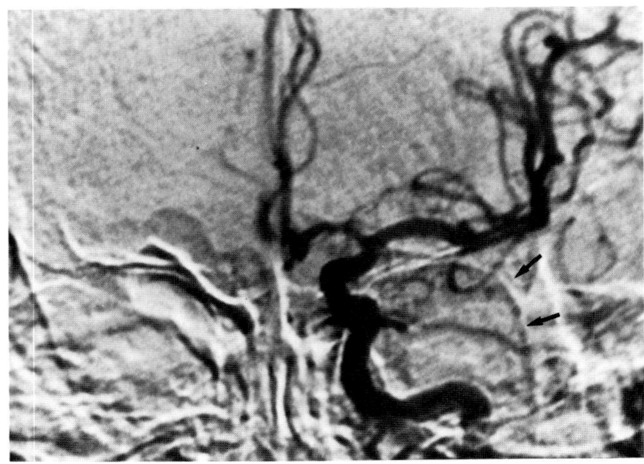

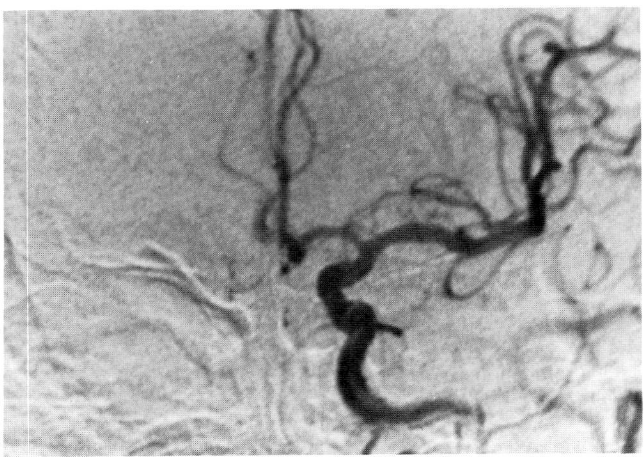

Fig. 36-3. Intraarterial DSA angiogram of the intercranial arteries, **A,** demonstrating misregistration artifacts. **B,** The same image after remasking. Notice the significant improvement in the misregistration artifacts, particularly in the region of the orbit *(arrows).*

IMAGE ZOOM

Another post-processing option is to magnify or *zoom* the image. Zooming the image increases the size of a part of the image to make some subtle feature more visible. Zooming can be performed by interpolation or by pixel duplication. Interpolation produces intermediate pixels by averaging adjacent pixels and has a more pleasing appearance. However, pixel duplication is usually faster. The duplication method is often called fast zoom, whereas the interpolation method is called interpolative zoom. It should be noted that neither of the methods increases the resolution of the image. They simply present the same information in a more obvious way (Fig. 36-4).

LANDMARKING

In landmarking, a small amount of the original image is put back into the subtraction image. This is commonly done to give surgeons anatomic landmarks so that they can more accurately locate structures in the image. Without the landmark information it is difficult to locate the structures because the background has been so effectively eliminated. Only a fraction of the mask is added, however, so that the mask does not overwhelm the subtraction image. As an alternative to landmarking, an unsubtracted image may be printed on the same film as the subtraction images and used as a reference.

ANALYTIC TOOLS

There are a wide variety of analytic tools available on most image processors, including methods to measure distances, quantitate vessel stenoses, calculate ventricular ejection fraction, and measure blood flow. These tools are more likely to be used in a research environment than in a routine clinical setting. However, in the proper hands these techniques can provide accurate quantitative data.

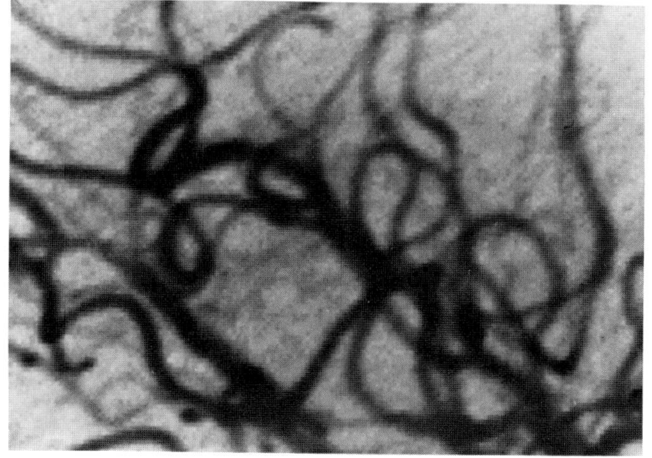

A

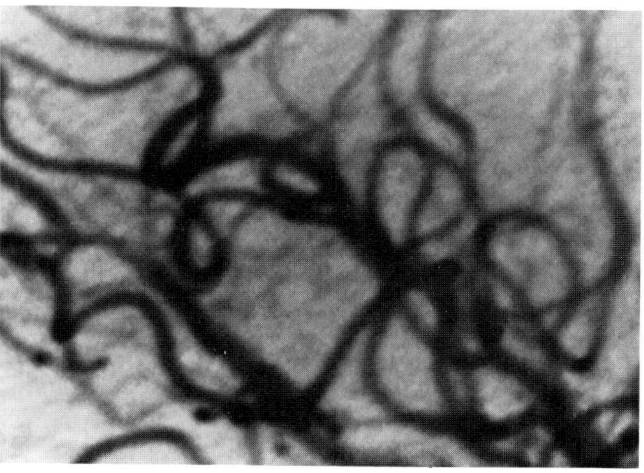

B

Fig. 36-4. A demonstration of the two types of image zoom on an intracranial DSA image; **A,** duplication and, **B,** interpolation. Notice the jagged appearance of the arteries when using the duplication method, **A.**

Clinical Uses

INTRAVENOUS DSA

Although most procedures are performed using the intraarterial approach, there are selected circumstances where the IV DSA approach is still applied. Specifically, the IV DSA approach is used to assess the patency of aorto-bifemoral grafts, femoral-popliteal bypass grafts, false aneurysms at arterial anastomotic sites, and indwelling Hickman catheters for upper limb venous thrombosis. In neurologic work, IV DSA is used to evaluate patients who are suspected of having superior sagittal sinus thrombosis (Fig. 36-5).

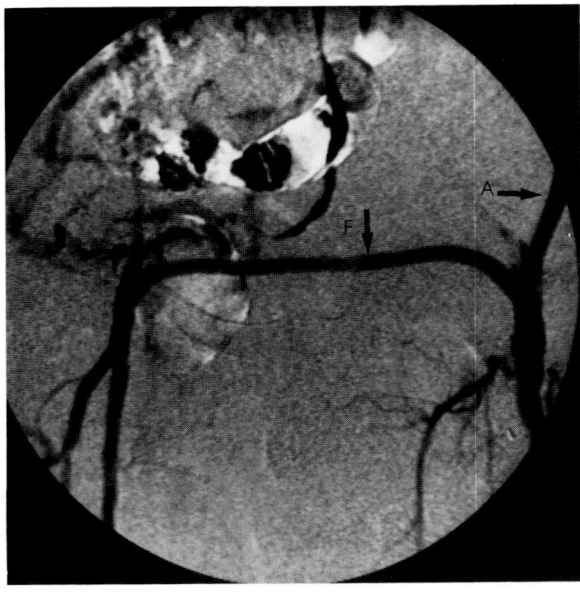

Fig. 36-5. An intravenous DSA image of the pelvic region showing a patent (unobstructed) *(A)* axillo-bifemoral *(F)* bypass graft.

INTRAARTERIAL DSA

Intraarterial DSA can be used for almost all cerebrovascular and peripheral examinations, except in patients scheduled for treatment with surgery or embolization when a subarachnoid hemorrhage or arteriovenous malformation is present. In such circumstances it is preferable to use the higher resolution of film angiography instead of DSA.

Patients with peripheral vascular disease typically will undergo an intraarterial DSA examination of the infrarenal abdominal aorta, pelvic vessels, and runoff vessels. Because DSA has considerably greater contrast sensitivity than film, the intraarterial DSA method permits the identification of small vessels in the lower limbs of patients with severe peripheral vascular disease. Some of these patients have been able to undergo a distal bypass procedure rather than amputation.

The intraarterial DSA approach can also be applied to pulmonary arteriography. To perform the examination, a catheter is placed within the main pulmonary artery, which permits the use of a small amount of contrast agent. In these situations, a rapid framing sequence (6 frames/sec to 15 frames/sec) is often used. Alternatively, ECG triggering can be used with lower imaging rates. This application of the intraarterial DSA approach is particularly helpful in a patient with severe pulmonary arterial hypertension who is at significant risk from the high-rate, high-volume contrast injection used for standard pulmonary arteriography (Figs. 36-6 to 36-9).

The intraarterial DSA approach has also resulted in the evolution of the road map technique. Most angiography/interventional radiologists use this technique routinely in the performance of angioplasty. The intraarterial road map technique provides the angiographer with a real-time continuous subtraction on the fluoroscopic monitor during a procedure. An injection is made while the subtraction mask is obtained, then the fluoroscopic images are subtracted continuously from the mask. The stationary anatomy is cancelled, but the iodinated arteries remain. When the catheter is advanced it also appears on the monitor along with the iodinated arteries, which act as a road map to guide the catheter. The road map technique is often used during the catheterization of a patient with a high-grade stenosis or an occlusion within a peripheral runoff vessel. Likewise, the intraarterial road map technique is also applied in superselective catheterization and as a monitor during the course of arterial embolization.

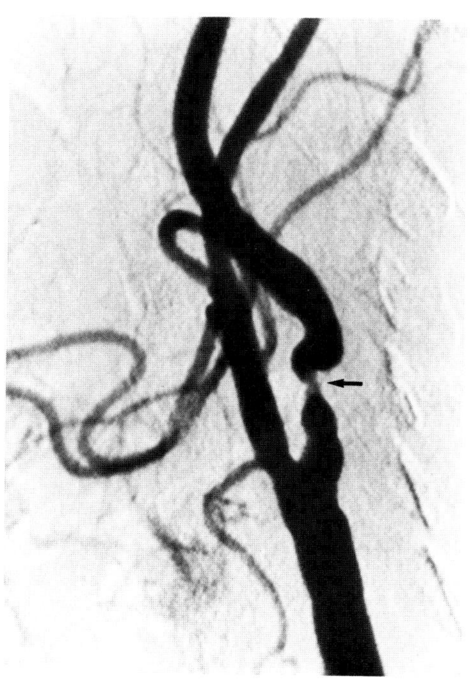

Fig. 36-6. Intraarterial DSA image of the common carotid artery demonstrating a severe stenosis of the internal carotid artery *(arrow).*

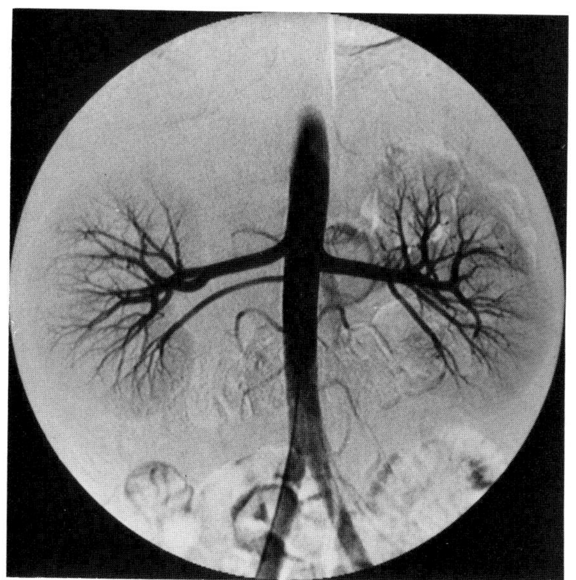

Fig. 36-7. Intraarterial DSA image of the abdominal aorta showing one renal artery on the left and two renal arteries on the right; all renal arteries are widely patent.

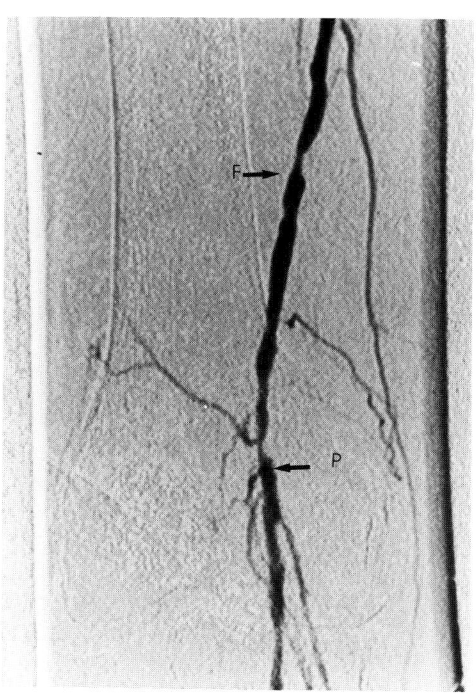

Fig. 36-8. Intraarterial DSA image of the distal superficial femoral *(F),* and popliteal *(P)* arteries showing diffuse, near occlusive disease.

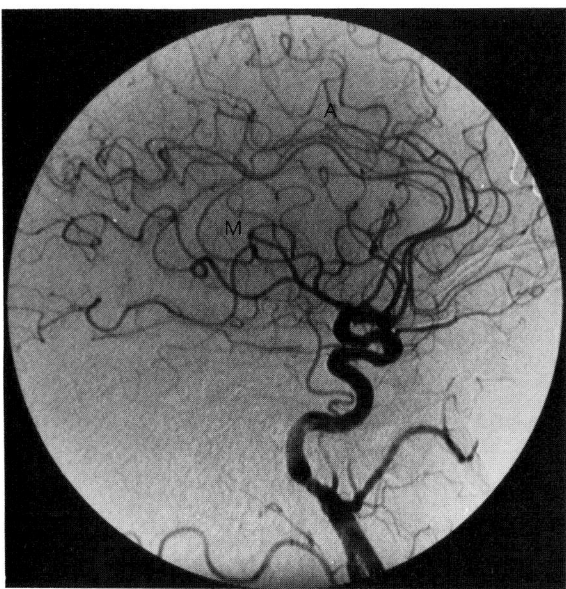

Fig. 36-9. Intraarterial DSA image of the intracranial vasculature showing patent anterior *(A)* and middle *(M)* cerebral arteries.

Conclusion

Digital subtraction angiography has had a great impact on diagnostic radiology. Its advantages over film angiography are that it has much greater contrast sensitivity, lower cost, and immediate availability of results. The digital nature of the data also permits quantitative analysis of DSA images. In some cases this has proven valuable, particularly in cardiac applications. The increased contrast sensitivity has permitted the use of lower total volumes and concentrations of contrast media; decreased patient discomfort and reduced toxicity are therefore obtained.

The early interest in intravenous injection of contrast medium has yielded to the intraarterial injection technique in most cases. Intraarterial DSA has been successfully used for imaging most major arteries, but there are still procedures where film angiography is the method of choice, particularly when maximum resolution is required. A properly equipped angiography suite will have the capability for both DSA and film angiography.

DEFINITION OF TERMS

angiography Producing x-ray images of the blood vessels after injection of contrast medium.

artifact Any undesirable side effect resulting from an image processing technique.

convolution matrix An array of values used in an operation called convolution when performing edge enhancement.

digital Information stored in discrete units, called bits. These bits are used to form a binary code for representing information.

digital disk A circular plate coated with magnetic material and used to store digital data.

digital subtraction angiography The use of digitally recorded x-ray images to produce subtraction images of the cardiovascular system.

digitize The process of converting a continuous analog voltage signal into a discrete digital value.

edge enhancement Making the edges of vessels more clearly visualized through intentional unsharp masking and/or computer manipulation.

frame A single image from a sequence of images.

hard copy A copy of a video image on film.

image intensifier An imaging device that converts an x-ray distribution (image) to an optical image with a large increase in brightness.

image processor A special-purpose computer designed to operate on images in a short time.

input phosphor A material that is coated on the input surface of an image intensifier tube, which emits light in response to the absorption of x-rays.

ionic contrast medium A contrast agent that ionizes in solution and causes more patient discomfort than nonionic contrast medium.

laser printer A device that uses a laser to produce a copy of an image on film.

mask An image in which the arteries do not contain iodine that is subtracted from images with iodine in the arteries.

matrix A two-dimensional array of pixel values that make up an image.

memory That portion of an image processor in which the numbers that represent an image are stored.

misregistration When the two images used to form a subtraction image are slightly displaced from one another.

multiformat camera A device that produces copies of several images on a single film.

nonionic contrast medium A contrast agent that does not ionize in solution and is safer, less painful, and better tolerated by the patient than ionic contrast medium.

output phosphor A material that is coated on the output surface of an image intensifier, which emits light (an image) in response to being struck by electrons.

pixel When an image is digitized, it is broken into a number of individual cells. Each cell, which represents only a small fraction of an entire picture, is called a pixel (*pic*ture *el*ement).

pixel shifting The digital image is shifted to compensate for misregistration marks caused by patient motion. It is an alternative to remasking.

post-processing Image processing operations performed when reviewing an imaging sequence.

real time Any image processing technique that can be performed within a time frame that is so short as to appear to be instantaneous.

remask Repeating the masking process, if necessary, to correct for misregistration marks.

semiconductor Solid-state material used in the construction of electronic devices, such as transistors or integrated circuits.

subtracted When the mask image is used to remove the scout image (via electronic superimposition) from the postinjection angiogram image.

video tape recorder A device that uses magnetic tape to record video images.

zoom Magnification of the image via interpolation or pixel duplication; resolving power remains unchanged.

SELECTED BIBLIOGRAPHY

American Association of Physicists in Medicine: Performance evaluation and quality assurance in digital subtraction angiography, report no 15, New York, 1985, American Institute of Physics Inc.

Brennecke R, et al: Computerized video-image preprocessing with applications to cardio-angiographic roentgen-image series. In Nagel HH, editor: Digital image processing, Berlin, 1977, Springer-Verlag.

Carmody RF, et al: Digital subtraction angiography: update 1986, Invest Radiol 21:899-905, 1986.

Christenson PC, et al: Intravenous angiography using digital video subtraction: intravenous cervicocerebrovascular angiography, AJR 135:1145-1152, 1980.

Coltman JW: Fluoroscopic image brightening by electronic means, Radiology 51:359-365, 1948.

Crummy AB, et al: Computerized fluoroscopy: digital subtraction for intravenous angiocardiography and arteriography, AJR 135:1131-1140, 1980.

Crummy AB: Digital subtraction angiography. In Taveras, JM and Ferrucci JT: Radiology: diagnosis-imaging-intervention, Philadelphia, 1987, JB Lippincott Co.

Crummy AB, et al: Digital subtraction angiography "road map" for transluminal angioplasty, Semin Intervent Radiol 1(4):247-250, 1984.

Digital subtraction angiography in clinical practice, Best, the Netherlands, 1986, Philips Medical Systems.

Foley WD, et al: Intravenous DSA examination of patients with suspected cerebral ischemia, Radiology 151:651-659, 1984.

Heintzen PH, Brennecke R and Bursch JH: Computer quantitation of angiocardiographic images. In Miller HA, Schmidt EV and Harrison DC, editors: Noninvasive cardiovascular measurements, vol 167, Bellingham, Wash, 1978, Society of Photooptical Industrial Engineers.

Hillman BJ: Digital radiology of the kidney, Radiol Clin North Am 23:211-226, 1985.

Kruger RA, et al: A digital video image processor for real time subtraction imaging, Optical Engineering 17:652-657, 1978.

Kruger RA, et al: Computerized fluoroscopy in real time for noninvasive visualization of the cardiovascular system, Radiology 130:49-57, 1979.

Krueger RA and Riederer SJ: Basic concepts of digital subtraction angiography, Boston, 1984, GK Hall Medical Publishers.

Meaney TF, et al: Digital subtraction angiography of the human cardiovascular system, AJR 135:1153-1160, 1980.

Mistretta CA and Crummy AB: Digital fluoroscopy. In Coulam CM, et al., editors: The physical basis of medical imaging, New York, 1981, Appleton-Century-Crofts.

Mistretta CA and Crummy AB: Diagnosis of cardiovascular disease by digital subtration angiography, Science 214:761-765, 1981.

Mistretta CA, et al: Multiple image subtraction technique for enhancing low contrast periodic objects, Invest Radiol 8:43-44, 1973.

Mistretta CA, et al: Digital subtraction arteriography: an application of computerized fluoroscopy, Chicago, 1982, Year Book Medical Publishers Inc.

Moodie DS and Yiannikas J: Digital subtraction angiography of the heart and lungs, Orlando, Fla, 1986, Grune & Stratton Inc.

Morgan RH and Sturm RE: Johns Hopkins fluoroscopic screen intensifier, Radiology 57:556-564, 1951.

Ovitt TW, et al: Intravenous angiography using digital video subtraction: x-ray imaging system, AJR 135:1141-1144, 1980.

Seeley GW, et al: Computer controlled video subtraction procedures for radiology, Proc Soc Photooptical Instrumentation Engineers 206:183-189, 1979.

Strother CM, et al: Clinical applications of computerized fluoroscopy: the extracranial carotid arteries, Radiology 136:781-783, 1980.

Zweibel WJ, et al: Comparison of ultrasound and IVDSA for carotid evaluation, Stroke 16:633-643, 1985.

Chapter 37

MAGNETIC RESONANCE IMAGING

JAMES H. ELLIS

Tremendous interest among medical workers and the general public has been generated by the appearance of *magnetic resonance (MR)** imaging as a technique for examining the human body. MR can provide both anatomic and physiologic information noninvasively. Like computed tomography (CT), MR is a computer-based cross-sectional imaging modality, but there the similarity to CT ends. The physical principles of MR image production are totally different from CT and conventional radiography; no x-rays, indeed no ionizing radiation of any kind, are used to generate the MR image. MR examines the interactions of magnetism and radio waves with tissue to obtain its images.

MR was originally called *nuclear magnetic resonance* or NMR. The word "nuclear" indicated that the nonradioactive atomic nucleus played an important role. The word "nuclear" has been disassociated from MR imaging because of public apprehension about nuclear energy and nuclear weapons, neither of which is associated with MR in any way (unless by coincidence a nuclear power plant is supplying electricity to an MR unit). In addition, there are forms of MR that do not involve the atomic nucleus and which may, in the future, be used for imaging under the "magnetic resonance" umbrella.

*All italicized terms are defined at the end of this chapter.

□The tireless efforts of Janet Roach and Becky Bertoia in manuscript preparation, review and suggestions by Mary Ann Helms, R.T., and photographic assistance from Peter Rothschild, M.D., are greatly appreciated.

Comparison of MR to Conventional Radiology

Since MR provides sectional images, it serves as a useful adjunct to conventional x-ray techniques. With a radiograph, all body structures exposed by the x-ray beam are superimposed into one "flat" image. Many times, multiple projections or contrast agents are required to clearly distinguish one anatomic structure or organ from another. However, sectional imaging techniques such as ultrasound, CT, and MR more easily separate the various organs, because there is no superimposition of structures. However, multiple *slices* (cross sections) are required to cover a single area of the body.

In addition to problems with overlapping shadows, conventional radiography is relatively limited in its ability to distinguish types of tissue. In radiographic techniques, *contrast,* the ability to discriminate two different substances, depends on differences in x-ray *attenuation* within the object and the ability of the recording medium (for example, film) to detect these differences.

Radiographs cannot detect small attenuation changes. In general, conventional radiographs can distinguish only air, fat, soft tissue, bone, and metal, where the difference in attenuation between each group is large. Most organs, for example, liver and kidneys, cannot be separated by differences in x-ray attenuation alone unless the differences are magnified through the use of contrast agents.

CT is much more sensitive than plain film radiography to small changes in x-ray attenuation. Thus CT can distinguish the liver from the kidneys on the basis of their different x-ray attenuation as well as by position.

MR can also resolve relatively small contrast differences among tissues. It should again be emphasized, however, that these tissue differences are independent from the differences in x-ray attenuation. Contrast in MR depends on the interaction of matter with electromagnetic forces other than x-rays.

Historical Development

The basic principle (discussed more fully below) of MR is that certain atomic nuclei, if placed in a magnetic field, can be stimulated by (absorb energy from) radio waves of the correct frequency. Following this stimulation, the nuclei release the extra absorbed energy by transmitting radio waves (the MR signal), which can be received by an *antenna* and analyzed. *Relaxation times* represent measurements of the rates of this energy release.

These properties of magnetic resonance were first discovered in the 1940s by separate research groups headed by Bloch and Purcell. Their work led to the use of MR *spectroscopy* for the analysis of complex molecular structure and dynamic chemical processes. Spectroscopic MR is still in use today. The Nobel Prize in physics was shared by Bloch and Purcell in 1952 in recognition of the importance of their discoveries.

Nearly 20 years later, Damadian showed that the relaxation time of the water in a tumor differed from the relaxation time of the water in normal tissue. This indication that the relaxation times varied from tissue to tissue suggested that images of the body might be obtained by producing maps of relaxation rates. In 1973, Lauterbur published the first cross-sectional images of objects obtained with MR techniques. These first images were crude and only large objects could be distinguished. Since then there has been an explosion in MR technology so that currently very small structures can be imaged rapidly, and the resolution of MR images is approaching that of computed tomography.

Physical Principles

MR SIGNAL PRODUCTION

The structure of the atom can be compared with the solar system, with the sun representing the central atomic *nucleus*. The planets orbiting the sun represent the electrons circling around the nucleus. MR imaging depends on the properties of the nucleus.

Many, but not all, atomic nuclei have magnetic properties; that is, they act like tiny bar magnets (Fig. 37-1). Normally the magnetic nuclei point in random directions as shown in Fig. 37-2. However, if these nuclei are placed in a strong, uniform magnetic field, they attempt to line up with the direction of the magnetic field, much as iron filings line up with the field of a toy magnet. The word "attempt" is appropriate because the nuclei do not line up precisely with the external field but at an angle to the field, and they rotate about the direction of the magnetic field similar to the wobbling of a spinning top. This wobbling motion, depicted in Fig. 37-3, is called *precession* and occurs at a specific *frequency* (rate) for a given atom's nucleus in a magnetic field of a specific strength. These precessing nuclei can absorb energy if they are exposed to *pulses* of radio waves, provided the radio waves are of the same frequency as the frequency of the nuclear precession. This absorption of energy occurs through the process of *resonance*.

After the external radio wave is turned off, the excited nuclei relax: they release their excess absorbed energy in the form of a radio wave. This radio wave transmitted by the nuclei represents the MR *signal* and is not pulsed. The MR signal can be picked up by a sensitive antenna, amplified, and processed by a computer to produce a sectional image of the body. This image, like the image produced by a CT scanner, represents an electronic image that can be viewed on a television monitor and adjusted to produce the most information. If desired, the image can be photographed for further study.

Most MR imaging currently involves the element hydrogen, the nucleus of which is a single proton. Hydrogen nuclei are the strongest nuclear magnets on a per-nucleus basis (thus giving the strongest MR radio signal). Also, hydrogen is the most common element in the body (again giving the strongest signal). Strong signals are important to produce satisfactory images. Nevertheless, many other nuclei in the body are potential candidates for imaging. Such nuclei as phosphorus and sodium may give more useful or diagnostic information than hydrogen, particularly in efforts to understand the metabolism of normal and abnormal tissues. Changes in metabolism may prove to be more sensitive and specific in the detection of abnormalities than the more physical and structural changes recognized by hydrogen imaging MR or by CT. However, the MR signal from nonhydrogen nuclei is very weak, their imaging requires more elaborate equipment, and anatomic detail is less (compared with hydrogen MR) in sodium and phosphorus images produced to date. Nonhydrogen nuclei may be of particular importance in combined MR imaging and spectroscopy, in which small volumes of tissue may be analyzed for chemical content.

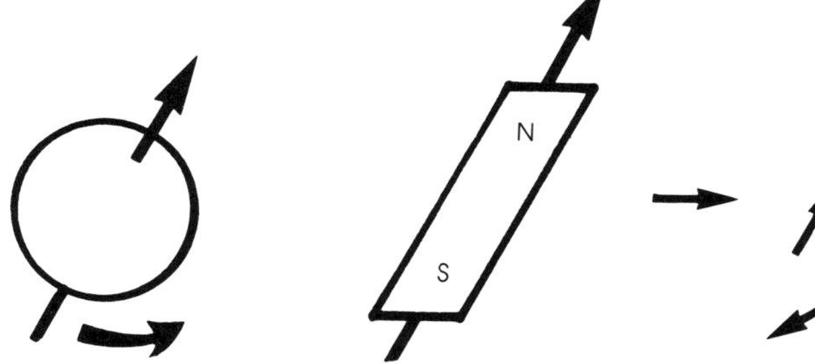

Fig. 37-1. A nucleus with magnetic properties can be compared to a tiny bar magnet. The *curved arrow* indicates that a nucleus spins on its own axis; this motion is different from that of precession.

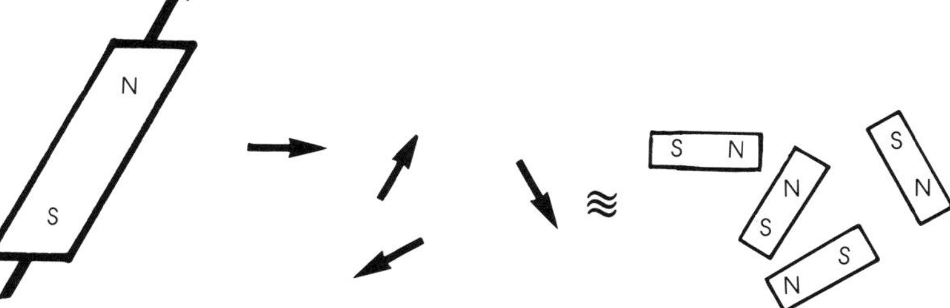

Fig. 37-2. In the absence of an external magnetic field, the nuclei *(arrows)* point in random directions and cannot be used for imaging.

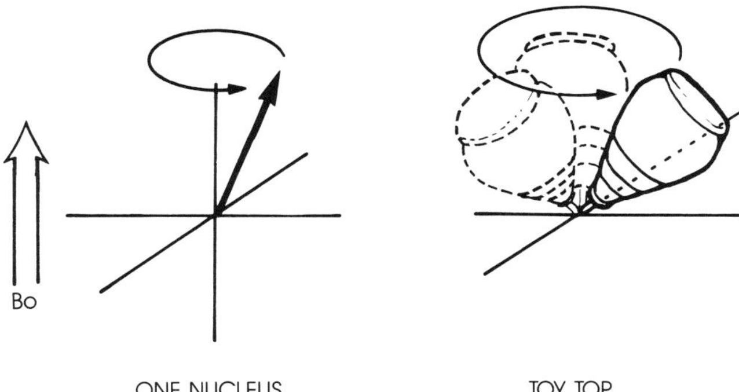

Fig. 37-3. Precession. Both the nucleus *(arrow)* and the toy top spin on their own axes. Both also rotate *(curved arrows)* around the direction of an external force in a wobbling motion called precession. Precessing nuclei can absorb energy through resonance. *Bo* represents the external magnetic field acting on the nucleus. The toy top precesses under the influence of gravity.

MR SIGNAL SIGNIFICANCE

Conventional radiographic techniques, including CT, produce images based on a single property of tissue: x-ray attenuation or density. MR images are more complex because they contain information about three properties of matter: nuclear density, relaxation rates, and flow phenomena. Each contributes to overall MR signal strength. The computer processing converts signal strength to a shade of gray on the image. Strong signals are represented as white in the image and weak signals are black.

One determinant of signal strength is the number of precessing nuclei *(spin density)* in a given volume of tissue. The signal released by the excited nuclei is proportional to the number of nuclei present. Therefore signal strength depends on the nuclear concentration, or density. Since the nucleus of hydrogen is a single proton, this is often referred to as *proton density*. Most soft tissues, including fat, have a similar number of protons per unit volume, so that proton density poorly separates most tissues. However, some tissues have very few hydrogen nuclei per unit of volume; examples include the cortex of bone and air in the lungs. These have a very weak signal as a result of low proton density, and can be easily distinguished from other tissues.

MR signal intensity also depends on the relaxation times of the nuclei. The process of energy release by the excited nuclei is called *relaxation,* and this can occur at different rates in different tissues. There are two processes by which excited nuclei relax. When the nuclei release their excess energy to the general environment (or lattice, the arrangement of atoms in a substance), this is called *spin-lattice relaxation*. The rate of this relaxation process is called *T1*. *Spin-spin relaxation* is the release of energy by excited nuclei through interaction among themselves. The rate of this process is measured by *T2*.

The rates of relaxation (T1 and T2) of a hydrogen nucleus depend on the chemical environment in which that nucleus is located. Chemical environment differs among tissues. For example, the chemical environment of a hydrogen nucleus in the spleen differs from that of a hydrogen nucleus in the liver. The relaxation rates of these nuclei differ, and the MR signals given off by these nuclei differ. Liver and spleen have a different signal intensity and a different appearance on the image, enabling the viewer to discriminate between them. Similarly, fat can be separated from muscle, and many tissues can be distinguished from others, based on the rates of the relaxation of their nuclei. Indeed, the most important factor in tissue discrimination is the relaxation times.

The signals produced by MR imaging techniques contain a combination of proton density, T1, and T2 information. By stimulating the nuclei with certain specific radiowave *pulse sequences,* the radio signal that the nuclei release may have more information about proton density, or about T1, or about T2. Therefore one can obtain images weighted toward any one of these three parameters. In most imaging schemes, a short T1 (fast spin-lattice relaxation rate) gives a high MR signal in T1 weighted images. Conversely, a long T2 (slow spin-spin relaxation rate) gives a high signal in T2 weighted images.

Using the data from two or more regular images, computer calculations of pure proton density, T1, or T2 images can be made. However, these calculated images have more *noise* and less resolution than regular MR images.

The final property that influences image appearance is flow. Moving substances, for complex physical reasons, usually have weak MR signals. (With some pulse sequences, this may not be true.) Flowing blood in vessels has a low signal, easily discriminated from surrounding stationary tissues without the need for the contrast agents required by regular radiographic techniques. Stagnant blood (such as an acute blood clot) typically has a high MR signal in most imaging schemes, as a result of its short T1 and long T2. It may be possible to assess vessel patency or determine the rate of blood flow through vessels by employing this property of MR (Fig. 37-4).

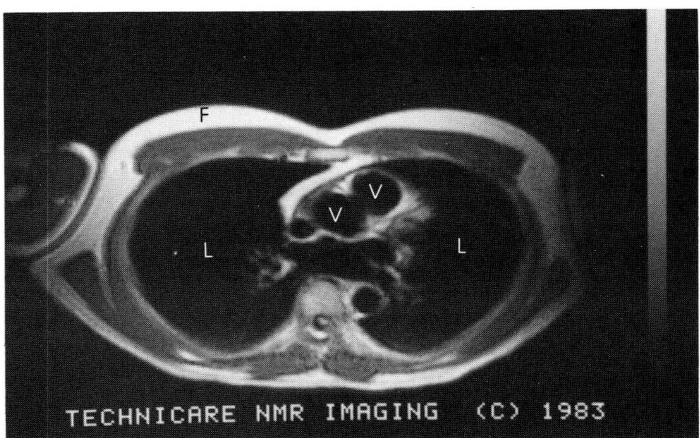

Fig. 37-4. Transverse 0.5 Tesla superconductive MR image through the heart and great vessels. Lungs *(L)* have low signal as a result of low proton density. Fat *(F)* has high signal because of its relaxation rates. Moving blood in vessels *(V)* has low signal from the flow phenomenon.

(Courtesy New York Hospital/Cornell University/Technicare Corp.)

Equipment

Similar to CT, MR requires a patient area (magnet room), a computer room, and an operator's console. A separate diagnostic viewing console is optional.

CONSOLE

The operator's console is used to control the computer. The computer then initiates the appropriate radiowave transmissions, receives the data, and analyzes it. Images are viewed on the operator's console to ensure that the proper part of the patient is being evaluated (Fig. 37-5). Images may be photographed, usually on radiographic films using a multi-image camera.

The diagnostic viewing console may perform the same functions as the operator's console, depending on system configuration, except that usually only the operator's console can control the actual imaging process.

COMPUTER ROOM

The computer room houses the electronics necessary for transmitting the radiowave pulse sequences and receiving and analyzing the MR signal. The *raw data* and the computer-constructed images can be stored on a computer disk temporarily, and are usually transferred to magnetic tape for permanent storage and retrieval.

MAGNET ROOM

The major component of the MR system in the magnet room is the magnet itself. This magnet must be large enough to surround the patient and any antennas that are required for radiowave transmission and reception. Antennas are frequently wound in the shape of a coil. Most often, the patient is placed within the coil, which itself lies within the magnet. Surface coils are placed directly on the patient and image superficial structures. However, the patient and coil must still be within the magnet to be exposed to the proper magnetic field for imaging. The patient lies on the table and is advanced into the magnetic field (Fig. 37-6).

Various magnet types and strengths may be used to provide the strong uniform magnetic field required for MR imaging.

Resistive magnets are simple, although large, electromagnets. They consist of coils of wire. A magnetic field is produced by passing an electric current through wire coils. High magnetic fields are produced by passing a large amount of current through a large number of coils. The electrical resistance of the wire produces heat and limits the maximum magnetic field strength of resistive magnets. The heat produced is conducted away from the magnet by a cooling system.

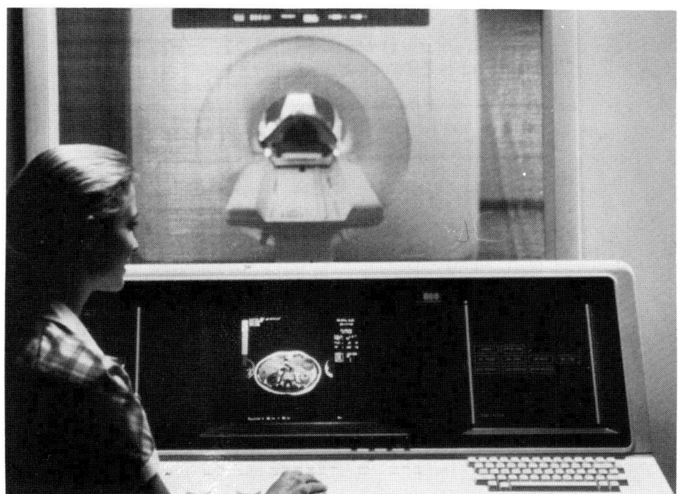

Fig. 37-5. Operator's console (foreground). This device controls the imaging process and allows visualization of images on a television monitor. The images may be manipulated to bring out the desired information. Patient within an MR imager is seen in the background through a screen shielding antenna from outside radio interference.

(Courtesy General Electric Co.)

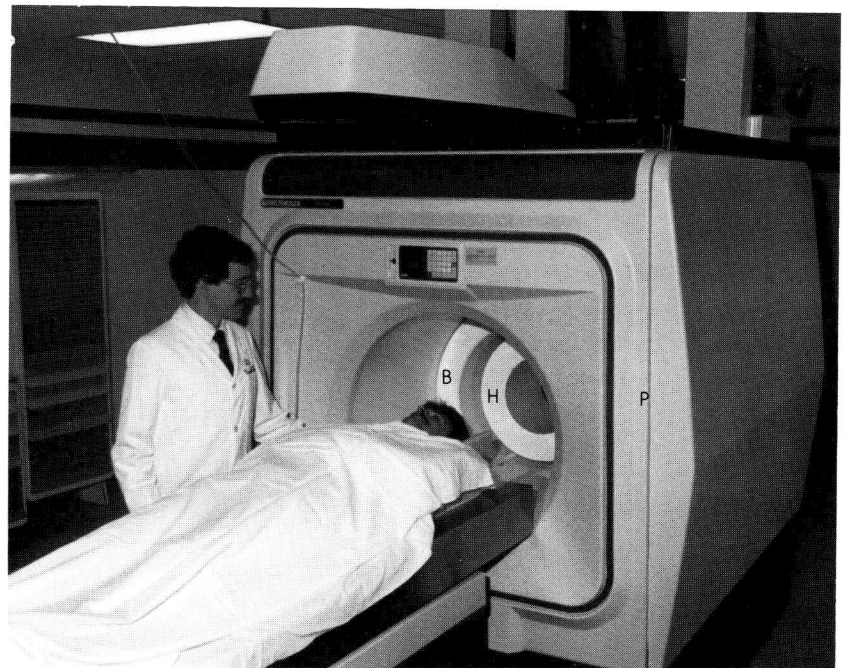

Fig. 37-6. Patient prepared for MR imaging. A protective housing *(P)* covers the magnet. The antenna coils for body *(B)* and head *(H)* imaging are seen within the magnet. The head coil is removed when body imaging is performed.

Superconductive (cryogenic) magnets are also electromagnets. However, their wire loops are cooled to very low temperatures with liquid helium and liquid nitrogen to reduce the electrical resistance. This permits higher magnetic field strengths with superconductive magnets than with resistive magnets.

Permanent magnets are a third method of producing the magnetic field. A permanent magnet has a constant field that does not require additional electricity or cooling to low temperatures. Early designs of permanent magnets were extremely heavy, even compared with the massive superconductive and resistive units, causing difficulties with placement in hospitals. With improvements in technology, permanent magnets may become more competitive with the other magnet types. Permanent magnets have the advantage that their magnetic field does not extend as far away from the magnet *(fringe field)* as do the magnetic fields of the other types. Fringe fields are a problem because of their effect on nearby electronic equipment.

Various MR systems operate at different magnetic field strengths. Magnetic field strength is measured in *Tesla* or *gauss*. Most MR imaging has been performed with field strengths ranging from 0.1 to 1.5 Tesla, although higher strength MR units are under development. Resistive systems generally do not exceed 0.15 Tesla, and permanent magnet systems do not exceed 0.3 Tesla. Higher field strengths require superconductive technology.

The choice of optimum field strength for imaging is controversial. Higher field strengths lead to increased MR signal, which can be used to improve image sharpness or obtain the image data faster. However, some authorities argue that higher field strengths lead to reduced tissue contrast.

Regardless of magnet type, MR imaging units are relatively difficult to locate in a hospital. Current units are quite heavy, in the neighborhood of up to 10 tons for resistive and superconductive magnets and approximately 100 tons for some permanent magnets. Some hospital structures will not support this weight without reinforcement. With resistive and superconductive magnets, the fringe field extends in all directions. These fringe fields may interfere with nearby electronic or computer equipment, such as television monitors and computer tapes. In addition, metal moving through the magnetic fringe field, such as automobiles or elevators, may cause ripples in the field, similar to the ripples occurring when a pebble is thrown into a pond. These ripples can be carried into the center of the magnet where they distort the field and ruin the images. Thus MR sites must be located far enough away from such moving metal objects to prevent this problem. Shielding of the magnetic fringe field to prevent its extension beyond the patient area continues to be developed to solve this difficulty.

The radiowaves used in MR imaging may be the same as those used for other nearby radio applications. These stray radiowaves from outside sources could be picked up by the MR antenna coils and interfere with normal image production. Many MR facilities require special room construction to shield the antenna from outside radio interference, which adds to the cost of the installation.

Biomedical Effects of MR

At the current levels of magnetic field strength and radiowave energy transmission, there are no known hazards intrinsic to patient exposure to MR imaging. However, the magnetic field itself is potentially hazardous to certain patients who have artificial metallic or electronic devices within them. For example, cardiac pacemakers may be adversely affected by the strong magnetic fields. Aneurysm clips on blood vessels within the skull could be twisted by the magnetic field and vessels could be torn. Therefore caution must be used in allowing patients or visitors to enter the magnet room.

Examination Protocols

INSTRUMENT PARAMETERS

The availability of many adjustable parameters makes MR a complex imaging technique. Knowledge of the patient's clinical condition or probable diseases is important in choosing the proper technique and imaging the correct area of the body.

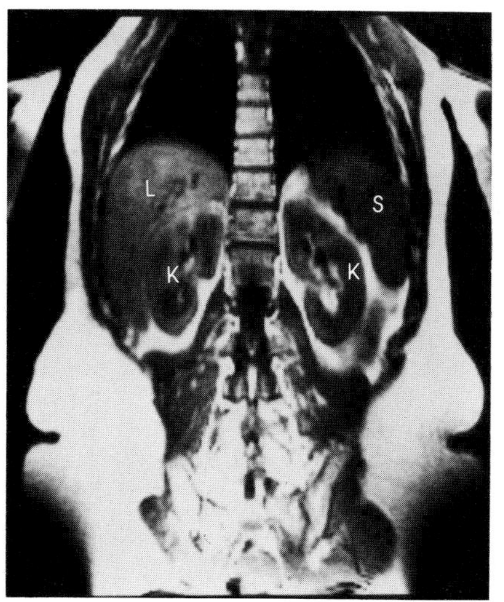

Fig. 37-7. Normal coronal 1.5 Tesla superconductive MR image. Excellent visualization of the liver *(L)*, kidneys *(K)*, and spleen *(S)*. This degree of resolution in a coronal image would be difficult to obtain by reformatting a series of transverse CT slices.

(Courtesy General Electric Co., 1984.)

A choice must be made whether to obtain a single slice image through a specific position in the body or to obtain multiple slices. Of course, a large area can be covered by making a series of single slices, just like CT. However, each MR slice requires considerable time to acquire, usually 2 to 5 minutes, compared with less than 1 minute for a CT slice. To improve throughput, MR units can obtain multiple slices in one data acquisition. Although it may take a long time to acquire this much data, the average time per slice is reduced.

The operator may choose to obtain MR images in the sagittal, coronal, or transverse planes. These are independently acquired images with equal resolution in any plane (Fig. 37-7). This differs from CT in which data can only be obtained in the transverse plane. Sagittal and coronal CT images can be generated by reformatting the data from a series of transverse slices, usually with a loss of resolution.

Slice thickness is important in the visualization of pathology. More MR signal is available from a thicker slice than a thinner slice so that thicker slices may provide more pleasing images that are less grainy. However, small pathologic lesions may be hidden by the surrounding tissues in the thicker slices. Therefore slice thickness may be adjusted, depending on the type of lesion under investigation.

Another important parameter is the overall imaging time. As imaging time (per slice) is lengthened, more MR signal is available for analysis. Image quality thus improves with increased signal. However, fewer patients can be imaged when extended data acquisitions are performed. In addition, patient motion increases with prolonged imaging times, reducing image quality.

The radiowave pulse sequence is a crucial parameter in MR imaging. Depending on the choice of pulse sequence, the resulting images may be more strongly weighted toward proton density, T1, or T2 information. A pathologic lesion may be easily recognized or difficult to see depending on the relative emphasis given to these factors. It is not unusual for a lesion to stand out dramatically when one pulse sequence is used, yet be nearly invisible (same MR signal as surrounding normal tissue) when a different pulse sequence is employed. Considerable research is in progress to determine the optimum pulse sequences for scanning various patient problems (Fig. 37-8).

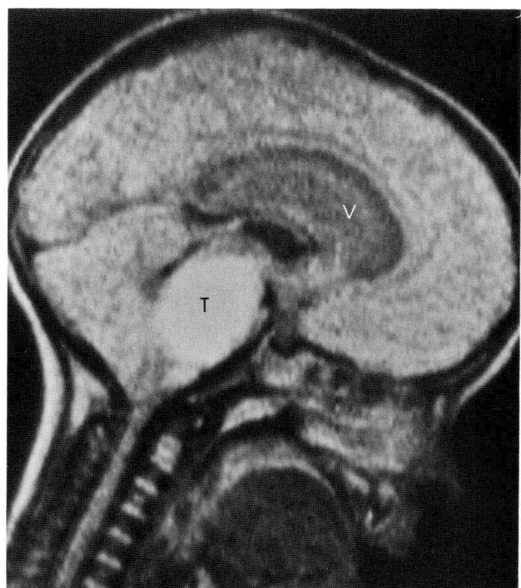

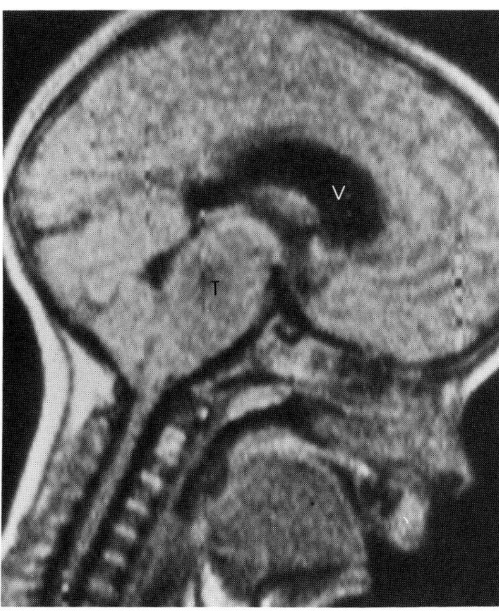

Fig. 37-8. Sagittal 0.15 Tesla resistive MR images using two different radiowave pulse sequences from a child with a brainstem glioma. There is dramatic contrast between the tumor *(T)* and normal brain in the left image; the lesion is much less obvious using the pulse sequence of the right image. Choice of pulse sequence is critical. These images also demonstrate the superiority of MR over CT in posterior fossa lesions due to lack of bone artifact. *V,* Cerebrospinal fluid in ventricle (which also changes appearance with change in pulse sequence).

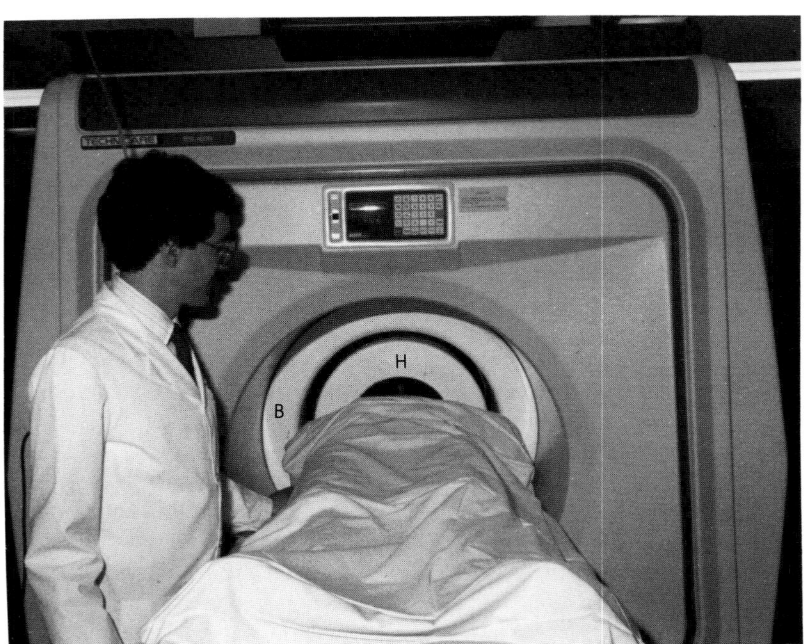

Fig. 37-9. Patient inside head *(H)* antenna coil. Body *(B)* antenna coil also shown. Some patients cannot be scanned because of claustrophobia.

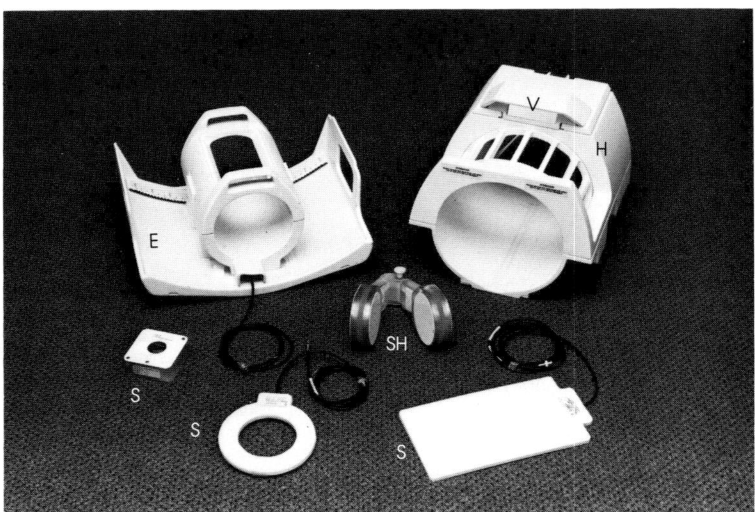

Fig. 37-10. Various coils used in MR imaging. Extremity coil *(E)* is used for knees and ankles. Head coil *(H)* has open construction and mirror *(arrowhead)*, allowing patient to see through coil to reduce claustrophobia. Shoulder coil *(SH)* fits over shoulder. Three shapes of general purpose surface coils *(S)* may be applied directly over the superficial part to be imaged, such as the wrist, orbit, or spine. The shoulder coil is a form of surface coil, because the antenna does not encircle the imaged part. Any coil can act as both a radio wave transmitter and a receiver, though often an encircling coil is used as transmitter when surface coils are employed as receivers.

POSITIONING

Patient positioning is usually straightforward with MR units. In general, the patient lies supine on a table that is subsequently advanced into the magnetic field. It is important to check that the patient has no contraindications to MR imaging such as a cardiac pacemaker or intracranial aneurysm clips. Occasionally, patient positions other than the supine position are employed. For example, the patient may be turned partly to the side to obtain oblique images. Prone or decubitus positioning also may be used to shift structures under the influence of gravity or for patient comfort. Claustrophobia may be a problem for some patients, because the imaging area is tunnel-shaped in most MR system configurations (Fig. 37-9).

COILS

The body part to be examined determines the shape of the antenna coil to be used for imaging. Most coils are round or oval shaped, and the body part to be examined is inserted into the coil's open center. Some coils, rather than encircling the body part, are placed directly on the patient over the area of interest. These "surface coils" are best for thin body parts, such as the extremities, or superficial portions of a larger body structure, such as the orbit within the head or the spine within the torso (Fig. 37-10).

CONTRAST AGENTS

Contrast agents that widen the signal differences in MR images between various normal and abnormal structures are a continuing area of research and development. The perfect agent for oral administration to identify bowel loops in MR scans has not yet been identified. In CT scanning, high-attenuation oral contrast clearly differentiates bowel from surrounding lower attenuation structures. However, in MR scans, the bowel may lie adjacent to normal or pathologic structures of low, medium, and high signal intensity, and these intensities may change as images of varying T1 and T2 weighting are obtained. It is difficult to develop an agent that provides good contrast between the bowel and all other structures under these circumstances. Air, water, fatty liquids (e.g., mineral oil), and solutions of dilute iron (e.g., Geritol) have all been employed, none with complete success.

As of this writing, the only intravenous MR contrast agent approved in the United States for routine clinical use is gadolinium-DTPA, although other gadolinium-containing compounds are under development. Gadolinium is a metal with *paramagnetic* effects. Pharmacologically, gadolinium-DTPA acts very much like radiographic iodinated intravenous agents: it distributes through the vascular system, its major route of excretion is the urine, and it respects the blood-brain barrier (that is, it does not leak out from the blood vessels into the brain substance unless the barrier has been damaged by a pathologic process). Gadolinium-DTPA has lower toxicity and fewer side effects than the intravenous iodinated contrast media used in radiography and CT.

Gadolinium compounds are used most frequently in evaluation of the central nervous system. The most important clinical action of gadolinium compounds is to shorten T1. In T1-weighted images, this provides a high-signal, high-contrast focus in areas where gadolinium has accumulated by leaking through the broken blood-brain barrier into the brain substance (Fig. 37-11). Since T1-weighted images can be obtained much faster than T2-weighted images, the use of gadolinium contrast agents can improve throughput if T2-weighted imaging sequences are eliminated. In addition, gadolinium-enhanced T1-weighted images are better at separating brain tumors or metastases from their surrounding edema than are routine T2-weighted images. Gadolinium improves the visualization of small tumors, or tumors that have signal intensity similar to normal brain, such as meningiomas.

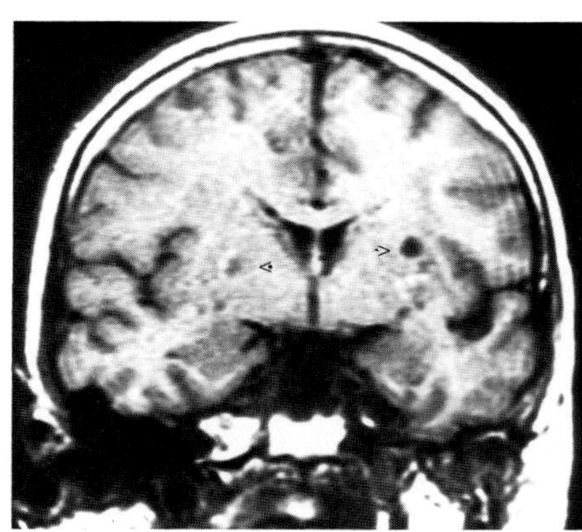

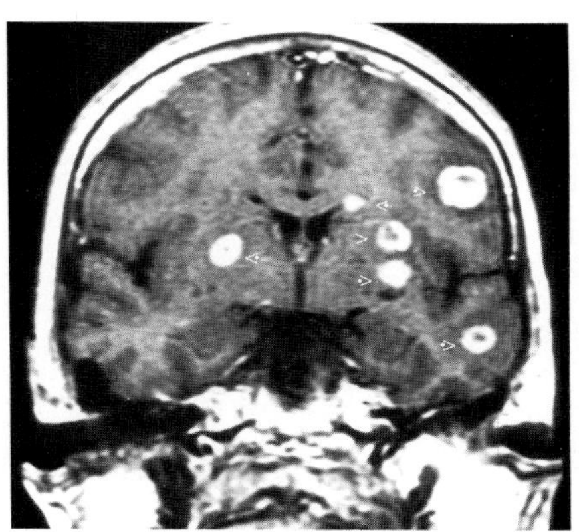

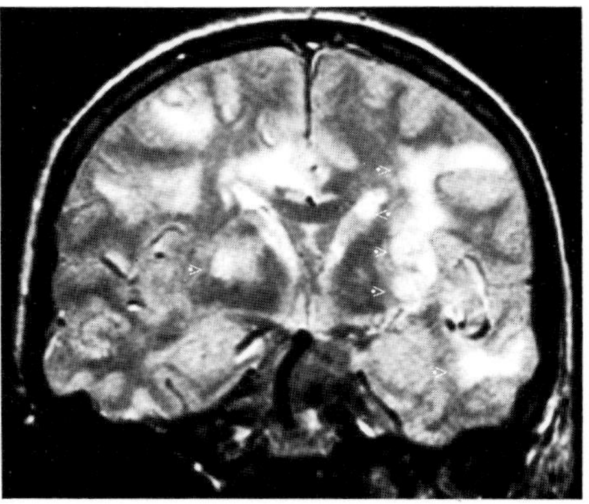

Fig. 37-11. Use of gadolinium intravenous contrast for lesion enhancement. Coronal 1.5 Tesla superconductive images of the brain. Left image shows relatively T1-weighted sequence. Two brain metastases *(arrowheads)* are identified as focal areas of low signal. Middle image employed same parameters after intravenous gadolinium contrast. Previously seen metastases are more conspicuous and additional metastases are recognized *(arrowheads)*. Right image is T2 weighted. High-signal areas *(arrowheads)* represent metastases and surrounding edema; identification of focal lesion size and precise location is more difficult. In addition, scanning of entire brain took three times as long with the T2-weighted sequence as with the T1-weighted sequence. Additional high-signal intensity areas on T2-weighted image represent edema from focal lesions seen on other slices in the gadolinium-enhanced series.

GATING

Gated images are another technique for improving image quality in areas of the body where involuntary patient motion is a problem. A patient can hold his head still for a prolonged data acquisition, but he cannot stop his heartbeat nor can he stop breathing for the several minutes required to obtain an image. This is a problem when images of the chest or upper abdomen are desired. If special techniques are not employed, part of the MR signal may be obtained when the heart is contracted (systole) and part when the heart is relaxed (diastole). If this information is combined into one image, the image of the heart will be blurred. This is analogous to photographing a moving subject with a long shutter speed. Similar problems occur with the different phases of respiration.

To solve this problem, *gating* techniques organize the signal so that only the signal received during a specific part of the cardiac or respiratory cycle is used for image production (Fig. 37-12).

OTHER CONSIDERATIONS

In the beginning of MR imaging, long imaging times were required to obtain enough information to reconstruct the sectional images, although later multiple images could be obtained during the course of one lengthy (measured in minutes) imaging run. For most routine imaging, this remains the standard. With advances in technology, however, it has become possible to quickly (within seconds) obtain enough data to reconstruct an image, using special fast-imaging pulse sequences. These fast-imaging pulse sequences are becoming more popular for specialized applications. In many such sequences, fluid has very high signal intensity. This can produce a myelogram-like effect in studies of the spine or an arthrogram-like effect when joint fluid is evaluated (Fig. 37-13).

Quality assurance is important in a complex technology such as MR. The calibration of the unit is generally performed by service personnel. However, routine scanning of phantoms can be useful to detect problems that may develop.

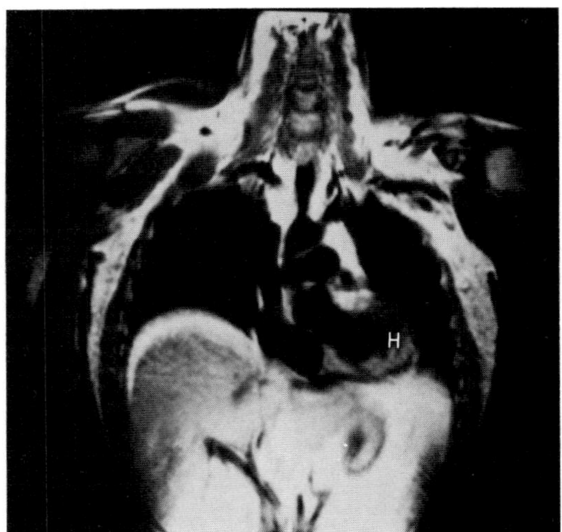

Fig. 37-12. Gated coronal 1.5 Tesla superconductive MR image of a normal heart. Heart muscle *(H)* is "frozen" in one phase of the cardiac cycle to ensure a sharp picture.

(Courtesy General Electric Co.)

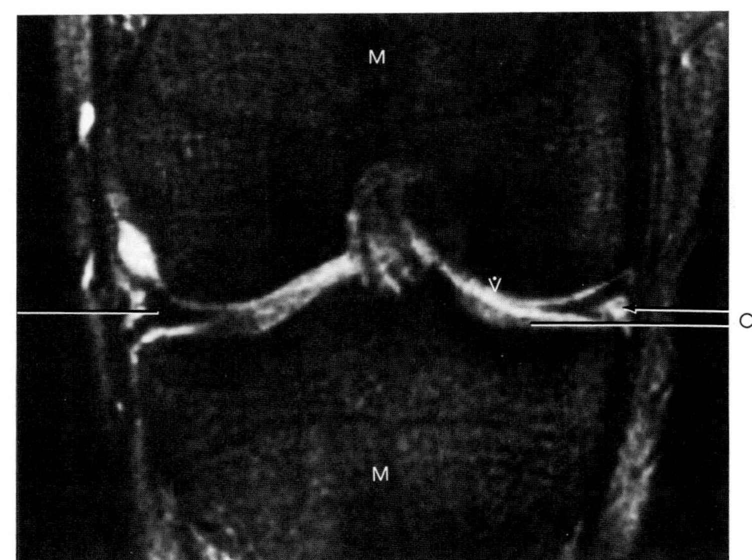

Fig. 37-13. Coronal 1.5 Tesla superconductive, fast-sequence image of the knee. Small amount of high-signal intensity joint fluid *(arrowhead)* outlines joint surfaces. Note articular cartilage *(C)* with slightly lower signal intensity and fibrocartilaginous lateral meniscus *(L)* with very low-signal intensity. Medial meniscus is torn as evidenced by high-signal intensity fluid within tear *(arrow)*. With fast sequences, fat may not show typical high intensity, as demonstrated by bone marrow *(M)*.

Clinical Applications

CENTRAL NERVOUS SYSTEM

MR imaging is superior to CT in imaging the posterior fossa, the portion of the brain that includes the cerebellum and brainstem. *Artifact* from the dense bone of the surrounding skull obscures this area with CT. There is very little MR signal from bone so that this area is artifact free with MR imaging.

In general, the absence of bone artifact with MR is a distinct advantage over CT. However, the inability to image calcified structures can be a disadvantage when the lesion is more easily recognized because of its calcium content. Lesions such as calcified granulomas of the lung or calcification in certain tumors are more difficult to detect with MR than with CT.

MR is playing an increasing role in the routine examination of the brain while reducing the role of CT in this area. Because there is more natural contrast among tissues with MR than with CT, the differentiation of gray matter from white matter in the brain is better with MR (Fig. 37-14). This enables MR to be more sensitive than CT in detecting white matter disease, such as multiple sclerosis.

Primary and metastatic brain tumors, pituitary tumors, and acoustic neuromas (tumors of the eighth cranial nerve) are generally better demonstrated by MR than CT. The use of gadolinium-based contrast agents has improved the ability of MR to identify meningiomas. MR can detect cerebral infarction earlier than can CT, but both tests provide similar information in subacute and chronic strokes.

MR has been successfully used to image the spinal cord. The absence of bone artifact allows excellent visualization of the contents of the neural canal. In addition, the technique can separate the spinal cord from the surrounding cerebrospinal fluid (CSF) without the necessity (as is required on CT) of contrast agents injected directly into the CSF (myelogram) (Fig. 37-15). MR is sensitive in the detection of spinal cord tumors and cystic changes of the spine (syringomyelia). MR is also valuable in the detection of degenerated and herniated spinal disks.

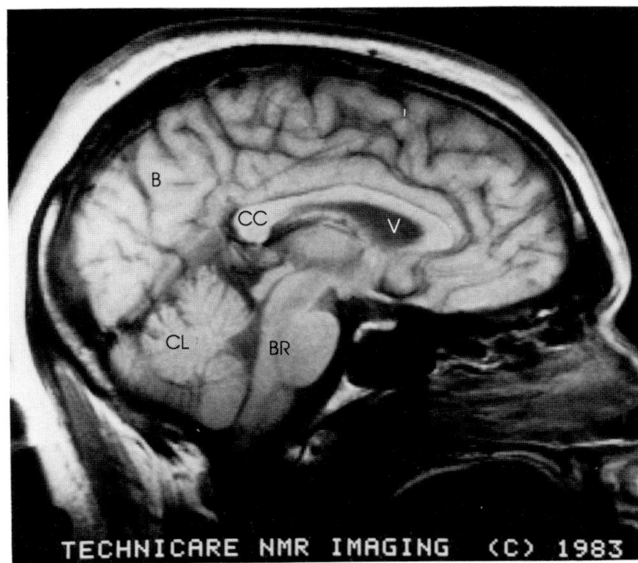

Fig. 37-14. Normal sagittal 1.5 Tesla superconductive MR image of the head. Excellent separation of white matter in corpus callosum *(CC)* from brain *(B)*. *CL*, Cerebellum; *BR*, brainstem; *V*, ventricle.

(Courtesy Technicare Corporation.)

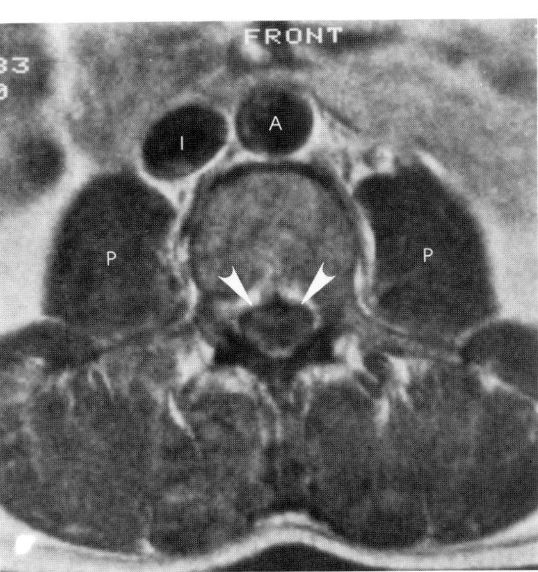

Fig. 37-15. Normal transverse 0.5 Tesla superconductive MR image through the spine. The spinal cord *(arrowheads)* is seen clearly without the use of contrast agents. *I*, Inferior vena cava; *A*, aorta; *P*, psoas muscle.

(Courtesy Siemens Medical Systems, Inc.)

CHEST

The chest would seem to be an ideal area for MR examination. The lungs have low signal as a result of low proton density, and the flowing blood in the great vessels of the chest also has a low MR signal. The heart muscle is well outlined by the lung and moving blood within the chambers. Furthermore, examination of the mediastinum is potentially fruitful since the normal structures of blood vessels and airways are of low signal. Any tumors of the mediastinum would be easily seen as areas of MR signal standing out against the normal low signal surroundings. The ability of MR to image in multiple planes may be helpful in evaluating tumor spread in the thoracic inlet, chest wall, or brachial plexus region.

However, difficulties with chest imaging remain because of cardiac and respiratory motion. Cardiac gating has markedly improved visualization of the heart with demonstration of septal defects and the cardiac valve leaflets. This is of great value in the study of congenital heart disease. Evaluation of the heart muscle for ischemia or infarction may require MR contrast agents. Respiratory gating should also help chest images.

ABDOMEN

Respiratory and cardiac motion also detract from upper abdominal images. Again, gating should be of assistance. There is evidence that MR is more sensitive than CT in detecting primary and metastatic tumors of the liver. The suprarenals (adrenals), kidneys, and retroperitoneal structures such as lymph nodes are well seen, but there is limited evidence that MR is superior to CT in this area. Visualization of the normal pancreas has been difficult with MR.

MR has some ability to predict the histologic diagnosis of certain abnormalities. For example, hepatic hemangiomas (common benign tumors of the liver) have a distinctive MR appearance that can be helpful in ruling out other causes of hepatic masses.

PELVIS

Respiratory motion has very little effect on the structures in the pelvis, leading to improved visualization compared to upper abdominal structures. The ability of MR to image in the coronal and sagittal planes is helpful in examining the curved surfaces in the pelvis. For example, bladder tumors are well shown, including those at the dome and the base of the bladder that can be difficult to evaluate in the transverse dimension (Fig. 37-16). In the prostate and female genital tract, MR is useful in detecting neoplasm and its spread.

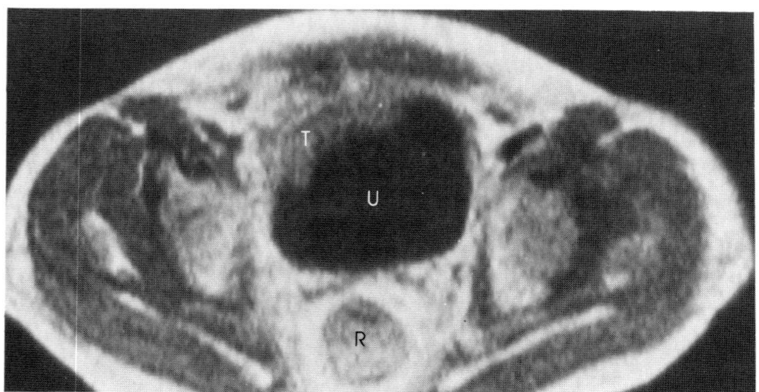

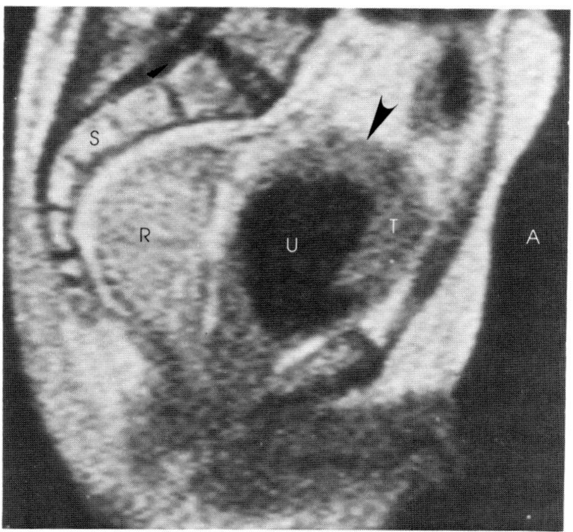

Fig. 37-16. Transverse *(upper image)* and sagittal *(lower image)* 0.15 Tesla resistive MR images of the pelvis. A bladder tumor *(T)* is easily seen against the lower-signal urine *(U)* in the bladder. The sagittal image shows extension of the tumor over the dome of the bladder *(arrowhead)*, a finding often difficult to see on transverse images alone. *R*, Rectum; *S*, sacrum; *A*, anterior surface of body.

LIMBS

MR produces excellent images of the limbs because they are free of involuntary motion and there is excellent MR contrast among the soft tissues. The lack of bone artifact on MR permits excellent visualization of the bone marrow (Fig. 37-17). Dense cortical bone frequently hides the marrow space from plain film evaluation and occasionally from CT. On the other hand, because of the lower MR signal from calcium, calcium within tumors is better seen with CT.

Overall, the ability to image in multiple planes, along with excellent visualization of soft tissues and bone marrow, has led to a rapidly expanding role for MR in musculoskeletal imaging. It is particularly valuable in studying joints and is replacing arthrography, and to a lesser extent, arthroscopy, in evaluation of the injured knee. Local staging of soft tissue and bone tumors is best accomplished with MR. Early detection of ischemic necrosis of bone is a strength of MR.

VESSELS

The contrast between soft tissue structures and the typical low signal of flowing blood gives MR the ability to visualize thrombosis within or tumor invasion of the major vessels, such as the venae cavae. Vascular anomalies, dissections, and coarctations also can be well evaluated by MR. Special pulse sequences under development allow MR visualization of moving blood within the vascular system, and may permit noninvasive angiogram-like images of the vessels.

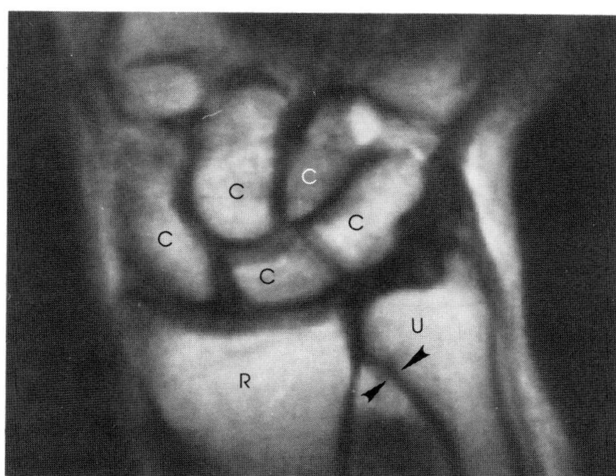

Fig. 37-17. Coronal 0.5 Tesla superconductive MR image of the wrist using a surface coil to improve visualization of superficial structures. Marrow within the carpal bones *(C)*, radius *(R)*, and ulna *(U)* has high signal as a result of its fat content. A thin black line of low-signal cortex *(arrowheads)* surrounds the marrow cavity of each bone.

(Courtesy Siemens Medical Systems, Inc.)

Spectroscopy

In general, for MR imaging, we assume that each nucleus in a specific small area in space is exposed to the same magnetic field, and thus precesses at and releases radiowaves of a particular frequency. If the magnetic field varies across the imaging volume in a known way, frequency can be used as one determinant of the location from which a signal is originating. There is a one-to-one relationship between frequency and location that is an integral part of creating the MR image. In actuality, however, each nucleus in a small area in space does not see precisely the same magnetic field. The externally imposed field is the same, but the magnetic environment of the nuclei differ, depending on the magnetic effects of other nearby atoms. These differences in frequencies are very small, and in general do not affect the image significantly; each signal is still placed in the correct position in the image. If we depart from imaging, however, and instead produce a detailed graph of signal strength against frequency, we are performing magnetic resonance spectroscopy and the graphs produced are called spectra.

Spectroscopy is essentially a tool for clinical analysis that can determine the relative quantity of chemical substances within a volume of tissue. Because the frequency differences are small, and electronic noise is relatively high, large volumes of tissue must be studied to receive enough total signal to produce useful spectra. In addition, magnetic field strengths of 1.5 Tesla or greater are required. Nevertheless, it is possible to obtain spectra from organs (e.g., muscle, liver) or large masses to examine normal physiologic changes (e.g., with exercise), chemical alterations in persons with metabolic diseases, or differences in chemical composition between normal tissue and tumors or other pathologic processes (Fig. 36-18).

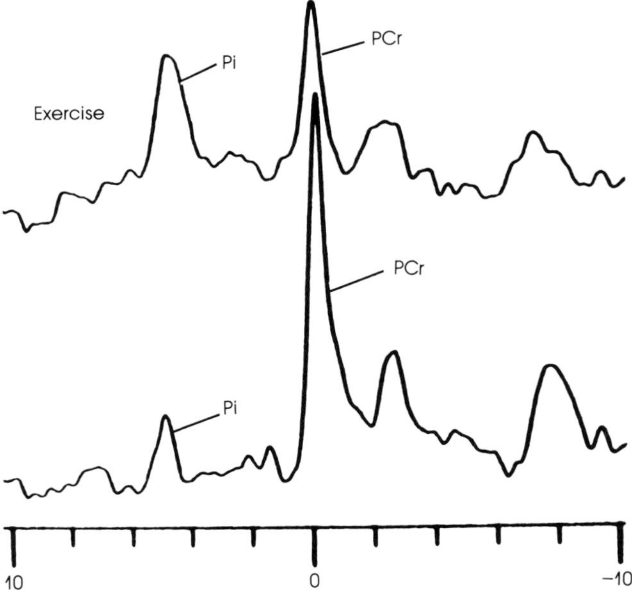

Fig. 37-18. Spectra from human muscle before *(lower line)* and during *(upper line)* exercise. Thin horizontal lines represent separate baselines for each spectrum. Each peak represents a different chemical species and the area under the peak down to the baseline indicates the amount of substance present. Inorganic phosphate (Pi) peak increases with exercise as energy-rich phosphocreatine (PCr) is used to provide energy for muscle contraction.

Summary

MR is an exciting new form of imaging that examines properties of tissue never before visualized. Dozens of publications have attested to MR's efficacy in evaluating various clinical conditions. However, it is more difficult to prove that MR is clinically superior to other imaging modalities; this analysis must await the completion of extensive research. In some cases, various modalities are complementary (Fig. 37-19).

MR is an expensive imaging technology. As a result of recent increased emphasis on cost constraints, MR will not spread as fast as it otherwise might have. MR also will have to compete with other modalities for an imaging "niche." Nevertheless, it is clear that MR will be the technique of choice in many clinical situations.

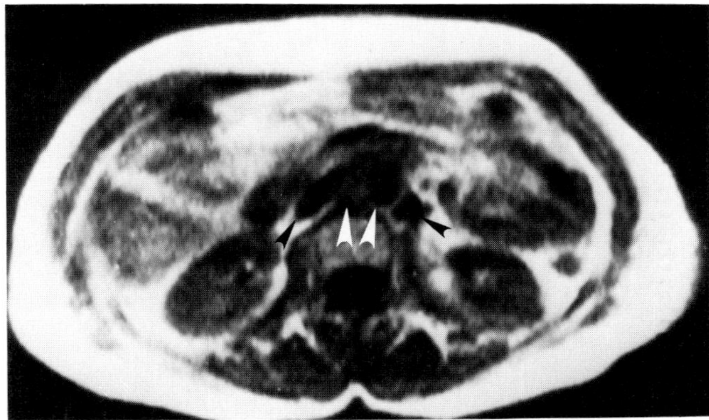

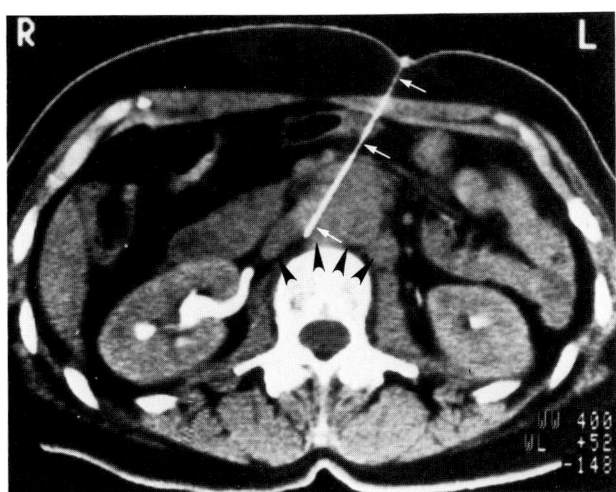

Fig. 37-19. Middle-aged woman with retroperitoneal lymph node metastases from ovarian cancer. From reader's left to right (patient's right to left), *arrowheads* represent inferior vena cava, metastatic tumor, aorta, and an anomalous vein. MR image *(upper)* better separates flowing blood (dark) from tumor (gray) and shows that anomalous vein is not a second site of metastasis. CT image *(lower)* indicates abnormal retroperitoneal structures but requires a bolus injection of intravenous contrast (not shown) to differentiate vessels from tumor. However, CT can more easily be used to guide a needle *(white arrows)* for biopsy under local anesthesia.

Definition of Terms

antenna A device for transmitting or receiving radio waves.

artifact A spurious finding in or distortion of an image.

attenuation The reduction in energy or amount of a beam of radiation when it passes through tissue or other substances.

contrast The degree of difference between two substances in some parameter. The parameter varies on the technique used, for example, attenuation in radiographic techniques or MR signal strength in MR imaging.

cryogenic Relating to extremely low temperature. See *superconductive magnet*.

frequency The number of times that a process repeats itself in a given period of time. For example, the frequency of a radio wave is the number of complete waves per second.

fringe field That portion of the magnetic field extending away from the confines of the magnet that cannot be used for imaging but can affect nearby equipment or personnel.

gating Organizing the data so that the information used to construct the image comes from the same point in the cycle of a repeating motion, such as a heartbeat. The moving object is "frozen" at that phase of its motion, reducing image blurring.

gauss A unit of magnetic field strength. See *Tesla*.

magnetic resonance (MR) The process by which certain nuclei, when placed in a magnetic field, can absorb and release energy in the form of radio waves. This technique can be used for chemical analysis or for the production of cross-sectional images of body parts. Computer analysis of the radio wave data is required.

noise Random contributions to the total signal that arise from stray external radio waves, imperfect electronic apparatus, etc. Noise cannot be eliminated, but it can be minimized. Noise tends to degrade the image by interfering with accurate measurement of the true MR signal, similar to the difficulty in maintaining a clear conversation in a noisy room.

nuclear magnetic resonance (NMR) Another name for *magnetic resonance*.

nucleus The central portion of an atom composed of protons and neutrons.

paramagnetic Referring to materials that alter the magnetic field of nearby nuclei. Paramagnetic substances are not themselves directly imaged by MR, but instead change the signal intensity of the tissue where they localize, thus acting as MR contrast agents. Paramagnetic agents shorten both the T1 and T2 of the tissues they affect, actions which tend to have opposing effects on signal intensity. In clinical practice, agents are administered in a concentration in which either T1 or T2 shortening predominates, usually the former to provide high signal on T1-weighted images.

permanent magnet An object that produces a magnetic field without requiring an external electricity supply.

precession The rotation of an object around the direction of a force acting on that object. This should not be confused with the axis of rotation of the object itself. For example, a spinning top rotates on its own axis, but it may also precess (wobble) around the direction of the force of gravity that is acting on it.

proton density A measure of proton (i.e., hydrogen, since its nucleus is a single proton) concentration (number of nuclei per given volume). One of the major determinants of MR signal strength in hydrogen imaging.

pulse A short burst of radio waves. If the radio waves are of the appropriate frequency, they can give energy to nuclei that are within a magnetic field by the process of *magnetic resonance*. The length of the pulse determines the amount of energy given to the nuclei.

pulse sequence A series of radio wave pulses designed to excite nuclei in such a way that their energy release has varying contribution from proton density, T1, or T2 processes.

raw data The information obtained by radio reception of the MR signal as stored by a computer. Specific computer manipulation of this data is required to construct an image from it.

relaxation Return of excited nuclei to their normal unexcited state by the release of energy.

relaxation time A measure of the rate at which nuclei, after stimulation, release their extra energy.

resistive magnet A simple electromagnet in which electricity passing through coils of wire produces a magnetic field.

resonance The process of energy absorption by an object that is tuned to absorb energy of a specific frequency only; all other frequencies will not affect the object. For example, if one tuning fork is struck in a room full of tuning forks, only those forks tuned to that identical frequency will vibrate (resonate).

signal In MR, the radio wave that is transmitted by nuclei on relaxation.

slice A cross-sectional image. Can also refer to the thin section of the body from which data is acquired to produce the image.

spectroscopy Science of analyzing the components of an electromagnetic wave, usually after its interaction with some substance (to obtain information about that substance).

spin density a measure of the concentration of nuclei (number of the nuclei per given volume) contributing to the MR signal by release of energy following *resonance*. One of the major determinants of MR signal strength.

spin-lattice relaxation The release of energy by excited nuclei to their general environment. One of the major determinants of MR signal strength. *T1* is a rate constant measuring spin-lattice relaxation.

spin-spin relaxation The release of energy by excited nuclei by interaction among themselves. One of the major determinants of MR signal strength. *T2* is a rate constant measuring spin-spin relaxation.

superconductive magnet An electromagnet in which the coils of wire are cooled to extremely low temperature so that the resistance to the conduction of electricity is nearly eliminated (superconductive).

T1 A rate constant measuring *spin-lattice relaxation*.

T2 A rate constant measuring *spin-spin relaxation*.

Tesla A unit of magnetic field strength. One Tesla equals 10,000 *gauss* or 10 kilogauss (other units of magnetic field strength). The earth's magnetic field approximates 0.5 gauss.

SELECTED BIBLIOGRAPHY

Alfidi RJ, et al: MR angiography of peripheral, carotid, and coronary arteries, AJR 149:1097-1109, 1987.

Axel L, editor: Glossary of MR terms, Reston, Va, 1986, American College of Radiology.

Bellon EM, et al: Magnetic resonance imaging of internal derangements of the knee, RadioGraphics 8:95-118, 1988.

Bloch F: Nuclear induction, Physiol Rev 70:460-473, 1946.

Boechat MI, et al: MR imaging of the abdomen in children, AJR 152:1245-1250, 1989.

Bottomley PA: Human in vivo NMR spectroscopy in diagnostic medicine: clinical tool or research probe? Radiology 170:1-15, 1989.

Brant-Zawadzki M: MR imaging of the brain, Radiology 166:1-10, 1988.

Chezmar JL, et al: Liver and abdominal screening in patients with cancer: CT versus MR imaging, Radiology 168:43-47, 1988.

Council on Scientific Affairs, American Medical Association: Magnetic resonance imaging of the abdomen and pelvis, JAMA 261:420-433, 1989.

Damadian R: Tumor detection by nuclear magnetic resonance, Science 171:1151-1153, 1971.

Ehman RL, et al: MR imaging of the musculoskeletal system: a 5-year appraisal, Radiology 166:313-320, 1988.

Ellis JH, et al: Resistive magnet systems: an MRI "whether" report, Diagn. Imaging 6:60-62, 1984.

Ellis JH, et al: NMR physics for physicians, Indiana Medicine 78:20-28, 1985.

Evens RG, et al: Economic and utilization analysis of MR imaging units in the United States in 1987, Radiology 166:27-30, 1988.

Gefter WB: Chest applications of magnetic resonance imaging: an update, Radiol Clin North Am 26:573-588, 1988.

Glazer GM: MR imaging of the liver, kidneys, and adrenal glands, Radiology 166:303-312, 1988.

Haughton VM: MR imaging of the spine, Radiology 166:297-301, 1988.

Heiken JP, et al: MR imaging of the pelvis, Radiology 166:11-16, 1988.

Kneeland JB, et al: High-resolution MR imaging with local coils, Radiology 171:1-7, 1989.

Lauterbur PC: Image formation by induced local interactions: examples employing nuclear magnetic resonance, Nature 242:190-191, 1973.

Lee SH, et al, editors: Imaging in neuroradiology, parts I and II, Radiol Clin North Am 26:701-1155, 1988.

Margulis AR, et al: Present and future status of MR imaging, AJR 150:487-492, 1988.

Mitchell DG, et al: The biophysical basis of tissue contrast in extracranial MR imaging, AJR 149:831-837, 1987.

Office of Medical Applications of Research, National Institutes of Health: Magnetic resonance imaging, JAMA 259:2132-2138, 1988.

Purcell EM, et al: Resonance absorption by nuclear magnetic moments in a solid, Physiol Rev 69:37-38, 1946.

Runge VM, et al: Gd DTPA clinical efficacy, RadioGraphics 8:147-159, 1988.

Sartoris DJ, et al: MR imaging of the musculoskeletal system: current and future status, AJR 149:457-467, 1987.

Stehling MJ, et al: Whole-body echo-planar MR imaging at 0.5 T, Radiology 170:257-263, 1989.

Young SW: Nuclear magnetic resonance imaging: basic principles, New York, 1984, Raven Press.

Chapter 38

DIAGNOSTIC ULTRASOUND

SANDRA L. HAGEN-ANSERT

Diagnostic *ultrasound,** sometimes called "diagnostic medical sonography," "sonography," or "echocardiography," has become a clinically valuable imaging technique over the past several decades. It differs from diagnostic radiology in that it uses nonionizing, high-frequency sound waves to generate an image of a particular structure. Radiography is useful in the visualization of dense bony structures and air- or contrast-filled structures, such as the lungs, stomach, colon, or small bowel. Ultrasound is employed in the visualization of soft tissue interfaces of homogeneous, fluid-filled, or "solid" organs, tumor masses, or muscles located throughout the body.

In addition, blood flow velocities may be calculated in the vascular and cardiac structures with the *Doppler* technique. The *pulsed-wave, continuous wave,* or color-flow mapping technique has proven to be very useful in determining direction of blood flow, resistance of flow, and regurgitation of flow from one structure to another.

*All italicized terms are defined at the end of this chapter.

The sonographer (an individual who performs ultrasound procedures) approaches the imaging of the body in a different manner than the conventional radiographer or nuclear medicine technologist. The principal difference lies in the knowledge of detailed anatomy and physiology and the three-dimensional understanding of the human body the sonographer must have to produce an adequate image.

Ultrasound has many advantages over other imaging techniques in medicine. One is the portability of most ultrasound equipment—it may be easily moved into the operating room, special care nursery, or intensive care unit or may be manually transported by means of a mobile van service to provide ultrasound coverage for smaller hospitals and clinics. Ultrasound is cost-effective. The versatility of the equipment allows flexibility in schedules; supplies are minimal; equipment price is low compared to other imaging modalities; and a minimal procedure time allows for a more rapid evaluation of patients. Ultrasound has always been known as a noninvasive examination; however, recent developments in transesophageal, transrectal, and endovaginal probe designs have somewhat changed that concept. Further development in high-frequency, millimeter-size *transducers* to be mounted on the tip of an angiographic catheter are likely to be the trend of the future. The advent of lithotripsy has used ultrasonic transducers to locate biliary and renal stones.

Historical Development

The development of materials, testing techniques, and sonar provided a major impetus for the development of diagnostic ultrasound. The equipment was constructed as a result of the defense effort during World War II, so the clinical development lay in the hands of various investigators who would later prove that ultrasound had a valid contribution to make to the medical community. These clinical investigations and the development of ultrasound are vividly described by one of the early pioneers, Joseph Holmes of the University of Colorado, in his article, "Perspectives in Ultrasonography: Early Diagnostic Ultrasonography."

In 1947 Dussick was one of the earliest to apply ultrasound to medical diagnosis when he positioned two transducers on opposite sides of the head to measure ultrasound transmission profiles. He also discovered that tumors and other intracranial lesions could be detected by this technique. In the early 1950s Dussick, with Heuter, Bolt, and Ballantyne, continued to use "through-transmission" techniques and computer analysis to diagnose brain lesions through the intact skull. However, they discontinued their studies after concluding that the technique was too complicated for routine clinical use.

Also in the 1950s William Fry used ultrasound to produce pin-point lesions within the central nervous system of animals by arranging several transducers to focus on a single point. Thus, a destructive lesion could be produced at a selected instance without destroying normal tissue along the path of the beam. Fry also observed that local heating by a second ultrasound beam enhanced echo reflection from adjacent structures. Fry and Russell Meyers applied his "pin-point" lesion technique to the human brain to treat Parkinson's syndrome and other brain lesions. Questions arose as to whether this destruction technique was the most suitable for patients with Parkinson's syndrome, and, again as a result of the requirement for highly skilled investigators to perform the procedure, the project was terminated.

In the late 1940s Douglass Howry (a radiologist), John Wild (a diagnostician interested in tissue characterization), and George Ludwig (interested in reflections from gallstones) independently demonstrated that when ultrasound waves generated by a *piezoelectric* crystal transducer were transmitted into the human body, ultrasound waves would be returned to the transducer from tissue interfaces of different acoustic impedances. At this time equipment development occurred in an effort to transform naval sonar equipment into a clinically useful tool.

In 1948 Howry developed the first ultrasound scanner, consisting of a cattle watering tank with a wooden rail anchored along the side. The transducer carriage moved along the rail in a horizontal plane, while the object to be scanned and the transducer were positioned inside the water tank. Howry also developed the *"compound"* (back and forth) double-scanning motion in an attempt to produce a more realistic anatomic image. The transducer carriage was moved in a 360-degree path around the object to produce reflections from all angular and curved surfaces. Many of the subjects were presurgical candidates, so actual comparison of the tissue could be made with the ultrasound image.

The water-bath equipment was modified for patient evaluation with a half-pan scanner with a plastic window along its flat side. The membrane was then oiled, and the patient pressed his abdomen flush against it. The transducer rotated through a 180-degree arc with a 4-inch compound sector.

Along with its medical applications, veterinarians also began using ultrasound to determine the lean to fat ratio of cattle and other animals ready for slaughter.

In 1954 echocardiographic techniques were developed by Hertz and Edler in Sweden. The investigators were able to distinguish normal heart valvular motion from the thickened, calcified valve motion seen in patients with rheumatic heart disease. In 1957 the early obstetric contact-compound scanner was built by Tom Brown and Ian Donald in Scotland. The development of the contact scanner in North America came in 1962 from the University of Colorado. This equipment had a transducer that moved in a mechanical sector scan 30 degrees to each side of the perpendicular, while the carriage moved over the surface to be scanned. The initial evaluation of the pregnant woman revealed the placenta localization, fetal age, and gross anomalies of the fetus. Shortly thereafter, the same engineers from the University of Colorado built the first commercial Physionics ultrasound system, which was later acquired by the Picker Corporation for distribution throughout the country (Fig. 38-1).

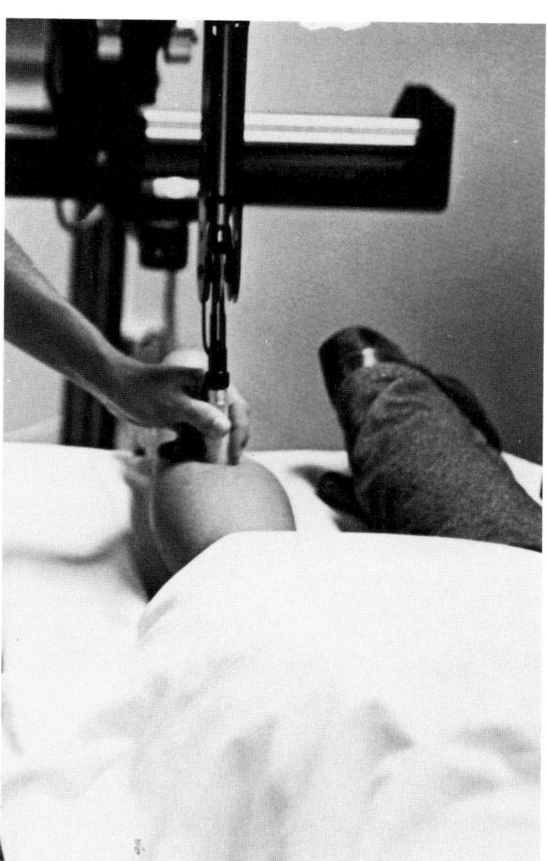

Fig. 38-1. The first commercially available diagnostic ultrasound equipment was produced by Physionics Corp., later to become part of Picker Medical Products. This is representative of the contact B-scan equipment. The transducer was mounted on a fixed carriage that was manually moved in small increments across the area to be scanned.

Meanwhile, in Australia in 1959, Kossoff, Robinson, and Garrett developed diagnostic B-scanners with the use of a water bath to improve *resolution* of the image. This group was also responsible for the introduction of *gray-scale* imaging with techniques first described in 1972 (Figs. 38-2 to 38-4).

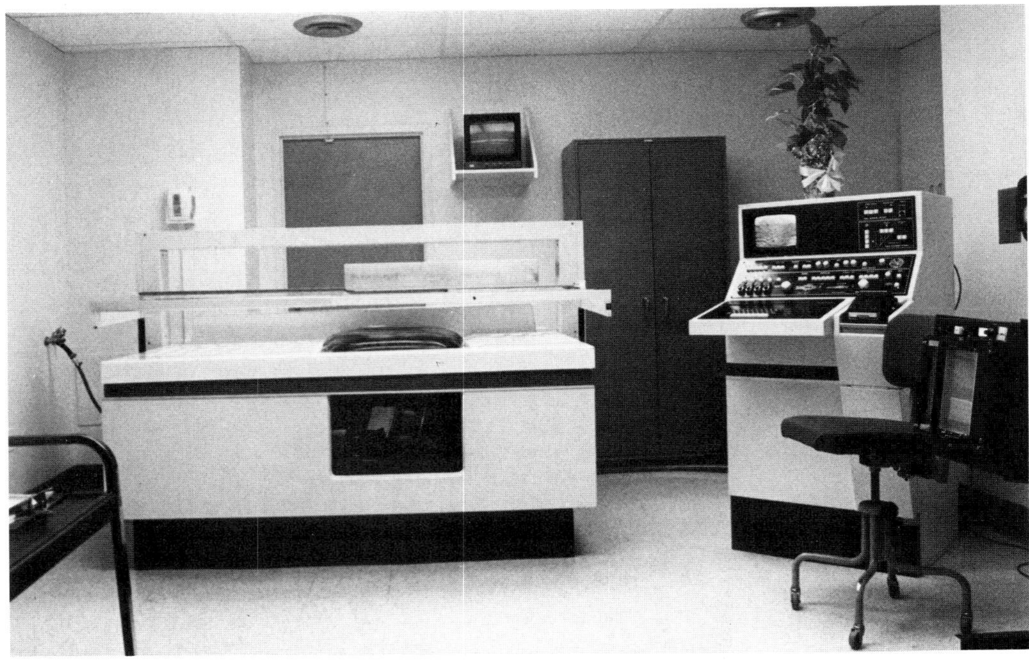

Fig. 38-2. The U.I. Octoson was developed in Australia. This unique ultrasound equipment had eight transducers mounted in a water bath. The patient was placed over the plastic membrane and scans were automatically made by an operator sitting at an independent control board to the right of the system.

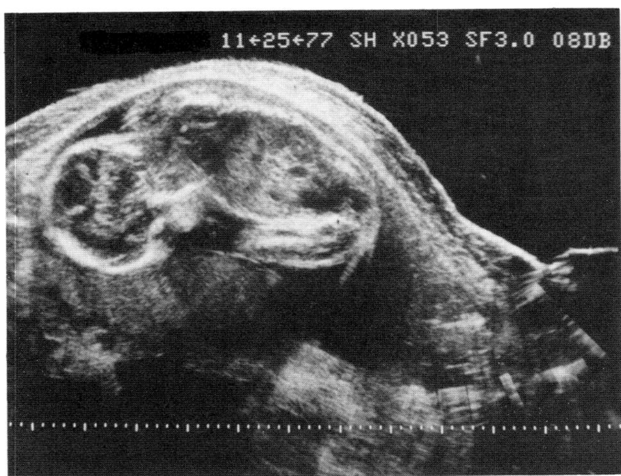

Fig. 38-3. The quality of scans made by the Octoson was very good in obstetrics, because the mother lay on her stomach, causing the fetus to be positioned flush against the uterine wall. This scan shows a fetus in the breech presentation.

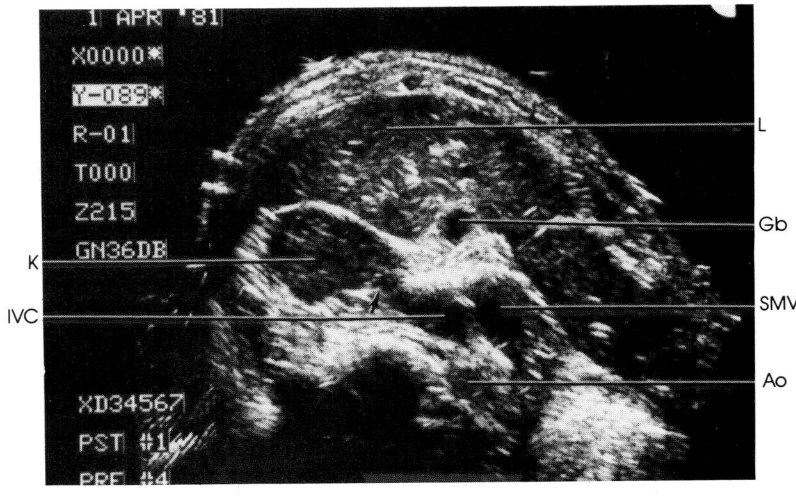

Fig. 38-4. The quality of the abdominal scans seemed to vary according to the patient's build. This scan over the right kidney *(K)*, inferior vena cava *(IVC)*, aorta *(Ao)*, superior mesenteric vein *(SMV)*, gallbladder *(Gb)*, and liver *(L)* was made with the patient lying in a right decubitus position.

The subsequent development of real-time equipment has virtually eliminated previously described ultrasound instrumentation (Figs. 38-5 and 38-6). High-frequency, high-resolution, small-diameter transducers are able to accumulate several images per second (depending on frequency and depth, as many as 30 frames per second). The flexibility of these small transducers affords the sonographer the opportunity to obtain high-quality images with the minimum of "overwrite."

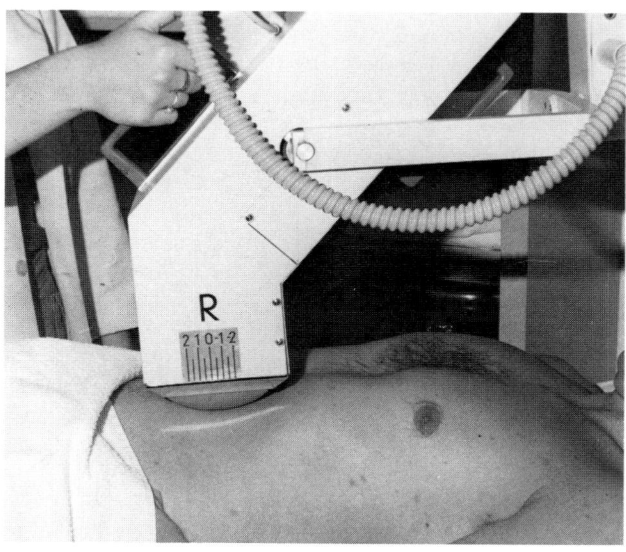

Fig. 38-5. Siemens Corp. developed a real-time system that was "hand" movable. A single large-diameter transducer was mounted inside the water tank and reflections were made off a parabolic mirror to obtain the real-time image.

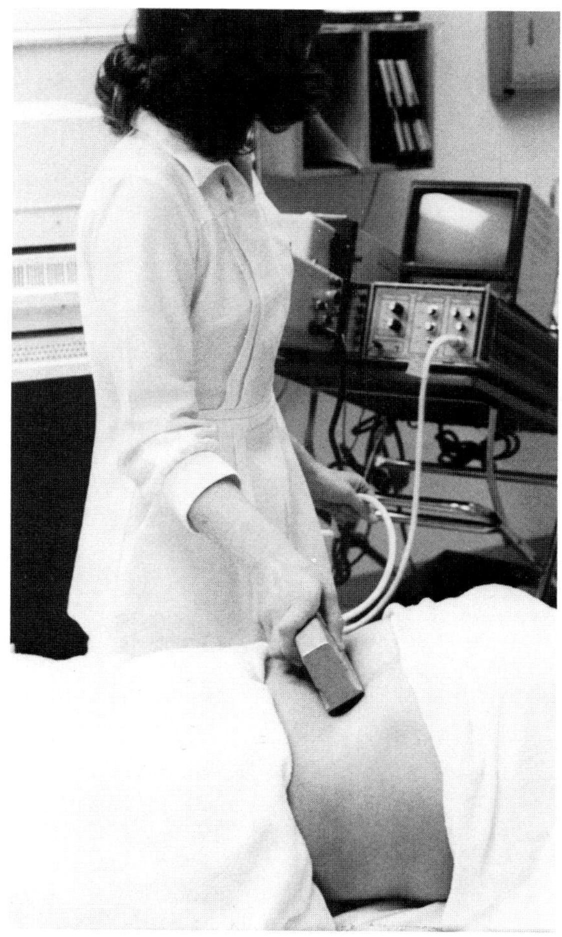

Fig. 38-6. Advanced Diagnostic Research developed a more flexible real-time system, in which the transducers (64 elements) were mounted inside the hand held apparatus. This was the first time sonographers were able to have more flexibility with the real-time transducer.

Physical Principles of the Modality

PROPERTIES OF SOUND WAVES

A *wave* is a propagation of energy that moves back and forth or vibrates at a steady rate. Sound waves are mechanical oscillations that are transmitted by particles in a gas, liquid, or solid medium. Generated by an external source, ultrasound is the transmission of high-frequency mechanical vibrations greater than 20 kHz through a medium.

Frequency may be explained by the following analogy. If a stick were moved in and out of a pond at a steady rate, the entire surface of the water would be covered with waves radiating from the stick. If the number of *vibrations* that were made in each second were counted, the frequency of vibration could be determined. In ultrasound, frequency refers to the number of oscillations per second performed by the particles of the medium in which the wave is propagating:

1 oscillation/sec = 1 cycle/second = 1 Hz
1000 oscillations/sec = 1 kilocycle/second = 1 kHz
1,000,000 oscillations/sec = 1 megacycle/second = 1 MHz

Ultrasound refers to sound waves beyond the audible (16,000 to 20,000 cycles/second) range. Diagnostic applications of ultrasound use frequencies of 1 to 10 million cycles/second, or 1 to 10 MHz (Table 38-1).

Table 38-1. Applications of sound frequency ranges

Frequency range	Manner of production	Application
Infrasound		
0 to 25 Hz	Electromagnetic vibrators	Vibration analysis of structures
Audible		
20 Hz to 20 kHz	Electromagnetic vibrators, musical instruments	Communications, signaling
Ultrasound		
20 to 100 kHz	Air whistles, electric devices	Biology, sonar
100 kHz to 1 MHz	Electric devices	Flaw detection, biology
1 to 20 MHz	Electric devices	Diagnostic medicine

Longitudinal waves

Ultrasound is a form of nonionizing radiation in which longitudinal pressure waves of high frequency are transmitted through a medium. These waves are formed by the oscillation of particles or molecules parallel to the axis of wave propagation. As illustrated in Fig. 38-7, part of the molecules are "squeezed" closer together, or *compressed,* and part undergo expansion, or rarefaction, by which the molecules are pulled farther apart. As sound travels through a material, alternate regions of compression and rarefaction occur.

Along with wave properties such as frequency and *intensity,* the *medium* that carries the sound is a major contributor in defining the ultrasound transmission properties. The medium can best be understood in forms of its bulk modulus and acoustic impedance characteristics. The bulk modulus is the amount of pressure required to compress a small volume of material a small amount. In part, the compressibility or density of a material determines the way sound is carried along with the material.

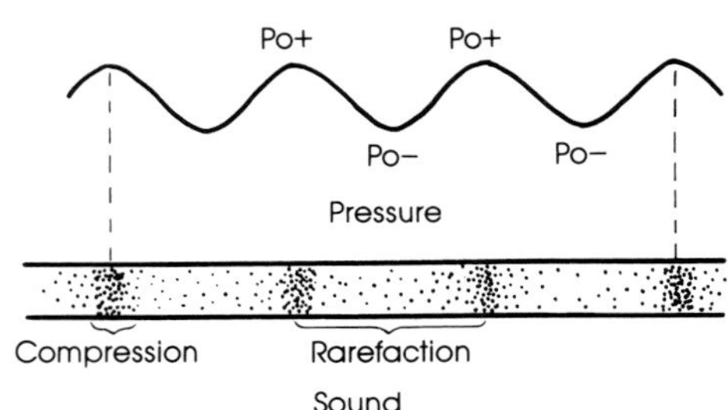

Fig. 38-7. Longitudinal wave formation occurs in pressure changes with fluctuating volume, causing compression and rarefaction.

Acoustic impedance

The ultrasound wave is very similar to a light beam in that it may be *focused, refracted, reflected,* or *scattered* at interfaces between different media. At the junction of two media of different acoustic properties, an ultrasound beam may be reflected depending on the difference in acoustic impedance between the two media and the angle at which the beam hits the interface *(angle of incidence)* (Fig. 38-8). In biologic tissues, with the exception of air-tissue and bone interfaces, the differences in acoustic impedance are slight so that only a small component of the ultrasound beam is reflected at each interface (Table 38-2). Most of the sound is passed into tissues deeper in the body and reflected at other interfaces. The acoustic impedance is the product of the *velocity of sound* in a medium and the *density* of that medium. The acoustic impedance increases if the density or propagation speed increases.

Table 38-2. Characteristic acoustic impedance

Material	Acoustic impedance ($gm/cm^2/sec \times 10^{-5}$)
Air	0.0001
Fat	1.38
Water	1.50
Blood	1.61
Kidney	1.62
Liver	1.65
Muscle	1.70
Skull	7.80

Table 38-3. Velocities of ultrasound

Material	Velocity (m/sec)
Air	331
Water	1430
Fat	1450
Liver	1550
Kidney	1560
Blood	1570
Skull	4080

From Hagen-Ansert SL: Textbook of diagnostic ultrasonography, St. Louis, 1983, The CV Mosby Co.

Velocity of sound

The velocity of sound in a medium is determined by the *density* and elastic properties of the medium. The velocity of sound differs greatly among air, bone, and soft tissue (Table 38-3). On the other hand, the velocity of sound varies by only a few percent from one soft tissue to another. Air-filled structures, such as the lungs and stomach, or gas-filled structures, such as the bowel, impede the sound transmission. Likewise, sound is *attenuated* through most bony structures. Small differences between fat, blood, and organ tissues, as seen on an ultrasound image, may be better delineated with high-frequency transducers that improve resolution.

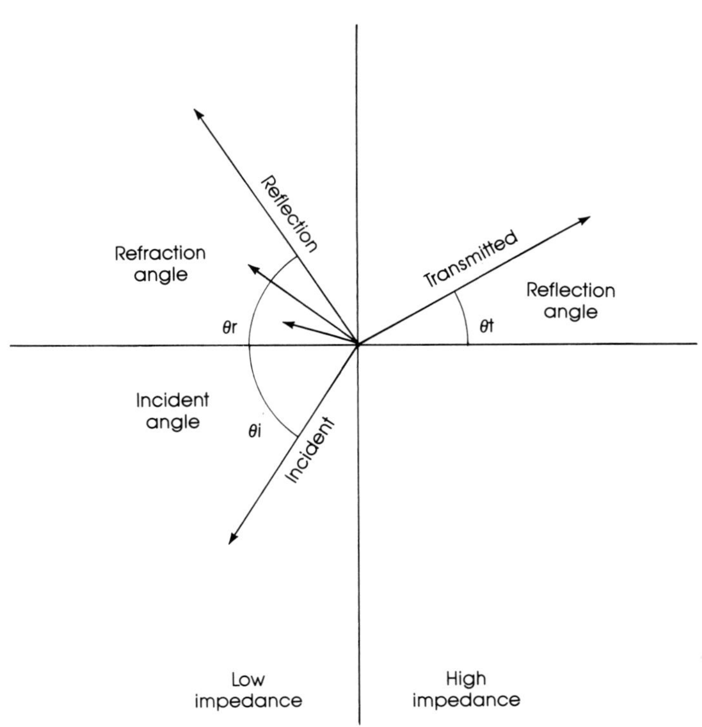

Fig. 38-8. Relationship among incident, reflected, and transmitted waves.

Physical principles of the modality

Measurement of sound

The *decibel* unit (dB) is often used to measure the strength or intensity of an ultrasound wave. The decibel unit allows for a quantitative statement to be made regarding the ratio of two intensities of two amplitudes. The signal level (in decibel units) is expressed as:

$$dB = 10 \log_{10} \frac{I_2}{I_1}$$

where I_2 and I_1 = any two intensity levels being compared. The intensity of the transmitted ultrasonic pulse on each ultrasound instrument may be varied by changing the size of excitation voltage applied to the transducer. Also, reduction of the sound beam intensity with depth or attenuation may be expressed as decibels per centimeter.

Attenuation is the sum of acoustic energy losses resulting from absorption, scattering, and reflection. If air or bone is coupled with soft tissue, more energy will be attenuated. Attenuation through a calcium interface such as a gallstone may produce a shadow on the B-scan image (Fig. 38-9).

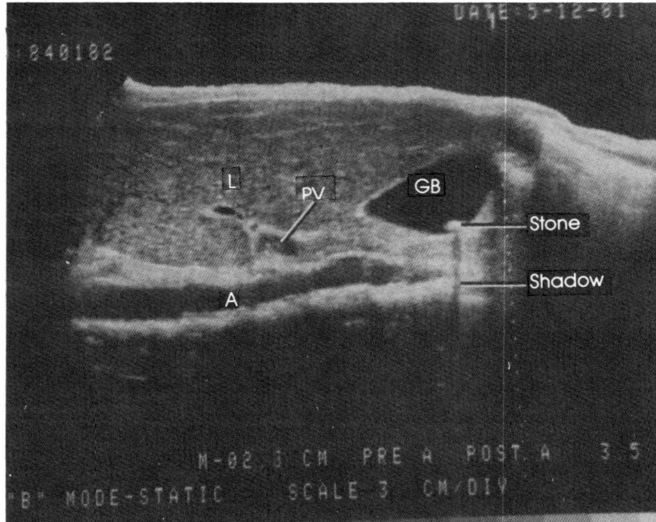

Fig. 38-9. Sagittal scan of the right upper quadrant. Anechoic gallbladder is well visualized with a solitary bright reflector along its posterior margin, representing a small gallstone. The acoustic shadow is seen posterior to the stone.

TRANSDUCERS

The sound beams used in diagnostic ultrasound are produced from a *transducer* by the *piezoelectric* effect. The transducer is a means for converting one form of energy into another (for example, electrical energy into mechanical sound waves). The Curies first described the piezoelectric effect in 1880. They observed that when certain crystals such as quartz undergo mechanical deformation, a potential difference develops across the two surfaces of the crystals. Synthetic ceramic crystals have been developed for medical use that can be molded into various shapes and sizes and focused for ultrasonic applications. Each ceramic crystal has a *resonant frequency* that depends on the thickness of the crystal.

Most diagnostic applications use short *pulsed ultrasound* waves for optimum resolution. As a pulse of ultrasound is emitted, the pulse travels through tissue. When the pulse strikes an interface, part of the energy is reflected. The returning echo is a sound pressure wave that causes a slight mechanical deformation of the ceramic as it impinges on the transducer face, resulting in an electrical pulse. Each transducer has a special damping material to "silence" any echo vibration return. The ringing is like a hammer striking a bell; the bell will continue to ring unless the vibrations are silenced by a stationary object.

DISPLAY MODES

A-mode

The *A-mode,* or amplitude modulation, display represents the time or distance it takes the beam to strike a particular interface and return its signal to the transducer. The greater the reflection at the interface, the larger the signal amplitude will appear on the A-mode screen (Fig. 38-10).

B-mode

If the tracing of the A-mode were rotated 90 degrees toward the observer, the spikes would be represented as dots. The brightness of the dots corresponds to the height of the spike. Gray-scale imaging refers to the condition of varying the brightness of the dot so that brightness is proportional to the echo-signal amplitude. Thus the greater the change in acoustic impedance at the interface of a medium, the taller the spike on the A-mode tracing, which in turn presents a brighter dot on the B-mode trace. As the transducer is moved across a plane, the echoes are imprinted on a screen to subsequently build up a two-dimensional image. The B-mode is the basis for all static and real-time images in ultrasound (Fig. 38-11).

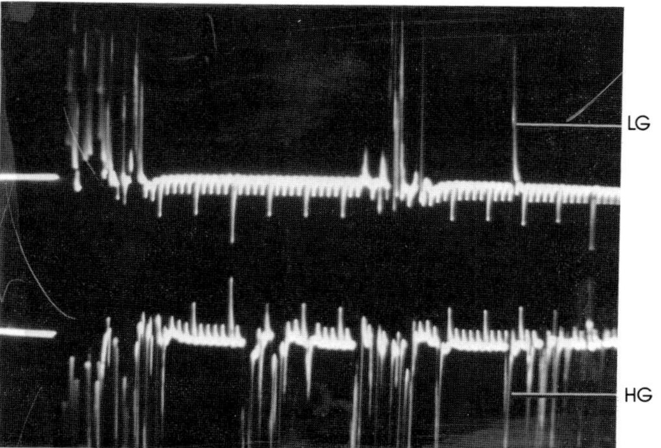

Fig. 38-10. A-mode tracing of a solid mass at low gain (upper tracing) and high gain (lower tracing). The solid mass attenuates the sound beam, giving a weak through transmission. As the gain is increased, there are multiple echoes seen within the solid mass.

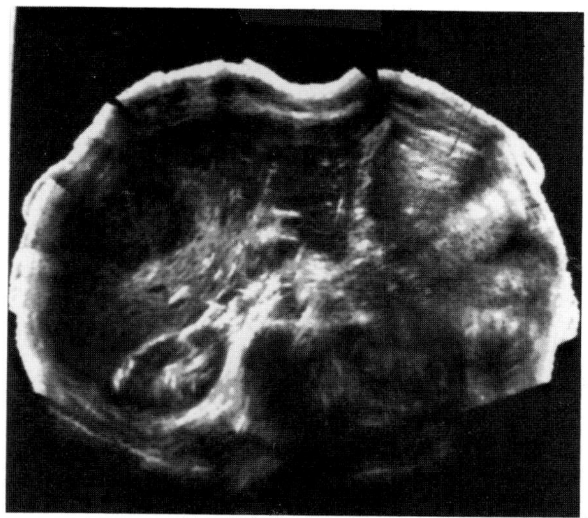

Fig. 38-11. B-mode tracing of a patient with a liver mass. The compound sector scan enabled the sonographer to outline the entire abdomen for a panoramic outline of the upper abdomen.

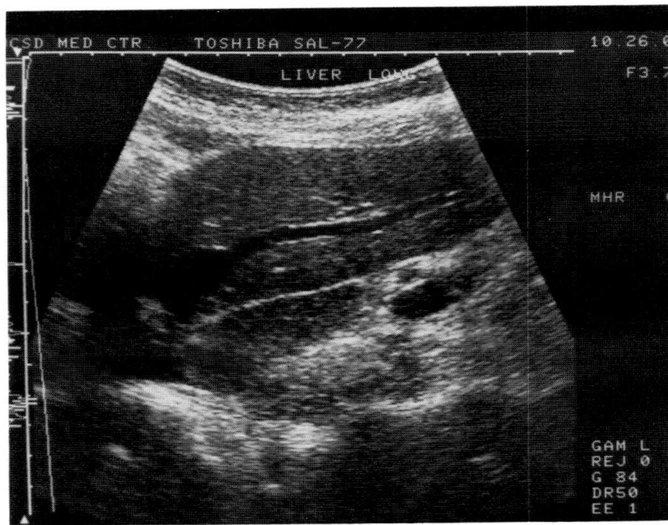

Fig. 38-12. Real-time tracing of the right upper quadrant provided a more dynamic image with greater flexibility in movement of the transducer. The panoramic "field of view" was lost with the real-time transducer and replaced with a narrow sector, or limited linear array view.

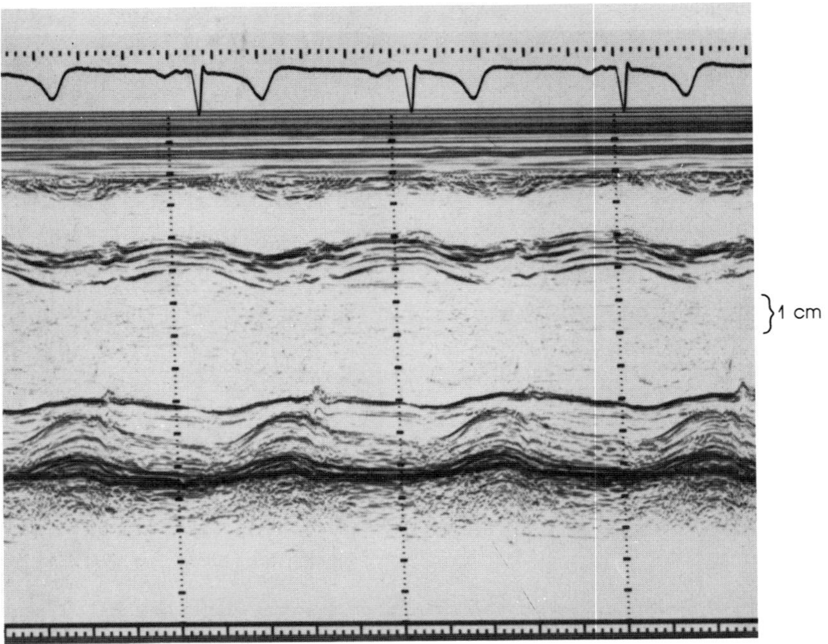

Fig. 38-13. M-mode tracing of the left ventricle is made by selecting one line of sight in the B-mode image, turning that image 90 degrees, and watching it over a period of time. Thus distance and time provided a means of calculating velocity and slope measurements of various cardiac structures.

Real time

Real time is the dynamic presentation of multiple-image frames per second over selected areas of the body (Fig. 38-12). The transducer may be a single crystal that mechanically wobbles back and forth, or it may be composed of several elements that can be electronically focused and fired in rapid sequence and in time to produce a real-time image. Thus structures are visible as they change position in time, such as the pulsatile arterial structures, diaphragm and cardiac motion, peristalsis in the bowel and stomach, and other organ structures that move with respiratory motion. This technique produces a high-quality image that is independent of operator hand-eye coordination.

M mode

The *"M-mode,"* or time-motion trace, uses the concepts of A- and B-modes as they are swept across the screen over a period of time. The M-mode is used to depict movement and is especially useful to record fetal heart motion and other cardiac valve and wall functions. The M-mode tracing can be recorded on paper, radiographic film, or video format for a permanent record and measurement analysis (Fig. 38-13).

Gray-scale imaging

"Gray-scale" imaging is able to selectively amplify and display the level of echoes from soft tissues at the expense of larger echoes. This signal processing is known as the compression amplication characteristic of gray-scale systems. Through digital scan converters, digital memory and circuitry converts echo signals into an image on a television monitor. This information then may be manipulated by the sonographer on a preprocessing or postprocessing basis, enabling the sonographer to change the presentation of the image from a softer shade of gray to a more contrasting image. Sometimes this technique is useful in imaging particular tumors or small masses within the abdomen or in visualizing the lower-level "soft" echoes.

Doppler principle

The *Doppler* principle refers to a change in frequency when the motion of laminar or turbulent flow is detected within a vascular structure (Fig. 38-14). In medical applications, a sound wave is bounced off moving red blood cells (RBCs). If the cell moves along the line of the ultrasound beam, the Doppler shift is directly proportional to the velocity of the RBC. If the RBC moves away from the transducer in the plane of the ultrasound beam, the fall in frequency is directly proportional to the velocity and direction of the RBC movement. The Doppler tracing is recorded on a type of M-mode format, with a baseline serving as the "zero" point. Movement towards the transducer is recorded as a positive (above the baseline) motion, while movement away from the transducer is recorded as negative (below the baseline) motion.

Instrumentation

The B-scan examination has been performed with the articulated arm (contact, static scanner), the water-bath system, or real-time instrumentation. Formerly, the most common B-scan instrument was the hand-held articulated arm, which required extensive operator experience and hand-eye coordination to produce a high-quality panoramic image. A modified compound-sector scanning motion was used to record the maximum number of interfaces. If too much sector was used, the scan was *"overwritten"* and lost its detail; therefore the sonographer had to judge during the performance of the scan when the information was complete.

Currently, high-resolution real-time instrumentation has replaced the static scanner in nearly all laboratories, primarily because it eliminates the requirement for tremendous skill in producing an acceptable image. Real-time instrumentation has added flexibility to obtaining quality images without "overwrite" features by enabling the sonographer to move freely about the abdomen, chest, and pelvis to find the best "windows" in which to visualize the soft tissue structures. The transducer size is generally small and is easily moved between intercostal margins and angles and in various directions to outline specific anatomic structures.

Real-time imaging has also added another dimension to cardiology by providing a two-dimensional image of pulsatile cardiac structures, with a simultaneous M-mode and Doppler capability for recording motion and function.

Regardless of the instrumentation employed, the sonographer must have a thorough knowledge of anatomy, physiology, pathology, and physical acoustic principles to produce an adequate scan. In addition, the sonographer must be familiar with special scanning techniques, artifacts, and equipment quality control.

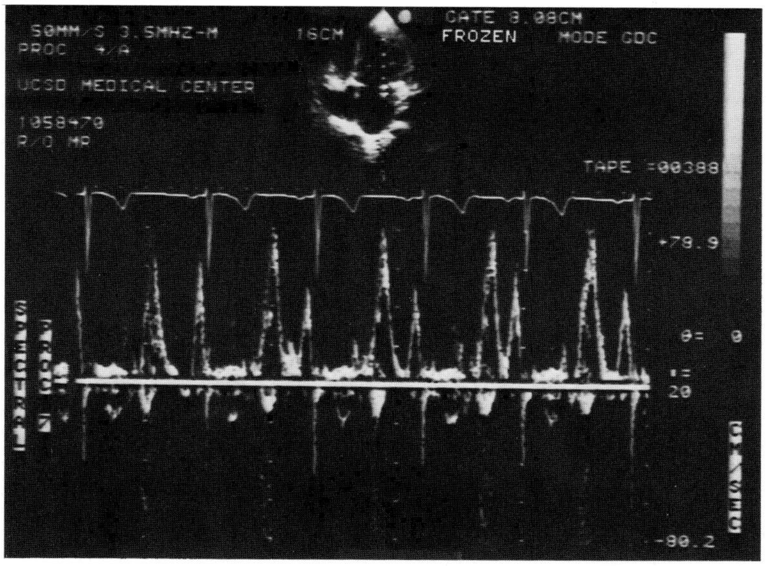

Fig. 38-14. Doppler tracing of the mitral valve shows a positive reflective above the baseline, representing the blood as it flows toward the transducer in diastole; as the atrium begins to relax, the flow drops off. At atrial contraction, the blood flows toward the transducer with less velocity than the initial flow. The end of diastole shows the flow back to the baseline.

Artifacts

Just as the sonographer must be able to distinguish anatomic and pathologic changes within the body, the recognition of *artifacts* is important for the production of adequate diagnostic images.

The sound beam must be perpendicular to the interface. A *rarefaction* artifact is produced by the bending of the beam at an interface where the beam is not perpendicular.

A *reverberation* can occur when the beam strikes a reflective structure, sending the beam in multiple pathways to produce many linear reflections. The sound striking a rib is a good example of reverberation in the upper abdomen. Bowel gas interference, barium in the gastrointestinal tract, dehydration of tissue, and adipose tissue all have an adverse effect on the image, yielding a suboptimal study. The sound wave is unable to penetrate these and often causes a shadow posterior to its highly absorbent or reflective material.

In addition, equipment malfunction (e.g., damaged transducer), poorly adjusted time-gain compensation, or misaligned calibration may have an adverse effect on the image, and the sonographer must be able to recognize these problems on a routine basis.

BIOLOGIC EFFECTS

Diagnostic ultrasound as used in clinical medicine has not been associated with any harmful biologic effects and ultrasound is generally accepted as a safe technique.

Much of the work on biologic effects has come about because of the wide use of ultrasound in obstetrics, largely because it is safe and without effect on the fetus. The rationale for this conclusion is based on: (1) the fact that the intensities normally used are too small to produce significant increases in temperature in exposed tissues, and (2) the tacit assumption that the pulses employed are too short to produce the selective, large-amplitude oscillation of microscopic gas bodies called *acoustic cavitation*.

Available information indicates that there are thresholds for transient cavitation that require peak intensities of 10W/cm^2 in microsecond-length pulses. It should be possible to be conservative and perform all diagnostic obstetric procedures with peak intensities substantially below these levels.

ANATOMIC RELATIONSHIPS AND LANDMARKS

The ability of the sonographer to understand anatomy as it relates to the cross-sectional, coronal, oblique, and sagittal projections is critical in performing a quality sonogram. Normal anatomy has many variations in size and position, and it is the responsibility of the sonographer to be able to demonstrate these findings on the sonogram. To complete this task the sonographer must have a thorough understanding of anatomy as it relates to the anteroposterior relationships, as well as the variations in sectional anatomy.

Liver

The diaphragmatic surface of the liver consists of the right, caudate, and left lobes, with the falciform ligament separating the left lobe from the rest of the liver (Figs. 38-15 and 38-16). Within this ligament is a round fibrous cord, the ligamentum teres, which represents the former umbilical vein.

Vascular access to the liver is through the porta hepatis via the portal vein and hepatic artery. The portal triad contains these two vessels and the common bile duct.

The bare area of the liver is where the peritoneal reflections from the liver onto the diaphragm leave an irregular triangle of liver without peritoneal covering. The peritoneal reflections around the bare area are called the coronary ligament. The caudal part of the coronary ligament is reflected onto the diaphragm and the right kidney and is called the hepatorenal ligament. Below this is a potential peritoneal space, the hepatorenal, or Morison's, pouch bounded by the liver, kidney, colon, and duodenum.

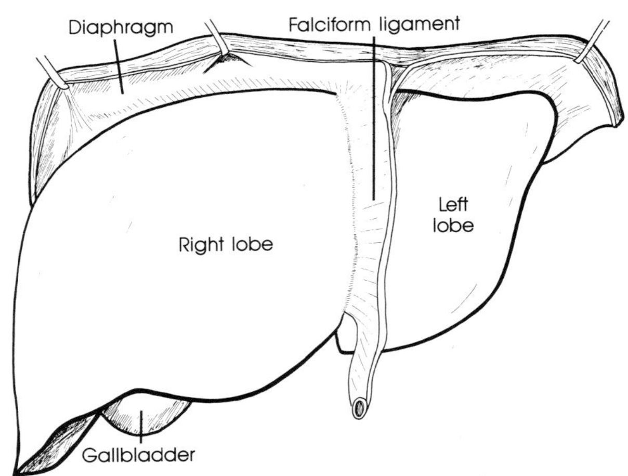

Fig. 38-15. Anterior view of the liver with the falciform ligament as it separates the left lobe from the rest of the liver. The falciform ligament is a well-visualized landmark in sonography.

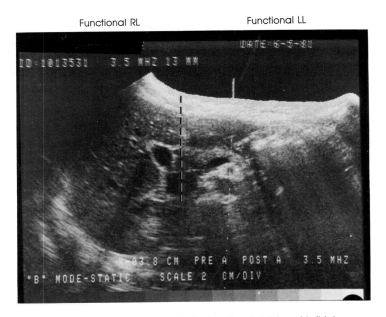

Fig. 38-16. The liver is divided into functional right and left lobes, according to its blood supply from the right and left portal veins.

Gallbladder

The gallbladder is attached to the inferior surface of the liver. The neck of the gallbladder empties into the cystic duct, which joins the common bile duct (along with the hepatic duct), to empty into the duodenum.

Vessels

The major great vessels are related to the posterior abdominal wall, with branches to the visceral organs (Fig. 38-17). The aorta arises from the left ventricle of the heart and descends through the thoracic cavity and abdominal cavity before branching into the iliac arteries. Major abdominal arteries are the celiac axis (splenic artery, left gastric artery, and hepatic artery), superior mesenteric artery, and renal arteries.

Pancreas

The pancreas is a retroperitoneal gland that is bounded anteriorly by the stomach and duodenum and posteriorly by the superior mesenteric artery and vein (Fig. 38-18).

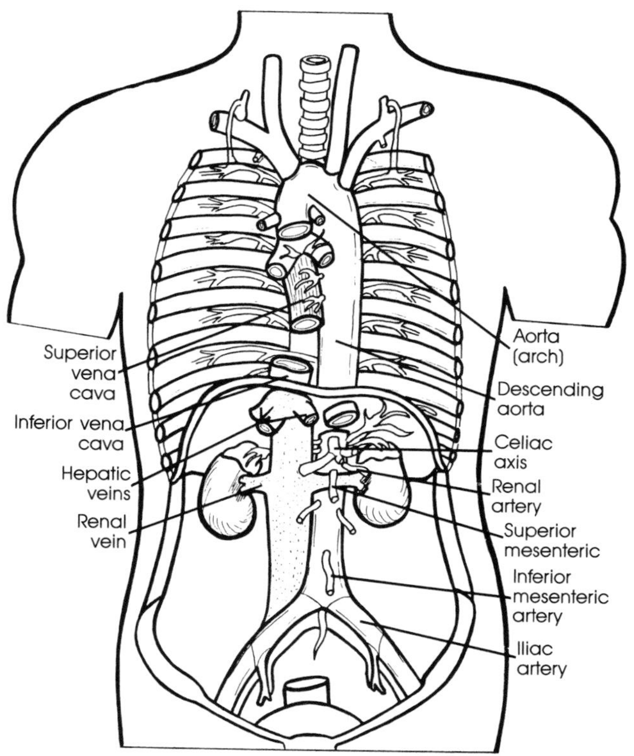

Fig. 38-17. The aorta may be visualized from its origin at the root of the vessel as it leaves the left ventricle, followed as it arches into the thoracic cavity and pierces the diaphragm to become the abdominal aorta. The major branches of the abdominal aorta (celiac trunk, superior mesenteric artery, and renal arteries) are well seen on the sonogram. The venous supply is imaged as the superior and inferior venae cavae enter the right atrium of the heart. The hepatic veins are seen to enter the inferior vena cava at the level of the diaphragm.

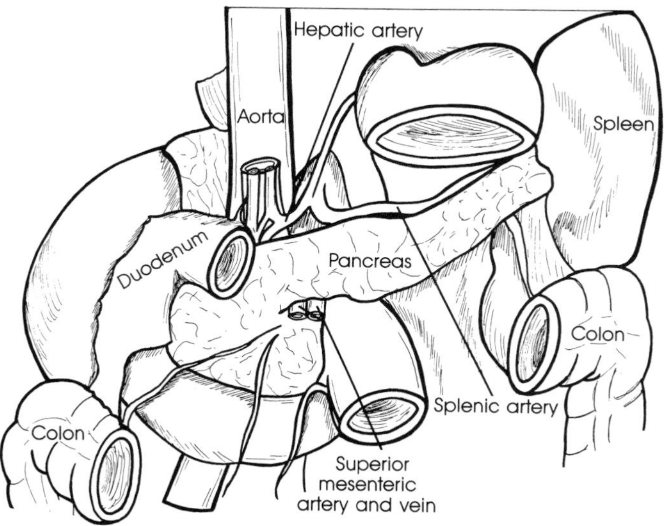

Fig. 38-18. The pancreas is a retroperitoneal structure that is recognized by locating the aorta and inferior vena cava, splenic artery, splenic vein, hepatic artery, and superior mesenteric vein. The stomach, when filled with fluid, may serve as a superior boundary of the pancreas as the fluid fills the duodenal loop that surrounds the pancreatic head.

Spleen

The spleen fits snugly under the diaphragm in the left upper quadrant. The hilum of the spleen contains the splenic artery and vein and tail of the pancreas. The left kidney is inferior to the spleen.

Kidneys

The kidneys lie along the psoas and quadratus lumborum muscles in the retroperitoneal cavity (Fig. 38-19). The left kidney borders the spleen, pancreas, colon, jejunum, and adrenal glands. The right kidney borders the liver, colon, and adrenal glands. On the medial surface of the kidney is the hilum, the point of exit of the renal vein and entrance of the renal artery. The renal pelvis is at the hilum and forms the ureter, which narrows to flow posteriorly into the bladder.

TRANSVERSE AND SAGITTAL ANATOMIC SECTIONS

The sonographer must be able to recognize vascular structures and know anatomic relationships to produce a complete abdominal study. Figs. 38-20 to 38-33 illustrate a complete scan in transverse and sagittal planes that shows these anatomic features. The patient is instructed to hold his or her breath during the study in an effort to move the liver into the abdominal cavity for better visualization.

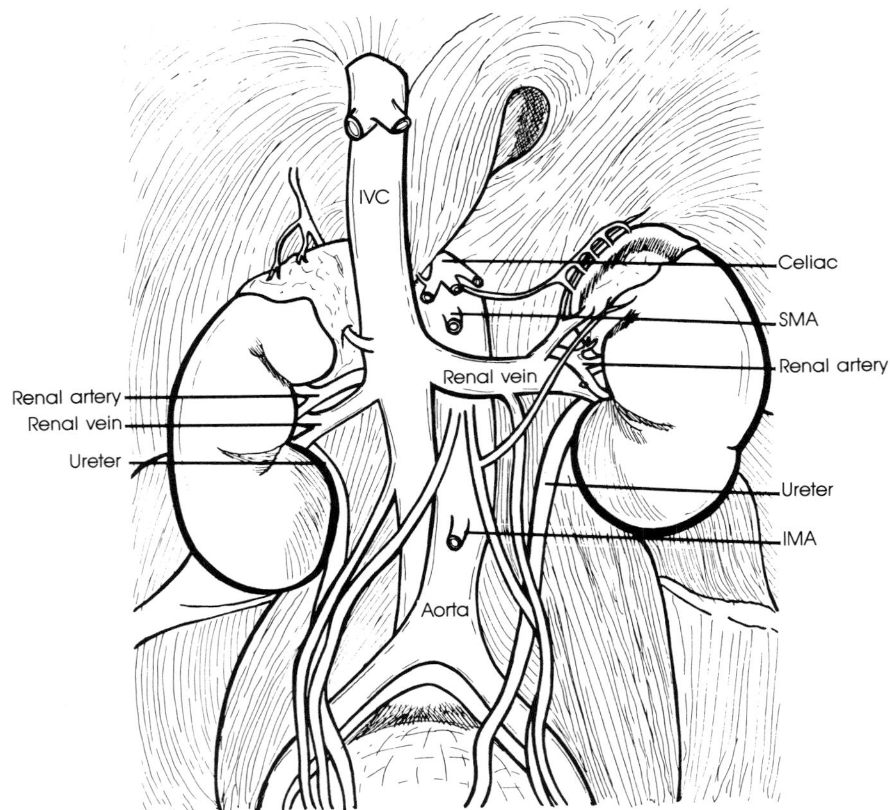

Fig. 38-19. The renals are best visualized by using the homogeneous liver or spleen to outline the kidneys as they lie along the psoas muscles.

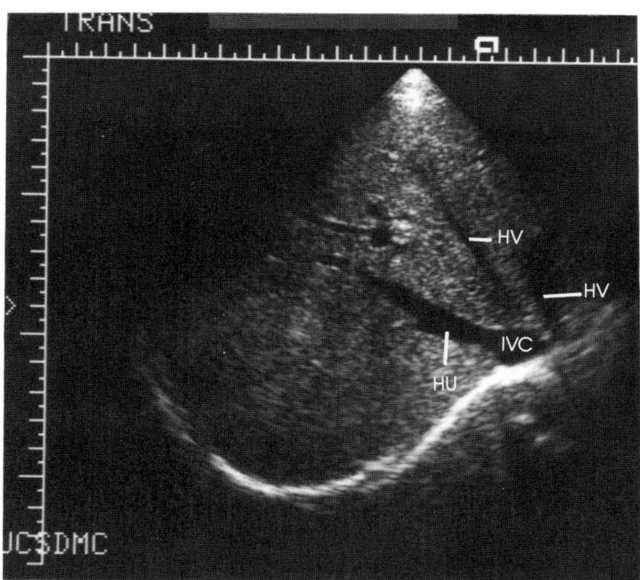

Fig. 38-20. Transverse scan high in the right upper quadrant shows the homogeneous liver with the hepatic veins *(HV)* draining into the inferior vena cava at the level of the diaphragm.

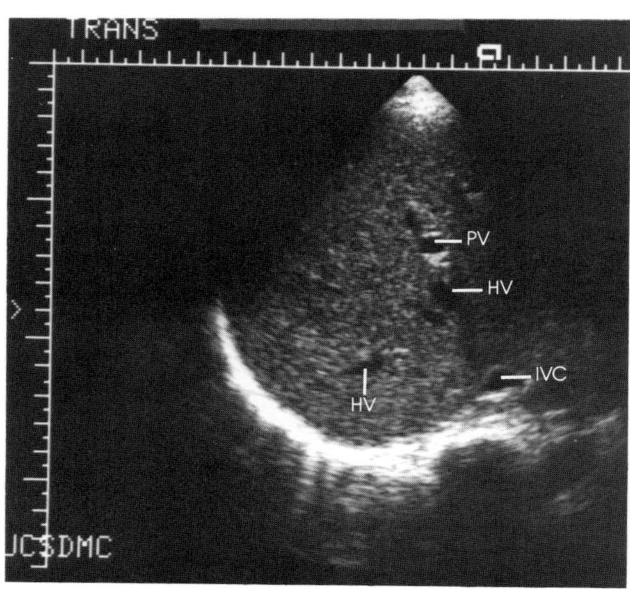

Fig. 38-21. Transverse scan slightly inferior to Fig. 38-20 shows the liver intermixed with hepatic and portal vein structures. The portal veins are more reflective than the hepatic veins.

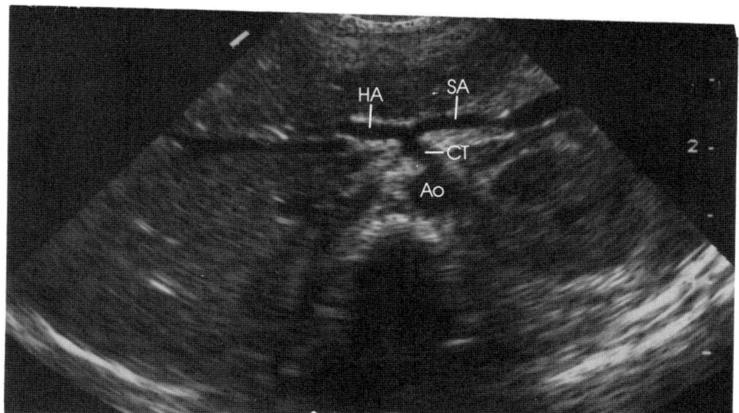

Fig. 38-22. Transverse scan over the area of the celiac trunk *(CT)* as it arises anteriorly from the aortic wall *(Ao)* to provide blood to the spleen (via the splenic artery *[SA]*), to the liver (via the hepatic artery *[HA]*), and to the stomach (via the left gastric artery—not shown).

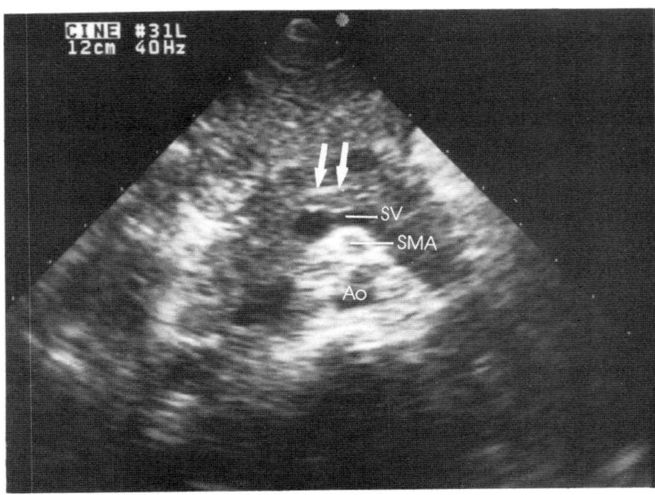

Fig. 38-23. Transverse scan at the level of the pancreas. The pancreatic duct is seen as a bright double echo *(arrows)* within the middle of the gland. The splenic vein *(SV)* is posterior to the pancreas, as are the superior mesenteric artery *(SMA)* and aorta *(Ao)*.

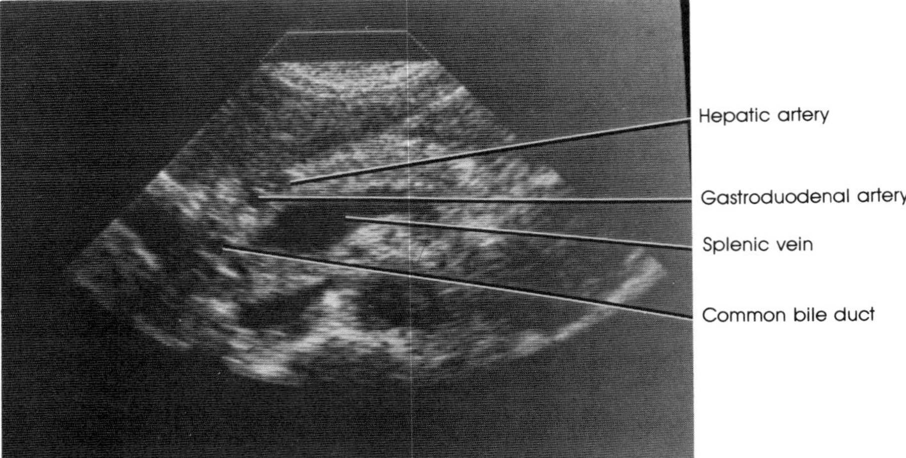

Fig. 38-24. Transverse scan over the area of the pancreas. The hepatic artery is the lateral margin of the gland. The gastroduodenal artery is also seen along the lateral margin of the head. The splenic vein is posterior to the body, whereas the common bile duct marks the lateral margin of the head.

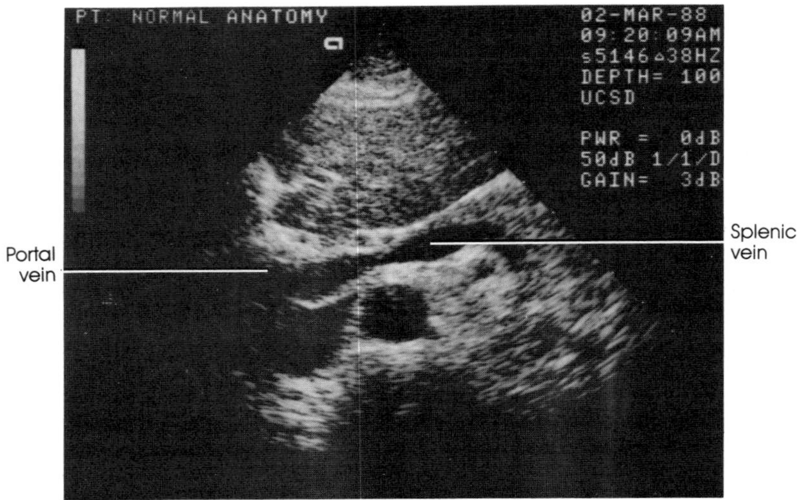

Fig. 38-25. Transverse scan showing the formation of the portal vein as the splenic vein arises from the hilum of the spleen to merge with the superior mesenteric vein to form the portal vein. (Superior mesenteric vein not shown since it has joined with splenic vein to form portal vein.)

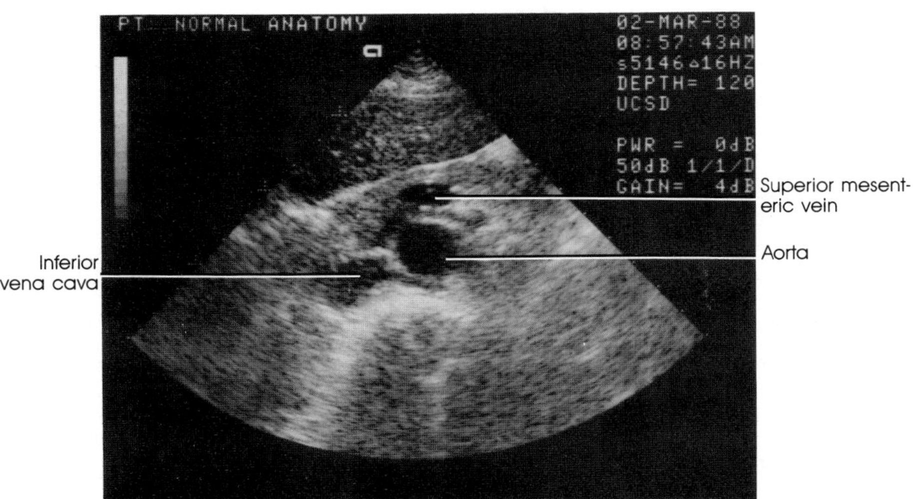

Fig. 38-26. The aorta, inferior vena cava, and superior mesenteric artery and vein should be demonstrated anterior to the spine to ensure adequate visualization of the pancreas. The duodenum often causes a shadow from the air within, thus the head of the pancreas may be difficult to see when this occurs and rotation of the patient must be done to move the air away from the gland.

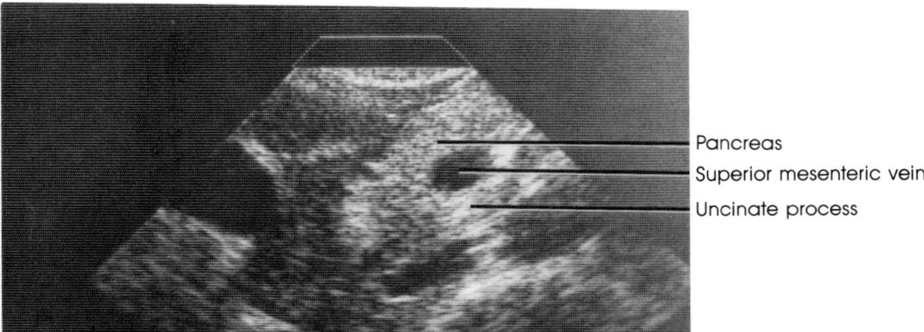

Fig. 38-27. The superior mesenteric vein is found posterior to the body of the pancreas and anterior to the uncinate process of the head.

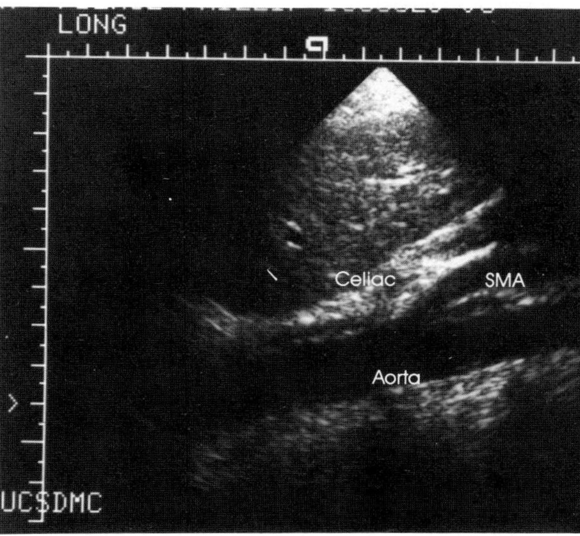

Fig. 38-28. Longitudinal scan over the left of the midline shows the aorta, celiac axis, and superior mesenteric artery as it arises from the anterior wall of the aorta.

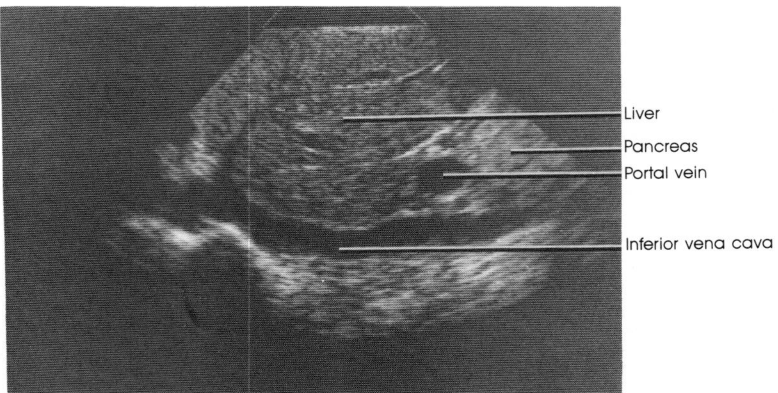

Fig. 38-29. Longitudinal scan over the inferior vena cava as it flows posterior to the liver to enter the right atrium. The portal vein is anterior to the IVC and superior to the pancreas.

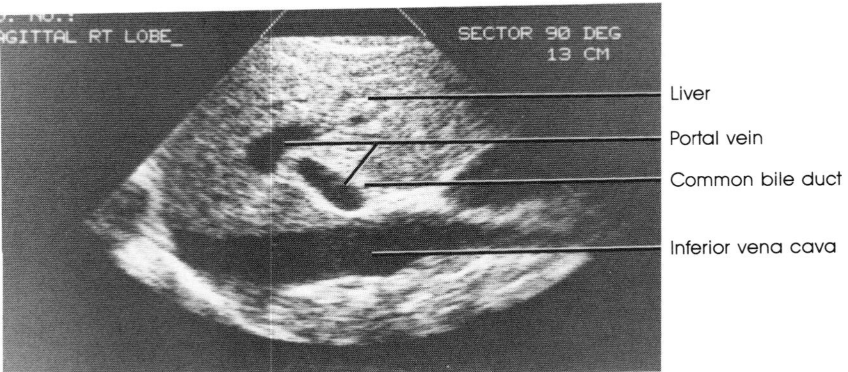

Fig. 38-30. Longitudinal scan taken slightly to the right of midline shows the inferior vena cava, portal vein, and common bile duct as it runs anterior to the portal vein before moving posterior to enter the head of the pancreas where it joins the pancreatic duct before emptying into the ampulla of Vater in the duodenum.

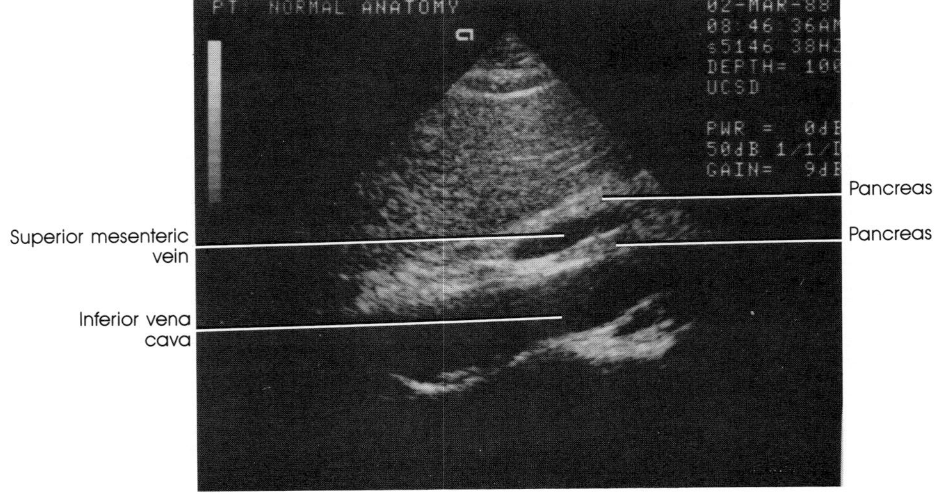

Fig. 38-31. Longitudinal scan taken slightly to the right of midline shows a long segment of the superior mesenteric vein as it flows up from the bowel to join the splenic vein.

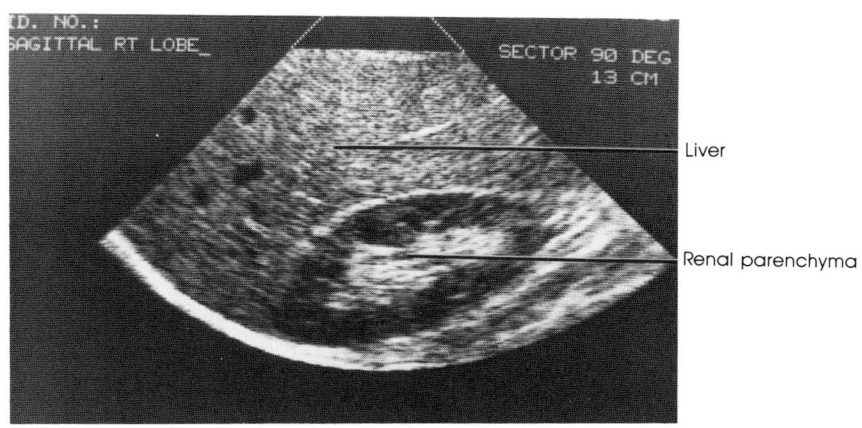

Fig. 38-32. Longitudinal scan taken along the mid to lateral right upper quadrant shows the homogeneous liver texture as compared with the more echolucent renal parenchyma.

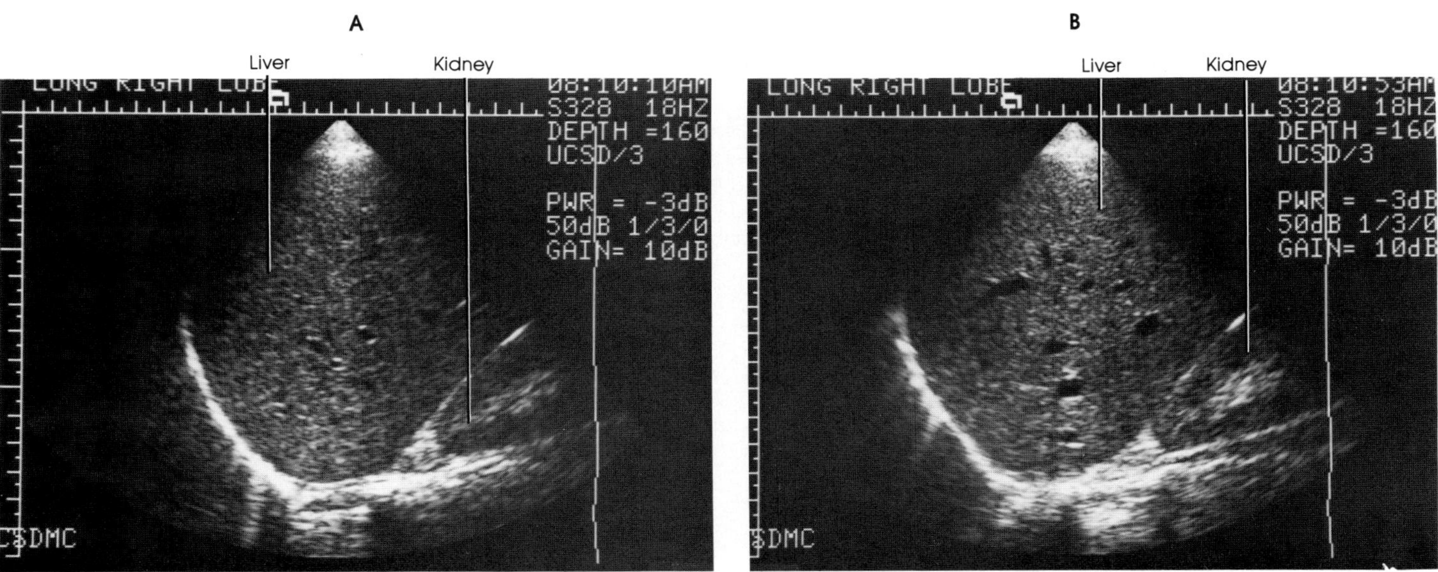

Fig. 38-33. A and **B,** Longitudinal scans taken along the right margin of the liver in different phases of inspiration show the uniform liver texture and right upper pole of the kidney.

Clinical Applications

ABDOMEN AND RETROPERITONEUM

The upper abdominal examination includes visualization of the liver, portal system, biliary system, prevertebral vessels, pancreas, spleen, kidneys, diaphragm, spine, and muscles. The patient is examined in the supine, decubitus, upright, or prone positions. Generally a high-frequency, 3.5 MHz, wide-diameter transducer is used for optimal resolution. In obese patients, a 2.25 MHz transducer may be used. In pediatric patients, a 5.0 MHz smaller diameter transducer is employed.

The patient does not eat or drink anything for several hours before the examination so that an adequate image of the biliary system may be obtained. The examination begins at the level of the xiphoid process with the patient's lungs fully expanded. Scanning may consist of transverse and sagittal planes, with additional scans made in the subcostal, coronal, and oblique planes.

For visualization of the left upper quadrant, a liquid such as water or tomato juice may be given to dilate the stomach and fill the duodenum to serve as a landmark for the visualization of the pancreas (Figs. 38-34 and 38-35).

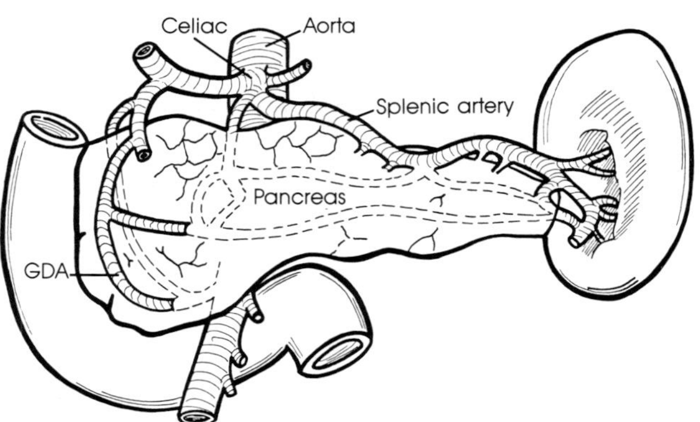

Fig. 38-34. The pancreas is visualized by demarcating the vascular structures that surround this gland. The tortuous splenic artery is the superior border of the pancreas *(SA),* whereas the gastroduodenal artery *(GDA)* is the lateral border of the head of the gland.

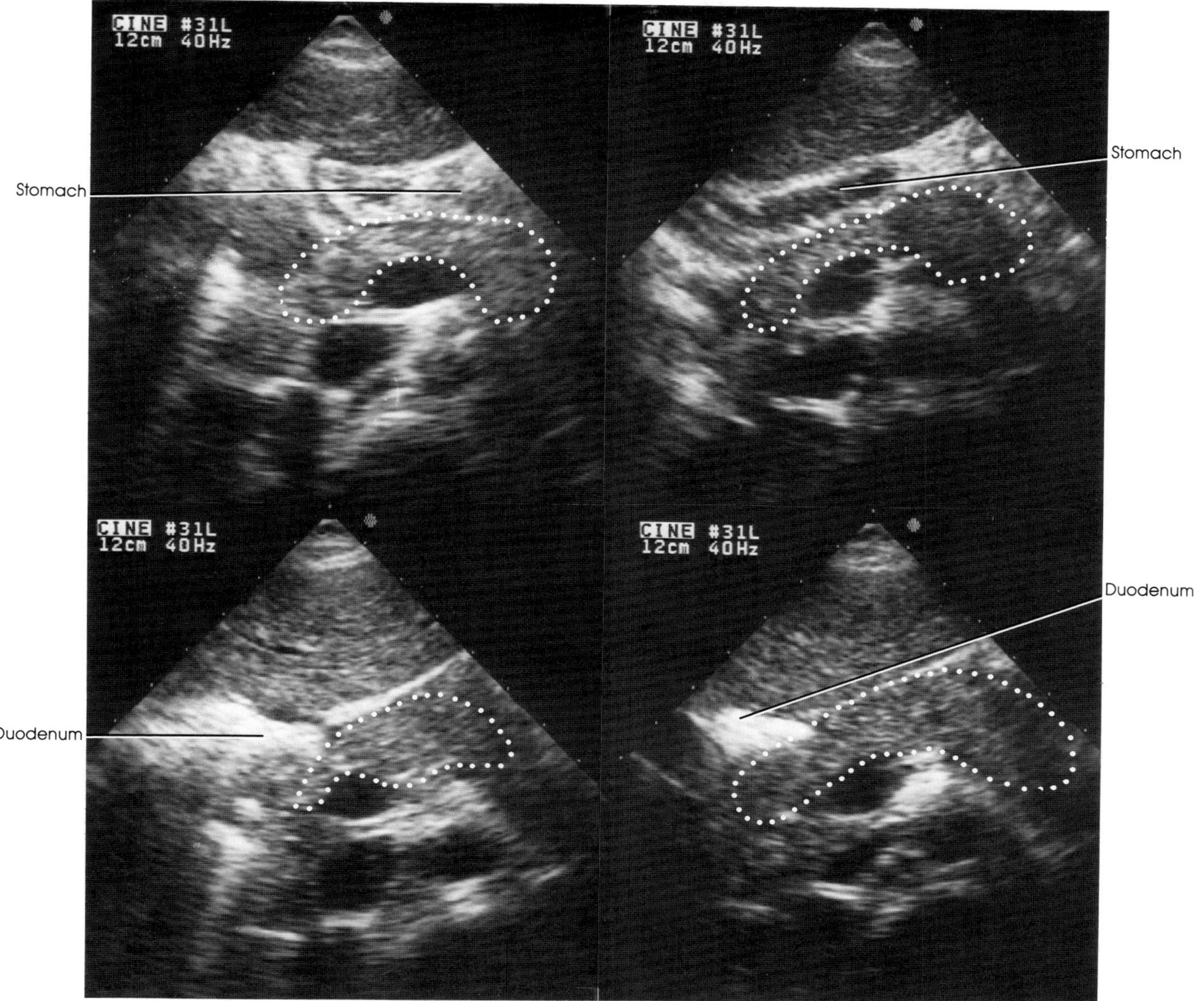

Fig. 38-35. Fluid in the stomach may help delineate the duodenum and thus outline the pancreas as one follows the duodenal loop surrounding the head of the gland. (Pancreas borders marked by broken line.)

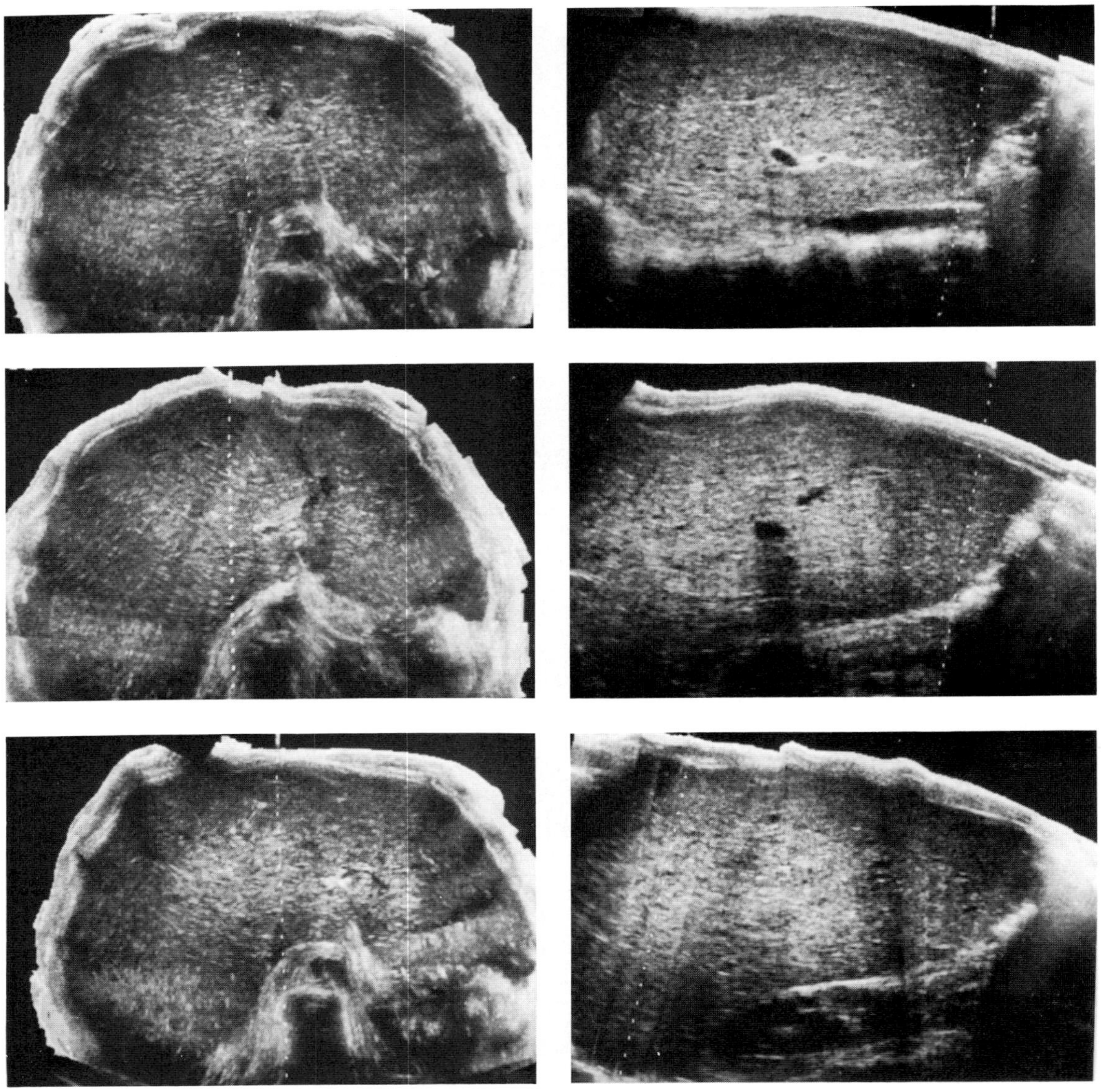

Fig. 38-36. A to **C,** Transverse, and **D** to **F,** longitudinal scans of the liver in a patient with acute cirrhosis of the liver. There is generalized enlargement of the organ with diffuse coarse echo texture throughout the liver parenchyma.

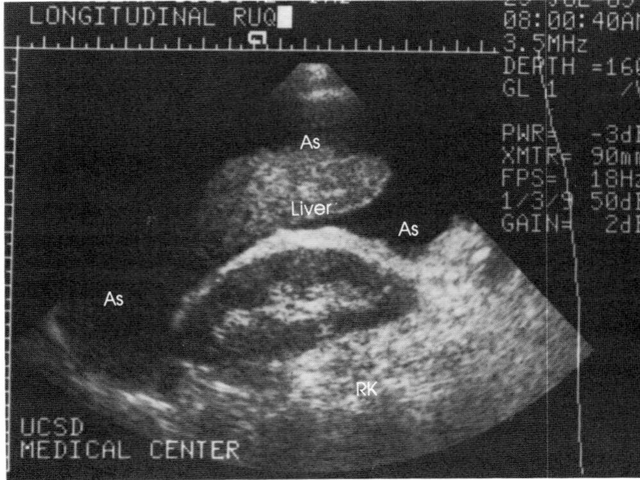

Fig. 38-37. Chronic cirrhosis as seen in this longitudinal scan shows a shrunken liver surrounded by ascites *(As)*. The right kidney *(RK)* is posterior.

The sonographer must understand the patient's clinical problem to produce an adequate scan for differential diagnosis. The normal sonographic patterns of organs and vessels must be recognizable to detect any pathologic condition that might require further investigation. Generally the liver, spleen, and pancreas are evaluated to assess size, homogeneity of tissue, and the presence of dilated vessels or ducts (Figs. 38-36 to 38-39). The gallbladder and biliary system are evaluated to assess size, wall thickness, and the presence of sludge, stones, polyps, or other masses (Figs. 38-40 to 38-45).

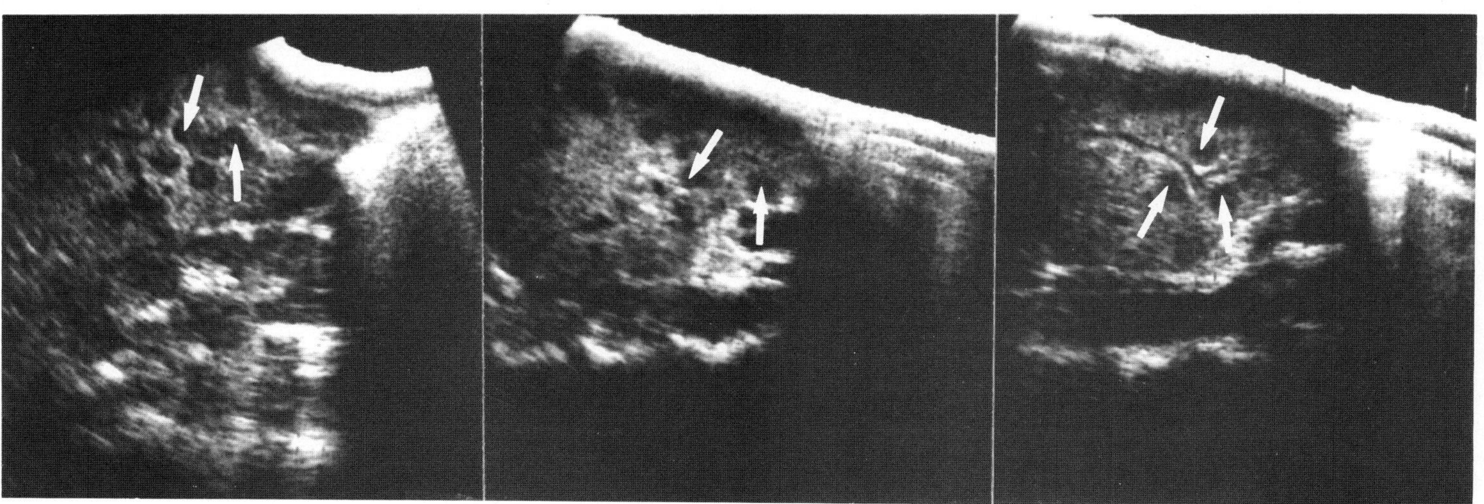

Fig. 38-38. Longitudinal scans of a patient with liver metastases show multiple, relatively sonolucent masses within the liver parenchyma *(arrows).*

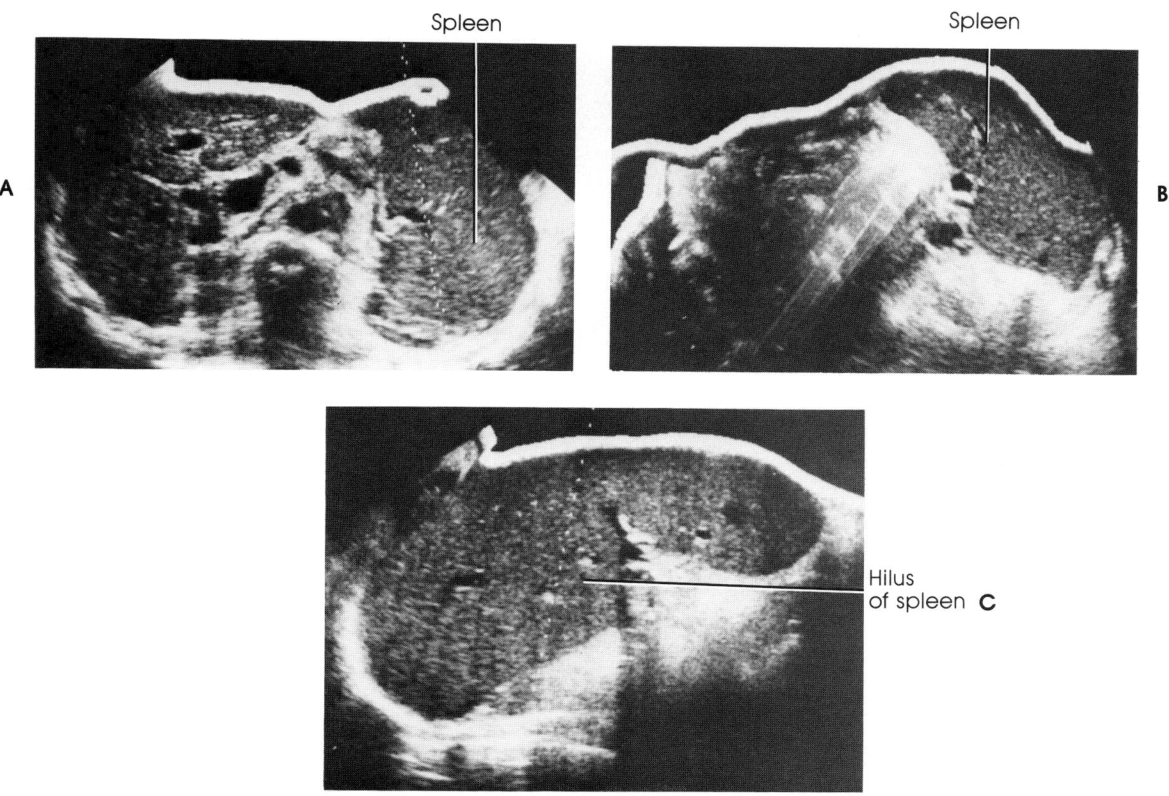

Fig. 38-39. A and **B,** Transverse, and **C,** longitudinal scans of a patient with massive splenomegaly. The splenic hilus is dilated as well. There are a number of causes of splenomegaly, namely leukemia, spirocytosis, anemia, sickle cell disease, and infection.

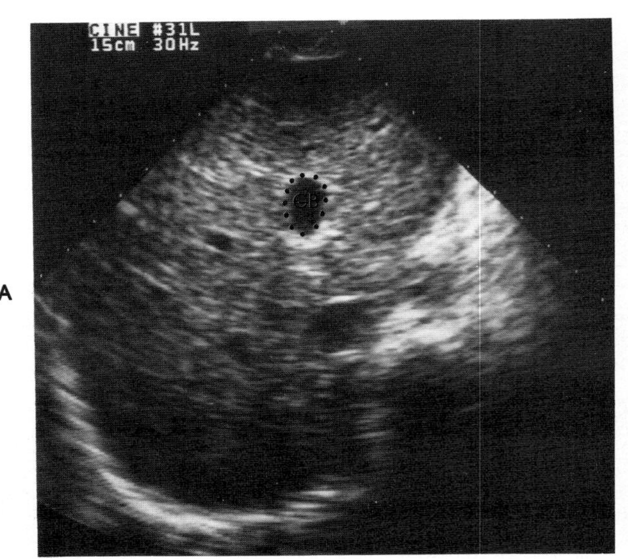

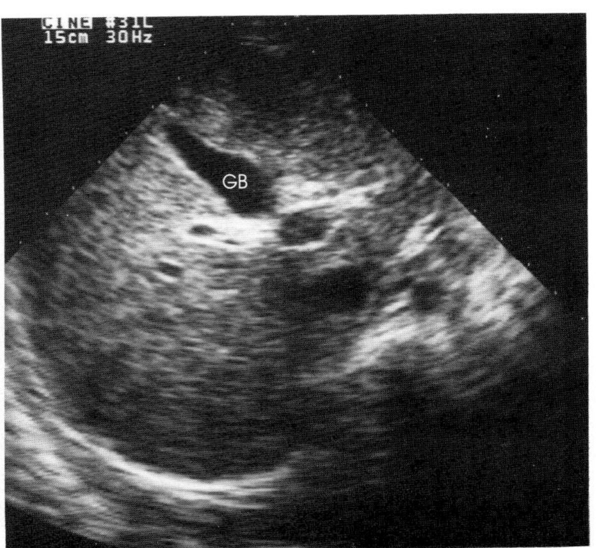

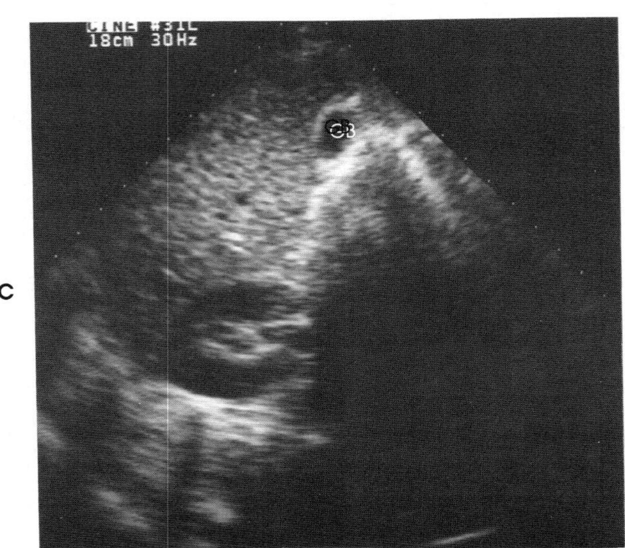

Fig. 38-40. A to **C,** Transverse scans over the right upper quadrant show a normal gallbladder.

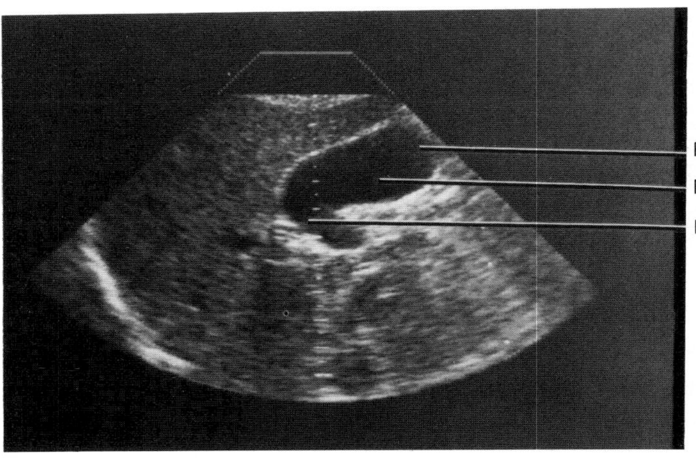

Fig. 38-41. Longitudinal scan of a normal gallbladder. An "artifactual" shadow may be seen to reflect off the neck of the gallbladder as the transducer reflects off the curved portion of the gallbladder.

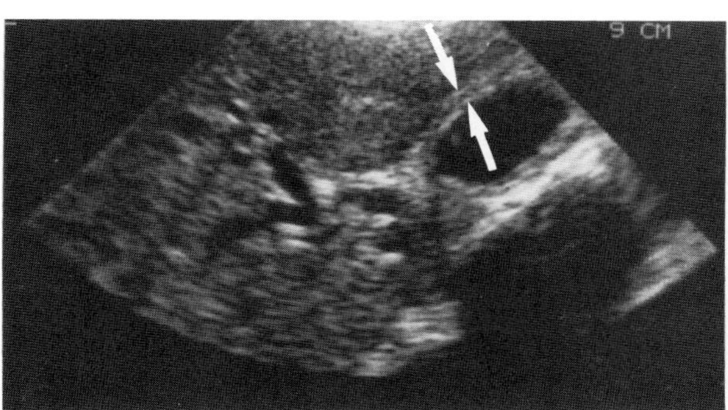

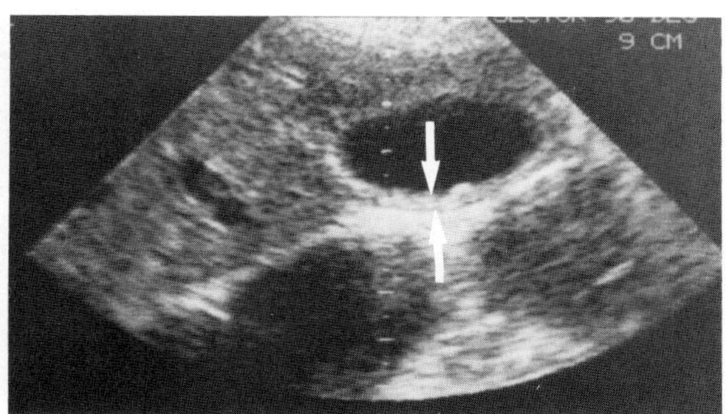

Fig. 38-42. Gallbladder wall thickness *(arrows)* is well seen in these scans. Normal wall thickness is less than 2 mm.

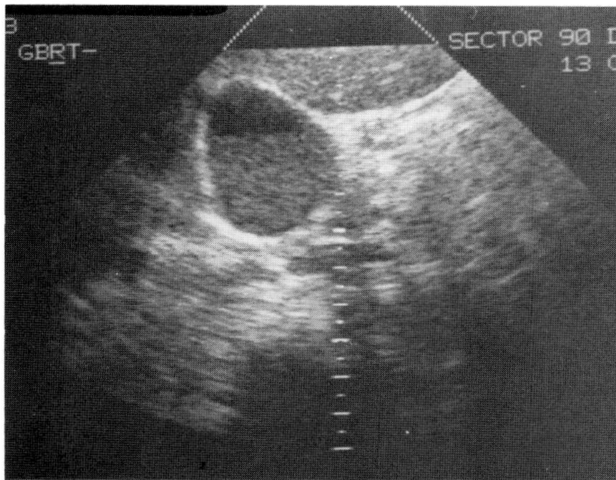

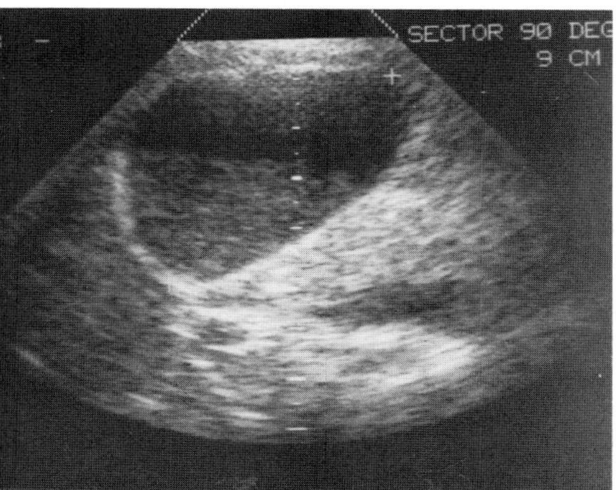

Fig. 38-43. Low-level echoes within the gallbladder represent sludge. This condition will not shadow; however, sludge may be a precursor to gallstones.

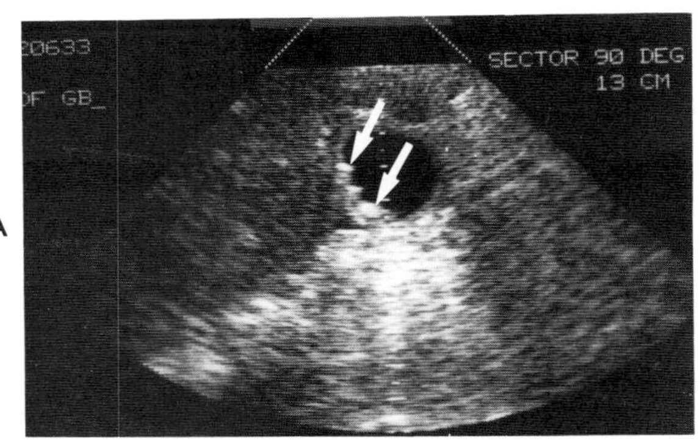

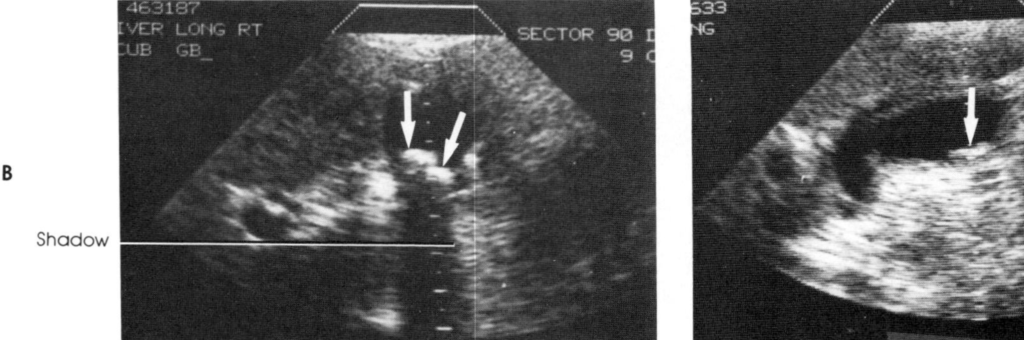

Fig. 38-44. Transverse scans **A** and **B** show a prominent gallbladder with bright interna. echoes. As the transducer is perpendicular to the echoes, the gallstones cast a posterior shadow. **C** is a longitudinal scan just at the edge of the gallstone *(arrows)*.

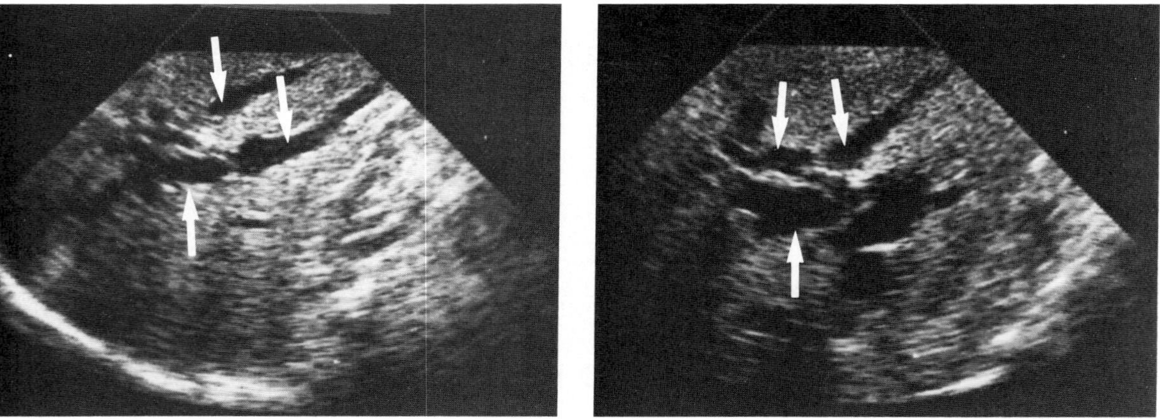

Fig. 38-45. Longitudinal scans over the liver show multiple tubes within the liver parenchyma that represent dilated intrahepatic ducts *(arrows)* caused by obstruction at the hepatic duct level.

The kidneys are assessed for size, normal calyceal pattern, abnormal texture pattern, and localization for renal biopsy (Figs. 38-46 to 38-48). Renal transplanted kidneys may be evaluated for size, presence of hydronephrosis, texture pattern (to rule out rejection), extrarenal fluid collections, and ureter size (Fig. 38-49). The retroperitoneal space is evaluated for the presence of mass lesions and abnormal omental or mesentary echo patterns.

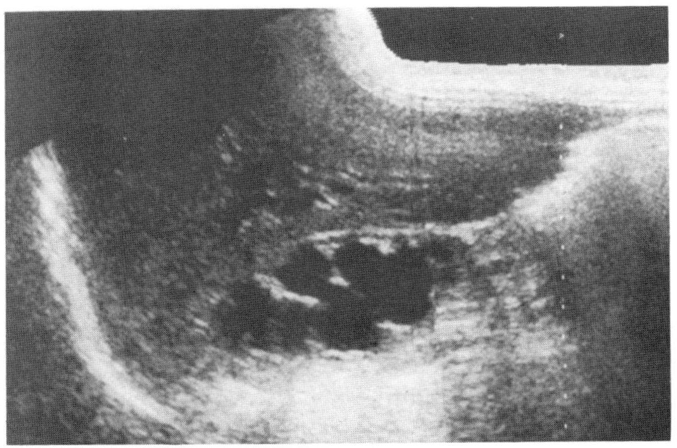

Fig. 38-46. Longitudinal scan of the right kidney shows a dark "cauliflower" appearance of the dilated renal collecting system representing renal hydronephrosis.

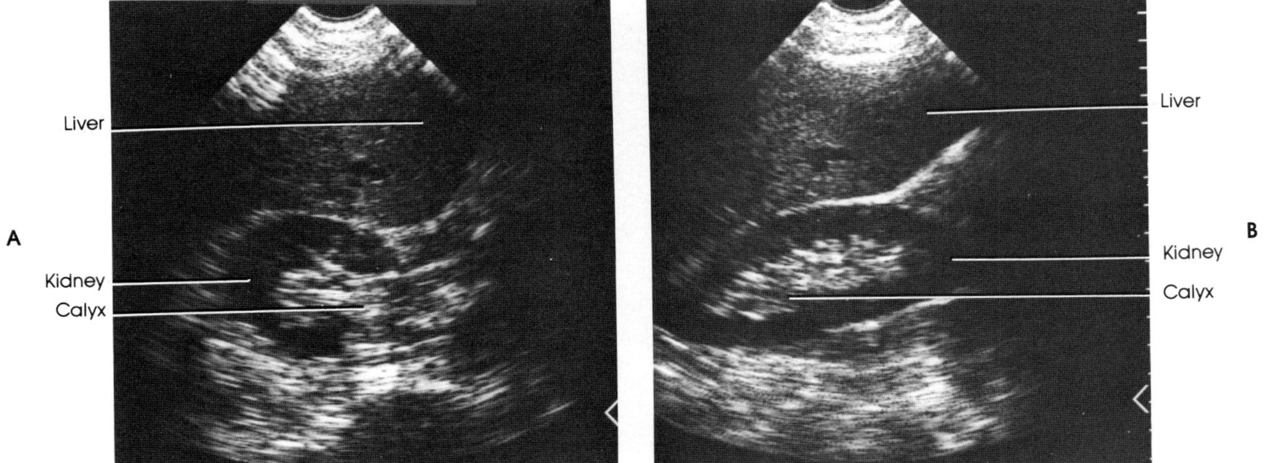

Fig. 38-47. A, Transverse and, **B,** longitudinal scans of the right kidney as visualized through the homogeneous liver parenchyma. The renal parenchyma is less echo producing than the liver except for the calyceal pattern seen in the middle of the kidney.

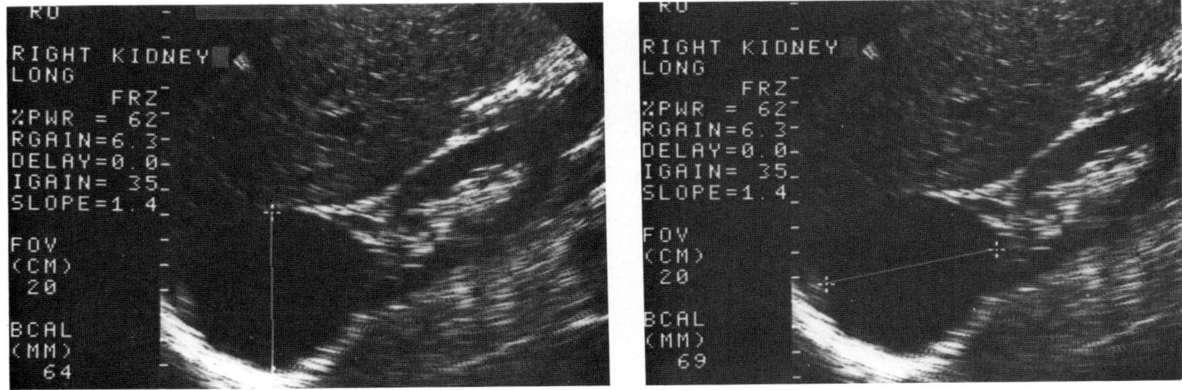

Fig. 38-48. Longitudinal scans of the right kidney show a large renal cyst at the upper pole. The cyst is seen measured in AP and longitudinal dimensions.

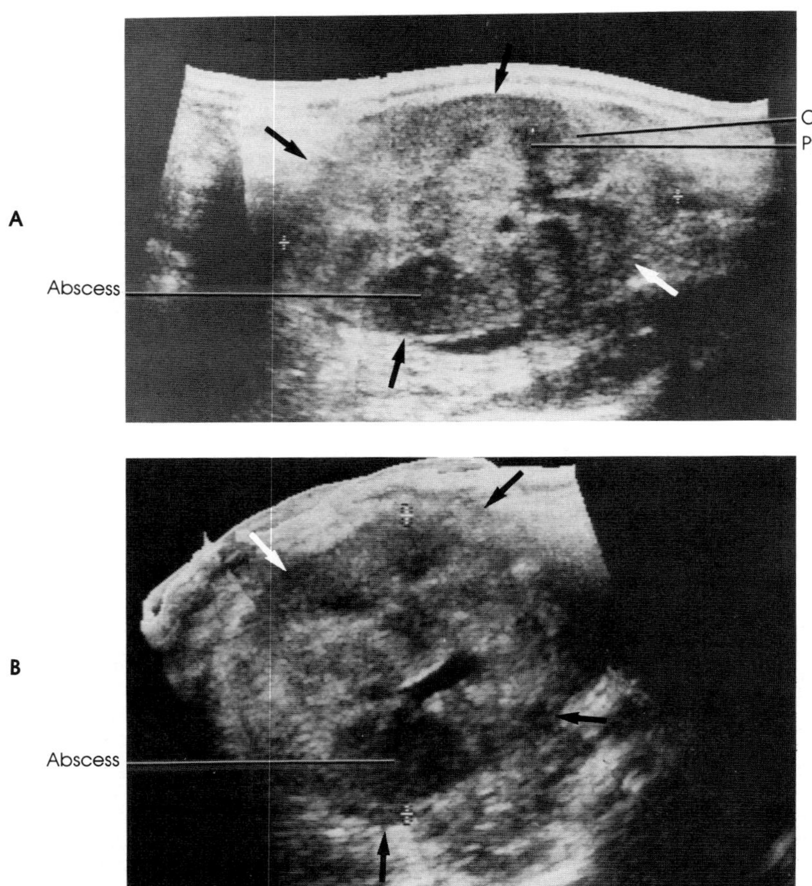

Fig. 38-49. A, Longitudinal and, **B,** transverse scans showing kidney border *(arrows)* of the renal transplant patient shows an area of decreased echogenicity that represents a renal abscess.

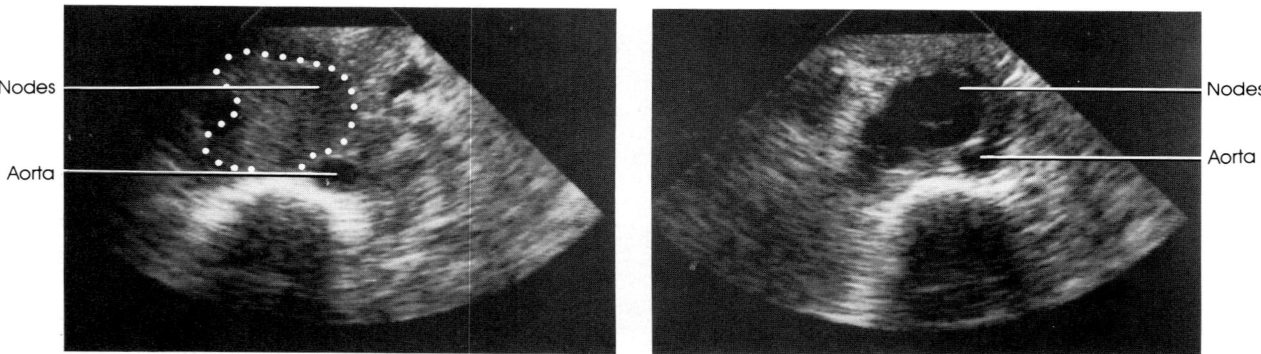

Fig. 38-50. A lymphoma patient, having undergone chemotherapy for several months, presented with fever. The question of an abscess was raised. Secondary to chemotherapy, the lymph nodes were in various stages of regression, which makes them difficult to distinguish from abscess formations. Transverse scans over the paravertebral vessels show a homogeneous and relatively low-level collection of echoes adjacent to the abdominal aorta. This represents enlarged lymph nodes.

Once a mass is suspected, the sonographer should evaluate its acoustic properties to determine if it is *hypoechoic* (fluid-filled, homogeneous, or necrotic tissue), *hyperechoic* (solid mass, thrombus, or calcification), or a combination of solid and cystic characteristics as seen in an abscess, necrotic tumor with hemorrhage, decomposing thrombus, complex tumor, or septated mass. The sonographer must additionally be able to determine the borders of a mass (whether it is smooth, irregular, ill-defined, thin, or thick) to further define its characteristics. A hyperechoic "attenuated" mass shows poor through-transmission, whereas a hypoechoic mass shows good through-transmission beyond the mass (Fig. 38-50).

A small calculus within a mass, such as a gallstone, may produce an *acoustic shadow* posterior to its border, depending on the angle of incidence and the diameter of the transducer (Fig. 38-51).

Thrombus within a vessel produces a low-level echo pattern within the dilated artery and is frequently detected in an aortic aneurysm (Fig. 38-52).

Once a mass has been localized, ultrasound can aid in the aspiration or biopsy procedure. The sonographer may locate the site of the lesion, calculate its depth, and determine the direction and angulation of needle placement for the procedure.

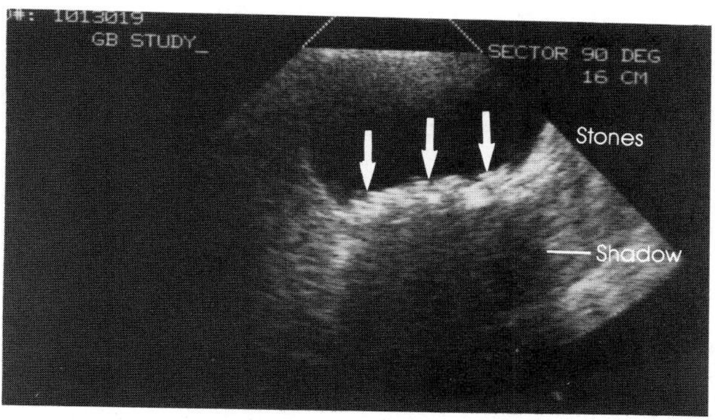

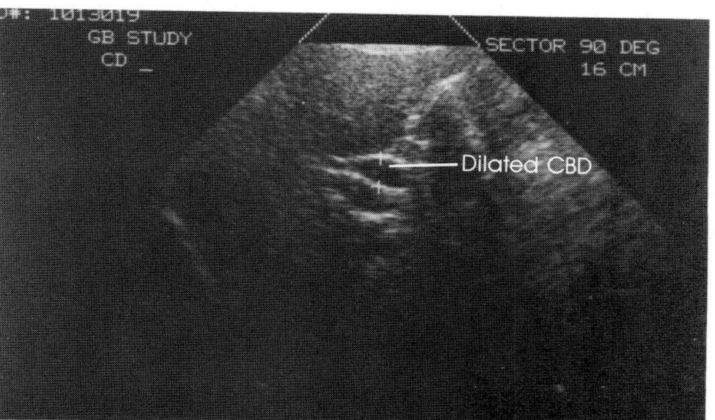

Fig. 38-51. An acoustic shadow is cast posterior to the multiple gallstones *(arrows)* in this transverse and longitudinal image (which also shows a dilated common bile duct).

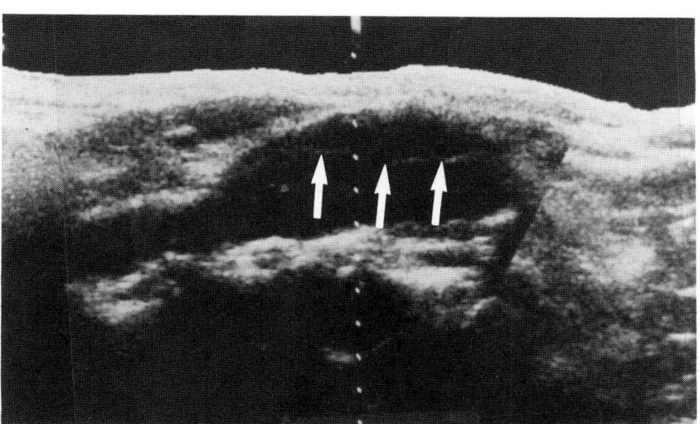

Fig. 38-52. Longitudinal scan of the abdominal aneurysm with clot formation along the anterior margin represented by a fine linear line *(arrows).*

PELVIS AND OBSTETRICS

Anatomic features of the pelvis

The pelvis is divided into the greater and lesser pelvic cavity with the pelvic brim being the circumference of a plane dividing these two portions. The greater, or false, pelvis is superior to the pelvic brim and is bounded on each side by the ilium. The lesser, or true, pelvis is situated caudal to the pelvic brim. The walls of the pelvic cavity are formed by muscles collectively called the pelvic diaphragm.

The female peritoneal cavity extends inferiorly into the lesser pelvis and is bounded by the peritoneum, which covers the rectum, bladder, and uterus (Fig. 38-53). In the female, the peritoneum descends from the anterior abdominal wall to the level of the pubic bone onto the superior surface of the bladder. It then passes from the bladder to the uterus to form the vesicouterine pouch. The pouch covers the fundus and body of the uterus and extends over the posterior fornix and the wall of the vagina. Between the uterus and the rectum the peritoneum forms the deep rectouterine pouch.

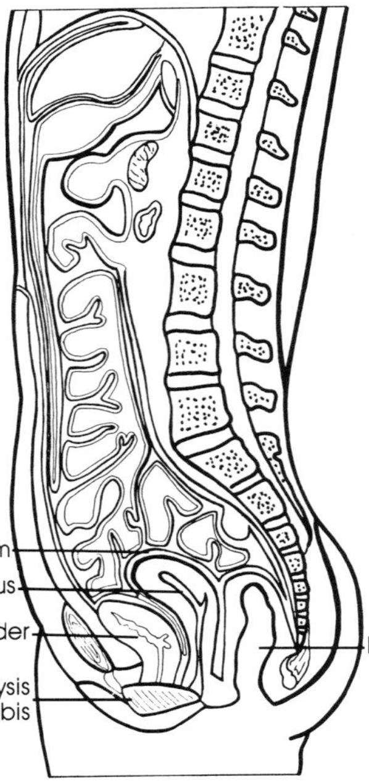

Fig. 38-53. Sagittal line drawing of the abdominal and pelvic cavity. The reflections of the peritoneal cavity are shown as it drapes over the rectum, uterus, and bladder.

Pelvis

Gynecologic examination. Examination of the female pelvis includes ultrasonic visualization of the distended urinary bladder, uterus, cervix, vagina, ovaries, and supporting pelvic musculature (Figs. 38-54 to 38-55). The rectum and other bowel structures are often visualized and, if necessary, filled by way of a water enema to separate normal structures from extra fluid or masses that may lie close to these structures. The fallopian tubes and broad ligament may be imaged, especially if the patient has excessive free fluid in the pelvic cavity.

Ultrasonic examination of the pelvis has been useful in localizing intrauterine or extrauterine pregnancies, in detecting masses or abscess collections, or in localizing an intrauterine contraceptive device.

To adequately visualize the pelvic anatomy, the patient must have a very full bladder. This allows the small bowel to be pushed superiorly out of the pelvic cavity, elevates the uterus somewhat, and serves as a *sonic window* to image the pelvic structures.

Distinct echo patterns of an enlarged uterus allow the sonographer to distinguish a leiomyoma from endometriosis or from an early gestational sac (Fig. 38-56). The sonographer is able to identify a cystic, solid, or complex mass within the ovaries or pelvic cavity, and with the use of a water enema, the sonographer can distinguish the mass from the bowel. The ultrasound interpretation, correlated with the patient's history and clinical symptoms, often allows for differential diagnosis.

Ultrasound also has been applied to women receiving fertility medication to monitor the serial growth of follicular cyst development within the ovaries. A large follicular cyst may be an indication that the egg is ready for stimulation with subsequent fertilization.

A new technique, called *endovaginal ultrasound,* allows the transducer to be inserted into the vagina to image the pelvic cavity in coronal and transverse planes. A higher frequency transducer (6 to 7.5 MHz) is employed for very high–resolution images. This technique has become a clinical aid in the visualization of the ovaries, follicles, and uterus. The gestational sac and yolk sac may be visualized very easily with this technique. A typical full bladder is not employed in this examination, although it is required with the transpelvic examination.

In postoperative patients who have developed a fever of unknown origin, ultrasound may play a role in excluding an abscess formation in the cul-de-sac of the pelvis (Douglas' pouch), the peripheral margins, or "gutters," of the abdomen, or the perirenal space.

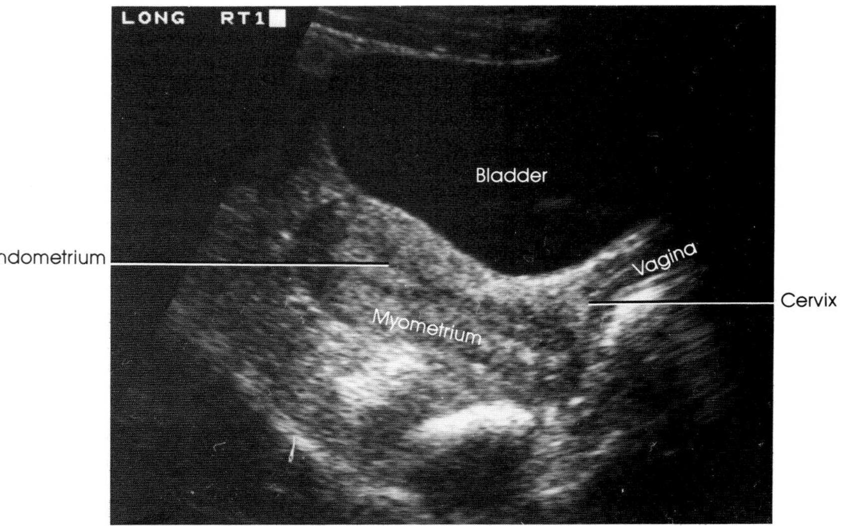

Fig. 38-54. Normal sagittal sonogram of the midline of the pelvic cavity. The distended urinary bladder is shown anterior to the uterus. The endometrium is shown as the bright linear echo within the uterus. The myometrium is the homogeneous smooth echo tissue surrounding the endometrium of the uterus. The cervix and vagina are well seen.

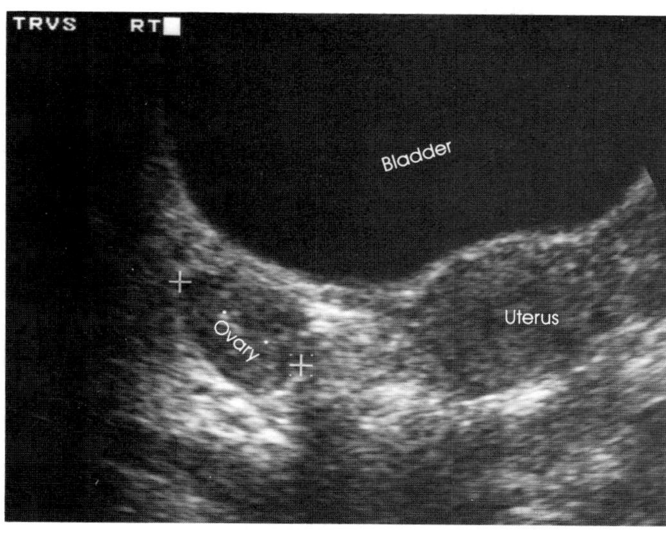

A

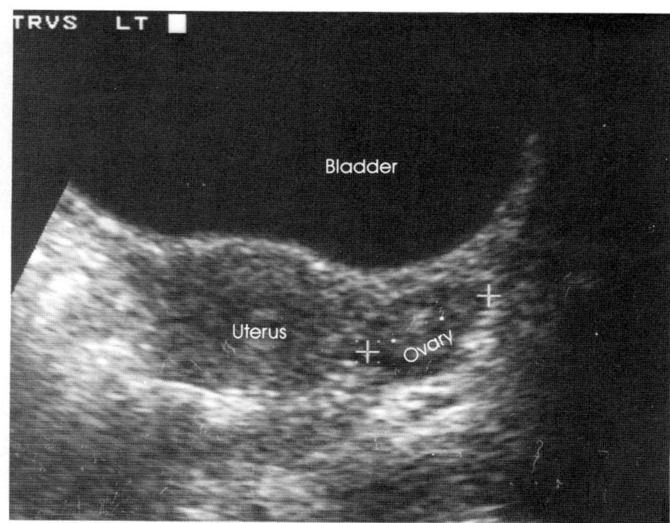

B

Pelvis and obstetrics

Fig. 38-55. A and **B,** Normal transverse scans over the lower pelvic segment show the distended bladder, uterus, and respective ovaries. If the ovaries are not visualized on transabdominal scans, the endovaginal technique is used.

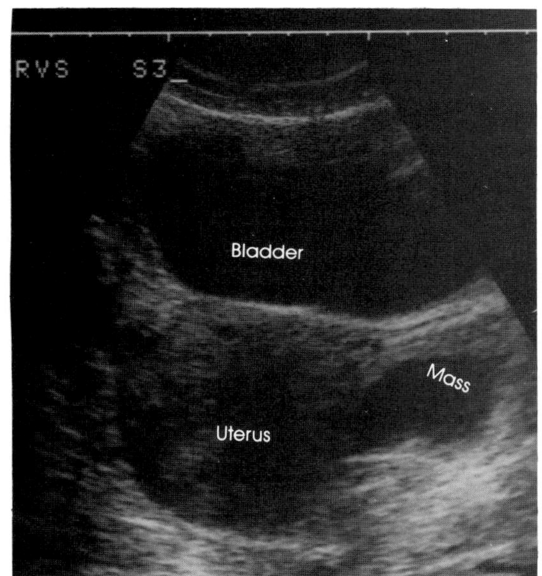

Fig. 38-56. Transverse scan in a 39-year-old female patient after undergoing dilation and curettage. The patient had bleeding and pain in the right lower quadrant. The left adnexal region shows a 2.9 × 2.4 cm complex mass. This may represent a complicated cyst with a hemorrhagic component, a chronic ectopic pregnancy, an endometrioma, or a dermoid tumor.

Obstetrics

Obstetric examination. The pregnant women is the ideal candidate for an ultrasound examination. The fluid-filled bladder acts as a sonic window to elevate the uterus out of the posterior pelvic cavity and push the small bowel away from the field of view. The amniotic fluid enhances sound penetration to differentiate fetal echo patterns from those of the placenta.

A gestational sac can be visualized as early as 4 weeks from the date of conception, and the embryo, heart, and placenta site can be seen at the tenth week of gestation. Heart motion (as well as chamber size, great vessel continuity, and valvular structure), fetal size, position, and anomalies can be assessed in the second trimester of pregnancy. Serial examinations provide information relevant to the normal or abnormal (intrauterine growth retardation) growth of the fetus. The location of the placenta can be accurately defined in diagnosing a patient with placenta previa or abruptio placentae or as an aid to the perinatologist in localization techniques for amniocentesis or other invasive procedures.

A pregnant patient whose uterus is too large for the calculated elapsed time allows the sonographer to assess for problems such as multiple gestation, hydatidiform mole development, a developing fibroid or other extrauterine mass, or simply a fetus that is more developed than the patient or physician suspected.

The fetal skull may be visualized around the eleventh week of gestation and, along with the fetal abdomen, femur, and chest, is useful in monitoring fetal growth by measurement of its *biparietal diameter* (Figs. 38-57 and 38-58). Abnormalities such as anencephaly, microcephaly, or hydrocephaly can be visualized by ultrasound in the second trimester (Figs. 38-59 to 38-63).

Other complications of pregnancy such as abnormal bleeding, an ectopic pregnancy, polyhydramnios, or oligohydramnios may also be assessed by ultrasound.

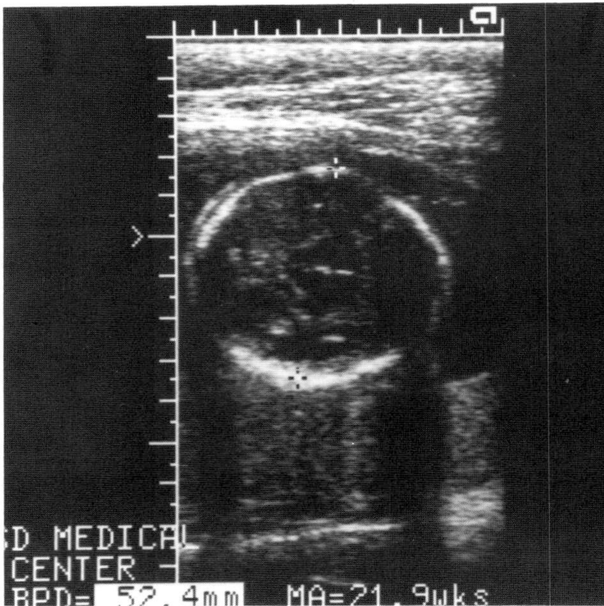

Fig. 38-57. Transverse sonogram of a fetal biparietal diameter measurement taken perpendicular to the falx of the midline. This particular measurement (marked on image) correlates with a gestational age of 21.9 weeks.

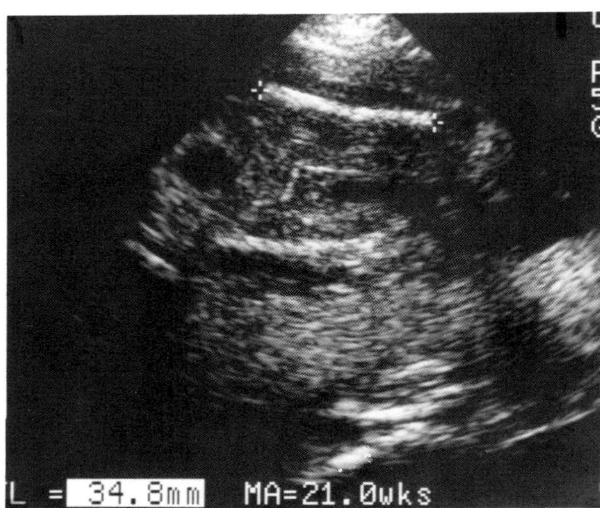

Fig. 38-58. Further correlation of the gestational age is made by taking measurements of the abdominal circumference and femur length as shown in this sagittal scan.

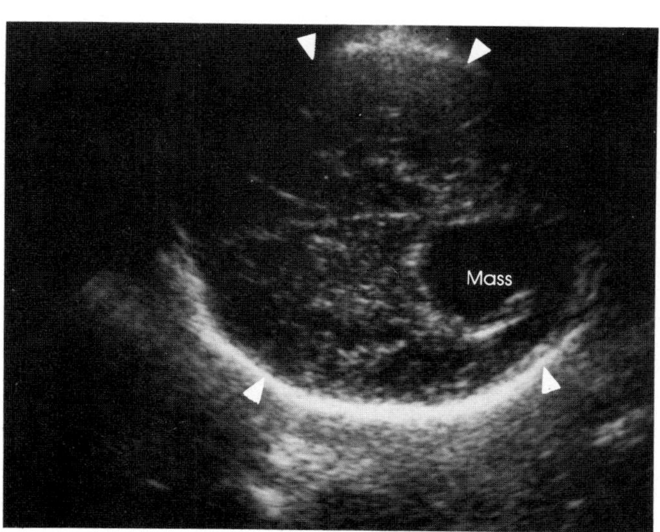

Fig. 38-59. Sonogram of the fetal skull *(arrowheads)* demonstrates a cystic mass within. This mass is located in the left supratentorial region and most likely represents an arachnoid cyst. No evidence of hydrocephalus was noted.

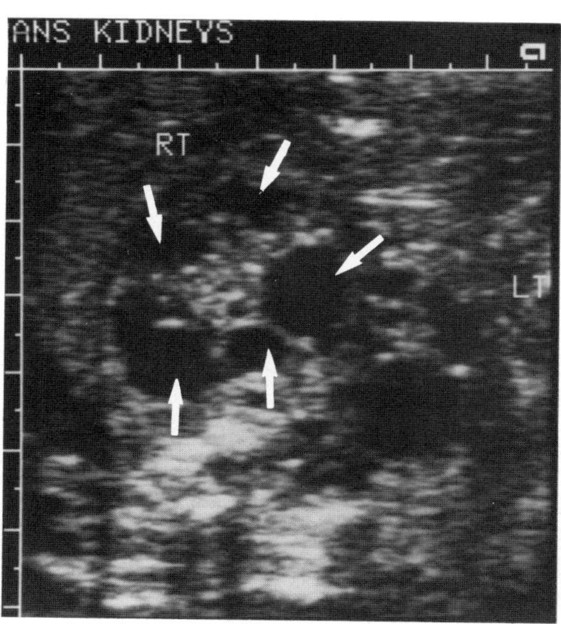

Fig. 38-60. Multiple scans on obstetric patient with severe oligohydramnios. Bilateral asymmetric renal cysts *(arrows)* were seen to occupy most of the fetal renal area with little or no renal parenchyma remaining.

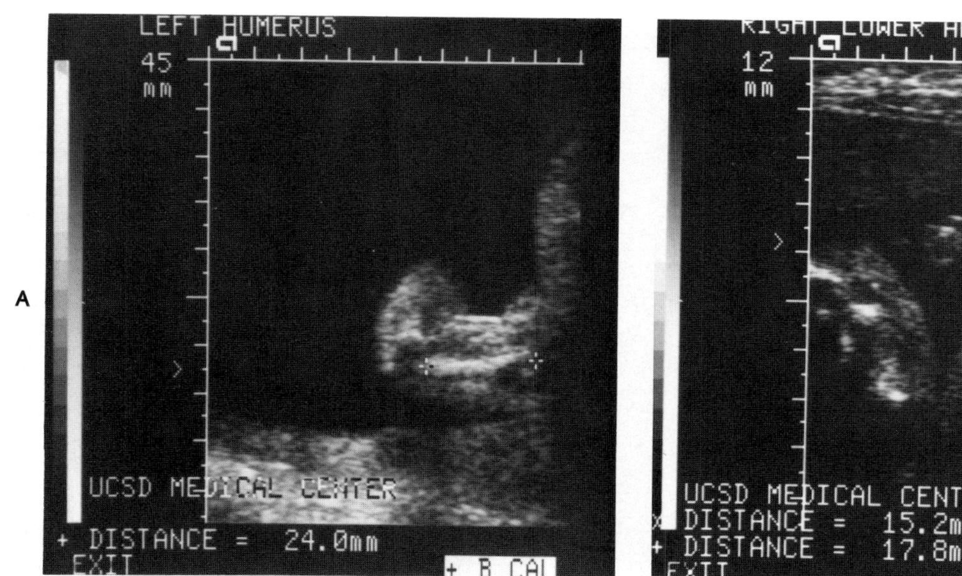

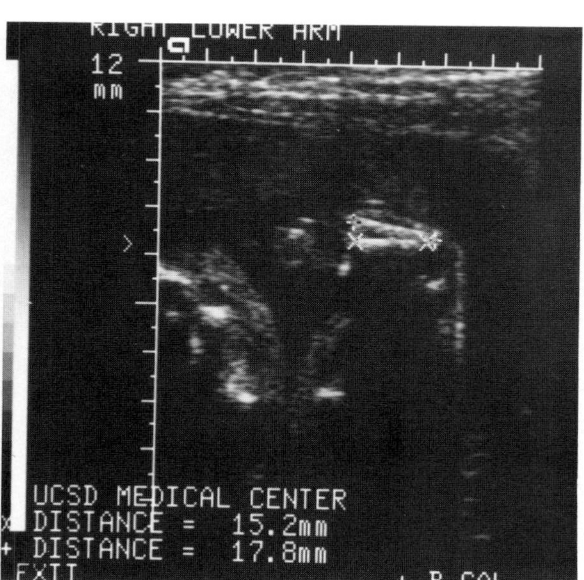

Fig. 38-61. Scans of, **A,** left humerus and, **B,** right radius and ulna taken in the second trimester of pregnancy. The extremity lengths corresponded to an 18-week gestation, whereas the other parameters indicated 29 weeks. These findings are representative of homozygous achondroplasia dwarf syndrome.

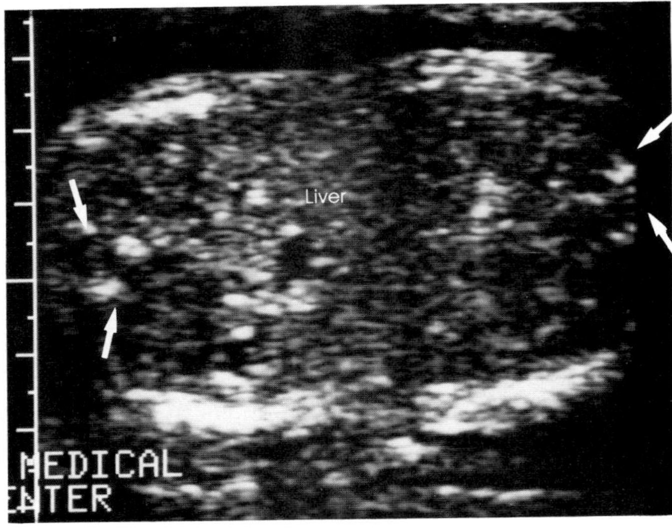

Fig. 38-62. Sonographic example of conjoined twins sharing an abnormal heart and a liver. The *arrows* point to the two respective spines in this transverse sonogram. (Scan was taken through the mid-abdomen below the level of the heart.)

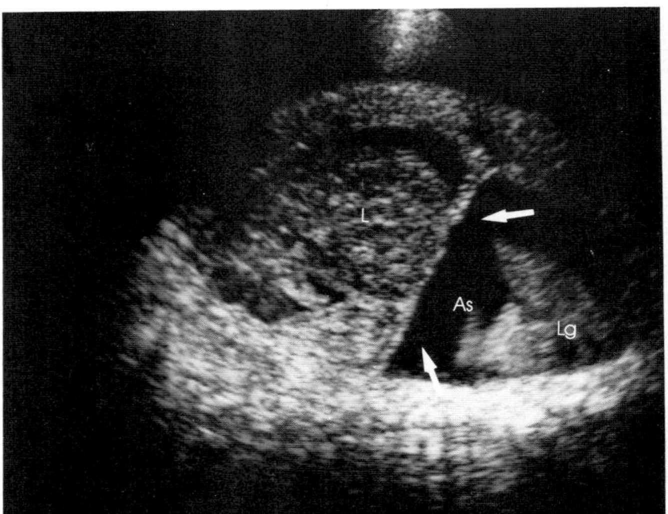

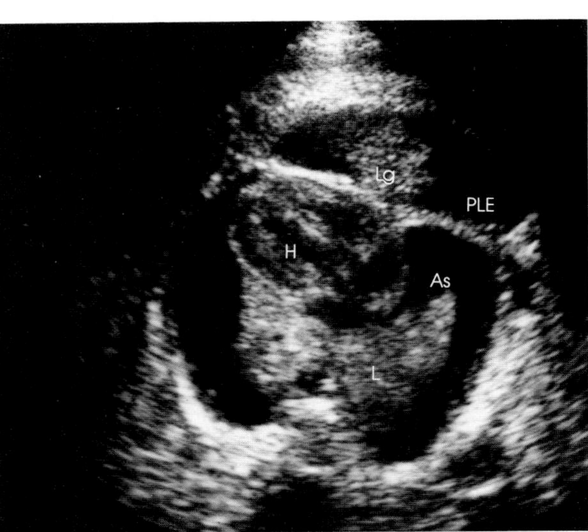

Fig. 38-63. Severe fetal hydrops shown with ascites, pleural effusion *(PLE)*, and diffuse skin thickening; liver *(L)*, diaphragm *(arrows)*, heart *(H)*, lung *(Lg)*, and ascites *(As)*.

Superficial structures

High-frequency (6 to 10 MHz) transducers have tremendously aided quality visualization of superficial structures such as the thyroid, scrotum, breast, carotid arteries, and other peripheral vascular vessels.

The visualization of minute structures such as the lactiferous ducts within the breast and spermatic cord within the testes are imaged in a routine ultrasound examination. Pathologic hypoechoic and hyperechoic areas (e.g., cyst, adenoma, carcinoma, or hydrocele) may be demonstrated on the sonogram.

The newest development in prostate imaging is the technological advance of *endorectal* transducers. This very high–resolution transducer is inserted into the rectum to visualize the anatomy of the prostate gland. If an abnormality is detected, guidance for the biopsy may be given with this ultrasound study.

Neonatal neurosonography

The B-mode evaluation of the infant head has been available since 1963; however, with technical advances in equipment, enthusiasm for this technique has grown rapidly.

The infant's head is evaluated with a series of scans performed at very small intervals across the entire head in several planes (coronal, sagittal, axial, occipital) (Figs. 38-64 to 38-66). The coronal and modified coronal sections are performed at 90 and 60 degrees from the canthomeatal line. The axial series is performed parallel to a line 10 degrees from the canthomeatal line starting 1 cm above the external auditory meatus and working toward the vertex of the cranium.

In addition, a posterior fossa (150 degrees) series perpendicular to the clivus is performed in cases in which posterior fossa abnormalities or a dilated fourth ventricle is suspected. A sagittal series is performed by scanning through the anterior fontanelle in the midline and through each lateral ventricle.

Abnormalities may be evaluated in meningomyelocele patients (Chiari II malformation), intracranial cystic abnormalities (for instance, hydrocephalus and Dandy-Walker syndrome) and other congenital malformations such as agenesis of the corpus callosum, holoprosencephaly, and arteriovenous malformations.

In addition, ultrasound is useful in evaluating the infant with intracranial infection, hemorrhage, tumor, or for following ventricular shunt function.

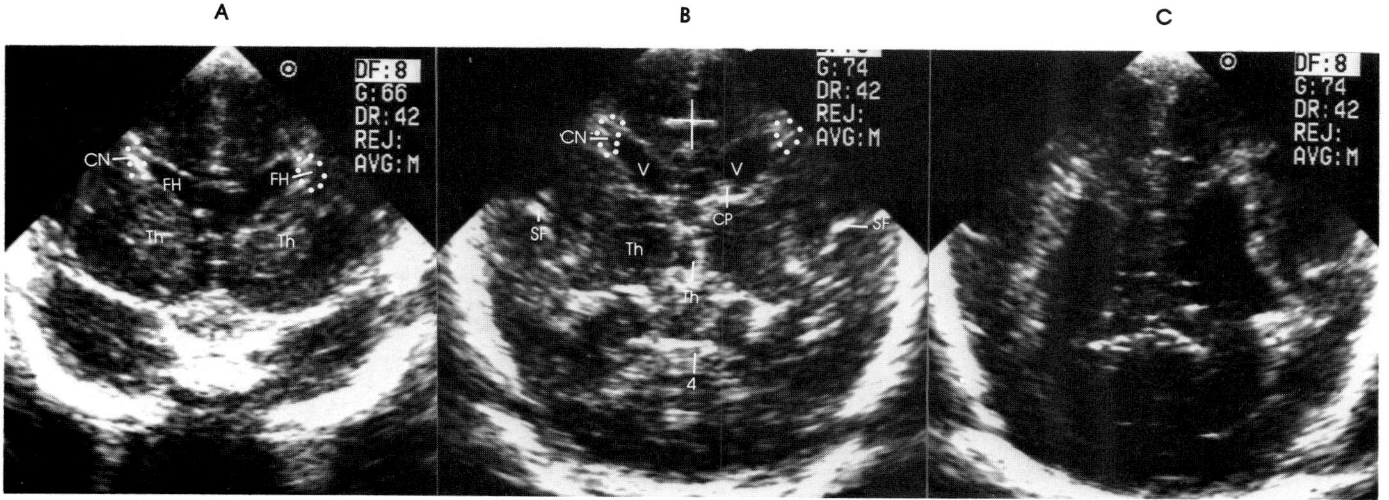

Fig. 38-64. Multiple coronal images of the neonatal skull; the coronal image is taken along the axis of the coronal suture. **A,** The transducer is angled toward the anterior skull (face); the small semilunar slits are anterior to the frontal horns *(FH)* of the lateral ventricle; the caudate nucleus *(CN)* is adjacent to the frontal horns, with the thalamus *(Th)* posterior. **B,** The transducer is perpendicular to the skull; the body of the ventricle *(V)* is seen, along with the third *(3)* and fourth *(4)* ventricles; the choroid plexus *(CP)* is the dense echogenic material found along the floor of the ventricle; the sylvian fissure *(SF)* is easily seen on the lateral aspect of the brain. **C,** The transducer is angled toward the posterior skull; the body of the lateral ventricles *(V)* is easily seen.

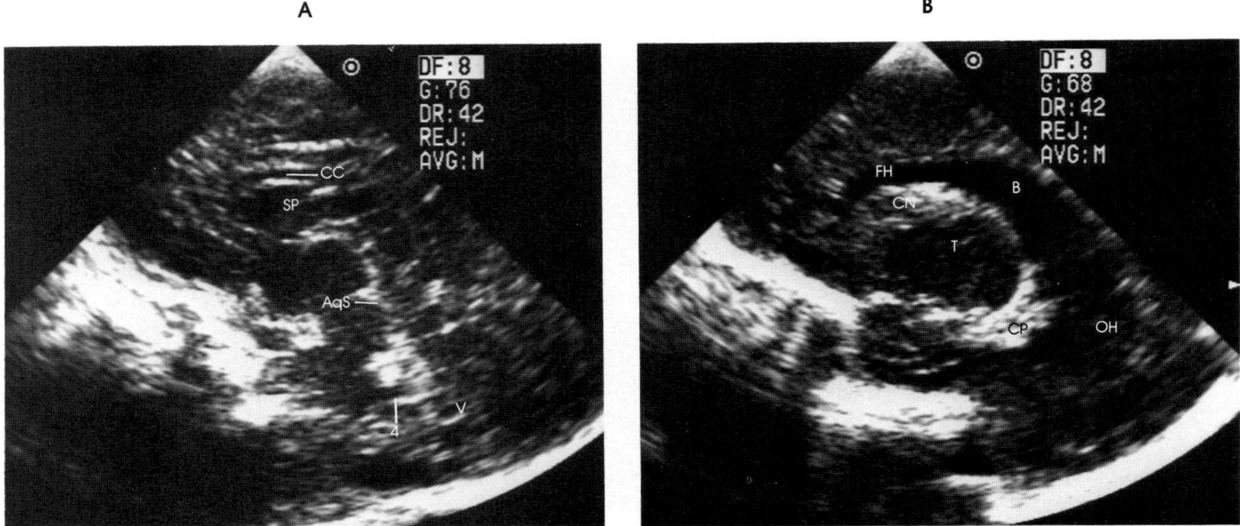

Fig. 38-65. Sagittal images of the neonatal skull. **A,** Midline sagittal view shows the cavum septi pellucidi *(SP)*, the corpus callosum *(CC)*, the aqueduct of Sylvius *(aqS)*, the fourth ventricle *(4)*, and the vermis of the cerebellum *(V)*. **B,** Sagittal scan shows the lateral ventricle (frontal horn *[FH]*, body *[B]*, occipital horn *[OH]*, and temporal horn *[TH]*); the caudate nucleus *(CN)* and choroid plexus *(CP)* are shown as echodense structures; the thalamus *(T)* is also seen.

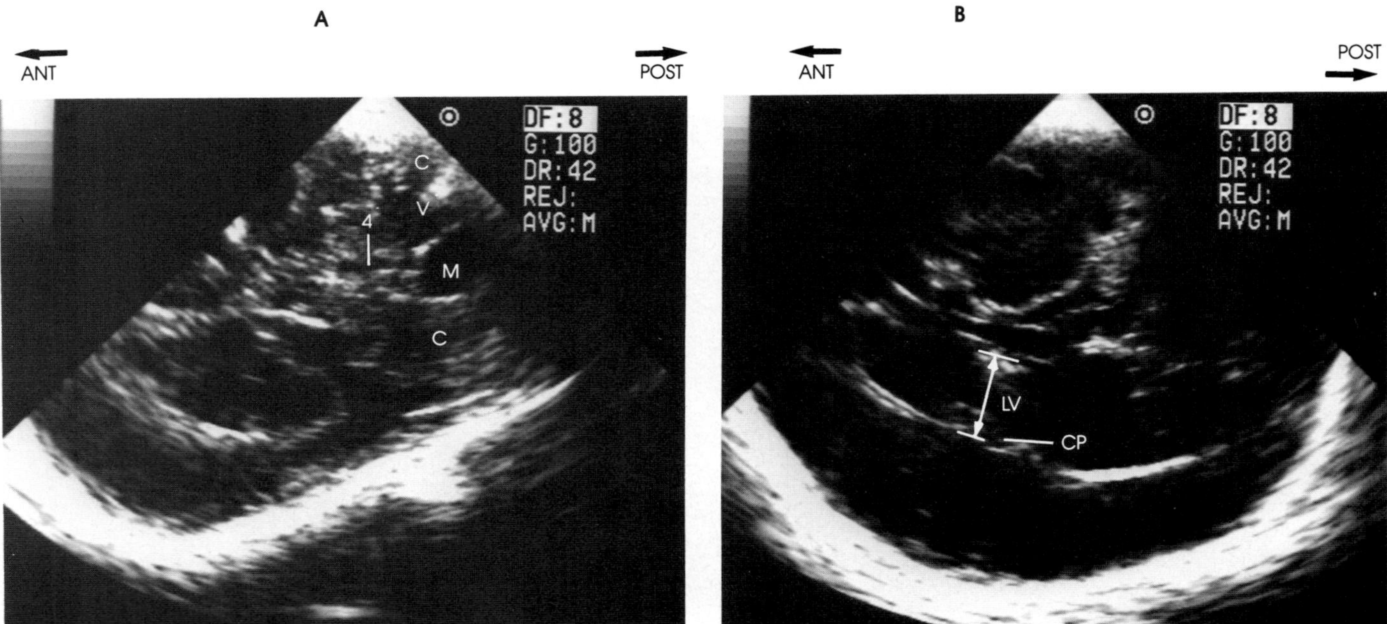

Fig. 38-66. Axial views of the neonatal skull obtained by placing the transducer on the lateral aspect of the neonatal head: anterior is to the left; posterior to the right. **A,** Axial view showing the area of the fourth ventricle *(4)*, cerebellum *(C)*, and medulla oblongata *(M)*. **B,** Axial view with a slight superior angulation shows the lateral ventricles *(LV)* with the choroid plexus lying along the far lateral edge; this is a good view to measure the size of the lateral ventricles.

Cardiology applications

The echocardiographic examination includes visualization of the four chambers of the heart (right and left ventricles, right and left atria), the four valvular structures (mitral, tricuspid, aortic, and pulmonic valves), the interatrial and interventricular septa, the delineation of cardiac musculature (endocardium, myocardium, epicardium), the papillary muscles and chorda tendineae cordis, and the pericardium (Fig. 38-67). The application of real-time two-dimensional ultrasound in the adult, pediatric, neonatal, and fetal patient has proven to be a tremendous diagnostic aid for the echocardiographer.

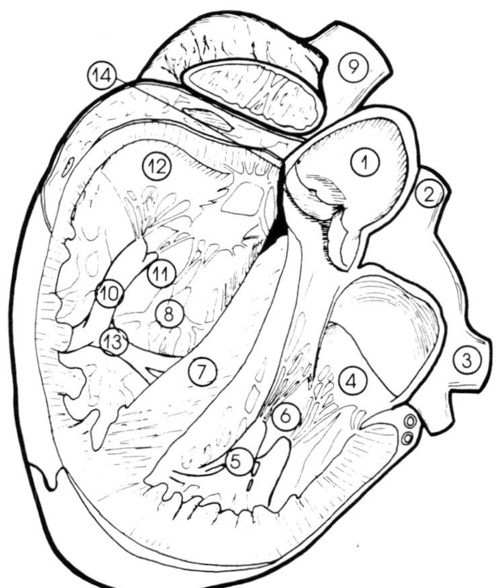

1 Ascending aorta
2 Right pulmonary vein
3 Left pulmonary vein
4 Mitral valve
5 Posterior papillary muscle
6 Left ventricle
7 Muscular interventricular septum
8 Right posterior papillary muscle
9 Superior vena cava
10 Septal band
11 Right ventricle
12 Tricuspid valve
13 Moderator band
14 Membranous interventricular septum

Fig. 38-67. Schematic drawing of the right and left ventricles of the heart. The left ventricle is slightly larger than the right. Its wall is thicker because of increased pressure on the left. The interventricular septum separates the two chambers.

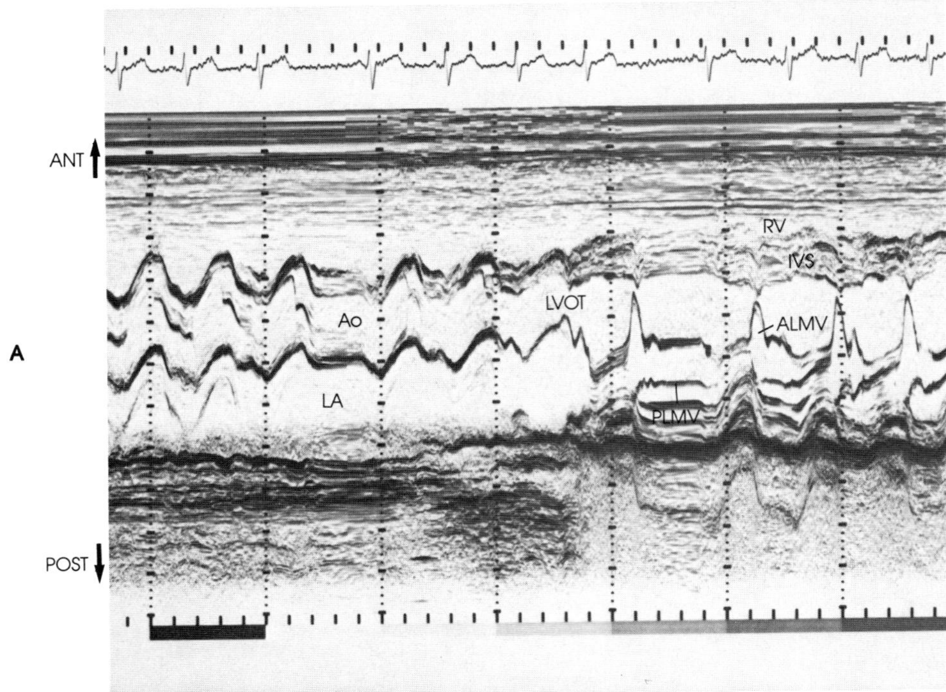

Fig. 38-68. A, M-mode tracing of a sweep from the aorta *(Ao)* and left atrium *(LA)*, to the left ventricular outflow tract *(LVOT)*, to the right ventricle *(RV)*, interventricular septum *(IVS)*, and anterior *(ALMV)* and posterior *(PLMV)* leaflets of the mitral valve. Continuity is shown between the anterior wall of the aorta and the interventricular septum; continuity is also shown between the posterior aortic wall and anterior leaflet of the mitral valve.

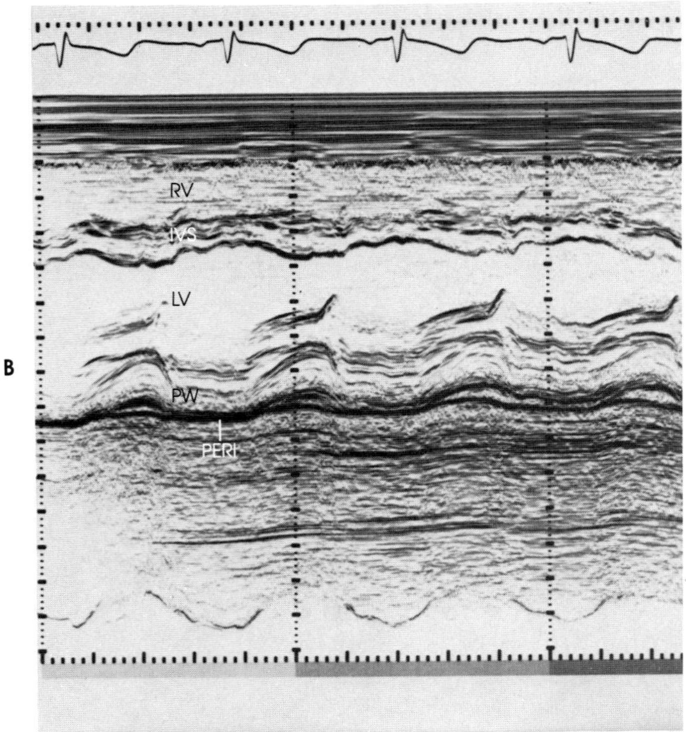

Fig. 38-68, cont'd. B, M-mode tracing of the right and left ventricles. The posterior wall of the left ventricle is easily seen. The pericardial *(Peri)* echo is very strongly reflected because of the change in acoustic impedance between the blood-filled ventricle and the lung interface.

Although M-mode recordings allow precise measurement of cardiac structures, they provide a very limited "ice pick" view of the total cardiac anatomy when used alone (Fig. 38-68). Thus two-dimensional ultrasound allows visualization of the cardiac activity and structures from the base of the heart to its apex with simultaneous M-mode tracings for subsequent measurements and analysis.

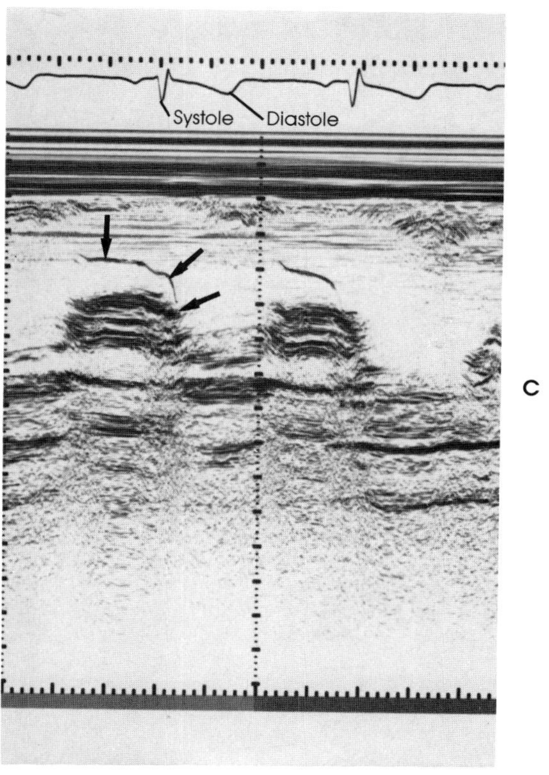

Fig. 38-68, cont'd. C, M-mode tracing of the pulmonic valve as it opens in systole and closes in diastole.

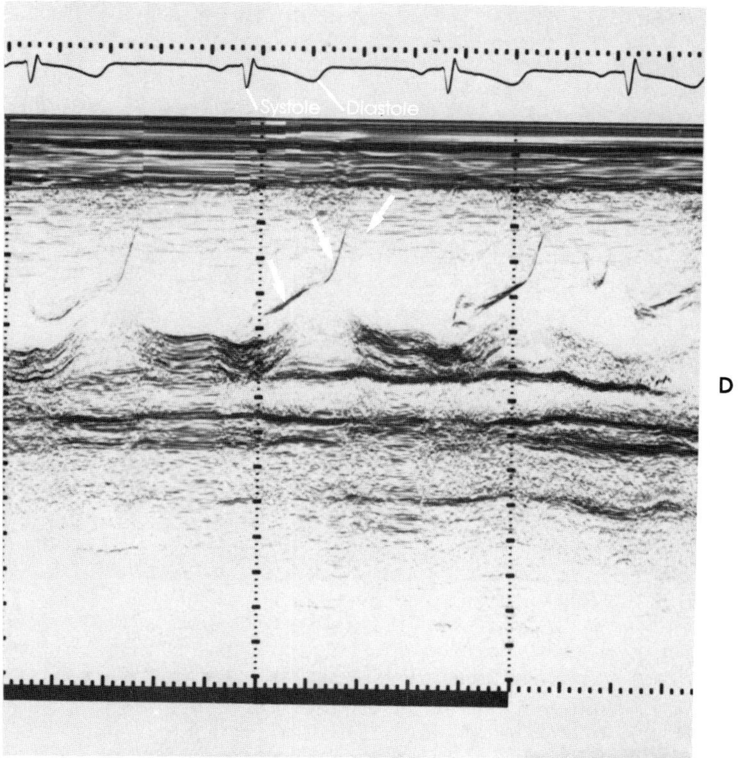

Fig. 38-68, cont'd. D, M-mode tracing of the anterior leaflet of the tricuspid valve located on the right side of the heart. The valve opens in diastole and closes in systole.

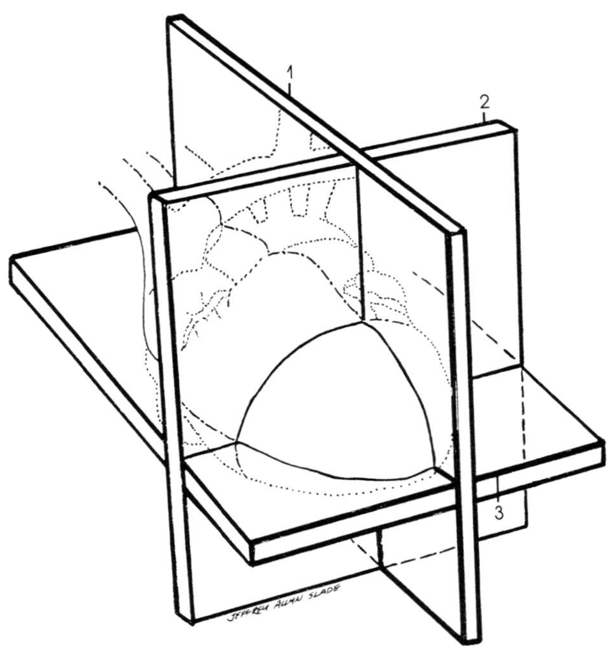

Fig. 38-69. Schematic drawing of the multiple planes of the heart used in echocardiography: *(1)* denotes the parasternal long axis, *(2)* denotes the parasternal short axis, and *(3)* denotes the apical four-chamber plane.

Procedure for echocardiography. The examination usually begins with the patient in a slightly left lateral, semidecubitus position, because this moves the heart away from the sternum and closer to the chest wall, thus producing a better cardiac window (Fig. 38-69). The transducer should be placed slightly to the left of the sternum in the third, fourth, or fifth intercostal space. The "cardiac window" is then located by noting the strong pulsatile reflection of the pericardial sac as a result of the change in acoustic impedance from the cardiac structures to the air-filled lung.

The real time procedure usually includes the following views:

1. Long-axis views: from the base of the heart to its apex (Fig. 38-70)
2. Multiple short-axis views (Figs. 38-71 and 38-72)
3. Apical or subxiphoid views: to image the four chambers and valves simultaneously (Figs. 38-73 and 38-74)
4. Suprasternal view: to image the aortic arch and tributaries, right pulmonary artery, left atrium, and left mainstem bronchus

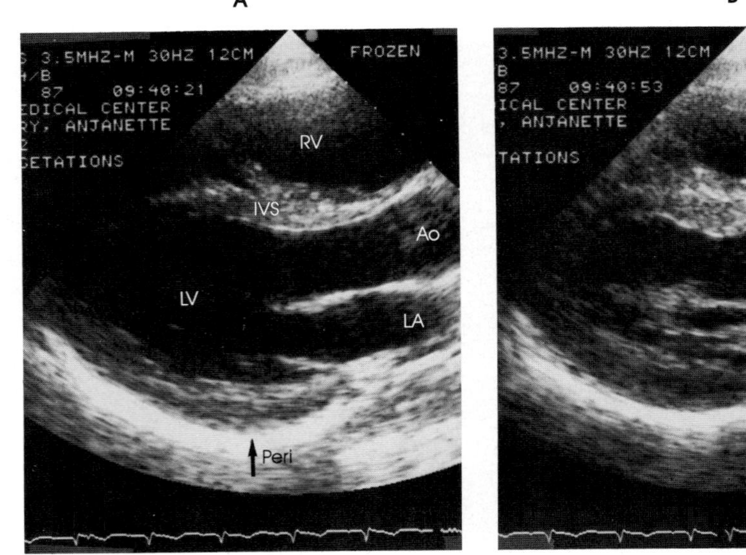

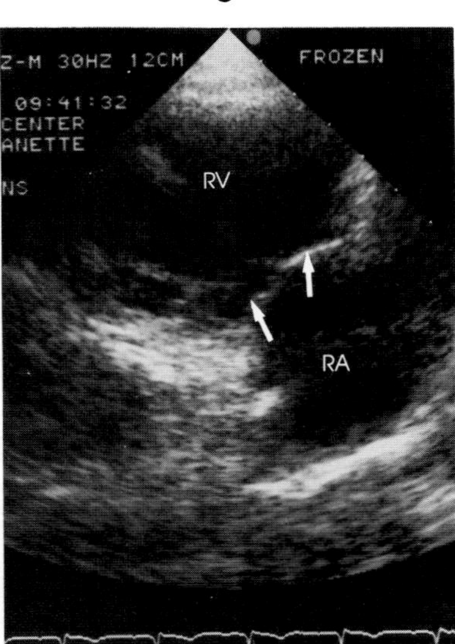

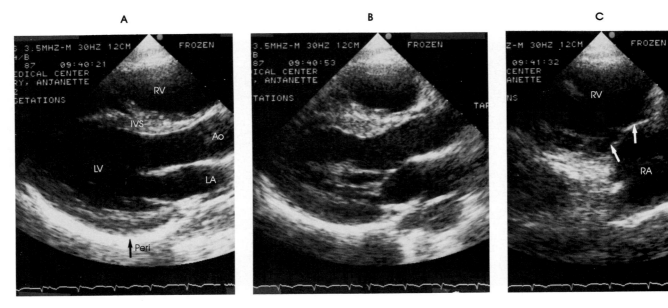

Fig. 38-70. **A,** Diastolic and, **B,** systolic frames of the parasternal long-axis view in the heart as the mitral valve opens in diastole to allow blood to fill the ventricular cavity as it flows through the orifice from the left atrium. When the mitral valve closes, the ventricle pumps blood through the aortic cusps into the ascending aorta. **C,** Parasternal long-axis view with the transducer angled medially and to the right shows the right ventricle *(RV)*, tricuspid valve *(arrows)*, and right atrium *(RA)*.

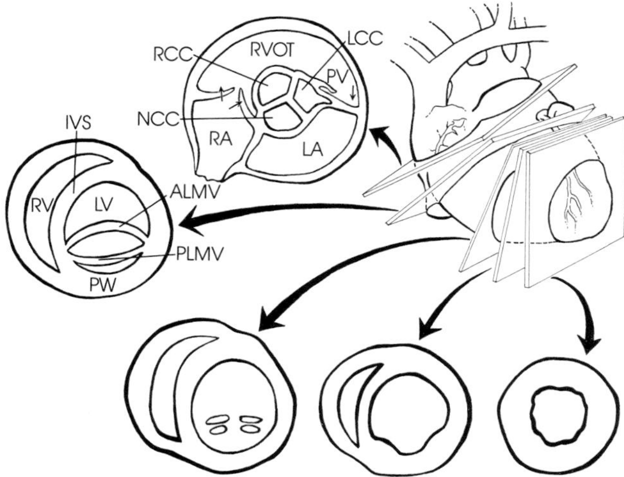

Fig. 38-71. Schematic drawings of multiple parasternal short-axis views of the heart. The transducer has been rotated 90 degrees from the long-axis plane. Right ventricle *(RV)*, interventricular septum *(IVS)*, left ventricle *(LV)*, anterior leaflet mitral valve *(ALMV)*, posterior leaflet mitral valve *(PLMV)*, and posterior wall of left ventricle *(PW)*, right ventricular outflow tract *(RVOT)*, right atrium *(RA)*, left atrium *(LA)*, aortic cusps *(RCC, LCC, NCC)*, pulmonary valve *(PV)*.

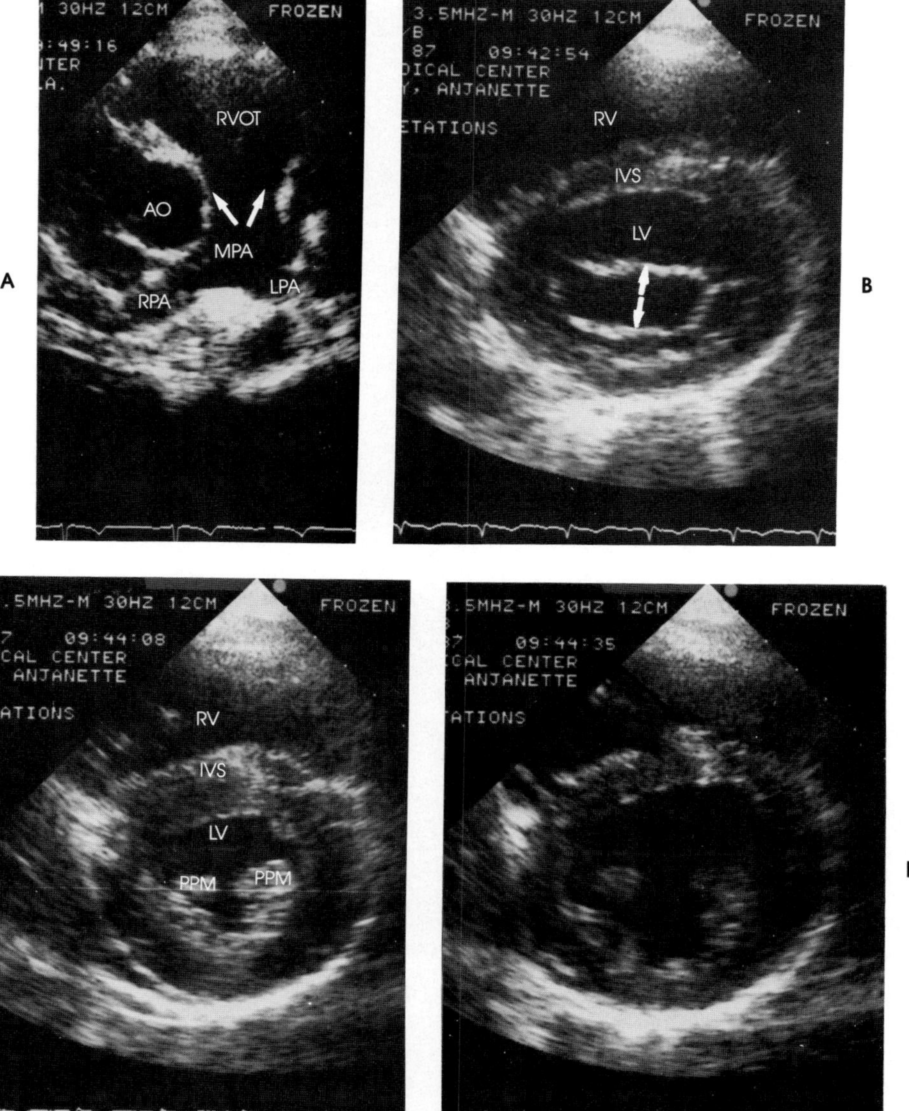

Fig. 38-72. A, High-parasternal short-axis view of the heart shows the right ventricular outflow tract wrapped anterior to the aorta. The main pulmonary artery *(MPA)* shows the pulmonary valve *(arrows)* before it bifurcates into right and left pulmonary arteries. **B,** Mid-parasternal short-axis view over the right ventricle, septum, and mitral valve within the left ventricle. **C** and **D,** Low-parasternal short-axis views of the heart show the right ventricle wrapped anterior to the septum and left ventricular cavity. The two prominent projections into the left ventricle represent the posterior papillary muscles *(PPM)*.

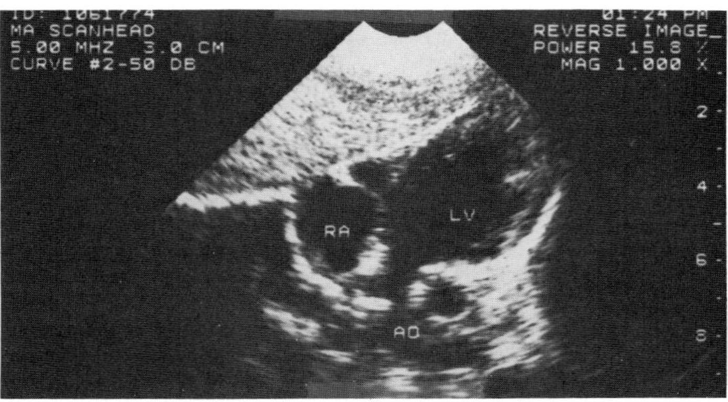

Fig. 38-73. Subcostal view with an anterior angulation clearly shows the left ventricular outflow tract and ascending aorta.

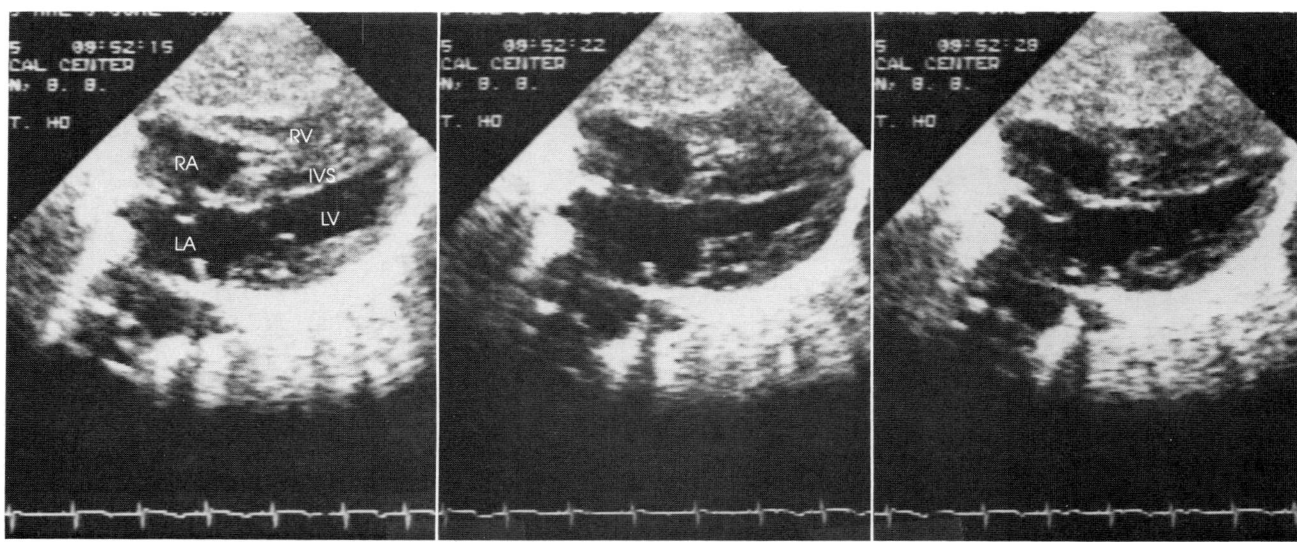

Fig. 38-74. Multiple subcostal four-chamber views taken in systole and diastole show the movement of the foramen ovale as it moves between the right and left atrial cavities.

Diagnosis of pathologic conditions. Pathologic conditions such as calcification, thickening, vegetation formation, clot, thrombus, rupture, tear, bulging, abnormal movement, or aneurysm can be detected to provide a diagnosis for the cardiac patient (Figs. 38-75 to 38-82).

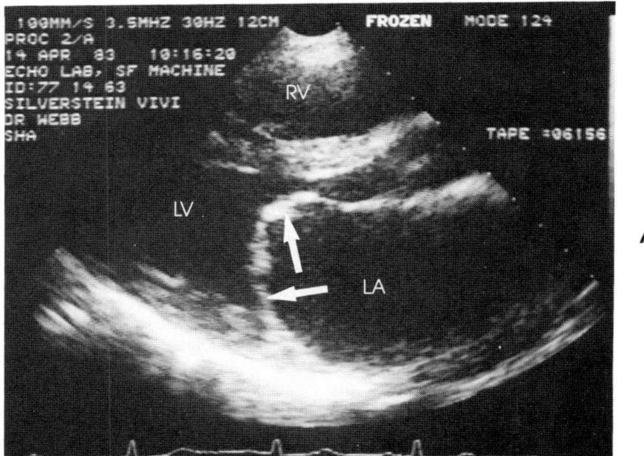

A

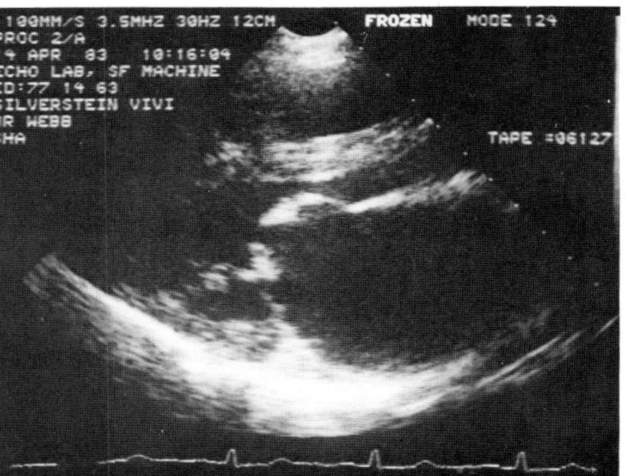

B

Fig. 38-75. A, Systolic and, **B,** diastolic frames taken in the parasternal long-axis view in a patient with severe mitral stenosis. The anterior leaflet *(arrows)* is thickened and does not open to its full excursion. The left atrium is dilated because of the calcified mitral valve, causing mitral regurgitation.

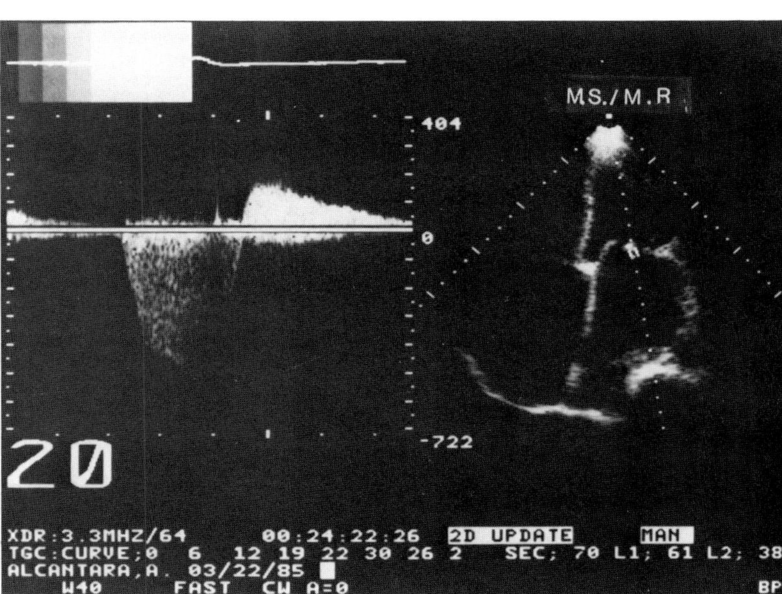

Fig. 38-76. Doppler tracing of a patient with severe mitral stenosis and regurgitation made in the apical four-chamber view. There is 5 m/sec velocity flow pattern of mitral regurgitation seen as a negative deflection from the baseline.

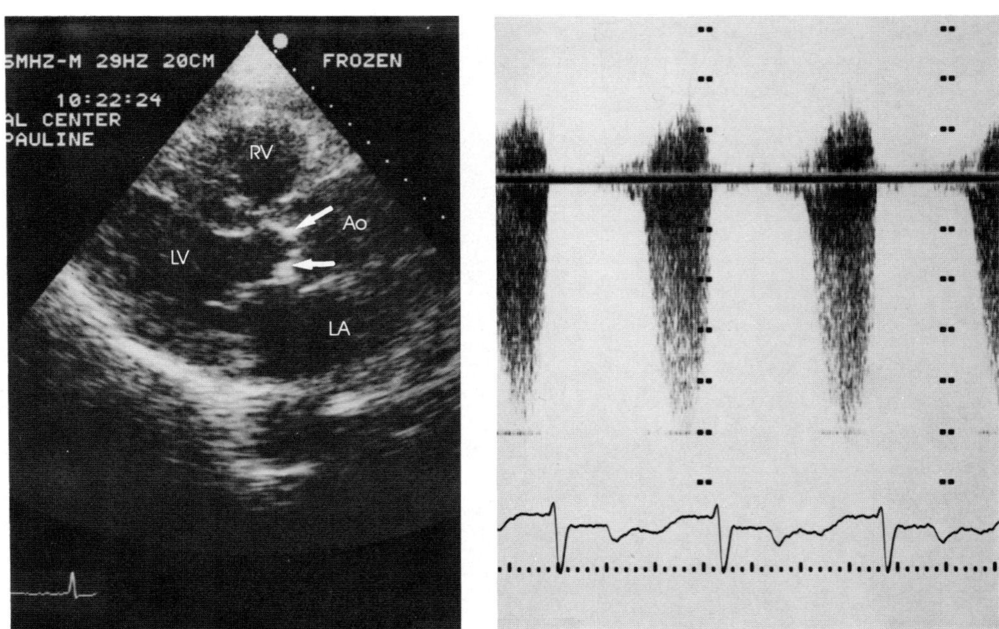

Fig. 38-77. Two-dimensional and Doppler tracings (from the apical five-chamber view) in a patient with significant aortic stenosis. The leaflets are thickened with restrictive opening. There is 4.5 m/sec of aortic stenosis.

A

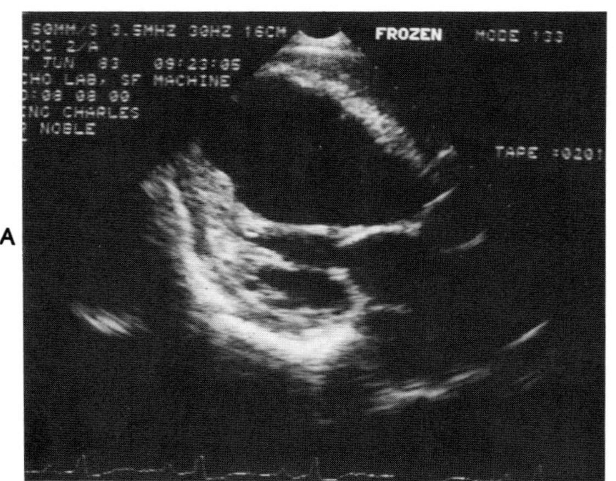

B

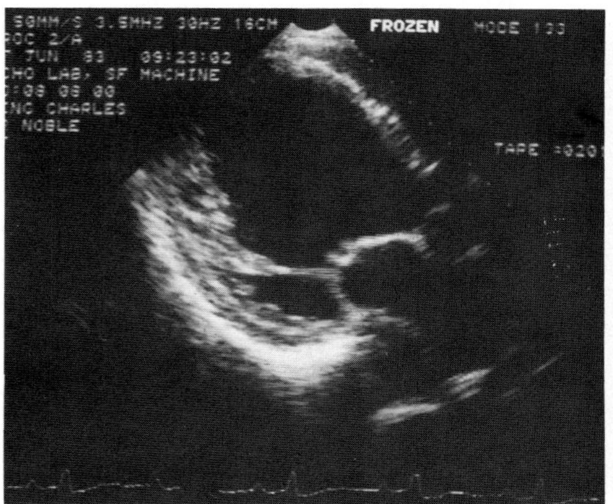

C

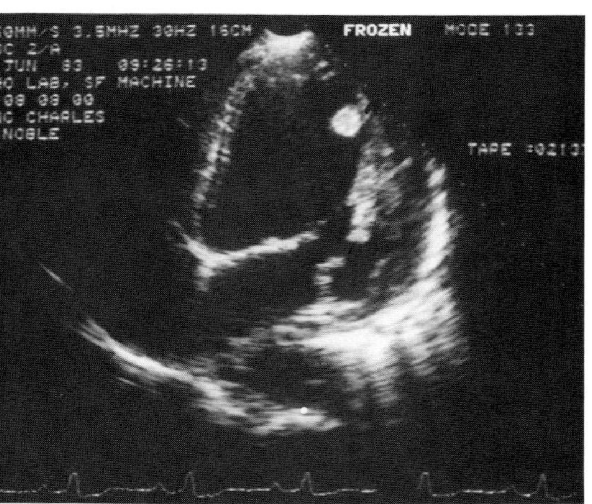

Fig. 38-78. A, Systolic and, **B,** diastolic long-axis views of a very dilated heart in a patient with congestive cardiomyopathy. **C** shows a four-chamber view of the cardiac dilation with a bright echo from a thrombus formation near the apex of the heart.

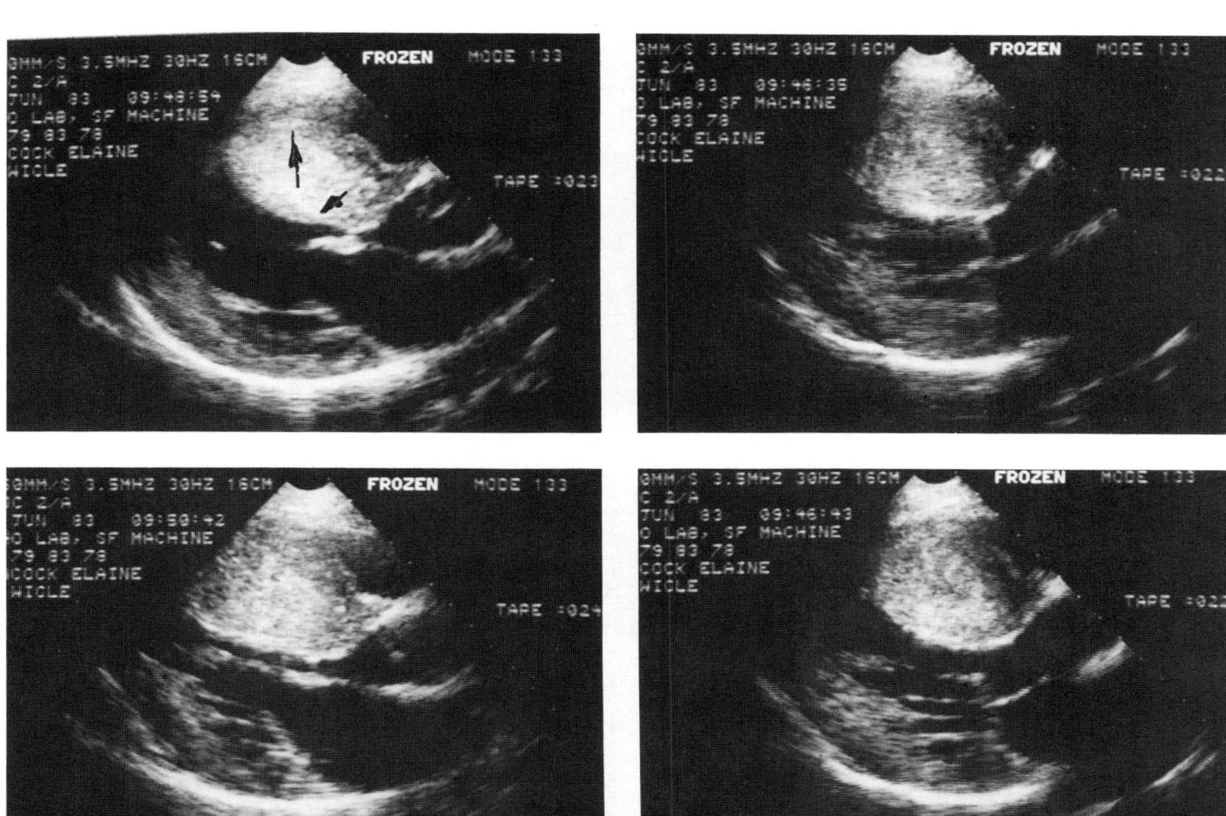

Fig. 38-79. Multiple parasternal long-axis views in a patient with hypertrophic cardiomyopathy show a huge septum *(arrows)* with bright echoes throughout.

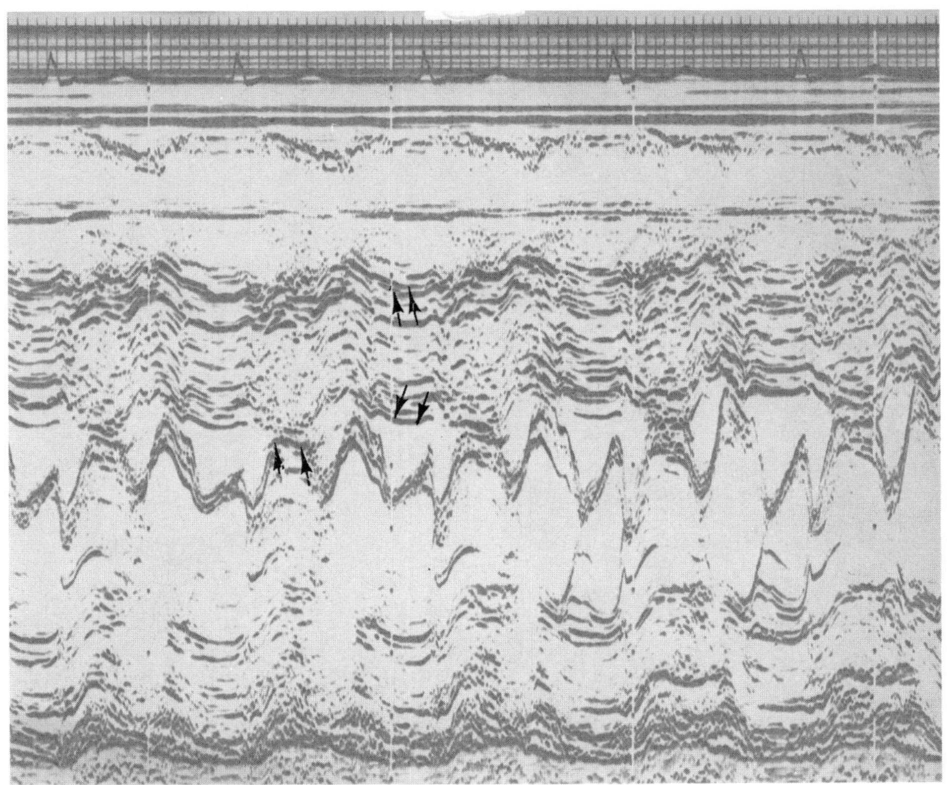

Fig. 38-80. One of the complications of hypertrophic cardiomyopathy is obstruction to the left ventricular outflow tract caused by a systolic anterior motion of the mitral leaflet *(arrows)*. The borders of the interventricular septum are highlighted by double sets of arrows. Normal septal thickness should not exceed 1.3 cm; this septum measures nearly 2.0 cm.

A

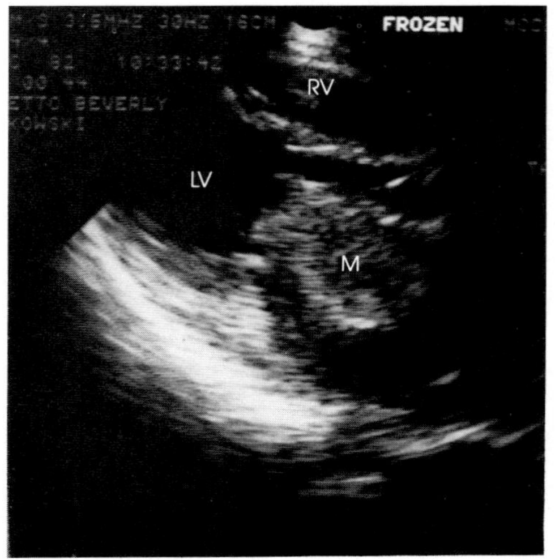

B

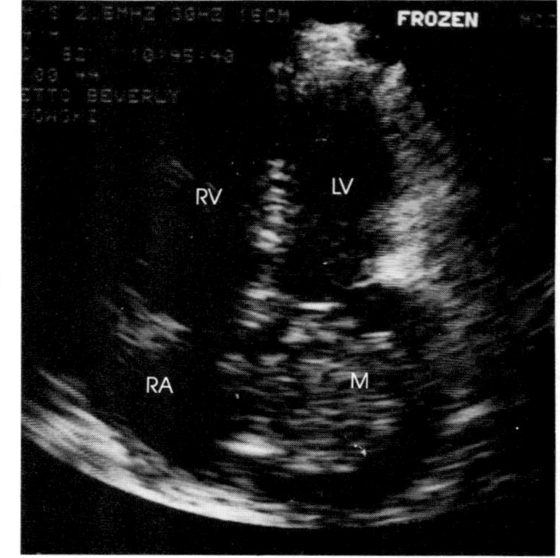

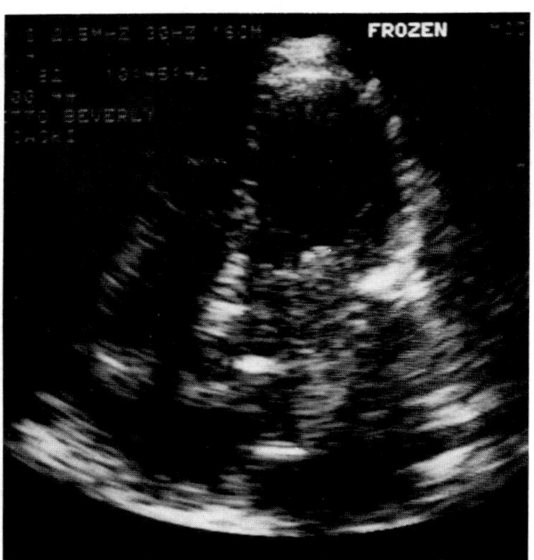

C

Fig. 38-81. A, Parasternal long-axis view and, **B** and **C,** apical four-chamber views of a patient with a large left atrial myxoma. The tumor mass is seen throughout the cardiac cycle as it flops behind the mitral valve and falls into the left atrial cavity.

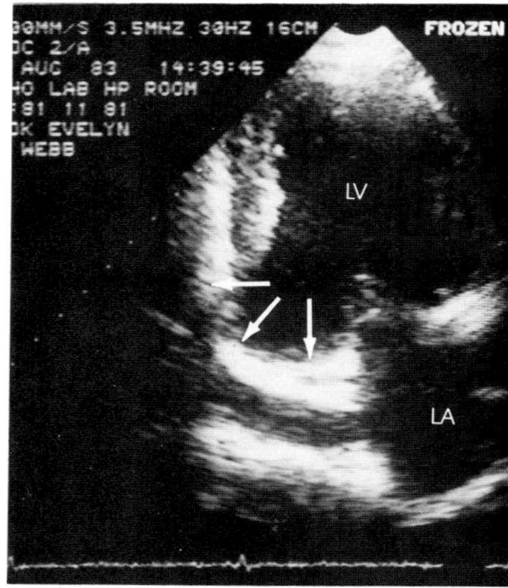

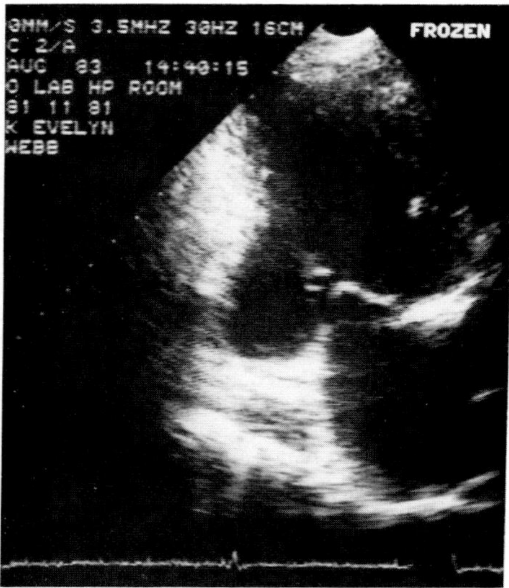

Fig. 38-82. Parasternal long-axis views of the left ventricle with an aneurysmal formation in the posterior basal segment *(arrows).* This condition may occur secondary to a myocardial infarction as the tissue becomes scarred and weakened.

The evaluation of pericardial effusion can be effectively monitored by ultrasound evaluation. In the event of a large effusion, the pericardiocentesis needle may be guided by the sonographer in a subxiphoid approach (Fig. 38-83).

The analysis of left ventricular function and the serial evaluation of patients after myocardial infarction are currently being investigated with the aid of computer analysis to measure change in the intraventricular and posterior left ventricular wall thickness and contractility. The gray-scale reflections of normal tissue, scar tissue, and newly infarcted tissues are also being evaluated through myocardial contrast studies for further understanding of the cardiac patient.

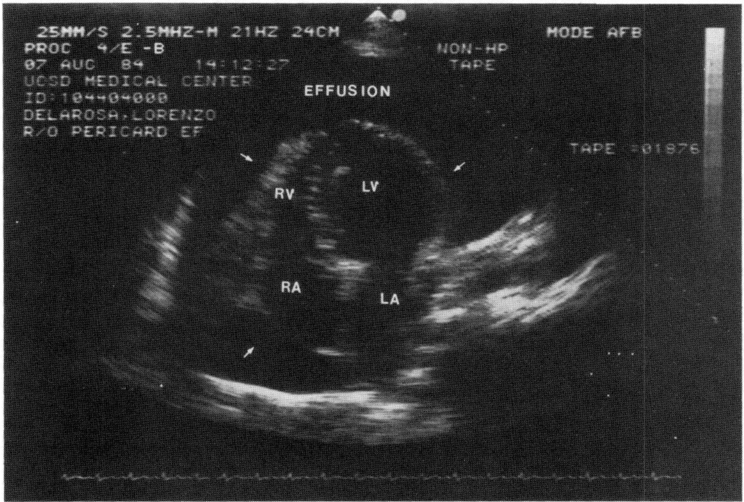

Fig. 38-83. In this apical four-chamber echocardiographic view, the four chambers of the heart are completely surrounded by the huge effusion *(arrows)* from the atrioventricular junction to the basal segment of the right atrium.

Simple and complex congenital lesions of the heart have been effectively diagnosed through the use of echocardiography. With careful evaluation, the sonographer can determine the size and number of chambers; the placement of valves (e.g., aortic-septal discontinuity represented by Fallot's tetralogy with a large ventricular septal defect and pulmonary stenosis); the size of the valves (e.g., agenesis, atresia, stenosis, deformed, domed, redundant); the size, thickness, and continuity among the chambers, walls, and interventricular and interatrial septa; and the orientation of the great vessels and their relationship to the ventricles (Figs. 38-84 to 38-89).

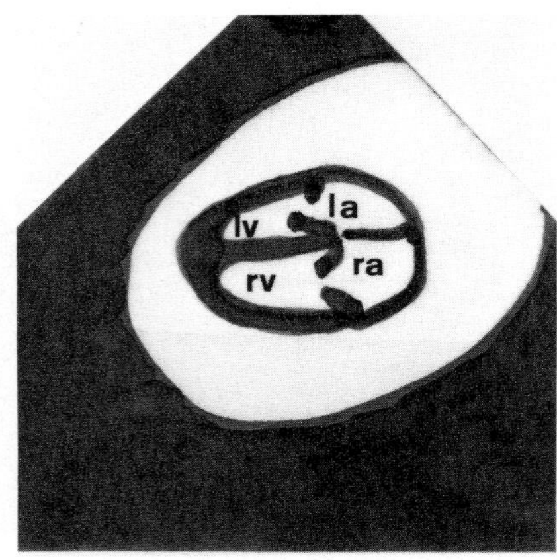

Fig. 38-84. Fetal echocardiography has become a useful diagnostic tool in high-risk obstetrical patients. This is an 18-week fetus with a normally developed four-chamber heart.

The critically ill newborn has a much better chance for survival if the correct diagnosis is made early. Thus, with the aid of a skilled sonographer, the condition of the cyanotic infant can be diagnosed as congenital heart disease or severe respiratory distress. Critical heart disease in a cyanotic infant includes a hypoplastic left heart, transposition of the great vessels, truncus arteriosus, or pulmonary atresia.

As a new addition to the cardiac examination, color-flow Doppler mapping has enabled the sonographer to assign specific flow maps to corresponding Doppler flow patterns. Thus, with the aid of audible Doppler flow, the pattern of flow may also be demonstrated on the two-dimensional image. Flow towards the transducer is coded in various shades of red, while flow away from the transducer is coded in various shades of blue.

The Doppler technique has added a new dimension to imaging flow patterns within the heart. Shunt flow across an ventricular or atrial septal defect is well defined with this technique. In addition, multiple defects may be detected with color mapping. Areas of narrowing, or stenosis, cause a specific turbulent pattern within the vessel, likewise areas that leak or regurgitate cause a smooth back flow from the valve into the chamber below.

A

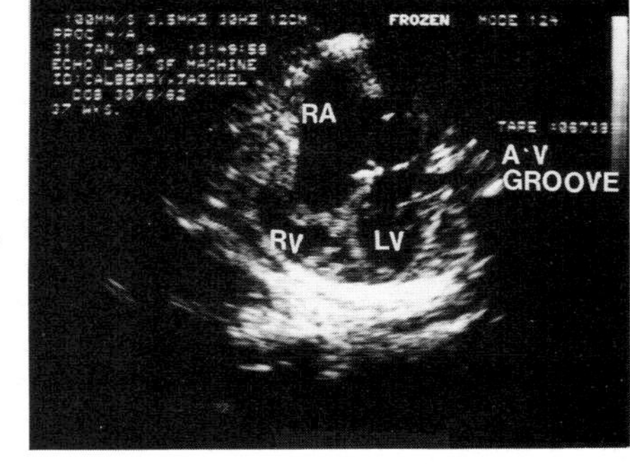

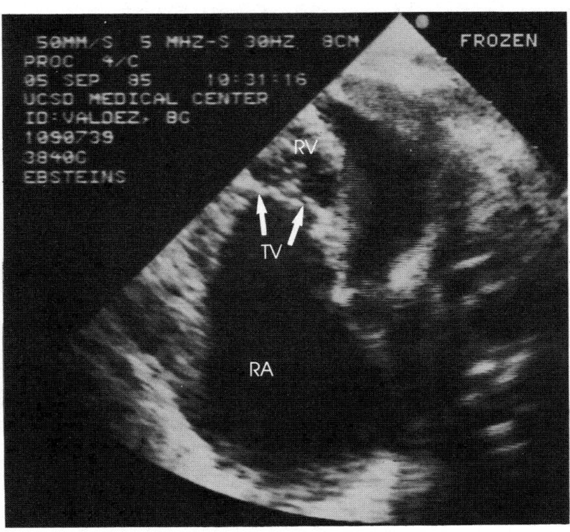

B

Fig. 38-85. Ebstein's anomaly of the heart in a fetus **(A)** and infant **(B)** show an apically displaced tricuspid valve *(TV)*, a large "atrialized right atrium" *(RA)*, and a small hypofunctioning right ventricle *(RV)*.

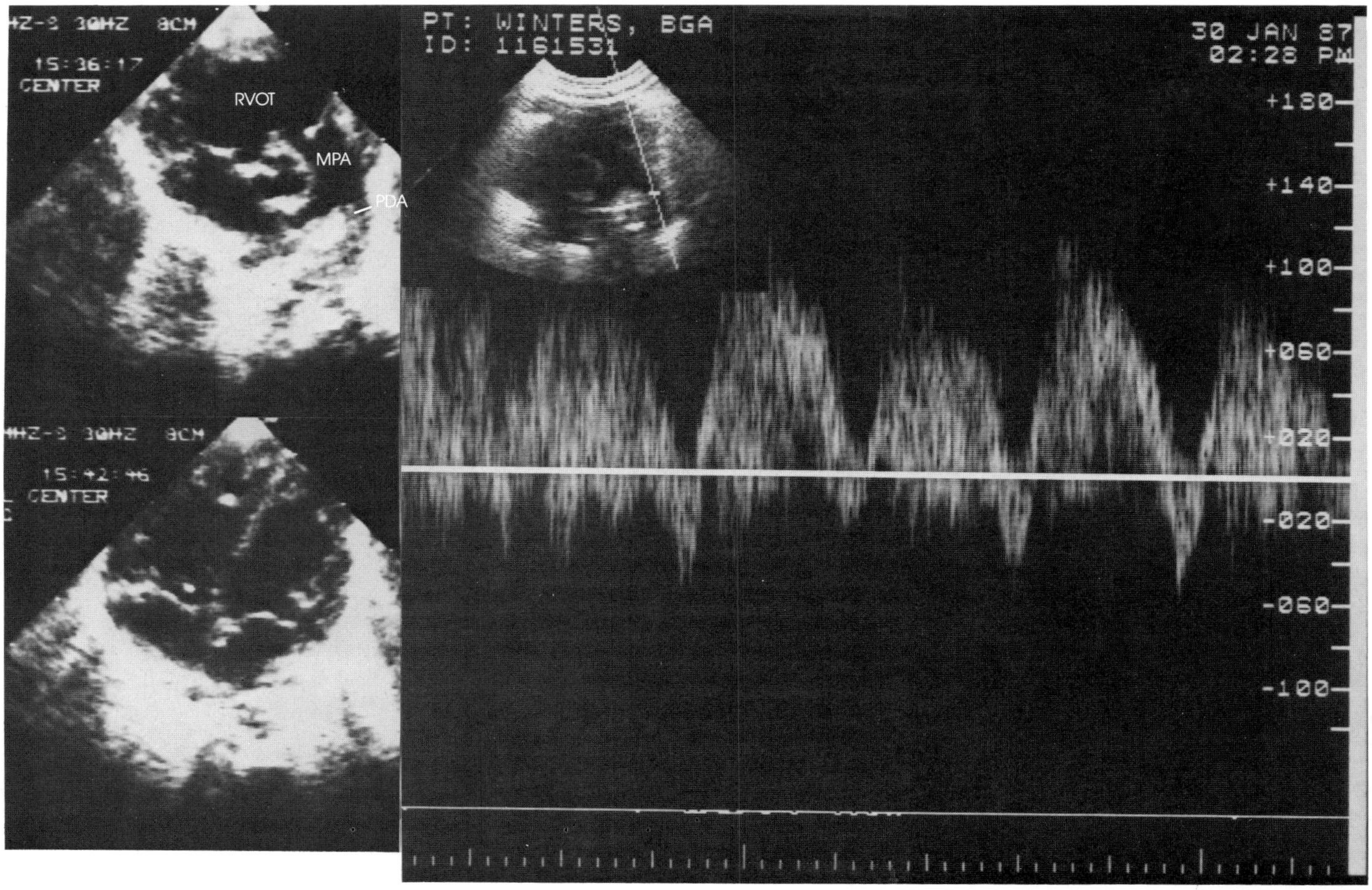

Fig. 38-86. Shunt occurrence in neonates can be a very critical management problem. A common left-to-right shunt seen in premature infants is the persistent patent ductus arteriosus (a communication between the pulmonary artery and aorta). The site of the ductus is best seen in a high-parasternal short-axis view. The Doppler tracing shows a positive reflection from the baseline, which indicates a left-to-right shunt.

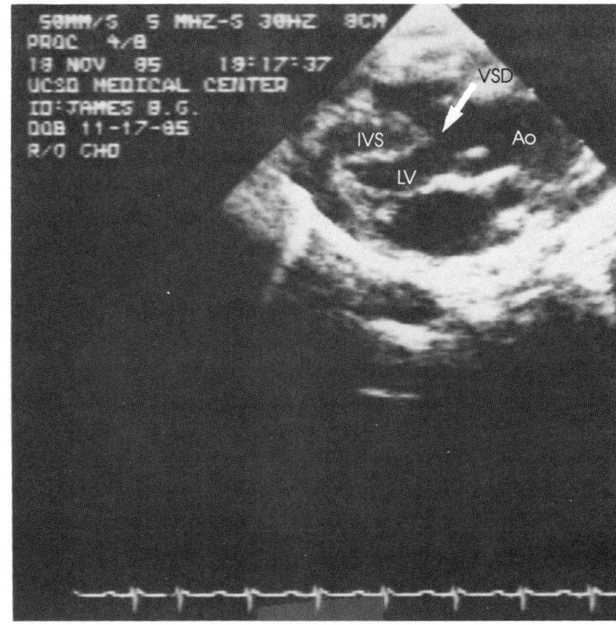

Fig. 38-87. A common congenital heart lesion in infants is tetralogy of Fallot. This syndrome is characterized by the presence of a ventricular septal defect *(VSD)*, overriding of the aorta *(Ao)*, pulmonary stenosis, and right ventricular hypertrophy.

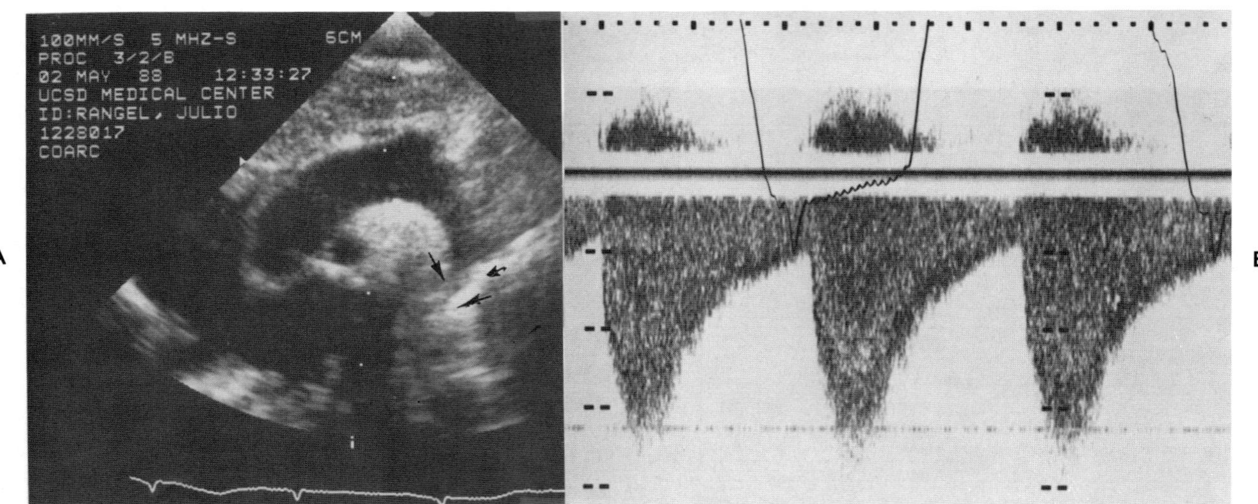

Fig. 38-88. A, Suprasternal view of the aortic arch shows the normal ascending aorta before it tapers as the level of the subclavian artery *(arrows);* this is a form of coarctation of the aorta. Doppler scan shows increased flow velocity across the point of narrowing that extends into diastole.

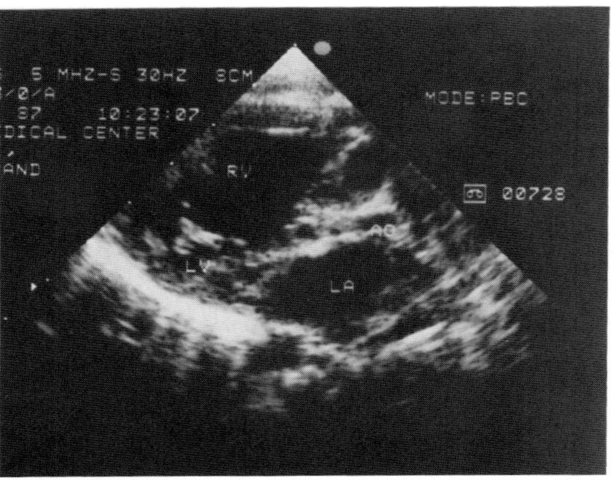

Fig. 38-89. Complex heart disease includes the syndrome of hypoplastic left heart, in which the left ventricle is severely underdeveloped, as is the mitral valve, ascending aorta, and arch of the aorta. This long-axis view shows the dilated right ventricle, small left ventricle, and hypoplastic aorta.

Summary

Diagnostic ultrasound has made significant progress during the last decade in the management and differential diagnosis of the patient. The advent of high-frequency transducers with endoscopic visualization (transvaginal, transrectal, and transesophageal) has aided the visualization of previously difficult areas. Better equipment design enables the sonographer to obtain more information and to process more data points to obtain a comprehensive report from the ultrasound or echocardiographic study. Color-flow mapping enables the sonographer to distinguish the direction and velocity of arterial and venous blood flow from other structures in the body and to determine areas of obstruction from areas of regurgitation and areas of normal flow. The cardiovascular applications of color-flow mapping are tremendous.

Improvements in resolution and transducer design has allowed for progress in resolving small structures within the abdomen, pelvis, heart, and neonatal head. Obstetric patients benefit from these improvements because of the increased ability to detect neural tube defects, cleft palates, shortened extremities, gastrointestinal and genitourinary abnormalities, in addition to other fetal anomalies. The examination of the fetal heart has become routine in high-risk obstetric patients and in patients with an increased risk for cardiac disease.

Continued research and development of computer analysis and tissue characterization of echo reflections should further contribute to the total diagnostic approach for the patient. Research into contrast agents for ultrasound is also being conducted in efforts to highlight various tumor masses with different scanning techniques.

Ultrasound has rapidly emerged into a useful, noninvasive, high-yield clinical diagnostic examination for various applications in medicine. It will continue to grow in importance with further development in resolution techniques and tissue characterization applications.

Definition of Terms*

acoustic cavitation Formation of partial vacuums in a liquid by high-frequency sound waves.

acoustic impedance The ratio of acoustic pressure to particle velocity at any point in the acoustic field.

acoustic shadow The loss of acoustic power of structures lying behind an attenuating or reflecting target.

adiabatic bulk modulus One of the elastic modules that is a measure of the volume elasticity of fluid media and is equal to the inverse of the adiabatic compressibility (Ba); the fractional change in volume (V) per unit change in pressure (P).

$$Ka = -V\left(\frac{dP}{dV_a}\right); Ka = \frac{1}{Ba}$$

adiabatic compressibility Adiabatic compressibility (Ba) is the inverse of adiabatic bulk modulus (Ka).

A-mode (amplitude) A method of acoustic echo display in which time is represented along the horizontal axis and echo amplitude is displayed along the vertical axis.

anechoic The property of being free of echoes or without echoes.

angle of incidence The angle at which the ultrasound beam strikes an interface with respect to normal (perpendicular) incidence.

array A spatial arrangement of two or more transducers.

artifact An echo that does not correspond in distance or direction to a real target.

attenuation Reduction of acoustic amplitude along the propagation pathway as a result of diffraction, absorption, scattering, reflections, or any other process that redirects the signal away from the receiver.

attenuation compensation The compensation for attenuation of acoustic signals along the propagation pathway as a result of losses and geometric divergence. When accomplished electronically this is called *time-gain compensation* (TGC).

backscatter The part of the acoustic energy reflected from a small (compared to the wavelength) target back toward the source.

biparietal diameter (BPD) The largest dimension of the fetal head perpendicular to the midsagittal plane. Measured by ultrasonic visualization; used to measure fetal development.

*Interim AIUM Standard Nomenclature, November, 1978. M Central Office, Washington, D.C. Kremkau, Frederick W, PhD: Diagnostic ultrasound. In Physical principles and exercises, 1980, Grune & Stratton. By permission.

B-mode (brightness) A method of acoustic display on an oscilloscope in which the intensity of the echo is represented by modulation of the brightness of the spot and in which the position of the echo is determined from the position of the transducer and the transit time of the acoustic pulse; displayed in the x-y plane.

cavitation Acoustic cavitation is an activity produced by sound in liquids or any medium with liquid content, involving bubbles or cavities containing gas or vapor.

characteristic acoustic impedance The impedance determined by the product of the undisturbed density and velocity (pc), which occurs in equations, describing plane progressive propagation in homogeneous media; hence, often regarded as "characteristic" of the medium.

compound scan A method of scanning that combines at least two basic scanning motions.

compression Process of decreasing the difference between the smallest and largest amplitudes.

continuous wave (CW) ultrasound A waveform in which the amplitude modulation factor is less than or equal to a small value.

coronal image plane An anatomic term used to describe a plane perpendicular to both the sagittal and transverse planes of the body.

cross-sectional display A display that presents ultrasound interaction echo data from a single plane within a tissue. It is produced by sweeping the ultrasound beam through a given angle, by translating it along a line, or by some combination of linear and angular motions. The depth in the tissue is represented along one coordinate and the position in the scan is represented by the second coordinate. The intensity of the echoes produced in echo ranging is displayed by modulation of the brightness of the image produced. The plane of the section may be sagittal, coronal, or transverse. The lateral resolution is determined by the beam width of the transducers.

decibel A unit used for expressing the ratio of two quantities of electrical signal or sound energy.

density Mass divided by volume.

Doppler effect A shift in frequency or wavelength, depending on the conditions of observation, caused by relative motions among sources, receivers, and the medium.

Doppler ultrasound Application of the Doppler effect to ultrasound to detect movement of a reflecting boundary relative to the source, resulting in a change of the wavelength of the reflected wave.

dynamic imaging Imaging of an object in motion at a frame rate sufficient to cause no significant blurring of any one image and at a repetition rate sufficient to adequately represent the movement pattern. This is frequently referred to as imaging at a real-time (frame) rate.

echo Reflection of acoustic energy received from scattering elements or a specular reflector.

echogenic A medium that contains echo-producing structures, in contrast to a structure that is free of echo-producing structures (anechoic).

endorectal Specially designed probe with high-frequency transducer (and decreased penetration) that can be inserted into the rectum to visualize the bladder and prostate gland.

endovaginal Specially designed probe with a high-frequency transducer (and decreased penetration) that can be inserted into the vagina to obtain high-resolution images of the pelvic structures. Technique often referred to as transvaginal sonography (TVS).

focal zone The distance along the beam axis of a focused transducer assembly, from the point where the beam area first becomes equal to four times the focal area to the point beyond the focal surface where the beam area again becomes equal to four times the focal area.

focus To concentrate the sound beam into a smaller beam area than would exist without focusing.

frequency Number of cycles per unit of time, usually expressed in Hertz (Hz), or megahertz (MHz—million cycles per second).

gray scale A term describing a property of the display in which intensity information is recorded as changes in the brightness of the display.

hard copy A method of image recording in which the data is stored on paper, film, or other recording material.

hyperechoic Producing more echoes than normal.

hypoechoic Producing fewer echoes than normal.

Intensity Power divided by beam area.

linear scan The motion of the transducer at a constant speed along a straight line at right angles to the beam.

longitudinal wave Wave in which the particle motion is parallel to the direction of wave travel.

matching layer Material placed in front of the face of a transducer element to reduce the reflection at the transducer surface.

medium Material through which a wave travels.

M-mode (motion) A method of display in which tissue depth is displayed along one axis and time is displayed along the second axis.

overwritten Refers to static scanners when there is manual control over the amount of information displayed on the screen; when the sonographer makes several passes over a particular area and "builds up" information on top of each pixel, losing anatomical detail in the process.

piezoelectric effect Conversion of pressure to electrical voltage.

power Rate at which work is done; rate at which energy is transferred.

pulsed ultrasound Ultrasound produced in pulse form by applying electrical pulses to the transducer.

rarefaction The state of minimum pressure in a medium transversed by compression waves.

real time Imaging with a real-time display whose output keeps pace with changes in input.

reflection Acoustic energy is reflected from a structure where there is a discontinuity in the characteristic acoustic impedance along the propagation path. The intensity of the reflection is related to the ratio of the characteristic acoustic impedance across the interface. The angle of reflection from a plane interface that is large compared to the acoustic wavelength is equal to the angle of the incident wave in accordance with Snell's Law.

refraction The phenomenon of bending wave fronts as the acoustic energy propagates from the medium of one acoustic velocity to a second medium of differing acoustic velocity.

resolution A measure of the ability to display two closely spaced structures as discrete targets.

resonant frequency Operating frequency.

reverberation The phenomenon of multiple reflections within a closed system.

scan A technique for moving an acoustic beam to produce an image for which both the transducer and the display movements are synchronized.

scan converter Device that stores a gray-scale image and allows it to be displayed on a television monitor.

scattering Diffusion or redirection of sound in several directions on encountering a particle suspension or a rough surface.

sector scan A system of scanning in which the transducer or transmitted beam is rotated through an angle, the center of rotation being near or behind the surface of the transducer.

sonic window Term used to denote the sonographer's ability to visualize a particular area. For example, the full urinary bladder is a good sonic window to image the uterus and ovaries in a transabdominal scan. The intercostal margins may be a good sonic window to image the liver parenchyma.

speed of sound The product of the frequency and the wavelength of the generated wave for a plane, longitudinal wave.

through transmission The process of imaging by transmitting the sound field through the specimen and picking up the transmitted energy on a far surface or a receiving transducer.

transducer Device that converts energy from one form to another.

transonic A term applied to a region of material, such as a cyst, or a tissue that is relatively unattenuating.

ultrasound Sound of frequency greater than 20 kHz.

velocity Speed with direction of motion specified.

velocity of sound Speed with direction of motion specified.

vibration Orderly movement of particles generated by an external source.

watt per square centimeter (W/cm^2) A unit of power density or intensity.

wave An acoustic wave is a mechanical disturbance that propagates through a medium.

SELECTED BIBLIOGRAPHY

Babcock DS and Han BK: Cranial ultrasonography of infants, Baltimore, 1981, Williams & Wilkins.

Bartrum RJ and Crow HC: Gray scale ultrasound: manual for physicians and technical personnel, Philadelphia, 1977, WB Saunders Co.

Callen PW: Ultrasonography in obstetrics and gynecology, Philadelphia, 1983, WB Saunders Co.

Carstensen EL and Gates AH: The effects of pulsed ultrasound on the fetus, J Ultrasound Med 3:145-147, 1984.

Coleman D et al: Ultrasonography of the eye and orbit, Philadelphia, 1977, Lea & Febiger.

Cooperberg P et al: Advances in ultrasonography of the gallbladder and biliary tract, Radiol Clin North Am 20(4):611-633, 1982.

Hagen AD et al: Two-dimensional echocardiography: clinical-pathological correlations in adult and congenital heart disease, Boston, 1983, Little, Brown & Co, Inc.

Hagen-Ansert SL: Textbook of diagnostic ultrasonography, ed 2, St Louis, 1983, The CV Mosby Co.

Hatle L and Angelsen B: Doppler ultrasound in cardiology: physical principles and clinical applications, Philadelphia, 1982, Lea & Febiger.

Holmes JH: Perspectives in ultrasonography: early diagnostic ultrasonography, J Ultrasound Med 2:33-43, 1983.

Johnson ML et al: The normal fetus, Semin Roentgenol 17(3):182-189, 1982.

Kurtz AB et al: Ultrasound and computed tomography of the liver, CRC Crit Rev Diagn Imaging 18(4):279-317, 1982.

Lerski RA: Ultrasonic tissue characterization, Diagn Imaging 51(5):238-248, 1982.

Lyons EA et al: The abnormal fetus, Semin Roentgenol 17(3):198-209, 1982.

Merritt CR et al: Intraoperative neurosurgical ultrasound: transdural and transfontanelle applications, Radiology 148(2):513-517, 1983.

McDicken WN: Diagnostic ultrasonics: principles and use of instruments, London, 1976, Granada Publishing, Inc.

Mossman KL: Ultrasound and x-rays in pregnancy: how safe are they? Contemp Ob-Gyn 23:175-196, 1984.

Pearlman AS et al: Clinical application of 2-D/Doppler echocardiography, Cardiovasc Clin 13(3):201-222, 1983.

Powis RL: Ultrasound physics for the fun of it, Denver, 1978, Unirad Corp.

Resnick MI and Sanders RC: Ultrasound in urology, Baltimore, 1979, Williams & Wilkins.

Sabbagha RE et al: The use of ultrasound in obstetrics, Clin Obstet Gynecol 25(4):735-752, 1982.

Sanders RC and James AE: The principles and practice of ultrasonography in obstetrics and gynecology, New York, 1980, Appleton-Century-Crofts.

Sickles EA et al: Breast cancer detection with sonography and mammography: comparison using state-of-the-art equipment, AJR 140(5):843-845, 1983.

Taylor KJW: Manual of ultrasonography, New York, 1980, Churchill Livingstone.

Zweibel WJ, editor: Introduction to vascular ultrasonography, New York, 1982, Grune & Stratton, Inc.

Chapter 39

NUCLEAR MEDICINE

PAUL J. EARLY

Shortly after the discovery of the x ray by Roentgen, Henri Becquerel was credited with discovering radioactivity. The year was 1896. Marie Curie, in her doctoral thesis, proved that these mysterious "rays" were different from those of Roentgen, and she actually identified three emissions from "pitchblend" (now known to be radium and its *daughters**). Madame Curie received the Nobel Prize for her work.

Curiously enough, the medical use of radioactivity did not occur until 1936 when radioactive phosphorus (^{32}P) was used to treat rats with leukemia and lymphomas; the tumors were destroyed. Treatment of humans gave similar results.

In 1951, Benedict Cassen gave nuclear medicine a boost with his development of the first nuclear (rectilinear) scanner. This device moved back and forth across the organ generating a picture of the organ based on the amount of radioactivity in it.

In 1958, Hal Anger took imaging one step farther with his development of the *scintillation camera*. This device allowed for the imaging of an entire organ at one time, creating the possibility of performing not only static images of organs but images of their dynamic functions as well. This discovery, timed with the discovery of technetium-99m (^{99m}Tc), allowed nuclear medicine to move into a position of prominence as a medical specialty in the early 1970s.

Since that time, much work and effort have been spent learning more about radiation, radioactivity, and radiobiologic effects. The field of nuclear medicine has expanded with the advent of sophisticated measuring equipment and imaging devices that have been interfaced with computers. Clinical nuclear medicine studies have become a standard inclusion in the modern day medical armamentarium.

*All italicized terms are defined at the end of this chapter.

Physics of Nuclear Medicine

To understand nuclear medicine, it is necessary to understand the constituent parts of the atom because these parts play an important role in understanding how nuclear medicine works. Not all parts of the atom are important to the world of nuclear medicine, but a few basic parts are and these are discussed here.

THE ATOM

The atom is composed of a centrally positioned, positively charged core known as the *nucleus*. Traveling around this nucleus in oval pathways at various distances from the nucleus are much smaller negatively charged *electrons*. This has been described by Bohr as similar to the solar system, with the nucleus representing the sun and the electrons representing the circling planets.

The nucleus is composed primarily of two particles; the *proton* and the *neutron*. Both particles are massive compared to the electron. The proton is a positively charged particle, approximately 1836 times the mass of the electron. The neutron is a neutrally charged particle slightly larger than the proton and 1840 times the size of the electron. Both of these intranuclear particles are referred to as *nucleons*.

The particles that provide the basis for the science of nuclear medicine are the alpha particle, beta particle, positron, and the neutrino. The alpha, beta, and neutrino particles are not directly used in nuclear medicine imaging. However, as a by-product of the alpha, beta, and neutrino decay process, gamma rays and radiation with discrete energies are produced and provide the radioactivity useful in nuclear medicine imaging. In each case, the resulting radiations arise from the nucleus but are not actual residents of the nucleus. Basically these are the particles and photons that occur during radioactive decay.

The *alpha particle* is a helium nucleus composed of two protons and two neutrons. Accordingly, it has a huge mass (approximately 7300 times the size of an electron) and a double-positive charge. It is these two facts that cause the alpha particle to be the single most damaging particle emitted from radioactive material, provided the radioactive atom is inside the body. The alpha particle does not penetrate the epidermis of the skin.

The *beta particle* is a high-velocity electron emitted from the nucleus. It has the same mass and charge as those of the orbital electrons. Once the beta particle is emitted from the nucleus, it passes through matter creating damage similar to, but much less than, that of the alpha particle.

A *positron* is a positively charged electron emitted from the nucleus of those atoms whose stability is disturbed by the existence of too many protons in the nucleus (neutron-poor). The positron, once emitted from the nucleus, has damaging properties similar to the particles listed above.

The *neutrino* occurs in all of the above reactions because it carries some of the excess energy away from the nucleus.

All of these particles play a role in nuclear medicine, whether they are a result of the normal constituents of the atom or are created by the radioactive atom in its search for stability. Thus radioactivity is the result of changing neutrons into protons or protons into neutrons and of the oftentimes subsequent emission of *gamma* rays from the nucleus and possibly even *x rays* (characteristic radiation) from the orbits. It is the emission of these gamma and x rays that allows their presence to be detected in nuclear medicine procedures.

ISOTOPES

An *isotope* may be defined as one of two or more forms of the same element having identical chemical properties. They have the same number of protons in their nuclei; therefore the number of electrons circling the nucleus is the same in all isotopes of that element. Having the same number of electrons in the orbits also dictates the chemical properties. It is for this reason that the use of radioisotopes in medicine is so meaningful. The injection of radioactive material that behaves in the same way as its stable counterpart biologically can reveal a great deal about the function and structure of many of the organs within the human body. These radioisotopes travel to the various organs, localize there, and demonstrate their presence by changes within the nucleus and the release of a gamma ray that is detected using nuclear medicine instrumentation. These radioactive isotopes can similarly be used therapeutically because the radioactive counterpart will be picked up by the various organs (euphemistically called the "magic bullet") and reside within that organ to irradiate the diseased tissue.

RADIATION

All human beings are exposed daily to a variety of radiations whether or not they recognize it. These radiations include radiowaves, visible light, sound, radio, television, and radar. There are other radiations that can neither be heard, seen, felt, nor otherwise perceived by the human senses. Examples of these are x rays and gamma rays.

All energy waves (called photons) have the same velocity, i.e., the speed of light or 3×10^{10} centimeters per second. They vary only in wavelength and frequency (Fig. 39-1). The wavelength is defined as the distance from one point on one wave to the same point on a subsequent wave, whereas the frequency is defined as the number of wave formations per unit of time. X rays and gamma rays fall into this highly energetic area of the *electromagnetic spectrum,* and it is because of their high energy that they are able to cause biologic damage to tissue in their paths.

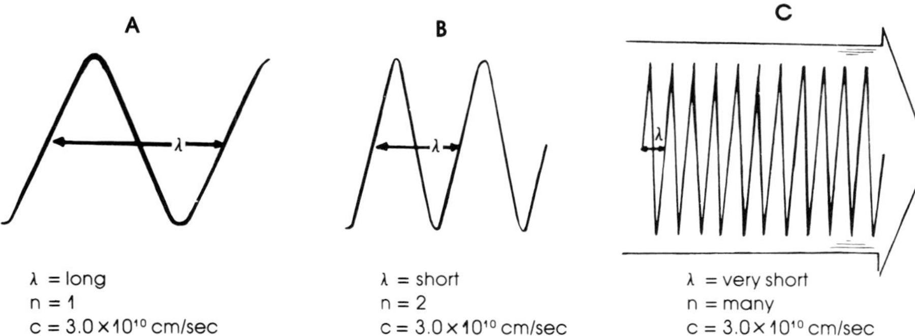

Fig. 39-1. Characteristics of electromagnetic waves. **A,** Wavelength, frequency, and velocity of a wave. **B,** As the wavelength decreases, the frequency increases, and velocity remains unchanged. **C,** Quantum nature of radiation; the wave behaves like a bundle of energy, having direction and traveling at the speed of light.

(From Early PJ and Sodee DB: Principles and practice of nuclear medicine, St Louis, 1985, The CV Mosby Co.)

RADIOACTIVE DECAY

The physical *half-life* ($T_{1/2}$ or T_p) is often called the radioactive half-life. It is defined as the length of time it takes for the original number of atoms in a given radioactive sample to disintegrate or decay to one half the original number. The rate of decay of any given isotope cannot be influenced by temperature, pressure, or chemical combination. Because of this decay process, all radioactivity decreases with time, because fewer atoms are left as some atoms decay. If one were to plot on linear paper the number of atoms present versus time for a given sample, the curve shown in Fig. 39-2, *A*, would be obtained. It is apparent that the same length of time is required for 100 atoms to decay to 50 atoms as is required for 50 atoms to decay to 25 atoms. The length of time during which the number of atoms is diminished to one half is referred to as the half-life. Half-lives range in value from thousandths of a second to millions of years. If the same curve were plotted on semilogarithmic paper with the number of atoms on the logarithmic scale and time on the linear scale, then the straight line would be obtained (Fig. 39-2, *B*). This rate of decay therefore can be said to have an exponential function. Formulas and tables are readily available for determining how much radioactive material is left at any given time or how much activity will be present before a certain time.

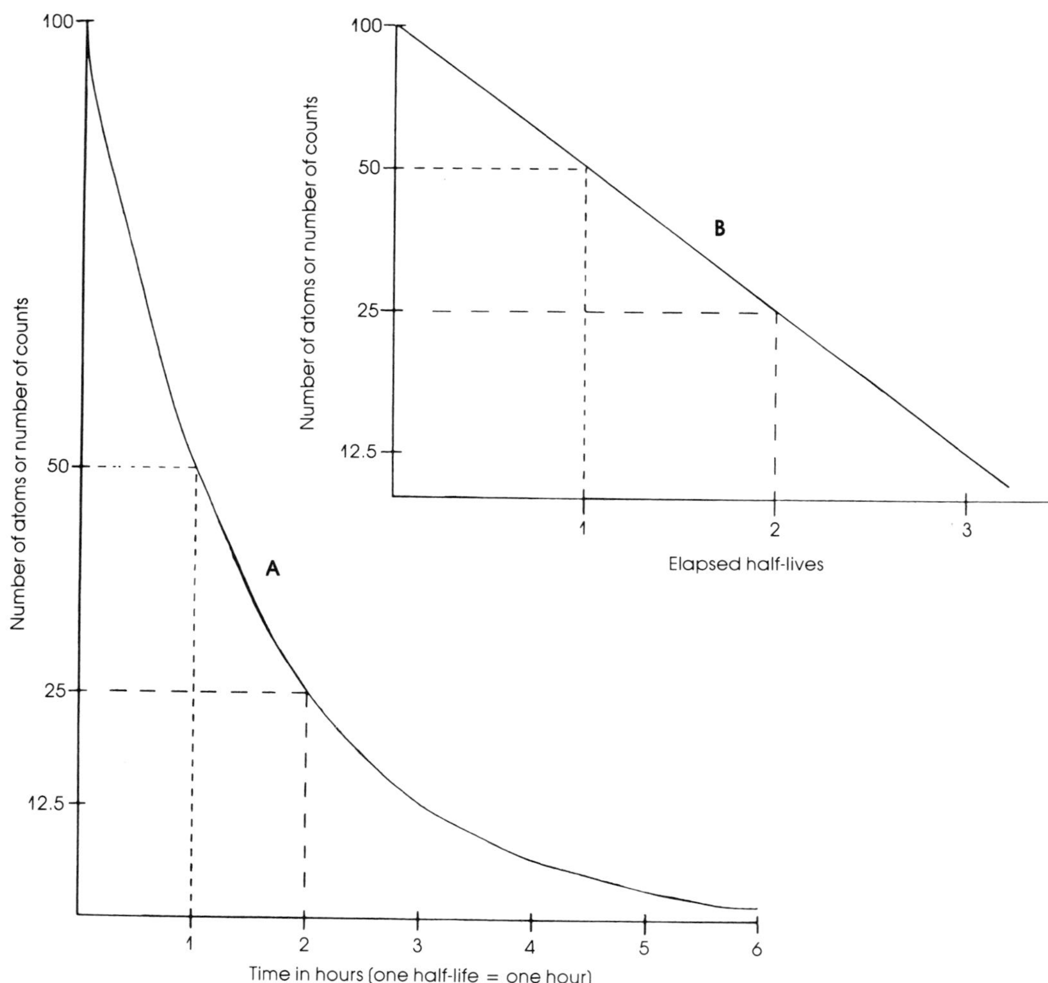

Fig. 39-2. Physical decay of radionuclide, plotting elapsed time versus number of atoms remaining or number of counts received. **A,** The relationship on linear graph paper. **B,** Semilogarithmic paper. **B** Can be used as a universal decay table, applying it to any radionuclide.

(From Early PJ and Sodee DB: Principles and practice of nuclear medicine, St Louis, 1985, The CV Mosby Co.)

Instrumentation

Because ionizing radiations cannot be perceived by human senses, it is advantageous to have some sensor device that can detect their presence. Furthermore, it is desirable to identify the different devices available and to understand their specific applications. The two main types of these devices are gas detectors and scintillation detectors.

GAS DETECTORS

The basic function of a *gas detector* depends on the collection of electrons produced in a gas volume by the passage of radiation through the detector. As the electrons are produced by the radiation passing through the gas, they migrate to the positive wall (anode) of the detector, provided an exterior voltage is applied. The general concept of the gas detector is that the electrons are collected by the anode, flow through a very sensitive current meter, and collect at the negative electrode. The measurement of this current flow is a function of the amount of ionization that has occurred inside the enclosed gas volume, which is in turn a measure of the amount of radiation to which the meter has been exposed. Examples of routine survey meters are seen in Fig. 39-3.

SCINTILLATION DETECTORS

Certain materials have the property of emitting a flash of light *("scintillation")* when struck by ionizing radiation. A *scintillation detector* is a sensitive device used to detect ionizing radiation by observing the scintillations induced in the material. This is accomplished by fixing a light-sensitive device to a special photo sensitive material that changes the flash of light into small electrical impulses. The electrical impulses are then amplified so they may be sorted and counted to determine the amount and nature of radiation striking the scintillating materials. Scintillators are used to determine the amount and/or distribution of *radionuclides* in one or more organs of a patient for diagnostic purposes.

The procedure for recording a scintillation involves several systems: the detector, a photomultiplier, a high-voltage power supply, the pulse height analyzer, and display modes.

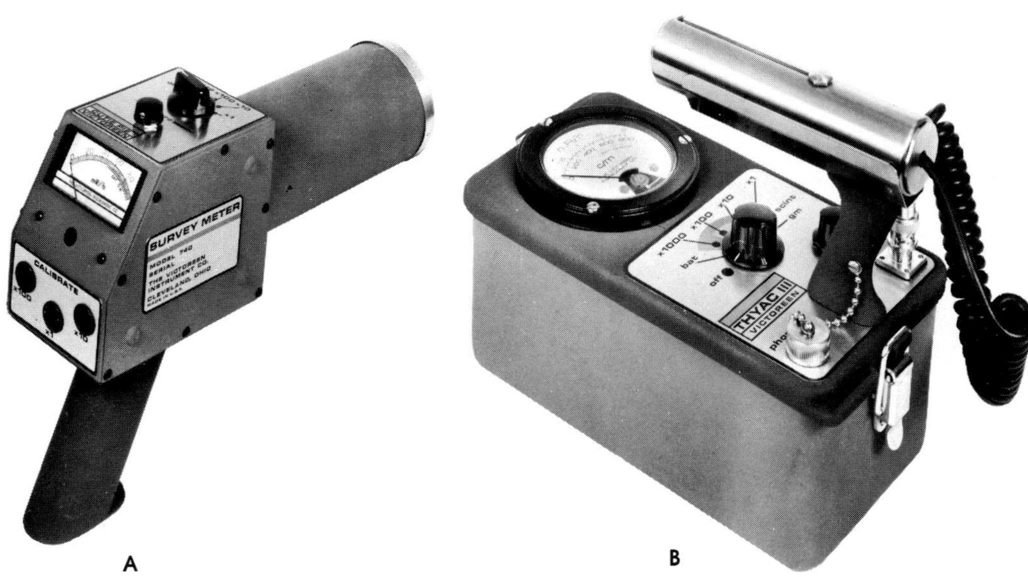

Fig. 39-3. A, Ionization-type dose rate survey meter. **B,** Geiger-Mueller–type dose rate survey meter.

(Courtesy Victoreen Instrument Co, Cleveland, Ohio.) (From Early PJ and Sodee DB: Principles and practice of nuclear medicine, St Louis, 1985, The CV Mosby Co.)

CRYSTAL DETECTOR

The most widely used scintillation detector in nuclear medicine is a sodium iodide (NaI) crystal. The detection process is initiated when a gamma ray enters the crystal. The energy eventually is absorbed totally inside the crystal. This is accomplished through a series of collisions. Each time a collision occurs, some of the energy of the gamma ray is transferred to an electron that produces luminous light. This flash of light eventually is directed to the photomultiplier tube.

Photomultiplier

The *photomultiplier* is a light-sensitive device that is connected optically to the sodium iodide crystal. Its purpose is to convert the light energy from the crystal to electrical energy and amplify the result to produce a pulse of electricity (Fig. 39-4).

Pulse height analyzer

The *pulse height analyzer* is an electronic device that enables the operator to select pulses of a certain height and reject all pulses of a different height. Another name for this is a spectrometer. The two levels that are set are called the *lower level discriminator* (LLD) and the *upper level discriminator* (ULD). By using this two level arrangement, both high-energy radionuclides and low-energy radionuclides can be separated from each other. Once the pulse passes through the pulse height analyzer, it is then ready to go to the display mode.

Display modes

The previous sequence of events provides a signal that the event finally has been recorded. This signal can be received by a *scaler* to count the pulse. A given number of pulses can be compared against a standard to calculate a percent function (e.g., thyroid uptake study); or the pulse can be accepted by an imaging device that allows it to be transformed into a flash of light from a *cathode ray tube* (CRT), where the flash of light is recorded on film. The latter approach gives us the images from scintillation cameras.

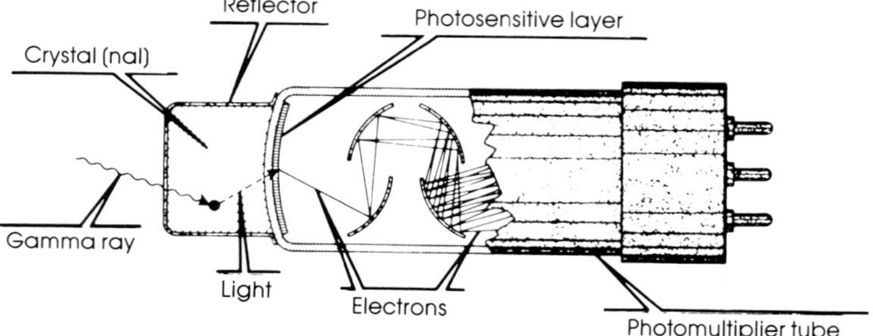

Total light to tube linearly proportional to gamma ray energy

If 1 electron ejects 5 from dynode, 11 dynodes result in 5 inches

or

about 50 million electrons output

Fig. 39-4. Crystal photomultiplier assembly illustrating the detection of a gamma ray by the crystal and its subsequent amplification through the photomultiplier tube.

(Courtesy US Nuclear Regulatory Commission.) (From Early PJ and Sodee DB: Principles and practice of nuclear medicine, St Louis, 1985, The CV Mosby Co.)

Scintillation camera

The *scintillation camera* is a device that uses all parts of the radiation field; it continuously employs a large single sodium iodide crystal measuring from 11 to 16 inches in diameter. This crystal is viewed by not just one but by as many as 91 photomultiplier tubes.

In the scintillation camera, gamma rays pass through the holes of the *collimator* and are totally absorbed in the scintillation crystal. The light that is produced is connected to an electrical pulse that goes directly to a resistor or capacitor network (Fig. 39-5) where all the pulses from all the photo tubes are modified, processed, and converted to X and Y position signals, which are displayed on an oscilloscope. The X and Y position signals (four of them) are used to place the event on the *oscilloscope* in a location commensurate with where it occurs on the organ. The oscilloscope produces a flash of light that is then recorded on film. Each dot of the oscilloscope is the result of a single gamma event occurring in the detector. Each change in location is produced by another event that occurred in the detector. The recording of these events over a period of time results in an image on film that displays the distribution of the radionuclide within an organ. This image is called a "planar image."

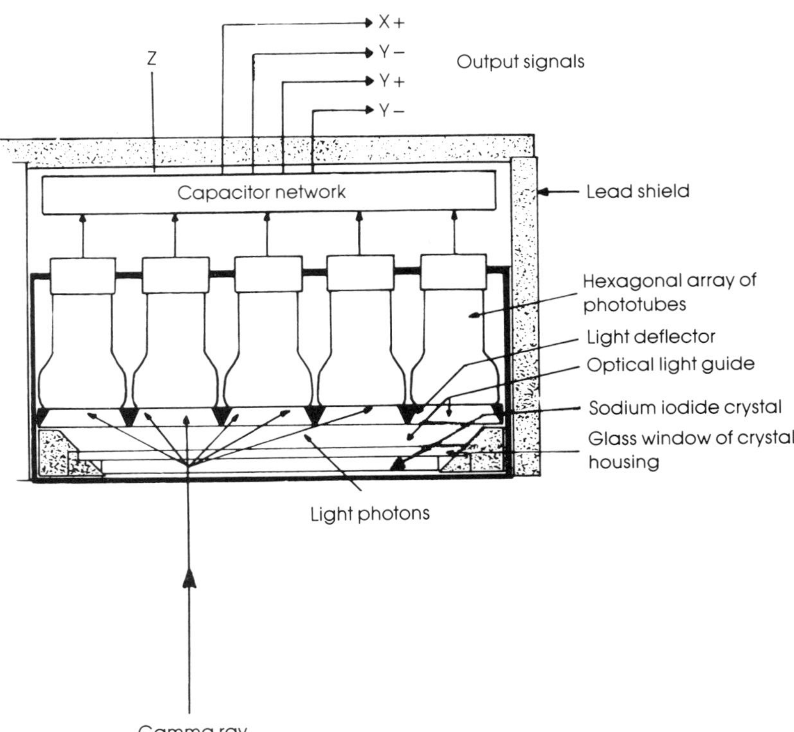

Fig. 39-5. Cut-away diagram of single crystal stationary imaging device.

(From Early PJ and Sodee DB: Principles and practice of nuclear medicine, St Louis, 1985, The CV Mosby Co.)

Instrumentation

Single photon emission computed tomography

The basic principle of the scintillation camera has been adapted to tomography called single photon emission computed tomography (SPECT). The concept of nuclear medicine tomography antedates x-ray computed tomography (CT) but not until the development of CT and its software programs (algorithms) were tremendous strides made in SPECT.

A SPECT system unit consists of a rotating scintillation camera mounted on a ring gantry (Fig. 39-6), which, with proper positioning, rotates around the subject's body at the level of the organ to be studied. As the detector rotates around the body, it stops for a preselected number of times and remains stationary for a preselected amount of time or number of counts, accumulating a planar image before continuing to the next position. Rather than generating an image for each of these stops (up to one stop per degree of rotation, or 360 hesitations), the information is retained in computer memory. When the rotation is completed, all the collected and stored data are subjected to traditional CT algorithm reconstruction. The resultant image is tomographic. The difference between SPECT and CT is that CT is a transmission tomographic study, whereas SPECT is an emission tomographic study. A CT image results from x rays from an x-ray tube, which are transmitted through the subject's body as the x-ray tube rotates around the body. A SPECT image results from the emission of gamma rays from inside the subject's body as a consequence of the concentration of radioactive pharmaceuticals within the organs of the body being investigated.

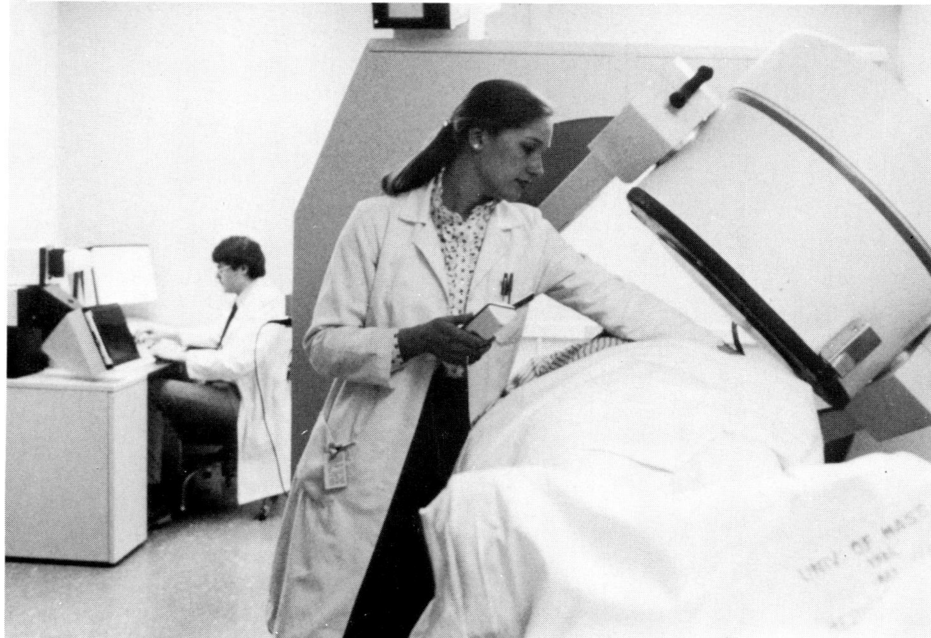

Fig. 39-6. Rotating tomographic camera, showing an oscilloscope in the background, being viewed by a cassette holding an x-ray film.

(Courtesy Picker International, Cleveland, Ohio.) (From Early PJ and Sodee DB: Principles and practice of nuclear medicine, St Louis, 1985, The CV Mosby Co.)

Positron emission tomography

Recent advances have been made in positron emission tomography (PET), another modality of nuclear medicine that can have much impact on the diagnosis and care of the patient (see Chapter 40 on PET). The basic component of PET is the positron. As stated in the section "Physics of Nuclear Medicine," the positron is a positively charged electron emitted from the nucleus of neutron-poor radionuclides. Once emitted, the particle ionizes nearby atoms until it loses all its energy. It then combines with a negative electron, and both particles annihilate, converting their entire mass to energy. This energy is displayed as two 0.511 meV photons, extending in exactly opposite directions from each other. It is the simultaneous detection of these two photons that gives PET its unique imaging capabilities.

Radiation Protection: Factors Unique to Nuclear Medicine

In nuclear medicine three types of emissions are of primary concern: alpha particles, beta particles, and gamma rays. X rays also result from several phenomena of interaction with matter, but most are generally very weak in nature and of no particular concern as far as radiation protection is concerned. One fact to be considered is that of external emission versus internal emission—whether the radiation comes from outside the body and penetrates the epidermis into the body or whether the emitters are already inside the body after being introduced by way of ingestion, inhalation, or intravenous injection. Gamma rays and x rays are able to penetrate the epidermis of the skin and therefore present approximately the same hazard whether they are externally or internally emitted. This is not the case with alpha and beta emitters. Alpha and beta emitters cannot ordinarily penetrate the outer layers of the skin. As external emitters they do not usually constitute a serious problem with radiation protection. If they are used as internal emitters, however, the problem of alpha and beta radiation damage becomes severe. The maximum permissible dose equivalents for occupational workers are summarized in Chapter 2 on "Radiation Protection" in Vol. I.

Clinical Nuclear Medicine

Clinical applications of nuclear medicine are based on two facts. First, a radionuclide is chemically identical to its stable isotope and follows the same physiologic pathways. Second, a radionuclide emits radiations that pass through matter, are detectable, and are measurable. As pointed out in an earlier section, these radionuclides have identical chemical properties and therefore follow identical physiologic pathways. Furthermore, the amounts of radioactive materials used in these clinical studies are so small that the physiologic balance is not altered in any way, and therefore these materials are called "tracers." A good example of this is iodine to the thyroid gland. It is a well-known fact that iodine is selectively removed from circulation by the thyroid gland. It is also easy to show that *radioactive* iodine also is selectively removed from circulation by the thyroid gland, which does not differ its normal physiologic response to proper quantities of this material. Therefore radioactive iodine serves as an excellent method of evaluating the thyroid gland.

The thyroid gland also provides a good example of "cold-spot" imaging. Cold-spot imaging refers to an area in any organ where the concentrations of radioactivity are significantly less than the surrounding tissue. Carcinoma of the thyroid gland demonstrates this phenomenon (Fig. 39-6). By contrast, "hot-spot" imaging refers to any area in any organ where the concentrations of radioactivity are significantly greater than the surrounding tissue. Brain tumors demonstrate this phenomenon (Fig. 39-10).

Another reason why radioactive materials are used in clinical studies is because the physiologic compounds can be manipulated chemically ("labeled" or "tagged") so that the material is not altered in any way. Technetium-99m (^{99m}Tc) can be added to a number of compounds so that the compound itself is not altered physiologically and therefore goes to the appropriate organ. If this labeled material is in the proper organ, the organ can be studied for size, shape, and function.

Another approach used in making radioactive materials function in a clinical setting is the use of various sized particles. In the instance of technetium-99m labeled MAA, the macroaggregated albumin particles are 30 to 40 microns in size, which prevents their passage through the pulmonary capillary bed, which is only about 8 microns in diameter. While these particles are held in that position, the lung can be studied.

Another particle with related use in radioactive materials is that of technetium-99m labeled sulfur colloid. In this instance the particles are small enough to go through the pulmonary capillaries but are selectively removed by the reticuloendothelial system of the liver and spleen. This trapping process allows some study of these organs.

Other approaches to the study of organ function include the use of radioactive gases to study movement of these gases into and out of the lung field. A large percentage of nuclear medicine procedures use technetium-99m. The reasons for this wide acceptance are that this radionuclide has an ideal energy of 140 keV (resulting in good detection and dosimetry characteristics) and an ideal physical half-life of 6 hours (resulting in good decay and dosimetry characteristics), and perhaps more importantly it can be produced within the nuclear medicine department via the ^{99}Mo/^{99m}Tc generator. All of these factors create a situation that allows for the use of radioactive materials in medicine.

Prominent organ systems that are currently studied routinely in nuclear medicine departments are those of the thyroid, brain, lungs, liver, spleen, kidney, bone, and heart. Each of these is discussed separately in the following sections.

THYROID

Rationale

It is a well-known fact that iodine is metabolized by the thyroid gland. Inorganic iodine is absorbed into the bloodstream from the gastrointestinal tract where the iodide is selectively removed by the thyroid gland to be organified and stored in the thyroid gland. Technetium-99m in the pertechnetate form can also be used to study the thyroid gland; however, this material is only trapped, not organified (i.e., not incorporated into the thyroid hormone molecule). For this reason, it does not act identically to iodine and therefore many clinicians feel that it should not be used for nuclear medicine studies of the thyroid gland.

Iodine-131 (^{131}I) is also used therapeutically in amounts of radioactivity approximately 1000 times that of diagnostic doses. In these quantities the radioactivity can alter the function of the thyroid.

Indications

The thyroid gland is studied when there is a suggested disturbance of function and/or of size.

Procedure

Function. Oral administration of 200 μCi of ^{123}I. Thyroid uptake measurements are collected at 2 hours, 6 hours, and/or 24 hours post administration. (One to two mCi^{99m}Tc can also be used with uptake measurements at 1 hour.)

Static images. Administer 200 to 400 μCi ^{123}I. Image at 24 hours.

Therapy. 20 to 30 mCi ^{131}I for hyperthyroidism; 100 to 200 mCi ^{131}I for thyroid carcinoma.

Results

Function. Normal uptake equals 10% to 30% at 24 hours. Any variations lower than 10% at 24 hours is considered hypothyroid; higher than 30% at 24 hours is considered hyperthyroidism. A 2- or 6-hour uptake is sometimes used to determine iodine deficiencies.

Static images. Normal imaging is based on size and shape (Fig. 39-7). Abnormal imaging is based on the presence of altered size, nodules, areas of deficiency, as well as areas of hyperactivity ruling out goiters, cancer (Fig. 39-8), and thyroiditis.

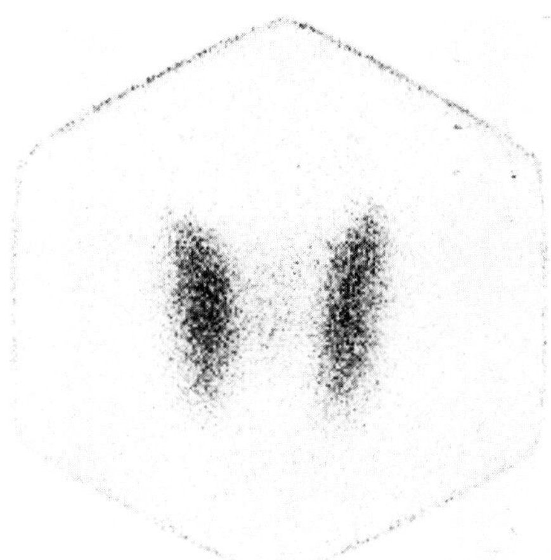

Fig. 39-7. Pinhole thyroid image 6 hours after 200 μCi dose of ^{123}I. Physical examination demonstrated no palpable nodules over the thyroid. The 6-hour thyroid uptake was within the normal range at 10%. There is a normal concentration and an even distribution of nuclide throughout both lobes of the gland. Diagnosis: normal thyroid.

(From Early PJ and Sodee DB: Principles and practice of nuclear medicine, St Louis, 1985, The CV Mosby Co.)

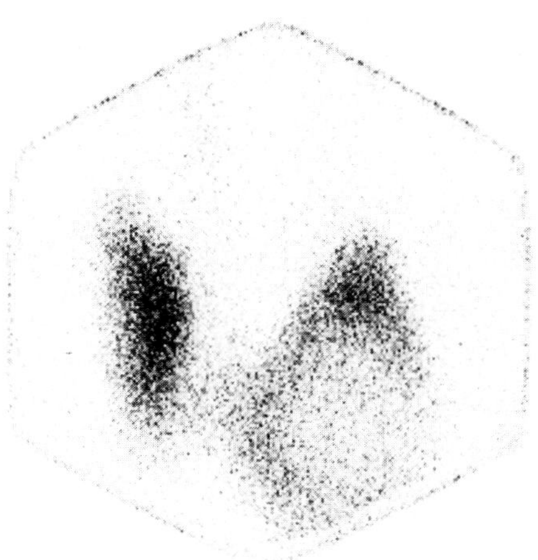

Fig. 39-8. Abnormal pinhole thyroid image 6 hours after 200 μCi dose of ^{123}I. Thyroid image demonstrates a 2.5 × 2.5 cm cold nodule expanding the inferior portion of the left lobe of the thyroid. There is a normal concentration and an even distribution over the right lobe with faint visualization of a pyramidal lobe. Diagnosis: cold nodule.

(From Early PJ and Sodee DB: Principles and practice of nuclear medicine, St Louis, 1985, The CV Mosby Co.)

BRAIN

Rationale

Many materials can be used for the study of brain lesions. Nuclear medicine is successful in brain tumor detection because the tumor itself creates a breakdown in the blood-brain barrier. Consequently, any materials that are in circulation will pool in any area where blood will pool. Because the nonpooled materials clear faster because they are in the main stream of blood flow, the pooled radionuclide remains behind to give a positive indication on a nuclear medicine imaging procedure.

Indications

The brain studies provided by nuclear medicine are used early detection of brain tumors and/or metastases. Subdural hematomas, cerebral vascular accidents, and abscesses are also indications for nuclear medicine brain studies.

Procedure

Dynamic. A bolus IV injection of 20 mCi of ^{99m}Tc diethylenetriamine pentaacetic acid (DTPA[sn]) is given with anterior images being taken every 3 seconds (Fig. 39-9).

Static. An IV injection of 20 mCi of ^{99m}Tc DTPA (Sn) is given with both immediate (Fig. 39-9, *D*) and delayed images taken from all four sides around the head (as well as vertex images in some instances) (Fig. 39-10).

Results

Dynamic. Changes in distribution on flow are seen in cerebral vascular accidents. Changes in timing on flow are seen in carotid artery obstruction.

Static. Areas of increased concentration of radioactivity are seen in brain tumors (Fig. 39-10).

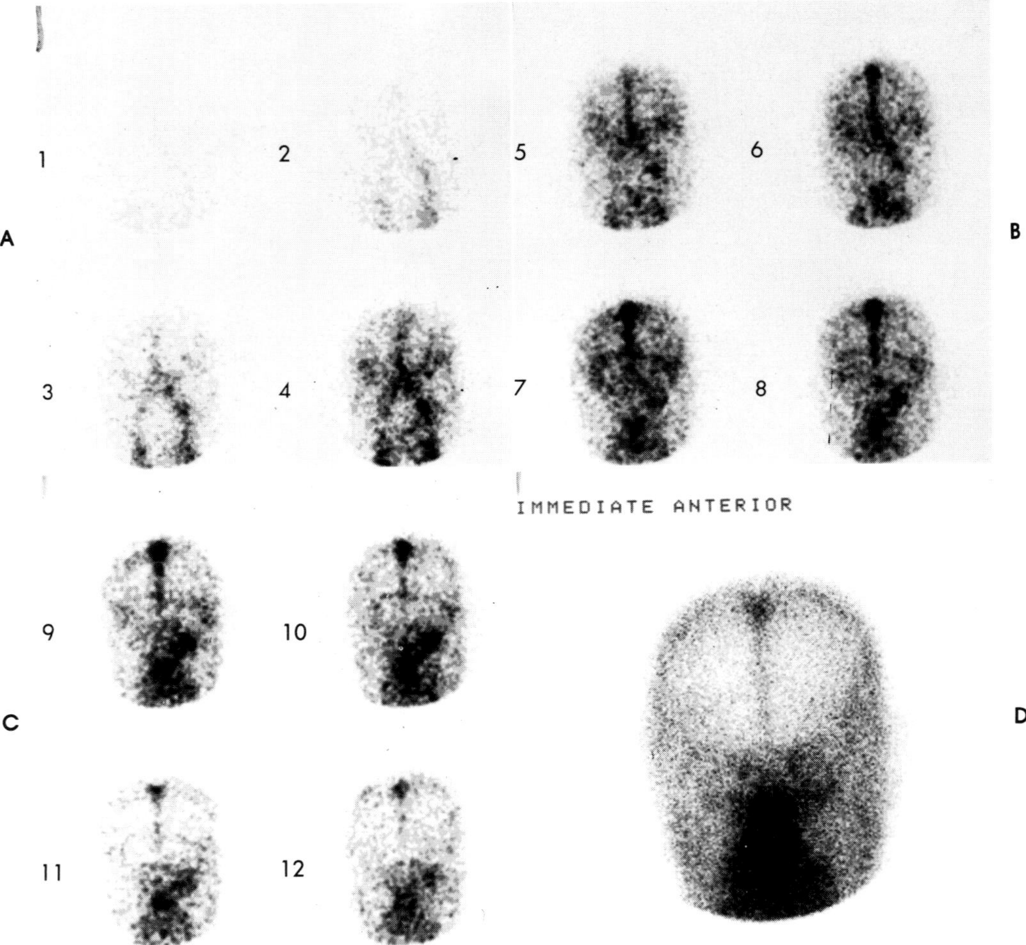

Fig. 39-9. Anterior cerebral perfusion study following injection of 20 mCi of ^{99m}Tc DTPA (Sn). **A,** Early arterial phase showing internal carotid arteries and anterior and middle cerebral arteries. **B,** Capillary venous phase. **C,** Venous phase. **D,** Immediate anterior static image after flow study. Diagnosis: normal anterior cerebral perfusion study.

(From Early PJ and Sodee DB: Principles and practice of nuclear medicine, St Louis, 1985, The CV Mosby Co.)

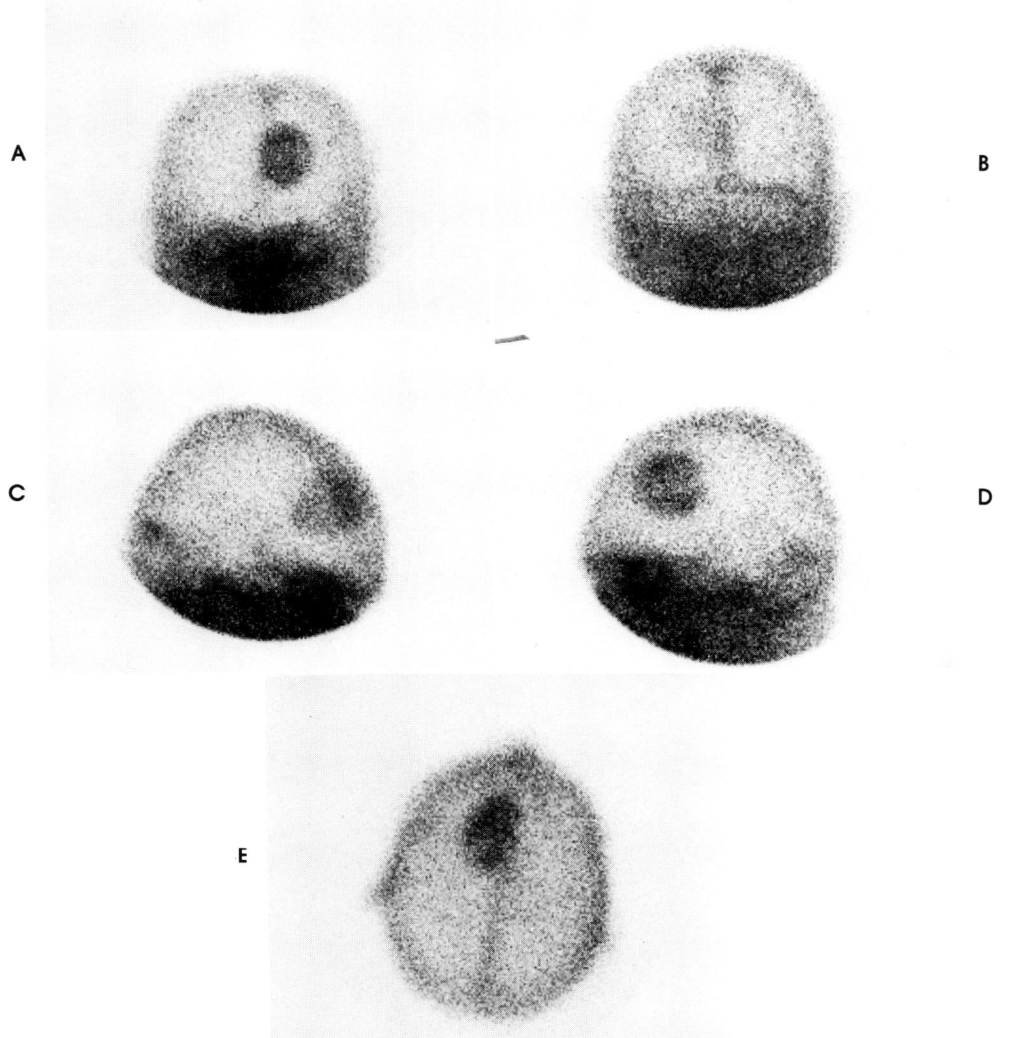

Fig. 39-10. Abnormal brain images; scan performed 2 hours after a 20 mCi dose of ^{99m}Tc DTPA (Sn) was injected. Images demonstrate 5 cm ovoid lesion located to left of midline in left frontal region. There is increased concentration of radionuclide around periphery of lesion. Centrally, lesion appears necrotic with decreased concentration of radionuclide. **A,** Anterior image. **B,** Reverse Towne's image. **C,** Right lateral image. **D,** Left lateral image. **E,** Vertex image. Diagnosis: solitary metastatic tumor of brain. Patient has history of primary breast carcinoma.

(From Early PJ and Sodee DB: Principles and practice of nuclear medicine, St Louis, 1985, The CV Mosby Co.)

LUNGS

Rationale

The study of the lungs has given considerable clinical information because almost all phases of lung function can be studied under nuclear medicine procedures. The lung has two functions: (1) the carbon dioxide (CO_2) laden blood goes to the lungs to replace its oxygen, and (2) the oxygen is exchanged with the CO_2. In the former situation, MAA labeled with ^{99m}Tc is used as a form of microembolization to study this function (Fig. 39-11). In the latter situation, radioactive xenon gas is used. Recently, ^{99m}Tc-DTPA aerosols are replacing radioactive xenon gas. By nebulizing the DTPA, particles can be made small enough to reach the alveoli. The larger particles (if any) adhere to the tracheobronchial tree. This new procedure has arisen because multiple images, which are not possible with xenon, are possible with ^{99m}Tc-DTPA aerosols. In addition, NRC regulations state that xenon must be used in a negative-pressure room, which precludes its use in any room except those specifically designed for xenon studies. ^{99m}Tc-DTPA aerosols are not bound by this regulation and therefore can be used in other places—for instance, intensive and cardiac care units and emergency rooms—where such studies of the lung are often indicated for patients for whom a move to the nuclear medicine department could be hazardous.

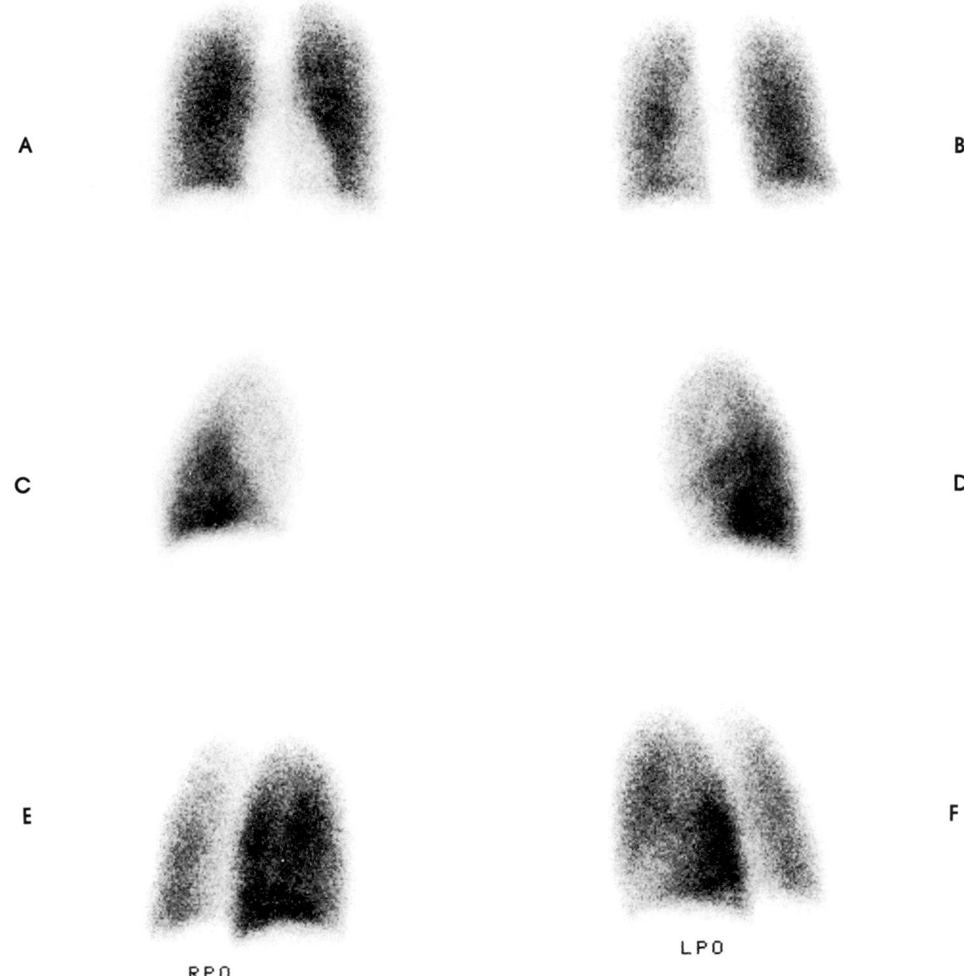

Fig. 39-11. Lung perfusion images using ^{99m}Tc MAA demonstrate normal distribution of radionuclide over both lung fields. **A,** Anterior image. **B,** Posterior image. **C,** Right lateral image. **D,** Left lateral image. **E,** Right posterior oblique image. **F,** Left posterior oblique image.

(From Early PJ and Sodee DB: Principles and practice of nuclear medicine, St Louis, 1985, The CV Mosby Co.)

Indications

These studies are used in suspected cases of pulmonary emboli, bronchiogenic carcinoma, and chronic obstructive pulmonary disease (COPD), such as emphysema and bronchitis.

Procedure

Dynamic. Ten to twenty mCi of ^{133}Xe is injected into a special breathing apparatus, and the patient is instructed to inhale and hold his breath for 15 seconds (if possible) for the image. The patient is asked to breath in and out normally until equilibrium is reached between the radioactive and nonradioactive gases in this breathing apparatus. Then an image is taken. Concluding this procedure is a washout phase in which the patient is imaged while breathing in normal room air and breathing out the radioactive gases until all xenon is removed from the lungs.

Static

^{99m}Tc-MAA. The patient is injected with 2 to 4 mCi of MAA, which proceeds through the heart to be stopped completely in the lungs. Images are taken on anterior, posterior, and both lateral aspects (Fig. 39-12).

^{99m}Tc-DTPA. After 25 to 35 mCi ^{99m}Tc-DTPA is introduced into the nebulizer, which is connected to an oxygen supply, the patient breathes through the nebulizer tubing for 2 to 3 minutes. Images are taken on anterior, posterior, and both lateral orientations.

Results

Xenon. Normal—uniform distribution of radioactive gases, symmetric clearance of gases with no activity after 3 minutes. Abnormal—ventilation defects plus retention of gases in the affected areas for greater than 3 minutes at the washout phase (Fig. 39-12).

MAA. Normal—uniform distribution of radioactivity. Abnormal—perfusion defects where areas of nonradioactivity exist (Fig. 39-12, *A*).

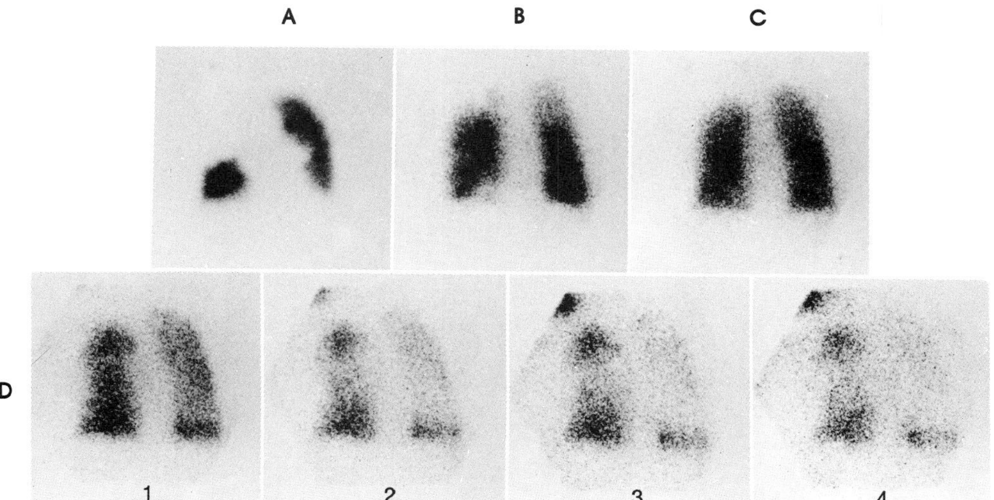

Fig. 39-12. Patient, 74 years of age, with moderately severe COPD (emphysema) and history of acute chest pain, increasing shortness of breath. **A,** Posterior perfusion (^{99m}Tc MAA) lung image reveals lower lobe as well as mediastinal region of right lung. **B,** ^{133}Xe ventilation study (posterior position). Inhalation phase: note ventilation of left lung and mediastinal portion of right lung. **C,** ^{133}Xe equilibrium phase. Even distribution of ^{133}Xe throughout both lung fields. **D,** Washout phase: note delayed washout of ^{133}Xe from areas of increased dead air space (emphysema). Combined studies imply that patient has pulmonary embolization superimposed on COPD.

(From Early PJ and Sodee DB: Principles and practice of nuclear medicine, St Louis, 1985, The CV Mosby Co.)

LIVER AND SPLEEN
Rationale

Dynamic. Liver function can be studied with the use of ^{131}I labeled rose bengal. This material is picked up and excreted by the parenchymal cells of the liver.

Static. Because one of the primary functions of the liver and spleen is phagocytosis through the reticuloendothelial system (RES), it is only necessary to introduce radioactive materials that will be phagocytosed by the liver to determine areas of damaged liver tissue. Such an agent is ^{99m}Tc labeled sulfur colloid.

Indications

Dynamic. This study is used to show biliary obstruction and evaluation of jaundice.

Static. This procedure is used to determine the size and shape of the liver, as well as to check for abnormal areas of tissue function; it also used with hepatomegaly or splenomegaly, mass evaluations, metastases, hepatomas, abscesses, jaundice, cirrhosis, hepatitis, and liver and/or splenic rupture.

Procedure

Dynamic. An I.V. injection of 250 μCi of ^{131}I labeled rose bengal is given, and anterior images are taken every 10 minutes following administration through the first hour. Images are taken again at 6 and 24 hours if necessary.

Static. An I.V. injection of 3 to 6 mCi of ^{99m}Tc labeled sulfur colloid is given, and images are taken after 5 to 15 minutes from the anterior, posterior, and right lateral images.

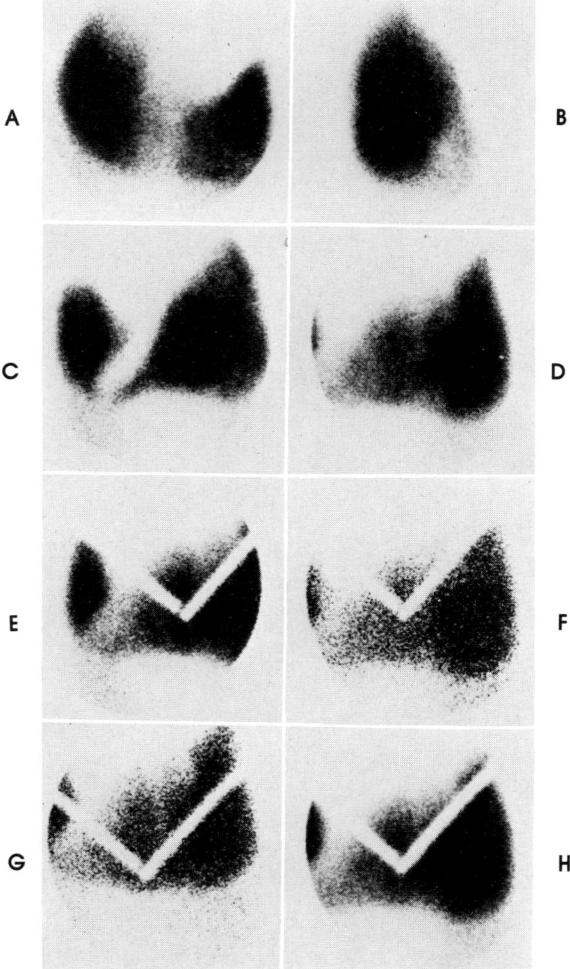

Fig. 39-13. Normal liver images. Study was performed with 6 mCi of ^{99m}Tc sulfur colloid administered intravenously. **A,** Anterior image with costal margin marker. **B** and **C,** Inspiration/expiration images. **D,** Anterior image of spleen with costal margin marker. **E,** Anterior image of liver without marker. **F,** LAO image of the spleen. **G,** Right lateral image. **H,** Posterior image of liver and spleen.

(From Early PJ and Sodee DB: Principles and practice of nuclear medicine, St Louis, 1985, The CV Mosby Co.)

Results

Dynamic. Normal—radiopharmaceutical should be visualized in the gastrointestinal tract by 30 to 60 minutes and cleared from the liver in no more than 4 hours. Abnormal—delayed visualization suggests a biliary obstruction.

Static. Normal—an equal distribution of all radioactivity in all areas of the liver and spleen, with the spleen having normally less activity (Fig. 39-13). Abnormal—an area of decreased activity suggests metastases or hepatomas (Fig. 39-14). Abnormal size is seen in instances of hepatomegaly and/or splenomegaly (Fig. 39-15).

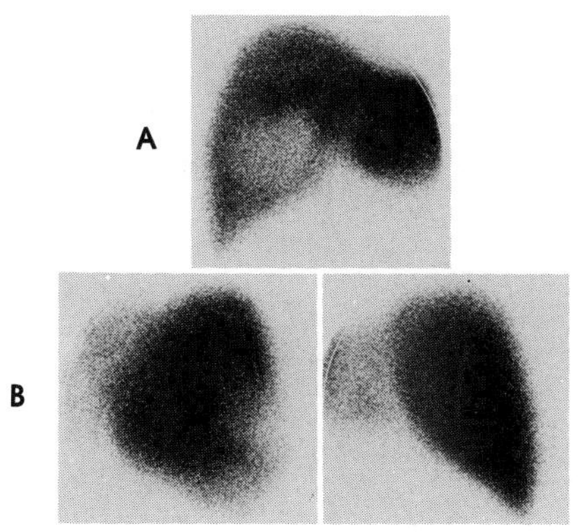

Fig. 39-14. Gallbladder carcinoma. **A,** Anterior image reveals right lobe with large space-occupying lesion extending from porta hepatis and gallbladder bed. Lesion is larger than dilated gallbladder. **B,** Lateral image shows anterior indentation of lesion. **C,** Lesion is not easily seen on posterior image.

(From Early PJ and Sodee DB: Principles and practice of nuclear medicine, St Louis, 1985, The CV Mosby Co.)

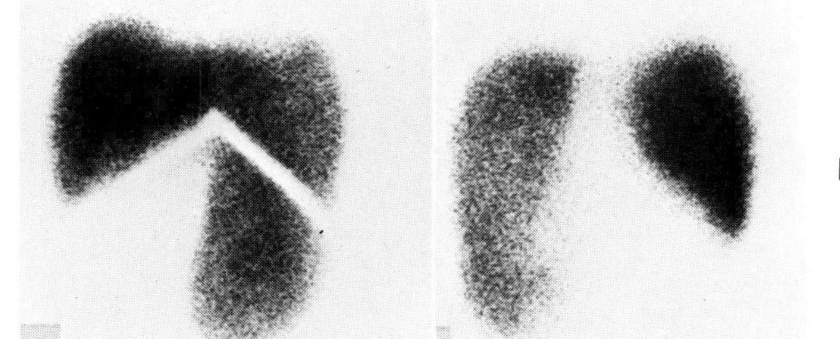

Fig. 39-15. Splenomegaly as a result of chronic lymphatic leukemia. **A,** Anterior image. **B,** Posterior image. Marked splenomegaly with even distribution of nuclide throughout spleen.

(From Early PJ and Sodee DB: Principles and practice of nuclear medicine, St Louis, 1985, The CV Mosby Co.)

KIDNEY

Rationale

Dynamic. ^{99m}Tc labeled DTPA (Sn) is cleared as a glomerular filtrate by the kidneys.

Static. Images are taken following dynamic studies to confirm the dynamic evaluation.

Indications

This procedure is used to evaluate hypertension, renal obstruction, congenital anomalies, tumors, cysts, and trauma.

Procedure

A 15 mCi dose of ^{99m}Tc labeled DTPA (Sn) is injected intravenously with immediate images on the flow from a posterior view. Static images are collected immediately following the dynamic study (Fig. 39-16).

Results

Dynamic functions show constrictions in the renal artery, whereas static images show areas of decreased radioactivity suggesting tumors, cysts, or polycystic kidney disease. Abnormalities in size and shape, such as horseshoe kidneys, can be detected by use of this procedure.

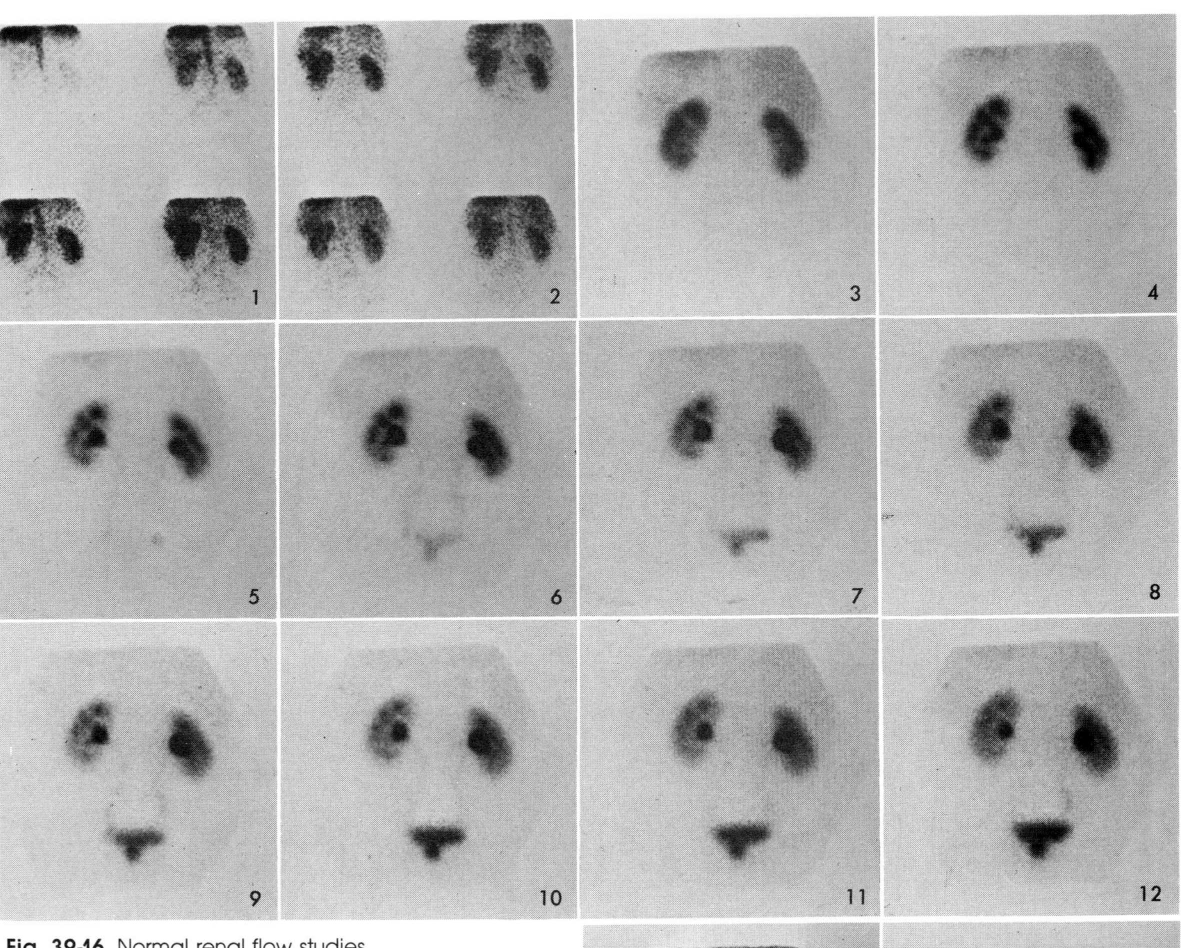

Fig. 39-16. Normal renal flow studies performed with 15 mCi of ^{99m}Tc glucoheptonate. *1* and *2*, Four-second interval renal perfusion study revealing symmetric perfusion of both kidneys. Sequential 1-minute images. *3*, Immediate 1-minute static image revealing even distribution throughout normal renal cortices. *4*, Visualization of calyces and pelves bilaterally. *5* through *12*, Continued increased visualization of renal excretory system. *13*, Image enhanced to bring out ureters. *14*, Five-hour delayed image of renal tubular retention of nuclide.

(From Early, P.J., and Sodee, D.B.: Principles and practice of nuclear medicine, St Louis, 1985, The C.V. Mosby Co.)

BONE

Rationale

Sometimes the exact elements used by an organ system are not available as a radionuclide. However, other elements that mimic those used by the system can be employed satisfactorily. Such is the case in bone studies. Bone utilizes calcium in making new bone or in repairing old bone. Phosphate complexes can mimic calcium and are therefore said to be calcomimetic. Bone studies are performed using these phosphate complexes labeled with ^{99m}Tc.

Indications

This procedure is used to evaluate metastases, tumors, arthritis, Paget's disease, and osteomyelitis.

Procedure

An I.V. injection of 20 mCi of ^{99m}Tc labeled phosphate complex is administered. Total body scans are performed in approximately 2 hours following administration (Fig. 39-17).

Results

"Hot spots" indicate a problem related to the history of the patient, for instance, metastases (Fig. 39-18), arthritis, or injury.

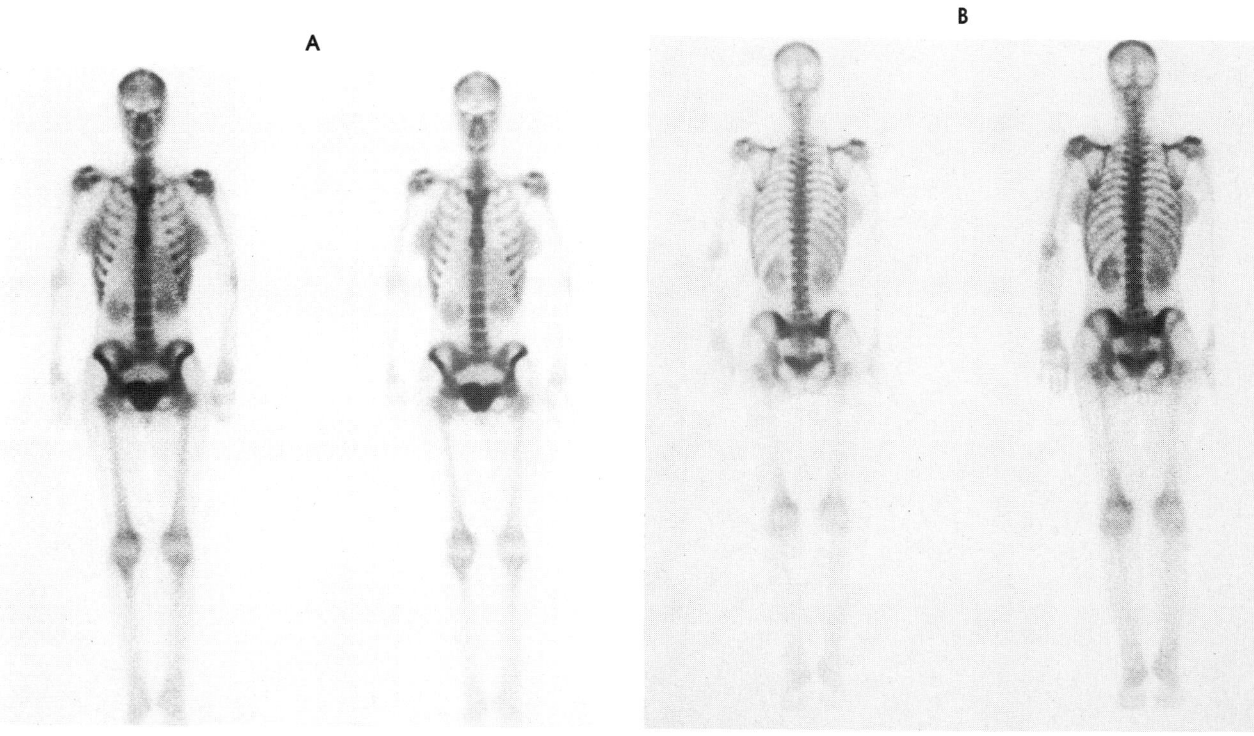

Fig. 39-17. Bone images taken 2 hours after administration of a 10 mCi dose of ^{99m}Tc medronate disodium. **A,** Anterior and, **B,** posterior whole body images. Diagnosis: normal bone study.

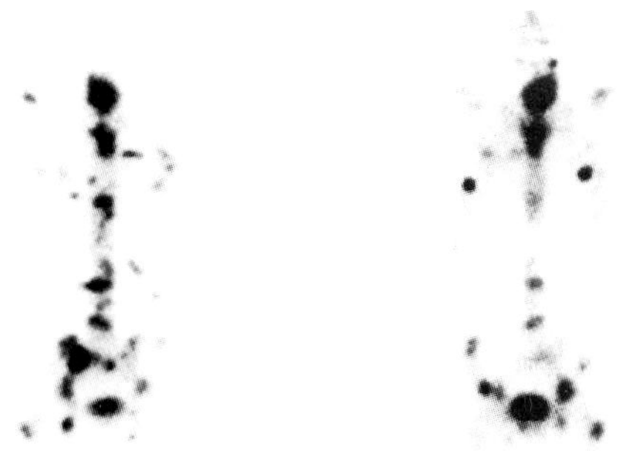

Fig. 39-18. Metastatic disease. Abnormal bone images taken 2 hours after administration of 20 mCi dose of ^{99m}Tc medronate disodium. There are multiple focal areas of increased concentration of radionuclide involving cervical, thoracic, and lumbar vertebral bodies as well as several ribs bilaterally, both sides of the pelvis, left shoulder, and proximal left femur. **A,** Posterior and, **B,** anterior whole-body images. Diagnosis: osseous metastasis secondary to prostate carcinoma.

(From Early PJ and Sodee DB: Principles and practice of nuclear medicine, St Louis, 1985, The CV Mosby Co.)

HEART
Rationale

Cardiovascular nuclear medicine is one of the fastest growing areas of the nuclear medicine field. Studies are performed both using "hot-spot" and "cold-spot" scanning techniques. Just as the phosphate complexes for bone are calcomimetic, thallium is potassiomimetic because thallium travels to the heart muscles in the same manner as potassium. "Cold-spot" imaging results from the use of ^{201}Tl, for example. "Hot-spot" imaging results from the use of ^{99m}Tc labeled pyrophosphate, which is used to show blood flow to the various organs of the body.

Dynamic. Normal ^{99m}Tc labeled pyrophosphate studies of the heart show no presence of radioactivity in the area of the heart (Fig. 39-19). Abnormal studies show a hot-spot image (Fig. 39-20).

Static. Because ^{201}Tl is potassiomimetic, a normal study is one in which the heart calls on the use of thallium in the same way it calls on the use of potassium in performing its normal function (Fig. 39-21). An area that is not functioning normally does not call for potassium and therefore is revealed as a "cold spot" on a thallium image.

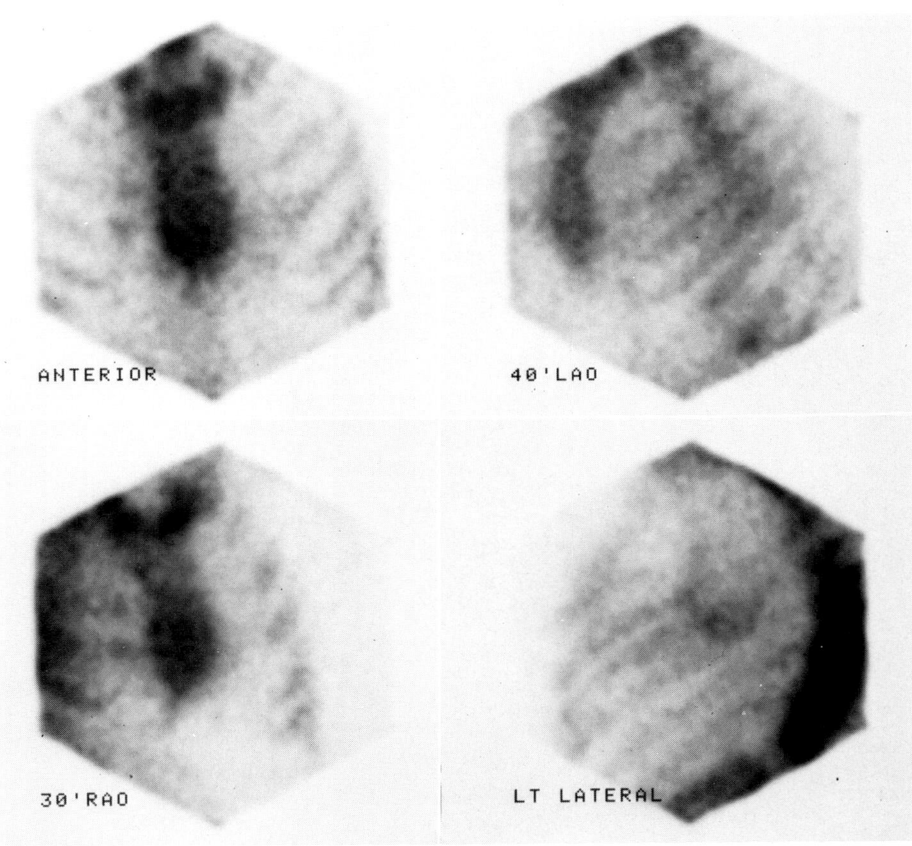

Fig. 39-19. Following intravenous administration of 15 mCi dose of ^{99m}Tc stannous pyrophosphate, images of thorax are negative. There is no concentration of nuclide in region of myocardium.

(From Early PJ and Sodee DB: Principles and practice of nuclear medicine, St Louis, 1985, The CV Mosby Co.)

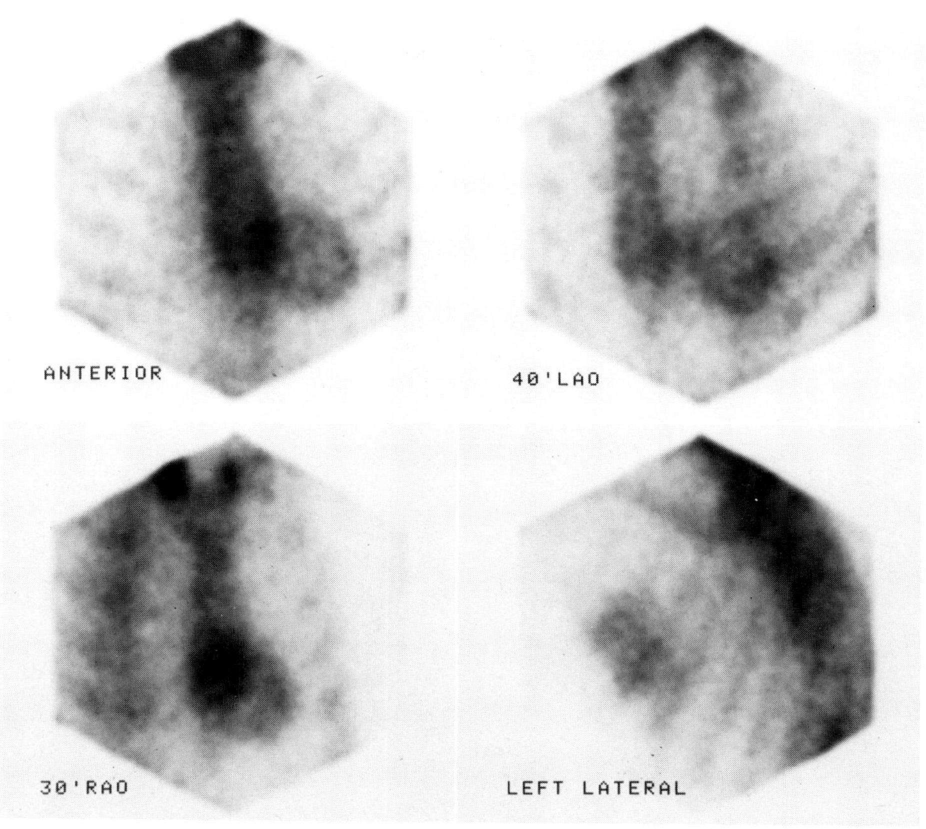

Fig. 39-20. Markedly abnormal pyrophosphate (PYP) ^{99m}Tc images of thorax in patient with clinical and laboratory evidence of anterior wall infarction. There is 4× increased concentration of PYP ^{99m}Tc in anterolateral left ventricular myocardium with central region of absent activity. This halo type of concentration implies a poor prognosis.

(From Early PJ and Sodee DB: Principles and practice of nuclear medicine, St Louis, 1985, The CV Mosby Co.)

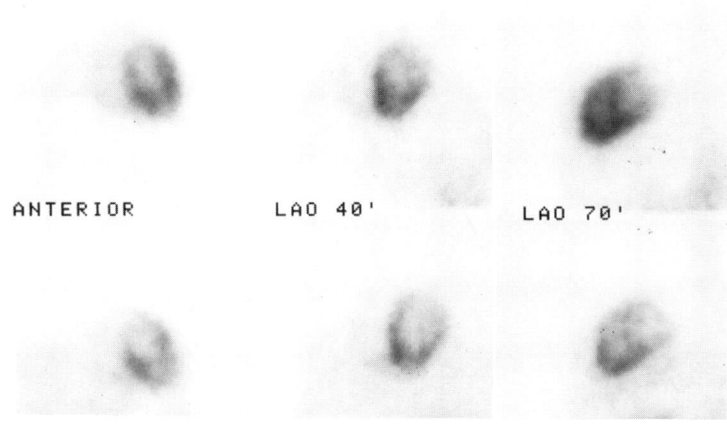

Fig. 39-21. Following intravenous administration of 2.0 mCi of ^{201}Tl chloride, post-stress and redistribution images are normal.

(From Early PJ and Sodee DB: Principles and practice of nuclear medicine, St Louis, 1985, The CV Mosby Co.)

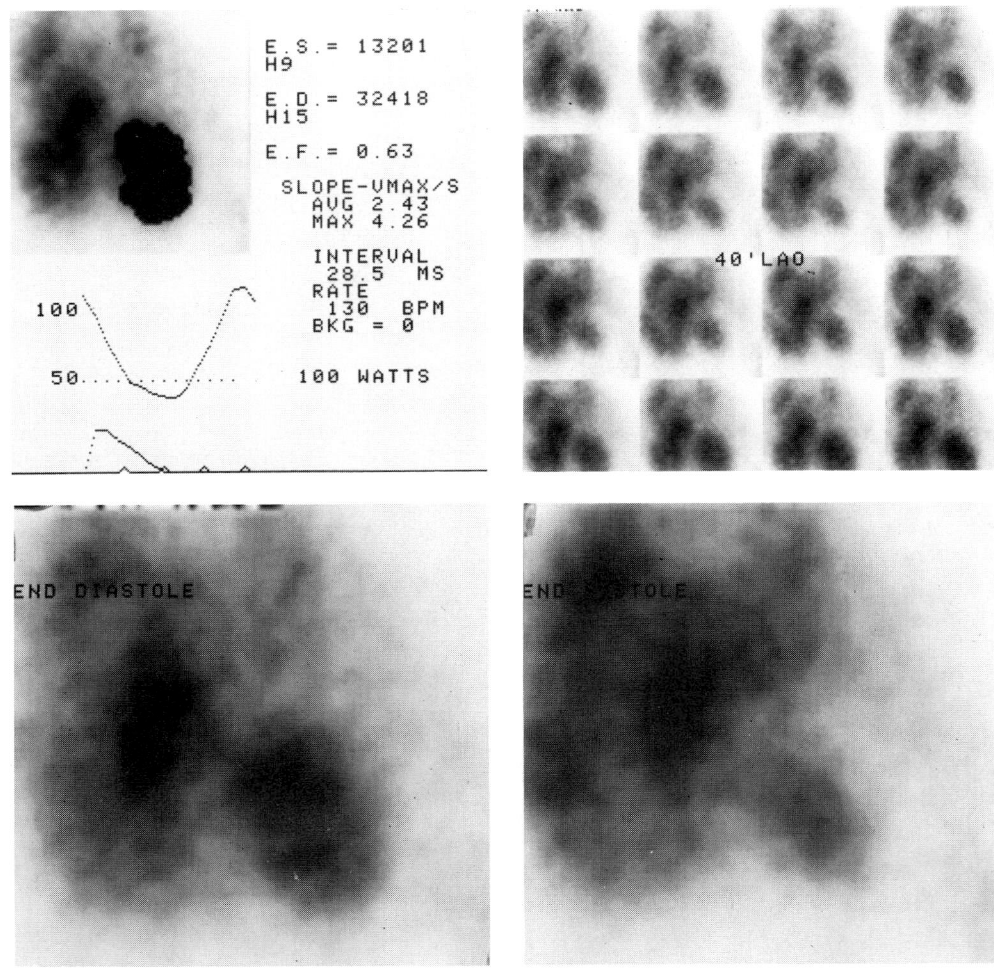

Fig. 39-22. A stress gated evaluation of patient with known aortic stenosis, illustrating ejection fraction and multigated acquisition results. End-systole and end-diastole segments are magnified.

Indications

This study is used to evaluate myocardial infarct, cardiac output, and coronary insufficiencies.

Procedure

Dynamic. The patient is injected with 20 mCi of ^{99m}Tc labeled pyrophosphate (labeled in vivo), and images are collected immediately to show cardiac function and wall motion. This procedure is commonly called a multigated acquisition (MUGA) study, and it incorporates the use of a computer, an electrocardiograph (ECG), and an internal (to the computer) clock so that the cardiac cycle can be framed into many segments. Each segment represents a certain phase of the heart's cycle. Because one heart cycle does not provide enough information for statistically significant data, many cycles are required. By partitioning the heart cycle into different segments (using the internal clock and the ECG), data from subsequent cycles can be segmented identically and each segment superimposed on its respective previous segment to achieve statistically valid results and images. Such a study is illustrated in Fig. 39-22, which shows the heart cycle divided into 16 segments with the end-systole and end-diastole segments magnified to show the extremes of ventricular wall motion. Also note in the data image that the cardiac output or ejection fraction (the average amount of blood expelled from the ventricle per contraction) is 63% (E.F. = 0.63).

Static. The patient exercises on a treadmill until he has achieved maximum stress, at which time he is injected with 2 mCi of ^{201}Tl. Immediate images (anterior, left anterior oblique, and left lateral) are taken of the heart and muscle function under stress conditions. The images are repeated at 2 to 3 hours post administration and post stress to determine if the thallium is redistributed under nonstress conditions.

Results

Dynamic. Poor wall-motion studies and poor cardiac outputs are consistent with myocardial infarcts.

Static. Normal—normal distribution in both stress and relaxation conditions. Abnormal—areas of nonperfusion on both stress and relaxation is suggestive of myocardial infarct; areas of abnormal perfusion on stress but normal distribution on relaxation is consistent with ischemia under stress.

• • •

Other studies using nuclear medicine are available, but those that are currently of major significance in nuclear medicine departments are described here. As advances are made in equipment design (e.g., tomography) and with the advent of new radiopharmaceuticals (e.g., monoclonal antibodies), the field of nuclear medicine will continue to expand and become an even greater force in diagnostic and therapeutic medicine.

Definition of Terms

alpha particle A particle that is identical to the helium nucleus, consisting of two protons and two neutrons. It carries a positive charge of 2.

beta decay The radioactive disintegration of a nucleus resulting in the emission of an electron (beta particle).

beta particle An electron, either positive or negative. Positive beta particles are called positrons B^+. Negative beta particles are sometimes called negatrons B^-. The term "beta particle" and the symbol "B" are reserved for electrons originating in a nucleus.

binding energy Amount of energy required to remove a particle from the nucleus or orbits of an atom.

cathode ray tube (CRT) Device used to record an event by exciting its phosphor.

collimator An apparatus, often consisting of a pair of slits, used to confine radiation to a narrow beam.

COPD Chronic obstructive pulmonary disease.

cutie-pie A "gun-type" portable instrument for measuring the radiation level.

cyclotron A device used to produce neutron-poor radionuclides.

daughter The decay product produced by a radioactive nuclide. When the *parent* nuclide undergoes decay, a *daughter* nuclide is produced.

decay The radioactive disintegration of a nucleus.

discriminator An electronic device capable of accepting or rejecting a pulse according to the pulse height of voltage.

dynodes Anodes used for amplification in a photomultiplier tube.

electromagnetic spectrum A listing of energy waves not affected by electrical or magnetic properties.

electron An elementary particle of nature having a charge of 1 and a mass of 9.1×10^{-28} grams.

film badge A piece of photographic film contained in a lightproof holder and worn by an individual to measure the amount of radiation to which he is exposed.

gamma rays Electromagnetic radiation having its origin in an atomic nucleus.

gas detector A device employing a gas plus a high-voltage power supply for detection of radiation.

Geiger-Mueller counter A small ionization chamber operated by gas amplification and used to detect small quantities of radioactivity.

generator A method of producing radioactivity in a nuclear medicine department.

half-life The time required for one half of a given number of radioactive atoms to undergo decay: symbol $T_{1/2}$.

half-value layer (HVL) Material necessary to reduce radiation intensity by one half.

isotope One of a group of nuclides of the same element (same Z) having the same number of protons in the nucleus but differing in the number of neutrons, resulting in different values of A.

linear accelerator A device used to produce neutron-poor radionuclides.

lower level discriminator (LLD) Device used to discriminate against all pulses whose heights are below an accepted level.

meV Symbol for one million electron volts, or 10^6 eV.

microcurie (μCi) One millionth of a curie.

millicurie (mCi) One thousandth of a curie.

negatron A negative electron or ordinary electron. Synonym for electron.

nucleon Any particle found within the nucleus.

neutrino An almost weightless particle smitten from the nucleus during the decay process.

neutron A neutral elementary particle having a mass number of 1. In the free state (outside the nucleus), it is unstable, having a half-life of about 12 minutes. It decays by the process $n = p + e + v$.

nuclear reactor A device for supporting a self-sustained nuclear chain reaction under controlled conditions.

nucleus The positively charged core of an atom in which almost all the mass is concentrated.

nuclide Any one of the more than 1000 species of atoms characterized by the number of protons and number of neutrons in the nucleus.

oscilloscope See cathode ray tube.

photocathode Photosensitive layer (cathode) of a photomultiplier tube.

photomultiplier tube A phototube of exceptionally high sensitivity, the electron or electrons released at the photocathode initiating a cascade from one dynode to another with a resultant electron amplification as high as 10.

positron A positive electron.

proportional gas detector A device for measuring primarily alpha and beta radioactivity.

proton A positively charged elementary particle having a mass number of 1. The nucleus of a hydrogen atom of mass 1.

pulse height analyzer (PHA) Device used to select some pulses and reject others.

radioactive Giving off radiant energy in the form of alpha, beta, or gamma rays by the breaking up of atoms.

radioisotope Synonym for radioactive isotope. Any isotope that is unstable, thus undergoing decay with the emission of a characteristic radiation.

radionuclide Synonym for radioactive nuclide.

radiopharmaceutical A radioactive substance used especially for diagnostic purposes or treatment of disease.

rectilinear scanner A device that generates an image of an organ by detecting radioactivity within that organ and recording it on film.

scaler An electronic device that produces an output pulse for a given number of input pulses. Term generally applied to a device for indicating the total number of observed pulses or events.

scintillation The flash of light produced in a phosphor by radiation.

scintillation camera An imaging device using all of the components of a scintillation counter.

scintillation counter A counter employing a phosphor, photomultiplier tube, and associated circuits for the detection of radiation.

scintillation detector Sensitive device used to detect ionizing radiation by electronically measuring the light (scintillation) produced.

thermoluminescent dosimetry (TLD) A method of measuring radiation exposure.

upper level discriminator (ULD) An electronic device used to discriminate against all pulses whose heights are above an accepted level.

x rays Electromagnetic radiation having its origin in the orbital shells of an atom.

SELECTED BIBLIOGRAPHY

Bernier DR, Langan JK and Wells LD: Nuclear medicine technology and techniques, St Louis, 1981, The CV Mosby Co.

Blahd WH: Nuclear medicine, New York, 1965, McGraw-Hill Book Co.

Bogardus CR Jr: Clinical applications of physics of radiology and nuclear medicine, St Louis, 1969, Warren H Green, Inc.

Casarett AP: Radiation biology, Englewood Cliffs, NJ, 1968, Prentice-Hall, Inc.

Chandra R: Introductory physics of nuclear medicine, Philadelphia, 1976, Lea & Febiger.

Dillman LT and von der Lage FC: Radionuclide decay schemes and nuclear parameters for use in radiation-dose estimation. MIRD Pamphlet No 10, New York, 1975, Society of Nuclear Medicine.

Goodwin PN and Rao DV: The physics of nuclear medicine, Springfield, Ill, 1977, Charles C Thomas, Publisher.

Gottschalk A and Potchen EJ: Diagnostic nuclear medicine, Baltimore, 1976, Williams & Wilkins.

Hendee WR: Medical radiation physics, ed 2, 1979, Chicago, 1979, Year Book Medical Publishers, Inc.

Johns HE: The physics of radiology, ed 2, revised ed, Springfield, Ill, 1964, Charles C Thomas, Publisher.

King ER and Mitchell TG: A manual for nuclear medicine, Springfield, Ill, 1961, Charles C Thomas, Publisher.

Quimby EH and Feitelberg S: Radioactive isotopes in medicine and biology, ed 2, Philadelphia, 1963, Lea & Febiger.

Rocha AFG and Harbert JE: Textbook of nuclear medicine: basic science, Philadelphia, 1978, Lea & Febiger.

Rollo FD: Nuclear medicine physics, instrumentation, and agents, St Louis, 1977, The CV Mosby Co.

Shapiro J: Radiation protection, Cambridge, Mass, 1972, Harvard University Press.

Shilling CW: Atomic energy encyclopedia in the life sciences, Philadelphia, 1964, WB Saunders Co.

Sorenson JA and Phelps ME: Physics in nuclear medicine, New York, 1980, Grune & Stratton, Inc.

Wagner HN: Principles of nuclear medicine, Philadelphia, 1968, WB Saunders Co.

Chapter 40

POSITRON EMISSION TOMOGRAPHY

RICHARD D. HICHWA

*Positron emission tomography** (PET) is a noninvasive nuclear imaging technique that involves the administration of a *radiopharmaceutical* and subsequent imaging of the distribution and *kinetics* of the radioactive material. PET imaging of the heart, brain, lungs, or other organs is possible if an appropriate radiopharmaceutical, also called a *radiotracer,* can be synthesized and administered to the patient.

Three important factors distinguish PET from all radiologic procedures and from other nuclear imaging procedures. The first factor is that the results of the data acquisition and analysis techniques yield an image related to a particular physiologic parameter, such as blood flow or metabolism. The ensuing image is aptly called a functional or *parametric image*.

Secondly, the images are created by the simultaneous detection of a pair of *annihilation* radiations that result from a *positron* annihilation occurrence as illustrated in Fig. 40-1.

*All italicized terms are defined at the end of this chapter.

The third feature distinguishing PET is the actual chemical and biologic form of the radiopharmaceutical. The radiopharmaceutical is specifically chosen for its similarity to naturally occurring biochemical constituents of the human body. Because very small amounts of the radiopharmaceutical are administered, equilibrium conditions within the body are not altered. If, for instance, the radiopharmaceutical is a form of sugar, it will behave very much like the natural sugar in the body. The kinetics of uptake and distribution of the radioactive sugar within the body are followed by measuring the distribution of the radioactivity concentration with the PET scanner as a function of time. From this, the distribution of metabolism of the sugar may be deduced by converting the many images that demonstrate the tracer kinetics into a single parametric image that indicates tissue function.

In this chapter, the basic concepts of PET are discussed and examples of neurologic studies are presented.

Comparison with Other Modalities

PET is predominantly used to measure human cellular, organ, or system function. That is, a parameter that characterizes a particular aspect of human physiology is determined from the measurement of the radioactivity emitted from a radiopharmaceutical in a given volume of tissue. In contrast, conventional radiography measures the structure of organs or human anatomy by determining x-ray transmission through a given volume of tissue. X-ray attenuation by structures interposed between the x-ray source and the radiographic film provides the contrast necessary to visualize an organ. Computed tomography (CT) creates cross-sectional tomographic images by computer reconstruction of multiple x-ray transmissions. A comparison among various modalities is given in Table 40-1.

Single photon emission computed tomography (SPECT) (also discussed in Chapter 39) uses nuclear imaging techniques to determine tissue function. However, the SPECT radiopharmaceutical form is substantially different from naturally occurring biomolecules within the body. Use of collimators and lower-energy photons from ^{99m}Tc offer reduced sensitivity and accuracy when compared with PET. Resolution with SPECT is much poorer than PET.

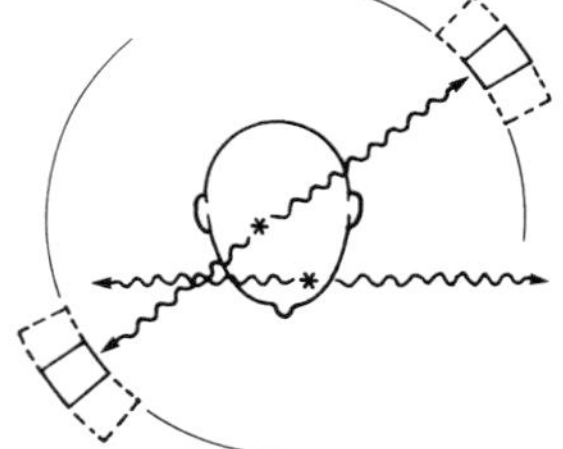

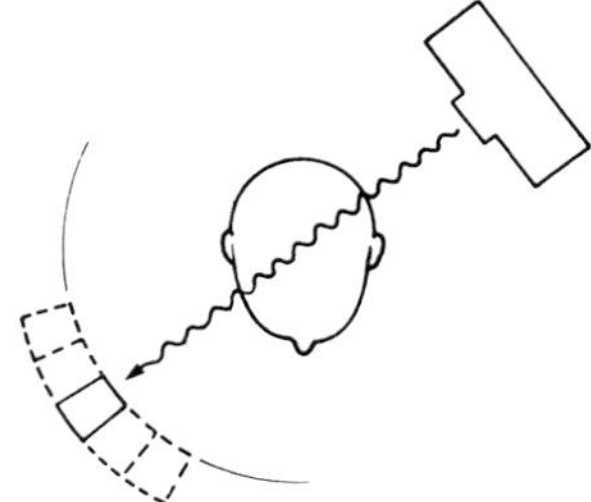

Fig. 40-1. Positron emission tomography relies on the simultaneous emission of a pair of annihilation radiations and their simultaneous detection for PET (left), compared with the transmission of x-rays for computed tomography (CT) (right). In both cases, detectors are used to measure photons exiting the body.

Table 40-1. Comparison of imaging modalities

	PET	SPECT	MRI	CT
Measures	Physiology	Physiology	Anatomy (physiology)	Anatomy
Resolution	5.5 mm	8-12 mm	2 mm	1 mm
Technique	Positron annihilation	Gamma emission	Nuclear magnetic resonance	Absorption of x-ray transmission
Harmful effects	Radiation exposure	Radiation exposure	None known	Radiation exposure
Use	Research	Clinical	Clinical (research)	Clinical
Number of examinations per day	3-6	4-8	7-10	10-15

To emphasize the differences between the various modalities, consider a study of the blood flow within the brain. Without an intact circulatory system, an IV injection of the radiopharmaceutical could not make its way into the brain and be distributed throughout the capillary network within the brain. Therefore a PET scan would not be possible. For radiographic procedures such as CT, structures within the brain may well be intact but there may be no blood flow to and through the brain tissues. A CT scan (see Chapter 34) under these circumstances may appear almost normal. The use of contrast materials for brain studies requires a working circulatory system for transport to the brain. Their use is, however, to help define structures of interest by providing increased x-ray absorption.

The contrast agents used in many of the radiographic studies to enhance image contrast are toxic. The x-ray dose to the patient from these radiographic studies is greater than in nuclear imaging studies. Radiopharmaceuticals used in PET studies are similar to the body's own biochemical constituents and are administered in very small amounts. Biochemical compatibility of the tracers with the body minimizes the risks to the patient because the tracers are not toxic. Trace amounts minimize the alteration of the body's *homeostasis*.

An imaging technique that augments both CT and PET is *magnetic resonance imaging* (MRI) (see Chapter 37). Images of each modality are shown in Fig. 40-2. MRI is primarily used to measure anatomy or morphology. Unlike CT, which derives its greatest image contrast from varying tissue densities (bone from soft tissue), MRI better differentiates tissues by their proton content and the degree to which these protons are bound in lattice structures. The tightly bound protons of bone make it virtually transparent to MRI. It is hoped that spectroscopic imaging of fluorine, phosphorus, and other elements will permit the determination of organ or cellular function. Measurement of large-vessel blood flow is already possible. Development of paramagnetic contrast agents, improved MRI imaging instrumentation, absolute quantification, and spectroscopy remain the major areas of MRI research.

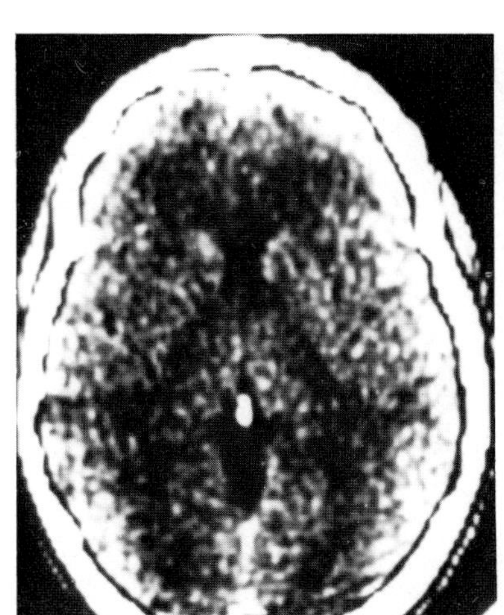
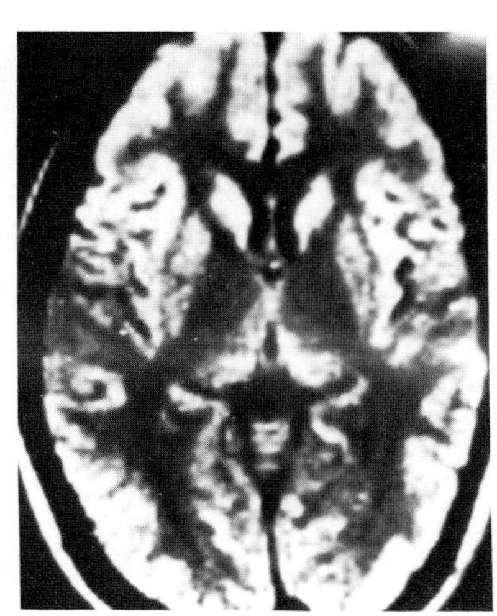
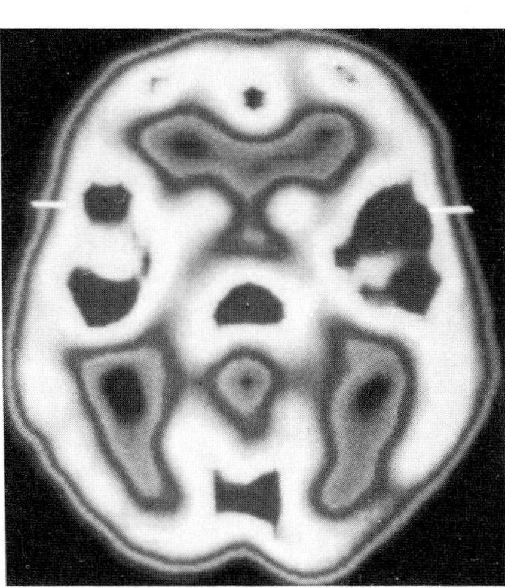

Fig. 40-2. Brain images of same patient in same position with CT (left), MRI (center), and PET (right).

Historical Development

The use of positron-emitting radiopharmaceuticals for medical purposes was first conceived by the inventor of the *cyclotron,* E.O. Lawrence, in the early 1930s. Simple compounds with positron-emitting radionuclides were synthesized, and Geiger counters were used to qualitatively measure the relative uptake in various parts of the body.

It was not until more suitable *scintillators* such as sodium iodide (NaI) and more sophisticated nuclear counting electronics became available that positron coincidence localization was possible. F.W. Wrenn demonstrated the use of positron-emitting radioisotopes for the localization of brain tumors in 1951. G.L. Brownell further developed instrumentation for similar studies in 1953.

The next major advance came in 1967 when G. Hounsfield demonstrated the clinical use of CT. The mathematics of PET image reconstruction are very similar to CT reconstruction techniques. Instead of x rays from a point source traversing the body and being detected by a single detector, PET imaging counts the resulting pairs of 0.511 meV photons from the positron-electron annihilation by using two opposing detectors.

During the next 8 years, significant developments were made in computer technology, scintillator design, and *photomultiplier tube* speed for the detection of high-energy photons. In 1975, the first closed-ring transverse positron tomograph was built for PET imaging by M.M. Ter-Pogossian and M.E. Phelps.

Since 1975, developments on two fronts have accelerated the use of PET. First, with vastly improved imaging instrumentation, scientists are nearing the theoretical limits (1 to 2 mm) of PET tomograph resolution by employing smaller, more efficient scintillators and photomultiplier tubes. Microprocessors now tune and adjust the entire ring of *detectors* that surround the patients, which may number as many as 500 to 600 detectors per ring. The second major area of development is in the design of new radiopharmaceuticals. Agents are being developed to measure blood flow, metabolism, protein synthesis, lipid content, receptor binding, and many other physiologic parameters. During the mid-1980s, PET was predominantly used as a research tool; but by the late 1980s clinical PET centers had been established, and PET was routinely used for diagnostic procedures on the brain and heart.

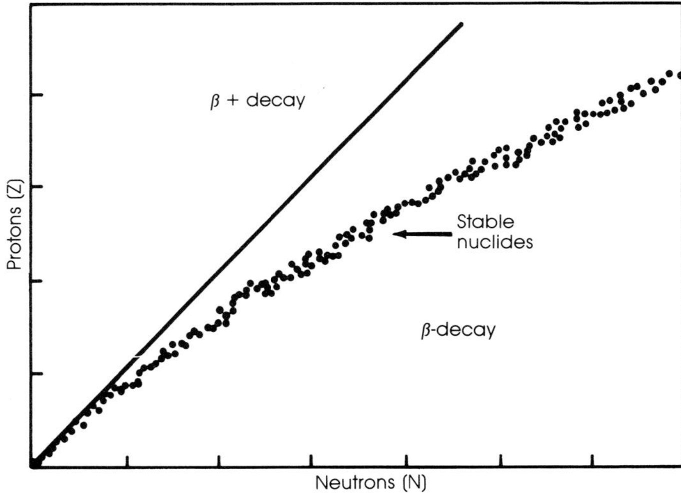

Fig. 40-3. Plot of stable nuclides (points) as a function of proton and neutron number. Nuclides with equal number of protons and neutrons are indicated by the solid line. Nuclides below stable species (neutron rich) predominantly decay by β^- emission, and nuclides above stable species (neutron deficient) more often decay by β^+ emission.

Underlying Principles and Necessary Facilities

In this section, the major concepts and facilities for the use of PET are discussed. To better understand the multidisciplinary nature of PET, four major functions are presented. These are radionuclide production, radiopharmaceutical production, data acquisition, and image reconstruction and image processing. A short discussion of the particles called positrons is presented.

POSITRONS

Living organisms are primarily composed of compounds containing the elements hydrogen, carbon, nitrogen, and oxygen. In PET, radiotracers are made by synthesizing compounds with radioactive isotopes of these elements. Chemically, the radioactive isotope is indistinguishable from their equivalent stable isotope. Neutron-rich (more neutrons than protons) radionuclides emit electrons or beta particles. The effective range or distance traveled for a 1 meV beta particle (β^-) in human tissue is only 4 mm. These radionuclides also do not emit other types of radiation that can be easily measured externally with counters or scintillation detectors. The only radioisotopes of these elements that can be detected outside the body are positron-emitting nuclides. Fig. 40-3 depicts the stable nuclides as a function of the number of neutrons and protons in the nucleus.

Positron-emitting radionuclides have a neutron-deficient nucleus (more protons than neutrons). Positrons (β^+) are identical in mass to electrons, but they possess positive instead of negative charges. The characteristics of positrons are given in Table 40-2. Positron decay occurs in un-

Table 40-2. Positron characteristics

Definition	Positively charged electron
Origin	Neutron-deficient nuclei
Production	Accelerators
Nuclide decay	$p = n + \beta^+ +$ neutrino
Positron decay	Annihilation to two 0.511 meV photons
Number	~240 known
Range	Proportional to kinetic energy of β^+
PET nuclides	^{11}C, ^{13}N, ^{15}O, ^{18}F

stable radioisotopes only if the nucleus possesses excess energy greater than the energy equivalent of two electron rest masses or a total of 1.022 meV. After a positron is emitted from the nucleus, it is rapidly slowed by interactions in the surrounding tissues until all of its kinetic energy is lost. At this point, the positron combines momentarily with an electron. The combination of particles totally annihilates or disintegrates, and the combined positron-electron mass of 1.022 meV is transformed into two equal energy photons of 0.511 meV, which are emitted at 180 degrees from each other as shown in Fig. 40-4. These annihilation photons behave like gamma rays, have sufficient energy to traverse the body tissues, and can be detected externally. Because two identical, or isoenergetic, photons are emitted at exactly 180 degrees from each other, the simultaneous detection of both photons defines a line passing through the body, and the line is located precisely between the two scintillators that detected the photons. A simplified block diagram for a single coincidence circuit is shown in Fig. 40-5. Creation of images from coincidence detection is discussed in the section on data acquisition. The important point to note is that the positron annihilation photons can be used for external detection from the positron-emitting radionuclides of carbon, nitrogen, and oxygen. Table 40-3 depicts the positron ranges for several energies in tissue, air, and lead. Hydrogen has no positron-emitting radioisotope, however, fluorine-18 (^{18}F) is a positron (β^+) emitter that is used as a hydrogen substitute in many compounds. This is accomplished because of its small size and strong bond with carbon.

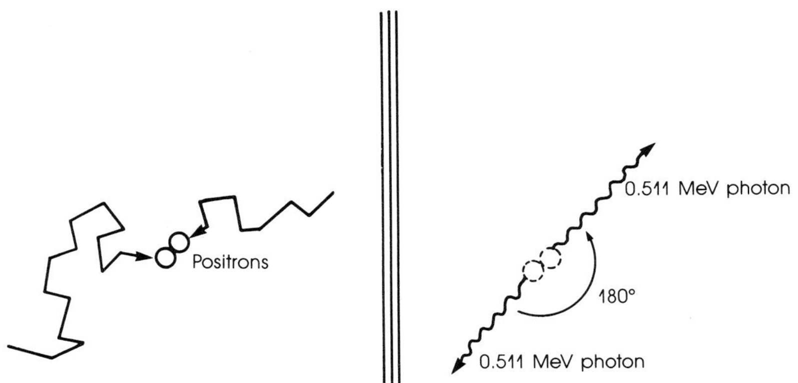

Fig. 40-4. Positron loses kinetic energy by scattering (erratic line) until coming to rest and interacting with an electron (left). Two photons of 0.511 meV ($E = M_oC^2$) result from the positron and electron annihilation (right).

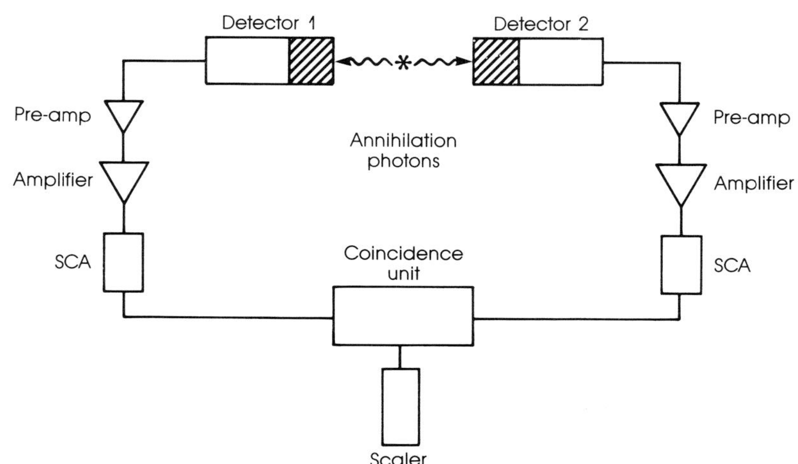

Fig. 40-5. Coincidence electronics for one pair of detectors in a PET ring tomograph.

Table 40-3. Range (R) of positrons in centimeters

	$\bar{E}$ (meV)	R_{tissue}	R_{air}	R_{lead}
β^+	0.5	0.15	127	0.01
	1.0	0.38	279	0.03
	1.5	0.64	508	0.05

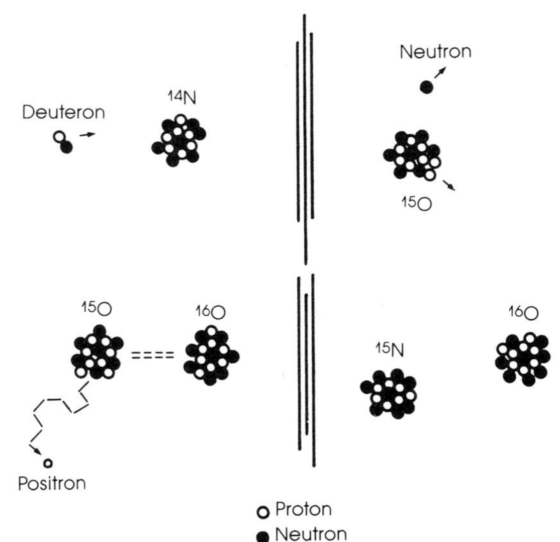

Fig. 40-6. Typical radionuclide production sequence. The $^{14}N(d,n)^{15}O$ reaction is used for making ^{15}O-^{16}O molecules. After positron decay, stable atoms of oxygen and nitrogen remain.

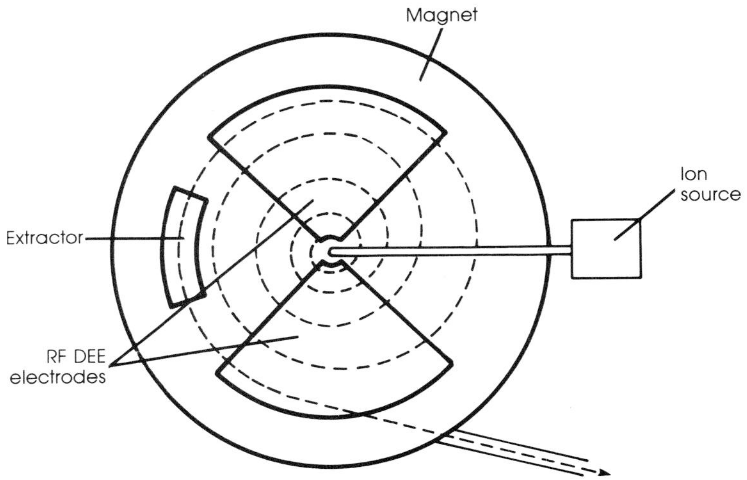

Fig. 40-7. Cyclotron schematic. *Dashed line* indicates path of accelerated particles for positive ion cyclotrons.

RADIONUCLIDE PRODUCTION

To produce positron-emitting radionuclides, a cyclotron is used to bombard appropriate nonradioactive *target* atoms with nuclei accelerated to high energies. The high energies are necessary to overcome the electrostatic and nuclear forces of the target nuclei so that a nuclear reaction can take place. An example is the production of oxygen-15 (^{15}O). Deuterons or heavy hydrogen ions (proton and neutron) are accelerated to approximately 10 meV. The target material is stable nitrogen-14 (^{14}N) gas. The resultant nuclear reaction yields a neutron and an ^{15}O atom. This ^{15}O atom is quickly associated with a stable ^{16}O atom also present in the target gas to produce a radioactive ^{15}O-^{16}O molecule. The ^{15}O atom emits a positron. This process transforms a proton into a neutron. Hence, the ^{15}O atom becomes a ^{15}N atom. This process is shown in Fig. 40-6. The half-life of ^{15}O is 122 seconds. To produce useful positron-emitting radionuclides such as ^{15}O with very short half-lives (seconds or minutes), a cyclotron or particle accelerator is needed nearby.

A cyclotron consists of four major parts as shown in Fig. 40-7. These are the ion source, the magnet, the radio-frequency high-voltage acceleration system, and the extractor.

The ion source, as the name suggests, is used to create ions for acceleration from simple stable gases. Carbon (C), nitrogen (N), oxygen (O), and fluorine (F) nuclides, as defined in Table 40-4, are produced from high-energy protons (ionized hydrogen gas) or deuterons (ionized deuterium gas). These ions, which are positive ions if their electrons have been stripped away or negative ions if an extra electron has been added, are extracted from the source and accelerated toward the outer rim of the cyclotron magnet. The cyclotron magnet is used to constrain the charged particles or ions to move in circular orbits. As one might expect, higher energy particles move with greater velocity and therefore travel in orbits of greater radii than lower energy particles. Fig. 40-8 shows a typical cyclotron used for radionuclide production. This cyclotron is located in a concrete vault. Some newer cyclotrons have shielding material located directly on the machine exterior and are called self-shielded cyclotrons.

Ions are accelerated by traversing the electric field gradient between the "dee" electrodes; these structures resemble the capital letter D. This gradient is created by charging the dees to a high voltage, much like charging a large capacitor. As an ion is repelled by the polarity of the charge on one dee and attracted toward the opposite polarity of the charge on the other dee, it gains kinetic energy and its velocity increases. Once an ion is inside the conducting dee structure, it no longer experiences electrostatic forces and is constrained to move in a circular orbit toward the opposite dee by the magnetic field. During this time, the polarity of the dees is automatically reversed. The alternating voltage cycle occurs at radio frequencies (RF) of 10 to 30 MHz. Therefore each time the ion traverses the gap between the two dees, it is accelerated by the respective attractive and repulsive electrostatic forces. It gains approximately twice the voltage difference between the two dees for every orbit or complete circular path. If the dee-to-dee voltage is 100 kV, then a proton gains 200 keV per orbit and undergoes approximately 130 orbits before gaining its maximum energy, which is 26 meV for the cyclotron shown in Fig. 40-8. During this time, the ion increases its orbital radius from the center of the cyclotron to near the edge of the main magnetic field in a spiral path.

A high-voltage electrostatic deflector is used to nudge positive ions from the edge of the magnet field to a point where they can now be extracted from the cyclotron. Negative ions are extracted by removing the added electrons by passing the ions through a thin carbon foil. Because these ions were once negative and are now positive, they rotate in the opposite direction under the influence of the constant magnetic field. Hence, the particles are easily extracted from the cyclotron. Because the ion source emits ions with every cycle of the RF voltage applied to the dees, regardless of their polarity, ions arrive at the extractor in packets synchronized with the RF frequency. These packets, or a beam of particles, are then focused and directed toward the targets for production of the positron-emitting radioisotopes. The radioisotopes produced in the target may be solid, liquid, or gaseous and may be produced either continuously or in batches.

Table 40-4. Production of the most useful PET nuclides

Nuclide	Half-life	Reaction(s)	Target material
^{15}O	122 sec	$^{15}N(p,n)^{15}O$; $^{14}N(d,n)^{15}O$	$N_2+1\%O_2$
^{13}N	9.97 min	$^{16}O(p,\alpha)^{13}N$	H_2O
^{11}C	20.4 min	$^{14}N(p,\alpha)^{11}C$	N_2
^{18}F	109.8 min	$^{18}O(p,n)^{18}F$; $^{20}Ne(d,\alpha)^{18}F$	$95\%^{18}O-H_2O$;Ne+ 0.1% F_2

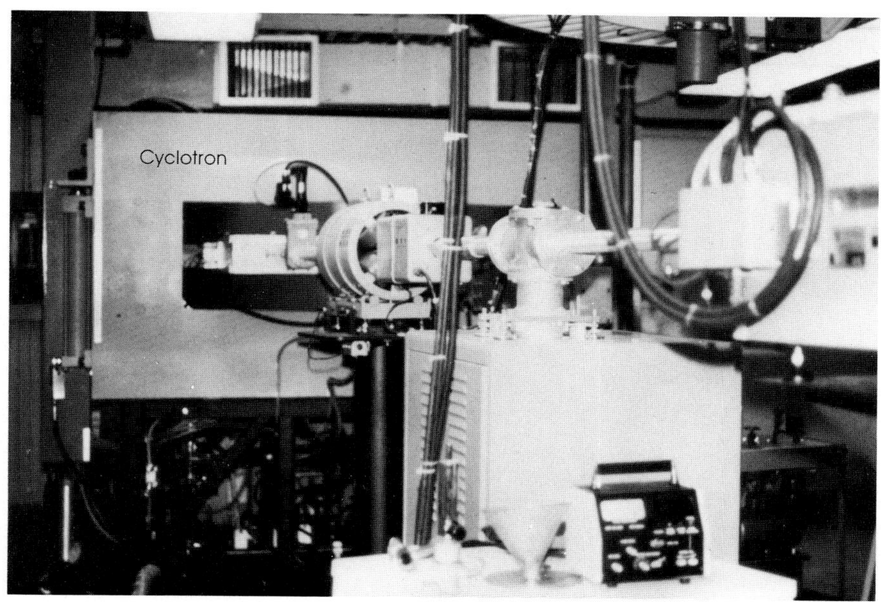

Fig. 40-8. Small cyclotron used for routine production of PET isotopes. The cyclotron is located in a concrete vault with 5-ft thick walls. Particles exit the cyclotron near the center of the figure and travel toward the right, all the while contained in a tube under high vacuum.

RADIOPHARMACEUTICAL PRODUCTION

Radiopharmaceuticals are synthesized from radionuclides derived from the target material. These agents may be very simple, as are the ^{15}O-^{16}O molecules described earlier, or they may be very complex.

There are two important radiopharmaceuticals presently used in many PET studies. Oxygen-15 water (^{15}O-H_2O) is produced continuously using the $^{14}N(d,n)^{15}O$ or $^{15}N(p,n)^{15}O$ nuclear reaction. This type of equation simply means that a deuteron beam irradiates a target of stable ^{14}N gas or a proton beam irradiates stable ^{15}N gas. A neutron is emitted by either reaction, leaving behind the ^{15}O radioactive atom. The radioactive oxygen quickly combines with a stable ^{16}O atom to form an oxygen molecule. The ^{15}O-^{16}O molecule is combusted over a platinum catalyst with small amounts of H_2 and N_2 gas. Radioactive water vapor is produced and cooled to yield a *specific activity* of 20 to 100 mCi/ml. A typical bolus injection of ^{15}O-H_2O is approximately 30 to 50 mCi in a volume of 1 to 2 ml. A dose of radioactive water can be prepared every 10 minutes. Radioactive ^{15}O-H_2O is used for determination of *local cerebral blood flow* (LCBF). A PET LCBF image and MRI image at the same slice of brain from the same subject are shown in Fig. 40-9.

The second major radiopharmaceutical used routinely in PET employs ^{18}F-^{19}F molecules to form a sugar analog called [^{18}F]-2-fluoro-2-deoxy-D-glucose or *^{18}F-FDG* for short. This agent is used to determine the *local cerebral metabolic rate of glucose* (LCMRG). Glucose, obtained from the foods we eat, is metabolized by the brain to provide the adenosine triphosphate (ATP) necessary for maintaining the membrane potential of the neurons within the brain. The metabolism of glucose is proportional to the neural activity of the brain and hence brain metabolism. Radioactive ^{18}F-FDG and glucose enter the same biochemical pathways in the brain. However, ^{18}F-FDG cannot be completely metabolized in the brain, as is glucose, because its metabolism is blocked at the level of fluoro-deoxyglucose-6-phosphate (^{18}FDG-6-PO_4). Because ^{18}F-FDG follows the glucose pathway into the brain, the concentration of ^{18}F-FDG-6-PO_4 within the cell is proportional to brain metabolism. These pathways for glucose and ^{18}F-FDG are schematically drawn in Fig. 40-10.

^{18}F-FDG is synthesized by combining the target gas (^{18}F-^{19}F) with 3,4,6-tri-O-acetyl-D-glucal (TAG). Hydrolyzing the result yields ^{18}F-FDG, which is purified with high-pressure liquid chromatography. A standard dose of 5 to 10 mCi in a few ml of isotonic saline is administered intravenously. The total time for target irradiation and radiochemistry preparation for each dose is approximately 1½ hours.

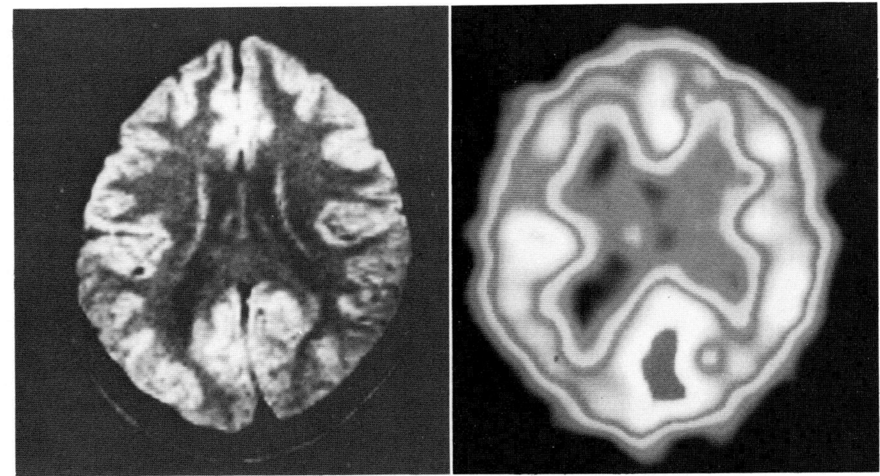

Fig. 40-9. MR image (left) and PET LCBF image (right) of the same normal, awake, 30-year-old male patient. Transverse images have the same slice thickness and are viewed from head to toe.

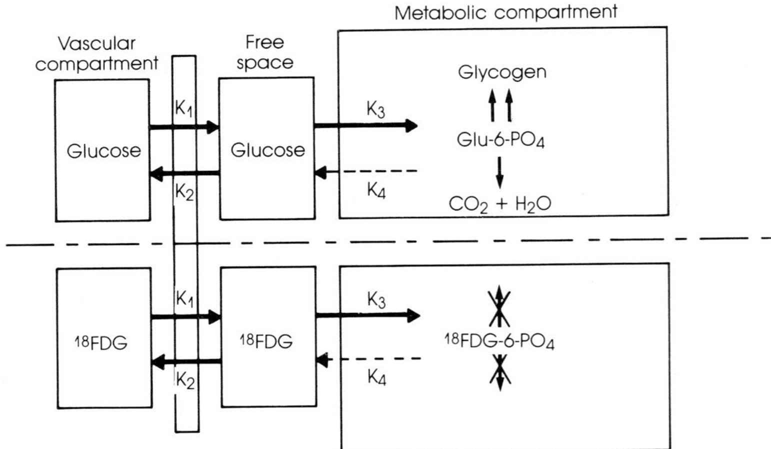

Fig. 40-10. Glucose compartmental model (above dashed line) versus ^{18}F-FDG model (below dashed line). Note that ^{18}F-FDG does not go to complete storage (glycogen) or metabolism (CO_2 + H_2O) as does glucose.

DATA ACQUISITION

The positron-electron annihilation photons are detected and counted with a PET scanner or tomograph as shown in Fig. 40-11. In general for neurologic PET scanners, the distance between detector faces is 70 cm. This is increased to 100 cm for whole body scanners. The field-of-view for these scanners is approximately 24 and 55 cm respectively. Typical scanners have between 400 and 500 detectors per ring. A detector module consists of scintillators organized into a matrix of small crystal cubes (4 × 4, 4 × 8, or 8 × 8 crystals/module). A light guide is used to couple the scintillator to the photomultiplier tubes. Individual tubes are no longer mated to single scintillator crystals but are arranged in an overlapping fashion similar to NaI crystals and PMTs in conventional gamma cameras. Coincidence count measures are obtained not only from detectors exactly opposite each other but also include activity from several detectors on either side of the opposite detector as shown in Fig. 40-12. Early scanners had only a single ring of detectors. Current tomographs are constructed of four to eight rings. Coincidence counts are not only collected for detector pairs within each ring (true-plane information), but data are also collected between adjacent rings (cross-plane information). Therefore seven to fifteen tomographic slices can be acquired simultaneously for four to eight ring tomographs. Fig. 40-13 shows the organization of rings. Dashed lines indicate the cross planes.

The *resolution* within the image plane for these scanners is approximately 5.5 mm FWHM (full width half maximum). Thus an image of a point source of radioactivity appears to be 5.5 mm wide at one-half the maximum intensity of the source image. The theoretical limit of resolution for PET tomographs is 1 to 2 mm and depends on the finite range of the positron in tissue for the particular radionuclide used. The resolution between tomographic planes or slices, that is, along the Z-axis, is about 6 mm.

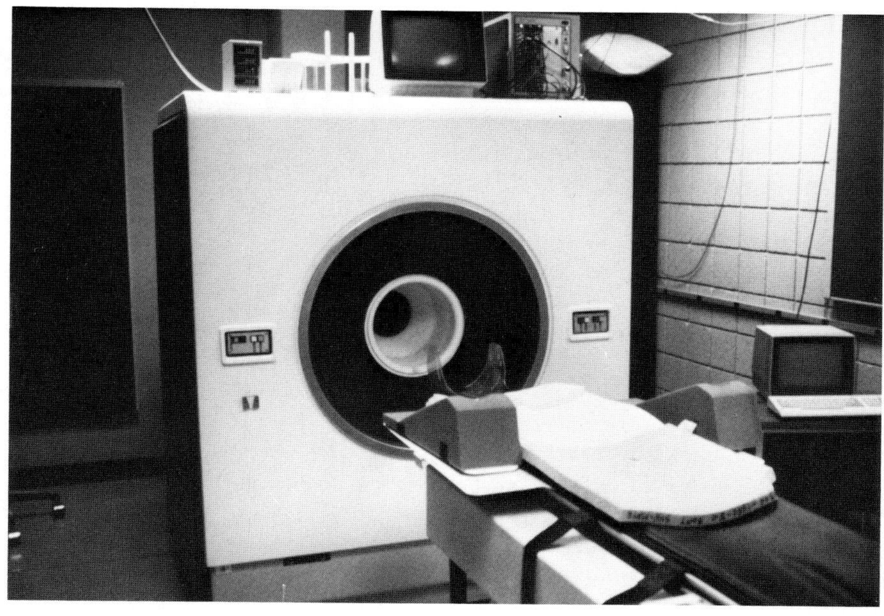

Fig. 40-11. Typical multi-ring neurologic PET scanner. Whole body scanners are similar to neurologic units but have a larger patient opening and more detectors. The bed travels through the patient opening to permit body scanning.

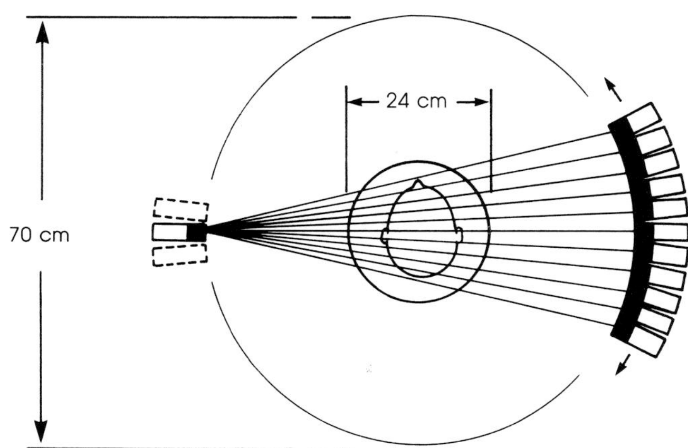

Fig. 40-12. Detector arrangement in neurologic PET ring. Coincidences from detector pairs are measured for each ray shown.

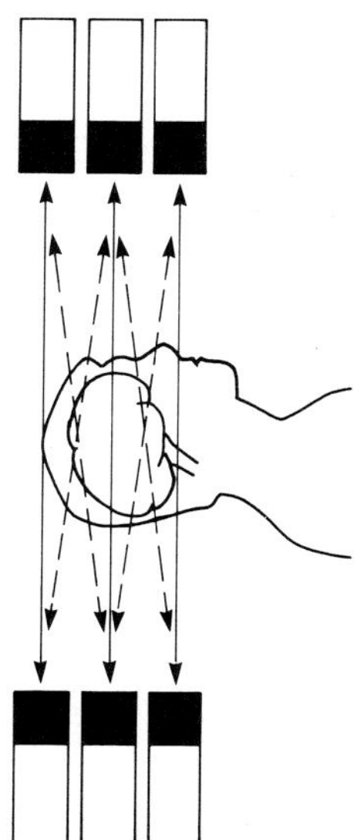

Fig. 40-13. An example of a multi-ring PET tomograph. Solid black squares indicate scintillator matrix. Photomultiplier tubes are attached to the rear of the scintillators. *Solid arrows* indicate true planes and *dashed arrows* depict cross planes.

Two techniques are used to improve image resolution. The first technique is to simply increase the number of detectors in each ring. To significantly increase the resolution, the number of detectors must be increased. On some devices now being constructed, over 800 detectors are being installed per ring. Of course, as the number of detectors in the tomograph increases, so does the complexity of acquiring and cataloging each annihilation event.

An alternate approach to improving resolution is to increase the number of effective detectors by simply rotating the detector array with respect to the patient. If we use the concept of a bicycle wheel as an example, one observes that the highest density of spokes is located at the hub. In the case of PET, *rays* between detectors correspond to the bicycle spokes. At the rim of the wheel, the density of spokes is reduced, and the number of detector rays is also reduced. That is why the field-of-view for these scanners is approximately one-third the distance from one detector face to another. Adequate ray density for the best resolution for image reconstruction is achieved only within this field of view (FOV).

If we take a picture of the wheel, then rotate the wheel a small amount (something less than an interspoke spacing) and take another picture as shown in Fig. 40-14, we can overlay the two pictures and observe that the total spoke density has increased by a factor of two. If we proceed to do this many times until the original interspoke spacing has been divided up into approximately four to eight equal parts, we now have a technique for increasing the total number of detector rays in a ring without actually increasing the number of detectors. From an engineering standpoint, rotating a detector array with high voltage and signal cables for 500 or more detectors creates a problem. The solution to this problem is achieved by *wobbling* the detectors continuously with an eccentricity of approximately 1 cm. This produces the equivalent detector motion as did the simple rotation scheme if viewed from any detector while looking directly toward its opposite detector. This is shown on the right in Fig. 40-14. The time required to complete one wobble cycle varies between scanners. A typical wobble time is 1 second.

Not all photons emitted from the patient can be detected. Some of the pairs of 0.511 meV photons from the positron annihilation impinge on detectors in the tomograph ring and are detected; most do not. Recall that the photon pairs are emitted 180 degrees from each other. The emission process is isotropic, which means that the gamma rays are emitted with equal probability in all directions so that only a small fraction (10%) of the total number of photons emitted from the patient actually strike the tomograph detectors as shown in Fig. 40-15.

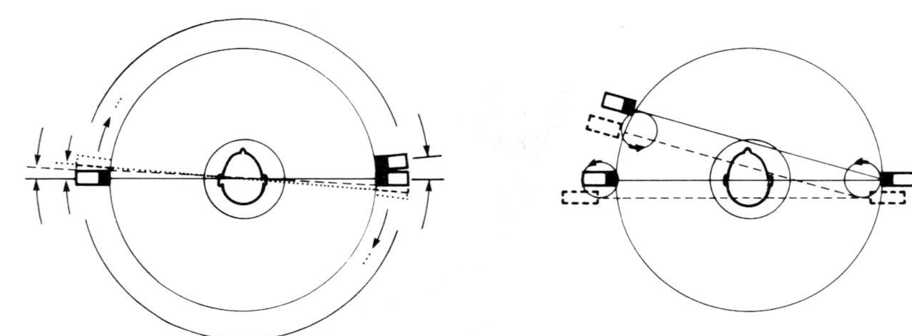

Fig. 40-14. Rotation of entire detector ring for improved resolution (left) versus wobble motion as an equivalent but more practical design (right).

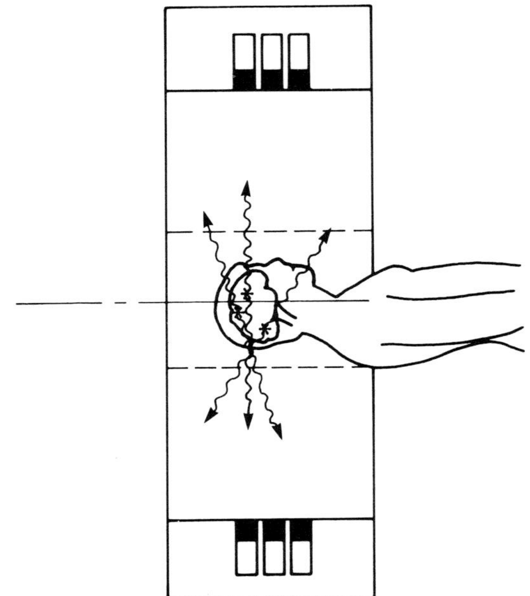

Fig. 40-15. Only 10% of the total number of emitted photons from the patient can be detected in a whole body tomograph. This is increased to 17% in a neurologic unit if Z-axis coverage is 10 cm and ring diameters are 100 cm and 60 cm respectively.

When pairs of photons are detected, they are counted as valid events, i.e., true positron annihilation, if and only if they appear at the detectors within the resolving time for the coincidence electronics. For many PET tomographs, this is typically 8 to 12 ns. If one photon is detected and no other photon is observed during that time window, the original event is discarded. This is essentially electronic collimation, hence, no lead collimators are used in PET scanners. These detector systems must also be able to handle very high count rates with minimal deadtime losses.

A raw data set, which is not yet a PET image, may be acquired in one wobble cycle for the highest temporal sampling of the tracer kinetics or may be integrated for many wobble cycles to improve statistics.

For PET procedures, data acquisition is not limited to just the tomographic count rates. To create parametric images of glucose metabolism, for example, the arterial blood concentrations of the radiopharmaceutical must be measured. This is accomplished by obtaining discrete samples of blood from an indwelling radial artery catheter and counting a known volume of plasma from each sample in a gamma well counter. A typical set of curves is given in Fig. 40-16. The curve created from the plasma data, as well as other blood data, is supplied to a mathematical model from which the parametric or functional image is created.

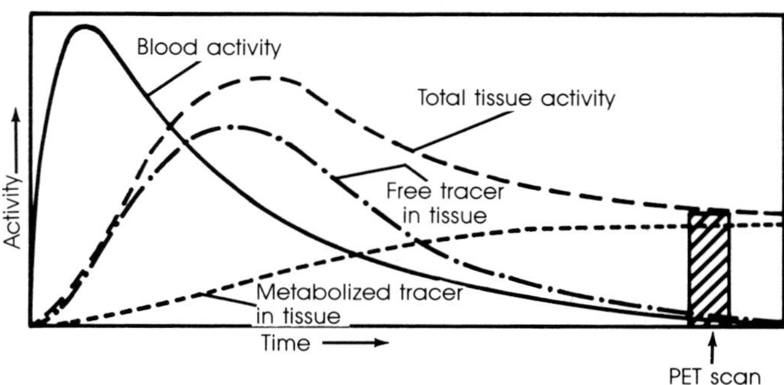

Fig. 40-16. Decay-corrected radioactivity curves for ^{18}F-FDG in brain tissue and blood (plasma).

IMAGE RECONSTRUCTION AND IMAGE PROCESSING

Images are created from the raw data collected as rays corresponding to each detected annihilation event. Typical images have 128 or 256 picture elements or pixels on a side. For brain studies, 30 slices of brain separated by approximately 0.5 cm adequately sample the entire volume of the brain from the top of the cerebral cortex to the base of the cerebellum. Array processors are used to perform the filtered backprojection reconstruction, a technique similar to that employed for CT image reconstruction.

Each image must have several corrections applied before being put into the physiologic model. Because short-lived radiotracers are used, all data are half-life corrected to the time of injection.

The disintegration of radionuclides follows Poisson statistics. As a result of this random process, photons from the different annihilation events may strike the tomograph detectors simultaneously. This is registered as a true event because it occurs within the coincidence time window. A simple approximation allows for the subtraction of the random events after image acquisition and is based on the individual count rates for each detector and the coincidence resolving time (8 to 12 ns) of the tomograph electronics.

Photons traversing biologic tissues undergo absorption and scatter. An attenuation correction is applied to account for those photons that should have been detected but were not, as shown in Fig. 40-17. The correction is based on a transmission study acquired with a radioactive ring source that circumscribes the patient's head. Another attenuation correction technique that is less accurate is to approximate the skull with an ellipse that closely resembles the dimensions of the cross-sectional brain slice. The actual attenuation coefficient for tissue is 0.096 cm^2/gm. An effective coefficient of 0.085 cm^2/gm is used as a first order scatter correction and attenuation correction coefficient. The coincidence data for each plane are multiplied by a matrix of numerical values within the boundary of the ellipse to correct the observed count rates to the true count rates for losses that result from attenuation.

A wobble correction is applied to an image if a wobbled study was performed because each detector spends more time sampling the radioactivity distribution near the ends of its oscillatory excursion than when the detectors are traveling at their highest velocity near the middle of the wobble motion.

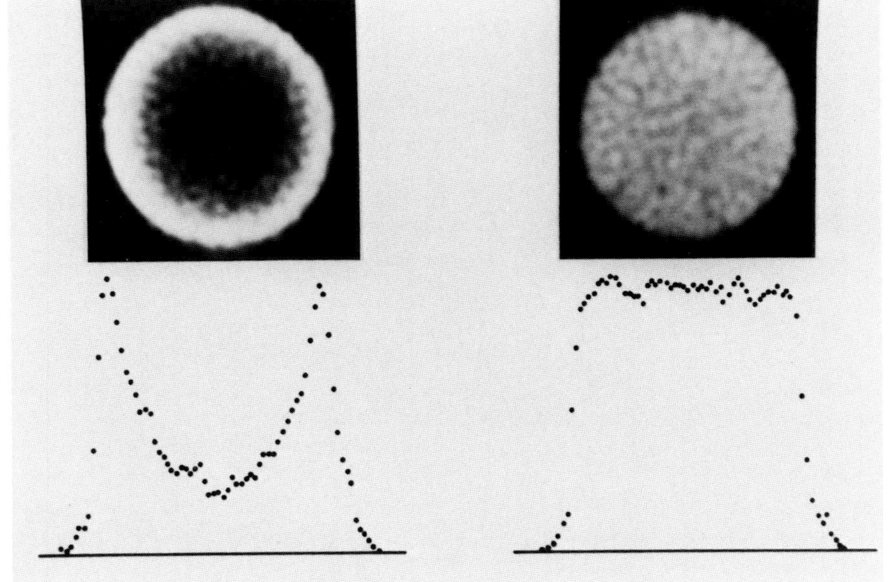

Fig. 40-17. Uncorrected image of a phantom homogeneously filled with a water-soluble PET nuclide (left) versus an attenuation-corrected image (right). Cross-sectional cuts through the center of each image are shown in the lower panels.

Count rates from the detectors are also corrected for deadtime losses. At high-count rates the detector electronics cannot process every event; therefore some of these events are lost. By measuring the tomograph response to known input count rates, empirical formulations for the losses are determined and applied to the image data.

Not every detector in the system responds exactly the same way to a uniform distribution of radioactivity. A calibration scan is performed to measure the count rate for each detector in the system from a homogenous source. A correction mask is created from this calibration scan and the raw data are multiplied by this mask to yield a uniform count-rate image from the homogenous (flood) source. This correction is then applied to all PET images.

Finally, the corrected images and the blood data are used as input to the physiologic model to create a parametric image. Each pixel in the parametric image represents a physiologic value for that volume of brain tissue. As an example, recall that a ^{18}F-FDG image represents local glucose metabolism of the brain (LCMRG). The pixel will contain a number between 0.0 and approximately 6 mg of glucose utilization per minute per 100 gm of brain tissue. For LCBF, each pixel represents blood flow in that particular volume of brain and possesses a value between 0.0 and 100 ml of blood flow per minute per 100 grams of brain tissue.

Once the raw data are converted to functional images, *regions of interest* (ROI) are drawn on the brain images. Average LCBF or LCMRG values are determined for each ROI. The data analysis task then is to correlate the physiologic value obtained from the PET image data of the patient to normative data. Intrinsically, biologic parameters have approximately a 15% standard deviation. To observe a true intersubject difference, variations in LCBF and LCMRG values must be greater than 15%. Intrasubject variability from PET studies has been shown to be about 7%. Therefore if a research or clinical protocol can be designed so that the patient serves as his or her own control, greater reliability and reduced errors are achieved.

Clinical Studies

It is necessary that patients and normal volunteers be selected according to very stringent protocols. Before each imaging procedure, all subjects receive a brief physical examination and laboratory blood tests. External landmarks (head diameter and distance from the top of the head to an imaginary line passing from the lateral canthus of the eye to the meatus of the ear, or *CM line* for brain studies) are measured. A radial artery is catheterized to obtain arterial blood samples that are used as input functions for the physiologic models. Patients are then positioned in the scanner in the supine position.

An intravenous bolus injection of the appropriate radiopharmaceutical is synchronized with the start of imaging. Arterial blood samples are collected according to the type of study being performed. For ^{18}F-FDG studies, a decay-corrected plasma activity curve is constructed. For $^{15}O\text{-}H_2O$ studies, arterial samples are continuously withdrawn at a rate of 5 to 7 ml per minute for 2 minutes with a peristaltic pump. Radioactivity detectors measure the whole blood $^{15}O\text{-}H_2O$ concentration while the blood is being withdrawn.

^{18}F-FDG studies require a 40-minute incorporation period after which 10- to 15-minute scans are acquired to measure the almost static distribution of ^{18}F-FDG glucose metabolism in tissue. The scanning procedure including incorporation takes about 1½ to 2 hours for a single injection of ^{18}F-FDG.

For $^{15}O\text{-}H_2O$ LCBF studies, a separate injection is necessary for each set of brain slices. This requires three to four injections to obtain the 30 or so brain images that encompass the entire brain volume. A scanning procedure only takes 40 seconds to 4 minutes for the blood flow studies. From one injection to the next, a total of 15 minutes are required for the ^{15}O radioactivity to reach low enough levels to repeat the study.

After the scanning procedures, the arterial catheter is removed and the patients are permitted to leave the facility.

NORMAL SUBJECTS

Normal volunteers studied using PET provide a database of normal LCMRG and LCBF values for comparison with patient data. Table 40-5 depicts local cerebral glucose metabolic rates for seven normal subjects. Three primary areas of brain LCMRG are presented. The first area is associated with control and coordination of voluntary muscle movements (cerebellum), the second reflects the intact gray matter cortical regions (temporal cortex), which may be related to such functions as memory and fine motor movements, and the last region is responsible for decoding visual images (primary visual cortex). In virtually all cases the visual cortex depicts the highest glucose utilization rates and the cerebellum the lowest metabolic rates. The hemispheric averages do not differ significantly from each other nor do they differ from the cerebellar values.

Table 40-5. LCMRG rates in normal test subjects (mg glucose utilization per minute per 100 gm tissue)

	Cerebellum	Temporal cortex	Visual cortex	Left hemisphere	Right hemisphere	Whole brain
Mean (7)	4.65	5.12	6.56	4.58	4.54	4.59
Standard deviation	0.53	1.17	0.97	0.87	0.83	0.85
Coefficient of variation	11.5%	22.9%	14.8%	19.0%	18.1%	18.5%

Future Studies

Considerable research has been conducted to study brain function with radiopharmaceuticals to measure metabolism, flow, and receptor density. PET scanners have been specifically designed to optimally acquire data from the brain. Whole body scanners have been developed primarily to study the heart. As the technology matures, greater emphasis will be placed on clinical and research investigation of heart, lung, liver, tumor, and organ transplant imaging with PET.

Summary

PET is a very complex diagnostic imaging procedure. Consequently, it is both a clinical and a research tool. It involves the multidisciplinary support of the physician, physicist, physiologist, chemist, engineer, and technologist. PET permits the investigator to peer into the working human brain organ system to examine numerous biologic parameters without disturbing the normal equilibrium physiology. It measures regional function that cannot be determined by any other means including CT and MRI imaging. Current PET studies involve PET imaging of patients with epilepsy, Huntington's disease, stroke, brain tumors, Alzheimer's disease, and other disorders of the brain. PET studies of the heart are providing routine diagnostic information on patients with coronary artery disease. Our understanding of physiology will increase as the technology advances, yielding higher resolution instruments, new radiopharmaceuticals, and improved analysis of PET data.

Definition of Terms

analog A PET radiopharmaceutical biochemically equivalent to a naturally occurring compound in the body.

annihilation The total transformation of matter into energy. Occurs after the antimatter positron collides with an electron. Two photons are created; each equals the rest mass of the individual particles.

attenuation coefficient A number that represents the statistical reduction in photons that exit a material (N) from the value that entered (N_o) the material. The reduced flux is the result of scatter and absorption, which can be expressed in the following equation: $N = N_o e^{-\mu x}$ where μ is the attenuation coefficient and χ is the distance traversed by the photons.

beta decay Type of radioactive decay in which the nucleus emits a beta particle (electron) or positron.

CM line Canthomeatal line defined by an imaginary line drawn between the lateral canthus of the eye and meatus of the ear.

cyclotron Cyclic particle accelerator used to increase the kinetic energy of nuclei such as protons and deuterons so that radioactive materials may be produced from the resultant nuclear reactions of the ions on stable materials.

detector A device that is a combination of a scintillator and photomultiplier tube. It is used to detect x rays and gamma rays.

^{18}F-FDG Radioactive analog of naturally available glucose. It follows the same biochemical pathways as glucose but is not totally metabolized to CO_2 and H_2O as is glucose.

gamma ray Electromagnetic radiation or photon emitted from the decay of a radioactive nucleus. Its energy is expressed in the equivalent energy of the photon in units of electron volts (eV) or millions of electron volts (meV).

gliosis Proliferation of stromal tissue in the central nervous system.

homeostasis State of equilibrium of the body's internal environment.

kinetics The movement of materials into, out of, and through biologic spaces. A mathematic expression is often used to describe and quantify the substances traversing membranes or participating in biochemical reactions.

local cerebral blood flow (LCBF) Description of the parametric image of blood flow through the brain. It is expressed in units of ml blood flow per minute per 100 gm brain tissue.

local cerebral metabolic rate of glucose utilization (LCMRG) Used in conjunction with parametric images of the brain and expressed in units of mg glucose utilization per minute per 100 gm brain tissue.

magnetic resonance imaging (MRI) A term used to describe the technique of nuclear magnetic resonance (NMR) as it is applied to medical imaging. Also abbreviated MR.

parametric image An image that relates anatomic position (the x,y position on an image) to a determination of a physiologic parameter (image intensity or color). It may also be referred to as a functional image.

photomultiplier tube (PMT) Vacuum tube that transforms visible light photons into minute electron currents that are subsequently amplified by a factor of approximately 10^6. Typically the output current is proportional to the energy of the incident photon.

positron Positively charged particle emitted from neutron-deficient radioactive nuclei.

positron emission tomography (PET) Imaging technique that creates transaxial images of organ physiology from the simultaneous detection of positron annihilation photons.

radioisotope Synonym for radioactive isotope. Any isotope that is unstable undergoes decay with the emission of characteristic radiation.

radiopharmaceutical Term used to describe a radioactive material that is inhaled, ingested, or injected into humans or animals. Synonymous with radiotracer.

radiotracer Synonym of radiopharmaceutical.

ray The imaginary line drawn between a pair of detectors in the PET scanner or between the x-ray source and detector in a CT scanner.

region of interest (ROI) An area that circumscribes a desired anatomic location on a PET image. Image processing systems permit drawing of ROIs on images. The average parametric value is computed for all pixels within the ROI and retuned to the operator.

resolution Smallest separation of two point sources that can be distinguished.

SCA Single-channel analyzer used to determine the pulse height from an amplifier attached to a scintillator/PMT system.

scintillator Material either organic or inorganic that transforms high-energy photons such as x rays or gamma rays into visible or near visible light (UV) photons for easy measurement.

specific activity Activity of a radioactive agent per unit volume. Normally expressed in units of mCi/ml.

SPECT Single photon emission computed tomography. A nuclear medicine scanning procedure that measures conventional single photon gamma emissions (^{99m}Tc) with a specially designed rotating gamma camera.

target Device used to contain stable materials and subsequent radioactive materials during bombardment by high-energy nuclei from a cyclotron or other particle accelerator. The term is also applied to the material inside the device, which may be solid, liquid, or gaseous.

wobble Eccentric rotation that permits increased resolution of tomographic imaging devices composed of discrete detector systems. Typical eccentric excursions are only 1 to 2 cm.

SELECTED BIBLIOGRAPHY

Barnes WE, editor: Basic physics of radiotracers, vols I and II, Boca Raton, Fla, 1983, CRC Press, Inc.

Bergstrom M et al: Correction for scattered radiation in a ring detector positron camera by integral transformation of the projections, J Comput Assist Tomogr 7:42-50, 1983.

Burns HD et al: (3-N-[^{11}C] Methyl) Spiperone, a ligand binding to dopamine receptors: radiochemical synthesis and biodistribution studies in mice, J Nucl Med 25:1222-1227, 1984.

Clark JC et al: Short-lived radioactive gases for clinical use, Boston, 1975, Butterworth Publishers.

Frackowiak RSJ et al: Quantitative measurement of cerebral blood flow and oxygen metabolism in man using ^{15}O and positron emission tomography: theory, procedure and normal values, J Comput Assist Tomogr 4:727-736, 1980.

Freedman GS, editor: Tomographic imaging in nuclear medicine, New York, 1973, The Society of Nuclear Medicine, Inc.

Heiss WD et al: Regional kinetic constants and cerebral metabolic rate for glucose in normal human volunteers determined by dynamic positron emission tomography of [^{18}F]-2-fluoro-2-deoxy-D-glucose, J Cereb Blood Flow Metab 4:212-223, 1984.

Helus F, editor: Radionuclides production, vols I and II, Boca Raton, Fla, 1983, CRC Press, Inc.

Hendee WR: The physical principles of computed tomography, Boston, 1983, Little, Brown & Co.

Herman TG, editor: Image reconstruction from projections—implementation and applications, New York, 1979, Springer-Verlag New York, Inc.

Hoffman EJ et al: Quantitation in positron emission computed tomography: 1. Effect of object size, J Comput Assist Tomogr 3:299-308, 1979.

Livingood JJ: Principles of cyclic particle accelerators, Princeton, NJ, 1961, D Van Nostrand Company, Inc.

Mazziotta JC et al: Tomographic mapping of human cerebral metabolism: normal unstimulated state, Neurology 31:503-516, 1981.

Minton MA et al: Brain oxygen utilization measured with 0-15 radiotracers and positron emission tomography, J Nucl Med 25:177-187, 1984.

Phelps ME et al: Tomographic measurements of local cerebral glucose metabolic rate in humans with (F-18)-2-fluoro-2-deoxy-D-glucose: validation of method, Ann Neurol 6:371-388, 1979.

Reivich M et al: The [^{18}F]Fluorodeoxyglucose method for the measurement of local cerebral glucose utilization in man, Circ Res 44:127-137, 1979.

Riggs DS: The mathematical approach to physiological problems, Cambridge, Mass, 1963, Williams & Wilkins.

Robertson JS, editor: Compartmental distribution of radiotracers, Boca Raton, Fla, 1983, CRC Press, Inc.

Schelbert HR et al: Regional myocardial perfusion assessed with N-13 labeled ammonia and positron emission computerized axial tomography, Am J Cardiol 43:209-218, 1979.

Sokoloff L et al: The ^{14}C-deoxyglucose method for the measurement of local cerebral glucose utilization: theory, procedure and normal values in conscious and anesthetized albino rats, J Neurochem 28:897-916, 1977.

Chapter 41

RADIATION ONCOLOGY

CHARLES H. MARSCHKE

*Radiation oncology**, radiation therapy, or radiotherapy, involves the treatment of cancerous tumors or lesions by the precise application of ionizing radiation. The radiation is usually administered by a *radiation therapy technologist* under the direct supervision of a *radiation oncologist,* a physician skilled in the art of applying radiation in the treatment of malignant disease.

Different specialists are routinely consulted in virtually all cases involving selection of a best plan of treatment for the patient. The individuals often consulted are specialists in tumor growth, spread, and response to treatment. Other specialists are usually the surgical and medical oncologists. As the name implies, the surgical oncologist is a surgeon who deals primarily with cancer patients. The medical oncologist is usually a certified physician in internal medicine who has gained additional expertise in the application of chemical agents in the treatment of cancer.

This coordinated "team approach" to the diagnosis, care, and treatment of cancer patients is essential to ensure the best possible therapeutic results.

Although radiation oncology may be used as the only method of treatment for malignant disease, a more common approach is to use radiation oncology in conjunction with surgery, chemotherapy, or a combination of the two. Some patients may be treated by only surgery or chemotherapy; however, approximately 70% of all diagnosed cancer patients are treated with radiation. The choice of treatment involves consideration of a number of patient variables such as the patient's overall physical and emotional condition, the histologic type of the disease, and the extent and anatomic position of the tumor. If a tumor is small and its margins are well defined, a surgical approach alone may be prescribed. On the other hand, if the disease is systemic, a chemotherapeutic approach may be chosen. Most tumors, however, exhibit degrees of size, invasion, and spread and require variations in the treatment approach that in all likelihood will include radiation oncology as an adjunct to or in conjunction with surgery or chemotherapy. These limitations determine the goal of treatment—definitive, palliation, or as an adjunct to surgery.

Once the patient has been fully evaluated and radiation oncology chosen as the form of treatment, the optimum therapeutic approach must be determined. Options include *teletherapy* versus *brachytherapy,* single-field versus multifield irradiation, temporary or permanent implant, particulate versus nonparticulate irradiation, and *fractionated* versus *protracted* dose application. Whatever treatment approach or regimen is decided, a number of variables must be considered, and the opportunities for error are many. The radiation therapy technologist participates in this decision-making process and is responsible for administering and keeping accurate records of the dose and monitoring the patient's physical and emotional well-being once the patient has begun the treatment schedule. The therapy technologist should have an understanding of *oncology,* radiobiology, radiation physics, anatomy, mathematics, and methods of patient care.

This chapter provides an overview of some of the aforementioned subject areas to enable the reader to have a greater understanding of the therapeutic approach. A complete and effective treatment plan is dependent on precise patient evaluation and diagnosis, excellent patient care, and meticulous attention to the patient setup throughout the course of treatment. The bibliography includes a list of references for further study.

Historical Development

Historically, ionizing radiation was applied to obtain a radiographic image of an individual's internal anatomy for diagnostic purposes. The resulting image depended on many variables, including the energy of the beam, processing techniques, the material on which the image was recorded, and most importantly, the amount of energy absorbed by the various organs of the body. This transfer of energy from the beam of radiation to the biologic system and the observation of the effects of this interaction became the foundation of radiation oncology.

Two of the most obvious, and sometimes immediate, biologic effects observed during the early diagnostic procedures were loss of hair (epilation) and a reddening of the patient's skin (erythema). Epilation and erythema resulted primarily from the great amount of energy absorbed by the skin of the patient during the radiographic procedure. These short-term radiation-induced effects afforded radiographic practitioners an opportunity to expand the use of radiation to treat conditions ranging from relatively benign maladies such as hypertrichosis (excessive hair), acne, and boils to grotesque and malignant diseases such as lupus vulgaris and skin cancer.

The first reported application of ionizing radiation to a patient for the treatment of a more in-depth lesion was begun on January 29, 1896, by Dr. Émile H. Grubbé (Table 41-1). Dr. Grubbé is

Table 41-1. Time line of development of radiation therapy

Dates	Persons	Events
1895	W.C. Roentgen	Discovery of x rays
1896	É. Grubbé	First use of ionizing radiation in treatment of cancer
	A.H. Becquerel	Discovery of radioactive emissions by uranium compounds
1898	M. and P. Curie	Discovery of radium
1902	C.E. Skinner	First documented case of cancer "cure" using ionizing radiation
1906	J. Bergonié and L. Tribondeau	Postulation of first law of radiosensitivity
1932	E.O. Lawrence	Invention of cyclotron
1934	F. Joliot and I. Joliot-Curie	Production of artificial radioactivity
1939	E.O. Lawrence and R.S. Stone	Treatment of cancer patient with neutron beam from cyclotron
1940	D.W. Kerst	Construction of betatron
1951		Installation of first cobalt 60 teletherapy units
1952		Installation of first linear accelerator (Hammersmith Hospital, London)

*All italicized words are defined at the end of this chapter.

reported to have irradiated for therapeutic purposes a woman with carcinoma of the left breast. This event occurred only 3 months after the discovery of x rays in November 1895 by Dr. W.C. Roentgen. Although Dr. Grubbé neither expected nor observed any dramatic results from irradiation of the patient, the event is significant simply because it occurred.

The first reported case of a patient being treated with ionizing radiation and considered to have been *cured* was performed by Dr. Clarence E. Skinner of New Haven, Connecticut, in January 1902. Dr. Skinner treated a woman who had a diagnosed malignant fibrosarcoma. During the next 2 years and 3 months the woman received a total of 136 applications of the x rays. In April 1909, 7 years after the initial application of the radiation, the woman was free of disease and considered to be "cured."

As more and more data were collected, the interest in radiation therapy grew. More sophisticated equipment, a greater understanding of the effects of ionizing radiation, an appreciation for time-dose relationships, and a number of other related medical breakthroughs gave impetus to the interest in radiation therapy that led to its evolution to a medical specialty.

Theory

The biologic effectiveness of ionizing radiation in living tissue is dependent partially on the amount of energy that is deposited within the tissue and partially on the condition of the biologic system. The terms used to describe this relationship are "linear energy transfer" (LET) and "relative biologic effectiveness" (RBE).

LET values are expressed in thousands of electron volts deposited per micron of tissue (keV/μm) and will vary, of course, depending on the type of radiation being considered. Particles, because of their mass and possible charge, tend to interact more readily with the material through which they are passing and therefore have a greater LET value. As an example, a 5-meV alpha particle has a LET value of 100 keV/μm in tissue. Nonparticulate radiations such as 250-kVp x rays and 1.2-meV gamma rays have much lower LET values: 1.5 and 0.3 respectively.

RBE values are determined by calculating the ratio of the dose from a standard beam of radiation to the dose required of the radiation beam in question to produce a similar biologic effect. The standard beam of radiation is usually 200- or 250-kV x rays, and the ratio is set up as follows:

$$\text{RBE} = \frac{\text{Standard beam dose to obtain effect}}{\text{Similar effect using beam in question}}$$

Table 41-2. RBE and LET values for certain forms of radiation

Radiation	RBE	LET
250-keV x rays	1.0	1.5
^{60}Co gamma rays	0.85	0.3
14-meV neurons	12.0	75.0
5-meV alpha particles	20.0	100.0

It is now accepted that, as the LET increases, so too will the RBE. Some RBE and LET values are listed in Table 41-2.

The effectiveness of ionizing radiation on a biologic system depends not only on the amount of radiation deposited but also on the state of the biologic system. One of the first laws of radiation biology, postulated by Bergonié and Tribondeau, stated in essence that the *radiosensitivity* of a tissue is dependent on the number of *undifferentiated* cells in the tissue, the degree of mitotic activity of the tissue, and the length of time that cells of the tissue remain in active proliferation. Although exceptions exist, the preceding is true in most tissues. The primary target of ionizing radiation is the DNA molecule, and the human cell is most radiosensitive during mitosis. Thus each group of cells or tissues may respond directly, relative to its radiosensitivity, depending on the aforementioned factors.

Because tissue cells comprise primarily water, most of the ionizing interactions occur with water molecules. These events are called indirect effects and result in the formation of free radicals such as OH·, H·, and HO_2·. These highly reactive free radicals may recombine, resulting in no biologic effect whatsoever, or they may combine with other atoms and molecules to produce biochemical changes that may be deleterious to the cell. The possibility also exists that the radiation may interact with an organic molecule or atom, which may result in the inactivation of the cell; this reaction is called the direct effect. Because ionizing radiation is nonspecific—i.e., it will interact with normal cells as readily as with tumor cells—it is obvious that cellular damage will occur in both normal and abnormal tissue. The deleterious effects, however, will be greater in the abnormal cells because a greater percentage of the abnormal cells are undergoing mitosis; they also tend to be more poorly differentiated. In addition, normal cells have a greater capability for repairing sublethal damage than do tumor cells. Because of these reasons, greater cell damage will occur to abnormal than to normal cells for any given increment of dose. The effects of the interactions in either normal or tumor cells may be expressed in a number of ways:

1. Loss of reproductive ability
2. Metabolic changes
3. Cell transformation
4. Acceleration of the aging process
5. Cell mutation

Certainly the greater the number of interactions that occur, the greater the possibility of cell death.

The preceding information leads to a categorization of tumors according to their radiosensitivity:

1. Very radiosensitive
   a. Gonadal germ cell tumors (seminoma of testis, dysgerminoma of ovary)
   b. Lymphoproliferative tumors (Hodgkin's disease, lymphoma)
   c. Embryonal tumors (Wilms' tumor of kidney, retinoblastoma)
2. Moderately radiosensitive
   a. Epithelial tumors (squamous and basal cell carcinomas of skin)
   b. Glandular tumors (adenocarcinoma of prostate)
3. Relatively radioresistant
   a. Mesenchymal tumors (sarcomas of bone, connective tissue, and muscle)
   b. Nerve tumors (glioma, melanoma)

Although many of the concepts originating in the laboratory have little practical application, they are beginning to influence the selection of treatment modalities and techniques of radiation oncology. The physician's understanding of cellular function and the effects of radiation on the cell have initiated research and interest in using drugs, or simply oxygen, to enhance the effectiveness of the radiation.

CANCER

Cancer has yet to be precisely defined; however, a number of attempts, such as the following, have been made:

1. Cells in which the normal growth-controlling mechanism is altered, permitting progressive growth
2. A group of diseases of unknown causes that occur in all human and animal populations and arise in all tissues that are composed of potentially dividing cells
3. A disease of tissue organization
4. A genetic disease of somatic cells resulting from a mutation of a previously normal cell into a new cell of enduring malignancy
5. So-called spontaneous autoaggressive disease of a tissue initiated by random gene mutation in a stem cell

Although the number of definitions may indicate confusion, some basic facts are known about cancer:

1. Cancers can arise from cells that have the ability to proliferate.
2. Tumor cells may mature inadequately and may be spoken of as *"anaplastic"* or "dedifferentiated."
3. Cancers may arise after a variety of stimuli (chemical, physical, or viral) but usually only after a prolonged latent period.
4. Cancer cells may lie dormant for prolonged periods.
5. No distinctive ultrastructural or biochemical difference between a cancer and a normal cell has been positively identified.
6. A few cancers regress spontaneously.

In addition to the preceding definitions and facts, more than 300 types of cancers have been recognized and defined histologically, and the degrees of variation within a single tumor type can be infinite. Finally, the physiologic, immunologic, and indeed the entire physical condition of the host will play an important part in the prevention or development of a cancer.

Malignant tumors, or cancers, are cells that have been influenced by a *carcinogen* to produce abnormal and uncontrolled growth. If the tumor is allowed to progress untreated, it will most likely result in the death of the host. The growth or spread of a malignant tumor is accomplished by invasion of the tumor into adjacent tissue, permeation of cancer cells into the blood or lymph vessels, and *metastasis*. The size of the tumor, its depth of penetration, whether it has invaded the lumina of the blood of lymph vessels, and whether it has metastasized determine the curability of the cancer.

Although cancers may arise in any human tissue, they are usually categorized under six general headings according to their tissue or origin as in the following examples:

Tissue of origin	Type of tumor
Epithelium	
Surface epithelium	Carcinoma
Glandular epithelium	Adenocarcinoma
Connective tissue	
Bone	Osteosarcoma
Fat	Liposarcoma
Hematopoietic tissue	
Plasma cells	Multiple myeloma
Erythrocytic tissue	Erythroleukemia
Nerve tissue	
Glial tissue	Glioma
Neuroectoderm	Neuroblastoma
Tumors of more than one tissue	
Embryonic kidney	Nephroblastoma
Tumors that do not fit into above categories	
Testis	Seminoma
Thymus	Thymoma

Table 41-3. Application of the TNM classification system*

Classification	Description of tumor
$T_0N_0M_0$	Occult lesion; no evidence clinically
$T_1N_0M_0$	Small lesion confined to organ of origin with no evidence of vascular and lymphatic spread or metastasis
$T_2N_1M_0$	Tumor of less than 5 cm invading surrounding tissue and first-station lymph nodes but no evidence of metastasis
$T_3N_2M_0$	Extensive lesion greater than 5 cm with fixation to deeper structure and with bone and lymph invasion but no evidence of metastasis
$T_4N_3M_+$	More extensive lesion than above with distant metastasis

*Although variations of the TNM classification system exist, the general description of the tumor does not change, that is, a T_1 lesion is confined to the organ of origin regardless of whether it is 0.5 or 1.5 cm in diameter.

To facilitate the exchange of patient information from one physician to another, a system of classifying tumors based on anatomic and histologic considerations was designed by the International Union Against Cancer (UICC) and the American Joint Committee for the Cancer Staging and End Results Reporting (AJC). The system designed was the "TNM" classification (Table 41-3), which describes a tumor according to (1) the size of the primary lesion, (2) the involvement of the regional lymph nodes, and (3) occurrence of metastasis.

Because of the various types of tumors, their sizes, the degree of spread, and symptoms exhibited by the patient, a number of classification and staging techniques are available. All have been designed to assist in describing the extent of the tumor for the purpose of treatment and prognosis.

Effective treatment of a malignant tumor with ionizing radiation depends on (1) the extent of the disease at diagnosis, (2) the histologic type of the tumor, (3) the general well-being of the patient, (4) the location of the tumor, and (5) whether the tumor is *radiocurable*. The first three concerns have been dealt with briefly in this chapter; the last two, however, will be expanded before discussion of treatment planning.

To treat a tumor definitively requires that the tumor be located in a tissue that is more radioresistant than the tumor itself. The therapeutic ratio (TR) was designed to assist in the determination of whether a tumor could be treated for cure, taking into account the normal tissue tolerance dose and the tumor lethal dose:

$$TR = \frac{\text{Normal tissue tolerance dose}}{\text{Tumor tissue lethal dose}}$$

If the TR is less than 1, the chances of cure are much less likely than if the TR is greater than 1.

A tumor must have some degree of radiosensitivity to be considered for radiation treatment; however, radiosensitivity does not necessarily imply radiocurability. The characteristics that make a tumor radiosensitive, for example, fast growth and vascularity, also cause it to spread more rapidly giving rise to a more extensive lesion (e.g., lymphosarcoma). This situation tends to compromise the treatment approach. Conversely some tumors that have been classified as radioresistant, for instance, carcinoma of the tongue, may be considered radiocurable.

BASIC PHYSICS

As stated earlier, the effectiveness of radiation oncology is partially dependent on the amount of energy that is deposited within the *tumor volume* while at the same time minimizing the amount of energy deposited in the normal surrounding tissue. If available, a beam of radiation with high LET and resulting RBE values, as well as the ability to deliver a cancericidal dose to only the lesion no matter what its anatomic depth, would be appropriate to use. Although beams of this nature are not available at present, research is being conducted in this area of radiation physics. Until the ideal beam can be produced and supplied for therapeutic purposes, currently available beams must be applied so that a cancercidal dose can be deposited to the lesion with a limited amount of damage to the surrounding normal tissue.

Most radiation oncology departments have available some or all of the following teletherapy units, the dose depositions of which are compared in Fig. 41-1.:

1. 120 keV superficial x-ray unit for treating lesions on or very near the surface of the patient.
2. 250 keV orthovoltage x-ray unit for more in-depth tumors
3. 4 to 35 meV linear *accelerator* or *betatron* to serve as a source of high-energy, or supervoltage, electrons and x rays
4. Cobalt 60 *gamma ray* source with an average energy of 1.25 meV

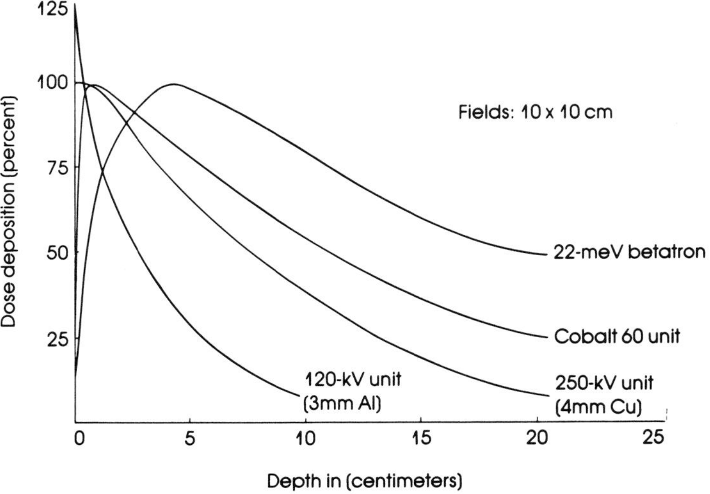

Fig. 41-1. Plot of percent depth of dose deposition versus depth in centimeters of tissue for various energies of photon beams.

Theory

Nonparticulate irradiations

The penetrability, or energy, of an x or gamma ray is totally dependent on its wavelength: the shorter the wavelength, the more penetrating the photon, and conversely the longer the wavelength, the less penetrating the photon. A low-energy beam (120 keV or less) of radiation tends to deposit all or most of its energy on or near the surface of the patient and thus is suitable for lesions on or near the skin surface. In addition, with the low-energy beam a greater amount of absorption or dose deposition takes place in bone than in soft tissue.

A high-energy beam of radiation (1 meV or greater) tends to deposit its energy throughout the entire volume of tissue irradiated, with a greater amount of dose deposition occurring at or near the entry port than at the exit port. In this energy range the dose is deposited equally in soft tissue and bone. The high-energy, or super-voltage, beam is most suitable for in-depth tumors.

The *skin-sparing* effect, a phenomenon that occurs as the energy of a beam of radiation is increased, is of value from a therapeutic standpoint. In the superficial and orthovoltage energy range the maximum dose occurs on the surface of the patient, with decreasing deposition of dose as the beam traverses the patient. As the energy of the beam increases into the supervoltage range, the maximum dose absorbed by the patient occurs at some point below the skin surface. The skin-sparing effect is of importance clinically because the skin is a radiosensitive organ and excessive dose deposition to the skin may compromise the treatment dose to a tumor that is at some depth within the patient. The greater the energy of the beam, the more in-depth the maximum dose will occur (see Fig. 41-2).

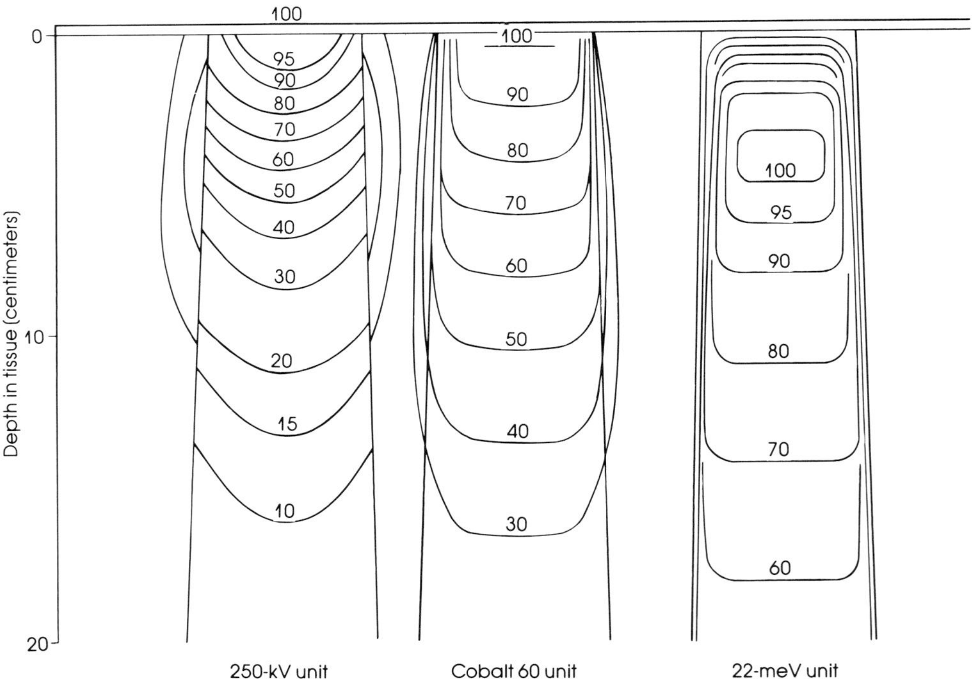

Fig. 41-2. Three isodose curves showing comparison of percent dose deposition from three x-ray units of different energies. As energy of beam is increased, percentage of dose deposited on surface of patient decreases.

Particulate irradiations

Particles in motion have kinetic energy; the greater their speed, the more kinetic energy they have, resulting in increased penetrability of the material irradiated. Once the particles have expended their kinetic energy and are no longer capable of *ionization,* they essentially cease to exist from a therapeutic standpoint.

Alpha particles (+2 charge and relatively large mass), when set in motion, have a large LET value but are virtually nonpenetrating and are essentially useless as a therapeutic tool. Moreover, they are a nuisance from a radiation protection standpoint.

Electron beam therapy, on the other hand, has become commonplace in most radiation oncology departments. Obtaining a beam of high-energy electrons involves removal of the transmission target from the path of the accelerated electrons, which are used for the production of x rays in the linear accelerators and betatrons. The usefulness of high-energy electrons is their deposition of energy within a given depth of tissue dependent on their kinetic energy (in million electron volts) and not any deeper. The general rule for determining the depth of tumor placement and depth of penetration in centimeters of a given beam of electrons is to divide the number of million electron volts of the beam by 3 and 2 respectively. For example, an 18 meV beam would be chosen for a tumor located 6 cm in depth (18 ÷ 3), and the resulting total depth of penetration of the beam would be 9 cm (18 ÷ 2). This phenomenon of the electrons depositing their energy within a given depth of tissue and no deeper allows the therapist to irradiate a tumor that may be in close proximity to a vital organ (Fig. 41-3). The LET values of electrons are dependent on their energy, but in the therapeutic ranges the value is similar to that of ^{60}Co.

Neutrons are of interest therapeutically for a variety of reasons, including the following:

1. The LET value for 20 meV neutrons is 7.
2. The biologic effectiveness of neutrons is not significantly altered by a lack of oxygen within the tumor cell.

However, only a few neutron therapy facilities are currently available, and research is still being conducted in this area.

Two other charged particles deserve mention: the proton and the pion. Although these particle beams are not available to most cancer centers in the United States, they are being investigated for their therapeutic use in a number of medical research facilities.

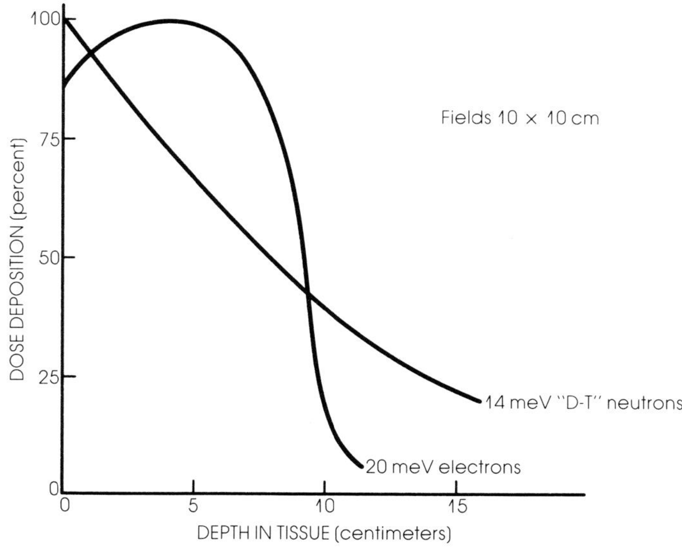

Fig. 41-3. Plot of percent dose deposition versus depth in centimeters of tissue for high-energy neutrons and electrons.

Most cancer patients are treated by teletherapy units; however, some may also be treated with an implant technique called plesiotherapy or brachytherapy. The theory behind brachytherapy is to deliver low-intensity radiation over an extended period of time to a relatively small volume of tissue. Brachytherapy may be accomplished in a number of ways:

1. Mould technique: placement of a *radioactive* source or sources on or in close proximity to the lesion
2. Implant technique: placement of a radioactive source or sources in a body cavity
3. Interstitial implant technique: placement of a radioactive source or sources directly into the tumor site

The majority of brachytherapy applications tend to be temporary; the sources are left in the patient until a designated tumor dose has been attained, possibly 3 to 4 days. The radioactive nuclides frequently used for this type of approach tend to have a long *half-life* and include *radium* 226, cesium 137, and iridium 192. The nuclides may be reused after being sterilized or disinfected.

Permanent implant therapy may also be accomplished. Examples of permanent implant nuclides are radon 222 seeds and iodine 125 seeds. Permanent implant nuclides have half-lives of hours or days and are left in the patient essentially forever. The amount and distribution of the radionuclide implanted in this manner are dependent on the total dose that the radiation oncologist is trying to deliver. In most if not all cases of brachytherapy implantation, the implant is applied as part of the patient's overall treatment plan and may be followed by more teletherapy or possibly a surgical approach.

Clinical Applications

TREATMENT PLAN

If a patient has been diagnosed as having a particular histologic type of cancer and the extensiveness of the tumor has been determined to include possible nodal involvement, extension into any adjacent tissues, and possible metastasis, the decision is made as to what part, if any, radiation oncology will play.

If radiation oncology is considered of value in offering the patient the best possible prognosis, a treatment plan must be outlined and implemented for the patient. The following variables must be determined:

1. Type and extent of tumor
2. Emotional and physical well-being of the patient
3. Time-dose fractions (size of dose over period of time)
4. Radiation oncology unit capabilities
5. Goal of treatment (cure or preoperative or postoperative palliation)

Each member of the radiation oncology department (e.g., radiation oncologist, radiation therapy technologist, oncology nurse, physicist, dosimetrist) plays an active and integral part in the planning and implementation of the optimum treatment plan.

DOSIMETRY

Dosimetry is the design and monitoring of a technique for the precise application of a dose of ionizing radiation to the tumor without irreparably damaging the surrounding normal tissue. Many approaches may be used to accomplish this purpose; following are some examples of teletherapy.

Single field

In some cases the entire tumor dose is delivered through only one treatment port or *field*. An example of this approach is the treatment of skin cancer.

Opposing ports

In this approach the tumor dose is the result of contributions from fields I and II (Fig. 41-4). In most cases, if the tumor dose is to be 200 rads per treatment day, 100 rads will be delivered through each of the treatment ports.

Multifield

This technique is basically an expansion of the opposing ports approach but employs the use of three or more fields to deliver the tumor dose (Fig. 41-5). Again, in most cases, the tumor dose will be delivered by equal contributions from the involved fields.

Rotational field

In this case the patient is positioned so that the tumor is located at the axis of rotation of the unit. When the unit is turned on, the source of radiation rotates around the patient until the dose has been delivered. This treatment technique is usually applied to centrally located lesions such as cancer of the esophagus. The advantage of this technique is that the maximum dose deposition is at the axis of rotation with minimal dose buildup to other parts of the anatomy.

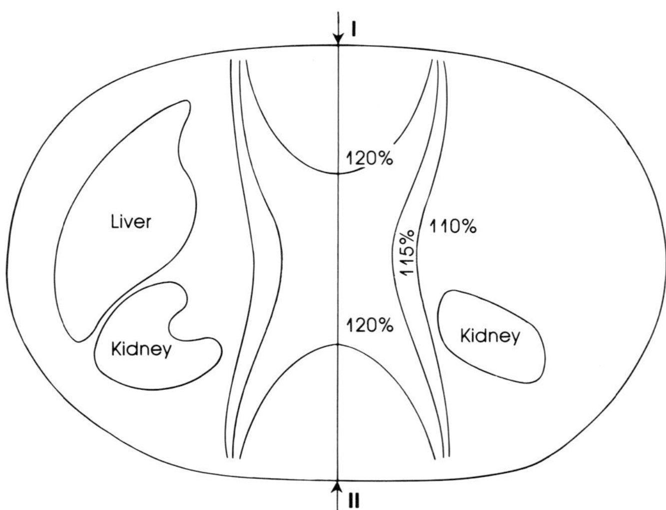

Fig. 41-4. Opposing ports teletherapy. Summated isodose lines represent equal dose contributions from fields I and II.

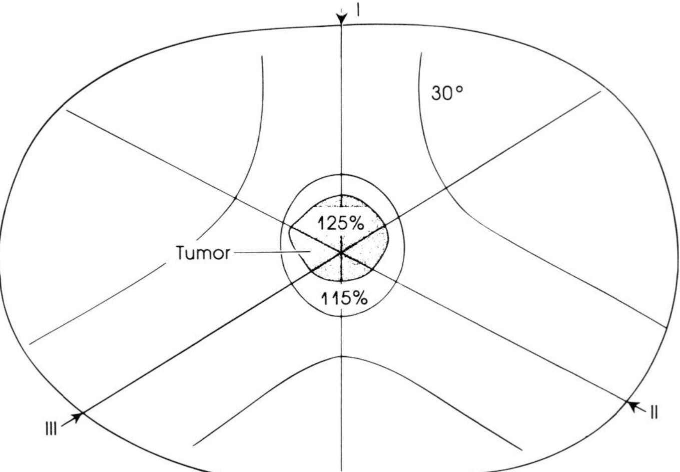

Fig. 41-5. Multifield teletherapy. Summated isodose lines represent equal dose contributions from fields I to III.

Fig. 41-6. Isodose curve obtained from cobalt 60 unit with wedge placed between source and absorbing material.

Wedge fields

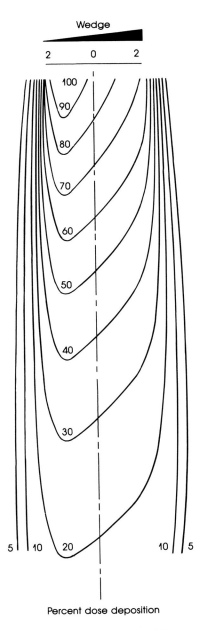

Occasionally, the primary beam must be altered to accomplish the treatment goal; one way is to apply a wedge field technique. To obtain the desired isodose distribution, a wedge-shaped device, usually made of lead, is placed in the beam approximately halfway between the source of radiation and the patient. When the wedge is correctly placed within the beam of radiation, an *isodose curve* similar to that illustrated is obtained (Fig. 41-6). The wedges, as well as the wedge fields they produce, must be oriented in a heel-to-heel manner with extreme care given to the daily setups. A combination of two wedge fields may be used to obtain the desired treatment plan. Although wedge fields may be used for tumors located at any anatomic site, they are usually employed in head and neck tumors (Fig. 41-7).

Shaped fields

Most radiation oncology units have field-defining *collimators* that are rectangular in nature. Often irradiation of the entire rectangular area is not necessary to deliver the tumor dose. To reduce the radiation exposure to only portions of the field, shaper blocks, such as those illustrated in Fig. 41-8, are placed at some point between the source and patient. The shaper blocks are generally lead or an equivalent material and reduce the intensity of the beam to between 5% and 10% of the original intensity.

• • •

The preceding examples do not exhaust the treatment options available to the therapist; others include the moving strip technique, tangential breast fields, and treatment techniques using *bolus* material and designed to deliver the precise tumor dose while limiting the amount of radiation to the uninvolved portions of the anatomy.

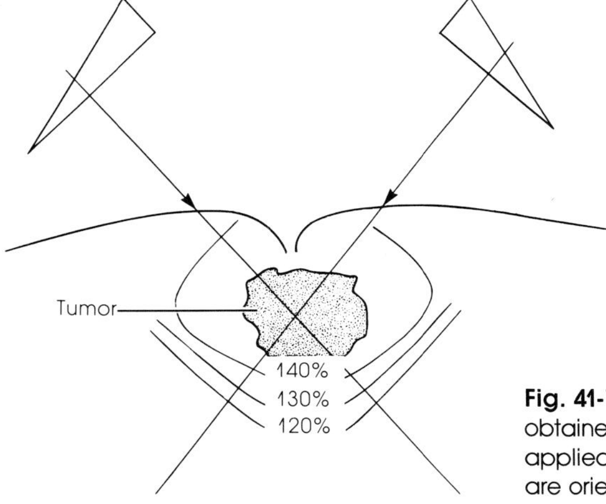

Fig. 41-7. Summated isodose curves obtained when pair of wedge fields are applied for therapeutic purposes. Wedges are oriented "heel to heel."

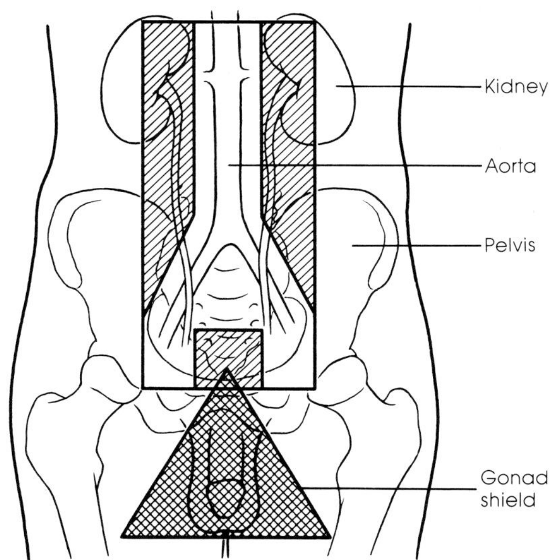

Fig. 41-8. "Inverted Y" radiation field frequently used to treat lymphatic disease below diaphragm. Darker area over gonads represents double thickness of lead shaper blocks.

To assist in the treatment planning and dosimetry of many treatment setups, computers, ultrasonography, and computed tomography are used not only to locate the tumor but also to localize the boundaries of noninvolved organs, to indicate doses outside the tumor volume, or possibly to evaluate the effectiveness of the treatment plan by recording tumor regression. In addition, new techniques are being investigated which, it is hoped, will enhance the effectiveness of cancer therapy. Specific areas of interest include intraoperative irradiation of selected tumors, the treatment of patients twice a day instead of the usual once-a-day regimen, and the use of radiosensitizing agents, hyperthermia, and high-energy particulate irradiation.

CLINICAL ENTITIES

Because the ability of the oncologist to treat any tumor for cure depends on early diagnosis of the disease, the following discussions assume that the disease process is in a beginning stage.

Carcinoma of the larynx

Lesions of this nature are best treated with super-voltage radiation. Tumors that are confined to the vocal cord, with normal cord mobility, have a 90% 5-year cure rate; in addition, the voice remains useful. The method of treatment is usually accomplished by opposing lateral fields of 4 × 5 or 5 × 5 cm and delivering a dose of 6000 to 6500 rads in a 6-week period.

Carcinoma of the skin

Carcinomas of the skin are usually squamous cell or basal cell lesions and are best treated with superficial radiation. Cure rates tend to run between 80% and 90%, and basal cell lesions less than 1 cm in diameter have a cure rate of almost 100%. The method of treatment is usually a single-field approach with attention given to shielding the uninvolved skin and delivering 4500 rads in a 3-week period.

Medulloblastoma

Children with this disease are usually referred to the radiation oncology department after a biopsy and shunt procedure. The tumor is radiosensitive, and patients who have had treatment of the entire cerebrospinal axis have a 5-year cure rate of 40% to 50%. The therapeutic approach tends to be complicated because the entire brain is irradiated with 4500 rads, the spinal cord receives a dose of between 3500 and 4500 rads, and the cerebellum an additional 1000 rads (Fig. 41-9). This irradiation is usually accomplished with parallel opposed fields to the cranial vault with an extended single field to the spinal cord. A megavoltage unit is often used with extreme care given to any areas of abutting fields.

Retinoblastoma

Retinoblastoma is an inherited disease that usually manifests itself before the individual is 3 years of age. If the tumor is diagnosed early and occurs in only one eye, the chances of controlling the disease are about 50%. The tumor dose of 3500 to 4500 rads in 3½ to 4½ weeks may be accomplished with either high-energy electrons or a megavoltage unit. Lateral ports are generally used with care given to dosimetry. Two important complications that often occur are radiation-induced cataracts and facial asymmetry caused by growth-retarding effects of radiation on bone.

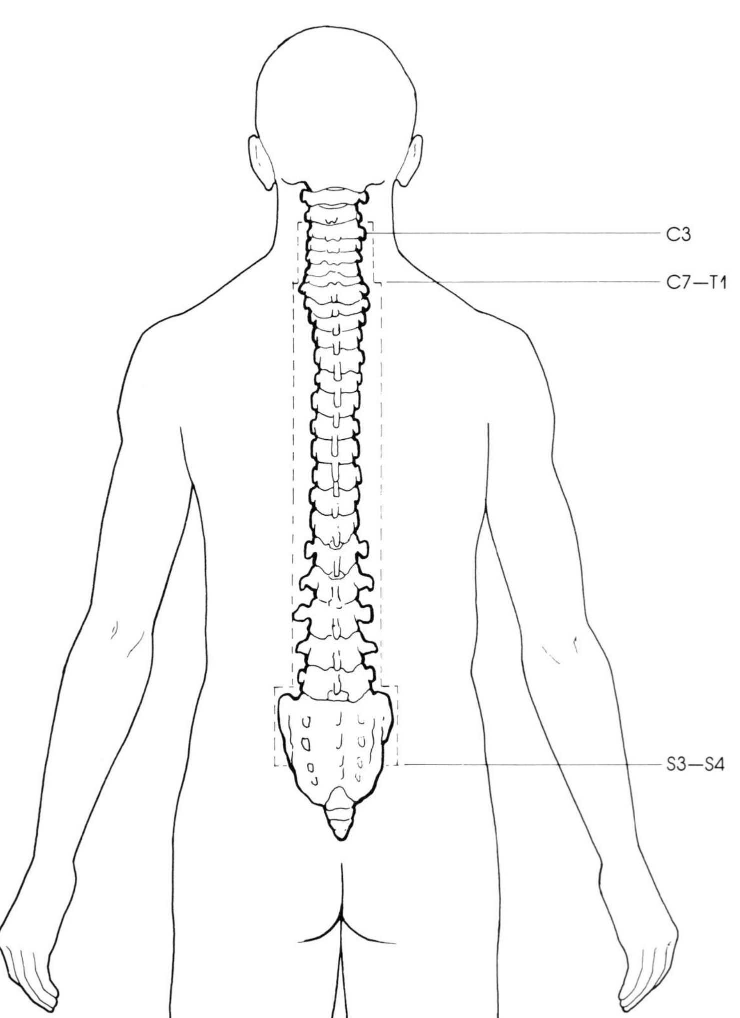

Fig. 41-9. Spinal treatment portal for medulloblastoma.

• • •

Radiation oncology may be the only therapeutic approach used in the treatment of some cancers, or it may be used in conjunction with chemotherapy or surgery. The decision of how a patient is treated is determined by weighing many factors and options and then integrating them with the capabilities of the medical facility. Following are some generally agreed on treatment factors (which may vary from institution to institution) for a number of frequently treated cancers.

Cancers treated primarily by radiation therapy

Cancer of the larynx: Irradiation from opposing lateral ports with small field sizes and possibly wedges is employed. A megavoltage unit delivers a total dose of 6500 rads in 6 weeks.

Cancer of the skin: This treatment involves a single field large enough to cover the lesion and any possible extension. The uninvolved tissue should be well protected. For lesions 2 to 3 cm in size, 5000 rads in 4 weeks are delivered by a superficial unit.

Cancer of the oral cavity: A number of approaches may be used depending on the size and the extent of the tumor. A peroral cone may be used to deliver 6000 rads in 4 weeks, with an orthovoltage beam for small lesions. Larger lesions may be treated with irradiation through opposing lateral ports from a megavoltage unit possibly followed by brachytherapy.

Cancer of the cervix: Early diagnosed lesions can be treated with either surgery or therapy. Opposing AP-PA ports using a megavoltage unit, preferably 10 meV or greater, deliver 4500 to 5000 rads in 5 weeks to an area of the primary and regional lymph nodes (Fig. 41-10). An intracavitary implant may also be indicated.

Hodgkin's disease and malignant lymphoma: The age of the patient and extent of the disease may determine the prognosis. Extended field therapy includes the lymphatic chain above and/or below the diaphragm and is applied by a megavoltage unit that delivers 4500 rads through AP-PA ports. Chemotherapy may also be indicated.

Cancer of the nasopharynx: Shaped lateral opposing ports are used to deliver 7000 rads in 6 to 8 weeks with the possibility of an intracavitary application (Fig. 41-11). The tumor dose is delivered by a megavoltage unit.

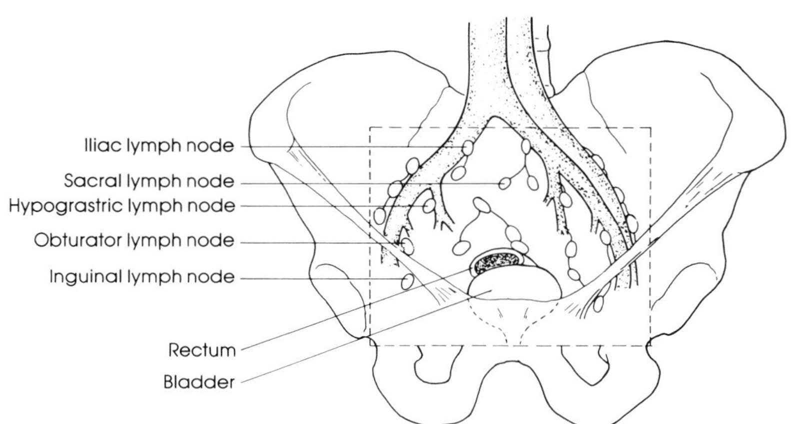

Fig. 41-10. Field employed for irradiation of primary tumor and adjacent lymph nodes.

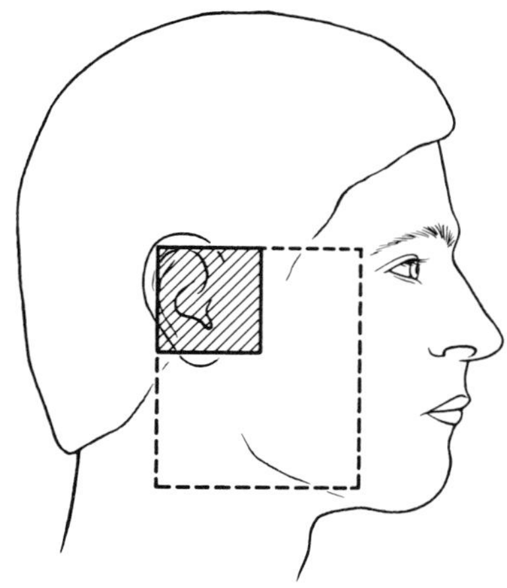

Fig. 41-11. Opposing ports for treatment of nasopharyngeal cancer. Shaded area represents the use of lead shaper blocks.

Cancers treated with radiation and surgery and/or chemotherapy

Cancer of the breast: Using two tangential fields to the chest wall or intact breast, megavoltage radiation delivers 5000 rads in 5 weeks (Fig. 41-12). Chemotherapy may also be indicated.

Cancer of the uterus: External megavoltage irradiation may be used preoperatively through AP-PA ports. After total hysterectomy an intracavitary implant may be indicated.

Cancer of the lung: Treatment for small lesions involves surgical resection followed by postoperative irradiation by a megavoltage unit that delivers 6000 to 7000 rads through opposing ports (Fig. 41-13). The total dose depends on the radiosensitivity of the surrounding tissue. Chemotherapy may also be indicated.

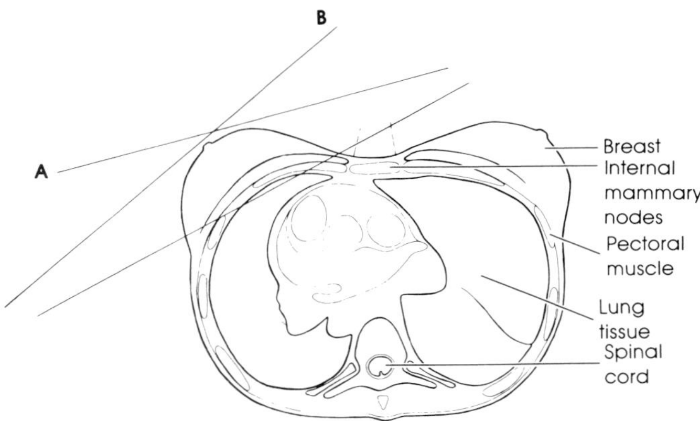

Fig. 41-12. Cross section of thorax. *A* and *B*, Field arrangements to tangentially irradiate intact breast.

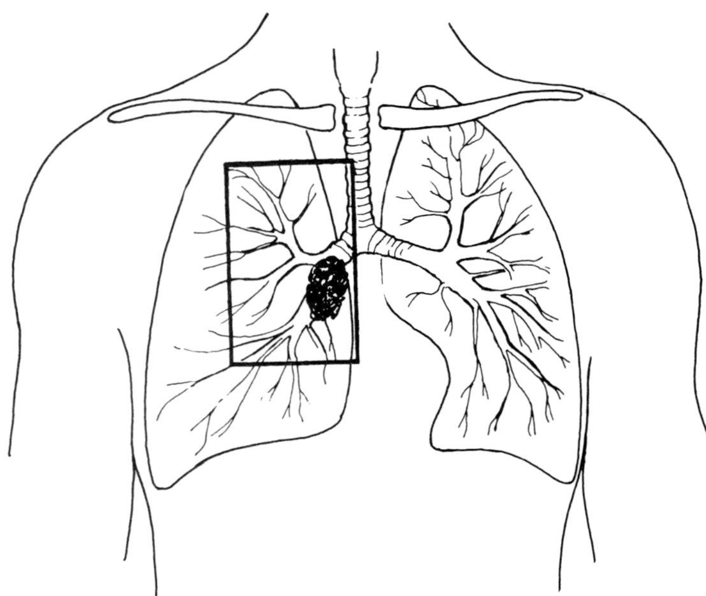

Fig. 41-13. Typical field for irradiation of carcinoma of the lung.

The Future

Because of the nature of cancer, it is wishful thinking to expect dramatic breakthroughs in research that will result in a cure for all cancers. A more realistic expectation is that research will continue to supply important bits of information that, when added to the present body of information, will afford a greater understanding of the disease and how to treat it effectively. The continued application of ionizing radiation as a treatment modality will not require the discovery of new radiation or the design of larger, more costly radiation-producing units. The future will more likely revolve around three specific questions: (1) when to irradiate, (2) under what altered biologic conditions, and (3) how much radiation over what period of time. It is not the usefulness of radiation that is the question—we know it works and we have a basic understanding of how it works. Instead, efforts will be directed toward effectively controlling and/or manipulating the biologic and physical environment to maximize the desired positive effects.

WHEN TO IRRADIATE

Evidence supports the argument that the earlier a tumor is diagnosed and treated the better the patient's prognosis will be. This truism will not change; however, it is hoped that, with increased public education efforts coupled with available screening programs, patients will be seen even earlier than at present. Additionally, increased diagnostic capabilities, such as those available with magnetic resonance imaging, CT scans, and newly devised medical laboratory examinations, allow for determinations of the extent and histologic type of a tumor far beyond the present capabilities.

ALTERING THE BIOLOGIC ENVIRONMENT

The effort to alter the biologic environment will be two pronged: (1) involving the immunotherapist approach, in which physicians will be able to trigger the body's own immune mechanism to recognize and destroy abnormal growth, and (2) incorporating the oncology effort to alter the biologic and/or physical environment to increase the radiosensitivity of the malignancy. Radiation oncology will be concerned with the latter effort.

Altering the biologic and physical environment will have much impact on therapists because it will require them to accommodate and become more knowledgeable in such diverse areas as hyperthermia, fractionated brachytherapy procedures, and possibly hyperbaric treatment techniques. These adaptations, coupled with a plethora of chemotherapeutic agents, will not only alter the tumor environment but will greatly increase the day-to-day patient care and treatment responsibilities of the radiation therapist.

HOW MUCH RADIATION AND IN WHAT TIME PERIOD

Finally, the appropriateness of delivering an established number of rads for a given type of tumor over a certain time frame is being questioned. Delivering 180 rads per day for 5 weeks for a total dose of 4500 rads (45 Gy) may no longer be the method of choice to obtain the desired biologic response. Radiation oncologists are investigating various therapeutic procedures that will enhance the biologic effects of radiation to tumors, while at the same time diminishing the deleterious effects to normal tissue. Techniques might include treating the patent twice a day, "tuning-down" linear accelerators to deliver fewer numbers of rads per monitor unit, and treating with greater (or lesser) total doses than those presently delivered.

There is little doubt that currently accepted radiation oncology treatment techniques will change. However, the changes will not take place overnight; rather, the changes will be subtle and well thought out. They will include some or all of the above three subject areas and hopefully will result in increased patient survival statistics.

The 1990s will be a decade of innovation and challenge in radiation oncology and should be entered with enthusiasm and a certain degree of cautious optimism.

Summary

From a somewhat questionable beginning, radiation therapy has emerged as one of the primary modalities employed in the treatment of malignant disease. Radiation therapy departments are currently examining and treating approximately 75% of all newly diagnosed cancer patients. The radiation oncologists and therapy technologists are integral members of the health team that discusses and selects the appropriate treatment regimens for all cancer patients.

As our understanding of those factors that initiate cellular change, growth, and spread increases, our ability to treat patients more effectively will also increase. The irradiation techniques presently used may change dramatically based on this new information. Additionally, new, more sophisticated, radiation-producing equipment is being designed that may cause us to reevaluate the presently accepted therapeutic techniques and dose levels. Finally, new chemotherapeutic agents are being produced that, when used by themselves or in combination with other drugs, may enhance tumor sensitivity when used in conjunction with radiation.

The positive role of radiation oncology in the treatment of cancer has been established. Certainly changes will occur, and if the present trend continues, it appears that radiation therapy will play an ever increasing and expanded role in cancer treatment.

Definition of Terms

absorbed dose Amount of ionizing radiation absorbed per unit of mass of irradiated material as it passes through matter.

accelerator (particle) Device that accelerates charged subatomic particles to great energies. These particles produce rays and neutrons and may be used for direct medical irradiation and basic physical research. Medical units include linear accelerators, Van de Graaff units, betatrons, and cyclotrons.

air dose Dose of radiation measured in roentgens in free air, uncorrected for absorption or backscatter.

anaplasia Alteration of cell to more embryonic state; may be used to describe particular type of tumor.

attenuation Removal of energy from beam of ionizing radiation when it traverses matter, by disposition of energy in matter and by deflection of energy out of beam.

betatron Electron accelerator that uses magnetic induction to accelerate electrons in circular path; also capable of producing photons.

bolus Tissue-equivalent material (e.g., rice, beeswax, petrolatum gauze, Silly Putty) placed around curved, irregularly shaped anatomic areas to obtain more uniform dosage distribution.

brachytherapy Placement of radioactive nuclide(s) in or on neoplasm to deliver cancericidal dose.

cancer Term frequently applied to malignant disease: neoplasm (new growth) or oma (tumor).

carcinogen Any cancer-producing substance or material such as nicotine, radiation, or ingested uranium.

chemical dosimeter Detector for indirect measurement of radiation by indicating extent to which radiation causes definite chemical change to take place (e.g., thermoluminescent dosimeter, TLD).

cobalt 60 (^{60}Co) Radioisotope with half-life of 5.25 years, average gamma-ray intensity of 1.25 meV (1.17 and 1.33), and ability to spare skin with buildup depth in tissue of 0.5 cm.

collimator Diaphragm or system of diaphragms made of radiation-absorbing material that define dimension and direction of beam.

compensating filter Filter designed to modify dose distribution within patient. Filters may be designed to account for patient shape, size, or position (e.g., wedge filter).

contamination Radioactivity in inappropriate places such as technologist's hands.

cure Usually, 5-year period after completion of treatment during which time patient exhibits no evidence of disease.

decay or disintegration Transformation of radioactive nucleus, resulting in emission of radiation.

differentiation Acquisition of cellular functions that differ from functions of original cell type.

dose rate Radiation dose delivered per unit of time, usually roentgens per minute.

dosimeter Device (e.g., film badge, ionization chamber, Geiger counter) that measures radiation exposure.

etiology Study of causes of diseases.

field Geometric area defined by collimator or radiotherapy unit at skin surface.

filter Attenuator inserted in beam near source to modify beam quality in desired way. Materials used most often are copper, aluminum, and lead.

fission Breaking apart of uranium 235 nucleus, liberating energy and neutrons, which are used in producing radioactive isotopes in reactor (^{60}Co).

fractionation Dividing of total planned dose into number of smaller doses to be given over longer period. Consideration must be given to biologic effectiveness of smaller doses.

gamma ray Electromagnetic radiation that originates from radioactive nucleus and causes ionization in matter; identical in properties to x ray.

grenz rays X rays generated at 20 kVp or less.

half-life Time (specific for each radioactive substance) required for radioactive material to decay to half its initial activity. Types are biologic and effective.

half-value layer Thickness of attenuating material inserted in beam to reduce beam intensity to half value.

ionization Process in which one or more electrons are added to or removed from atoms, creating ions. Can be caused by high temperatures, electrical discharges, or nuclear radiations.

isodose curve Curve or line drawn to connect points of identical amounts of radiation in given field.

metastasis Transmission of cells or groups of cells from primary tumor to site(s) elsewhere in body.

oncologist Doctor of medicine specializing in study of tumors.

oncology Study of tumors.

protraction Delivery of tumor dose over extended, uninterrupted time period.

radiation oncologist Doctor of medicine specializing in use of ionizing radiation in treatment of disease.

radiation oncology Medical specialty involving the treatment of cancerous lesions using ionizing radiation.

radiation therapy Older term used to define medical specialty of treatment with ionizing radiations.

radiation therapy technologist Person trained to assist and take directions from radiation therapist in use of ionizing radiations in treatment of disease.

radioactive Pertaining to atoms of elements that undergo spontaneous transformation, resulting in emission of radiation.

radiocurable Susceptibility of neoplastic cells to cure (destruction) by ionizing radiation.

radiosensitivity Responsiveness of cells to radiation.

radium (Ra) Radionuclide (atomic number, 88; atomic weight, 226; half-life, 1622 years) used clinically for radiation therapy. In conjunction with its subsequent transformations, radium emits alpha and beta particles and gamma rays. In encapsulated form it is used for various intracavitary radiation therapy applications such as that for cancer of cervix.

reactor Cubicle in which isotopes are artificially produced.

roentgen (R) Unit of exposure dose, based on extent of ionization in air and defined as 2.58×10^{-4} coulombs/kg of dry air, which is equivalent to 1 electrostatic unit of charge/cc or 0.001293 gm of dry air; 1.16×10^{12} ion pairs/gm of air; 2.08×10^{9} ion pairs/gm of air; or absorption of 87 ergs of energy/gm of air.

scattering Process in which trajectory of particle or photon is changed; caused by collision with atoms, nuclei, and other particles.

sequelae Reaction or side effects of ionizing radiation on tissue.

skin sparing In supervoltage beam therapy, reduced skin injury per roentgen exposure when electron equilibrium is not present at advance portal but occurs below skin. Occurs from 0.5 to 5.0 cm deep depending on energy.

teletherapy Radiation therapy technique for which source of radiation is at some distance from patient.

tumor volume Portion of anatomy that includes tumor and adjacent areas of invasion.

undifferentiation Lack or absence of normal cell differentiation.

unstable In excited, active state; with nucleus possessing excess energy.

Van de Graaff generator Electrostatic machine in which electronically charged particles are sprayed on moving belt and carried by it to build up high potential on insulated terminal. Charged particles are then accelerated along discharge path through vacuum tube by potential difference between insulated terminal and opposite end of machine. Often used to inject particles into larger accelerators.

SELECTED BIBLIOGRAPHY

Bental GC et al: Treatment planning and dose calculation in radiation oncology, ed 3, New York, 1982, Pergamon Press, Inc.

Cooper JS et al: Concepts in cancer care, Philadelphia, 1983, Lea & Febiger.

Hall EJ: Radiobiology for the radiologist, New York, 1973, Harper & Row Publishers, Inc.

Johns HE and Cunningham JR: The physics of radiology, ed 4, Springfield, Ill, 1983, Charles C Thomas, Publisher.

Meredith WJ et al: Fundamental physics of radiology, ed 3, Bristol, 1977, Wright & Sons.

Moss WT et al: Radiation oncology rationale, technique, and results, ed 5, St Louis, 1979, The CV Mosby Co.

Mould RF: Radiotherapy treatment planning, Bristol, 1981, Hilger.

Pizzarello DJ et al: Medical radiation biology, ed 2, Philadelphia, 1982, Lea & Febiger.

Rafla S et al: Introduction to radiotherapy, St Louis, 1974, The CV Mosby Co.

Rubin P et al: Clinical oncology for medical students and physicians, ed 6, 1983, American Cancer Society.

Selman J: The basic physics of radiation therapy, ed 2, Springfield, Ill, 1976, Charles C Thomas Publisher.

Walter J et al: A short textbook of radiotherapy for technicians and students, ed 3, Boston, 1969, Little, Brown & Co.

Chapter 42

INTRODUCTION TO RADIOGRAPHIC QUALITY ASSURANCE

WILLIAM F. FINNEY III

In a medical diagnostic radiographic imaging system there are numerous sources of variability. These sources can produce subquality images if they are not controlled. Most subquality radiographs often require repeat examinations resulting in additional radiation exposure to the patient and an increased cost to the department. A systematic and structured mechanism to control these variables is the foundation upon which radiographic quality assurance (QA) is built.

The intent of this chapter is to acquaint the reader with radiographic quality assurance. It is not designed to be a procedures manual for the various quality control tests but is written as an overview of the radiographic quality assurance concept. For those desiring additional information on any topic discussed in this chapter, please refer to the bibliography at the end of this chapter.

The information in this chapter draws heavily from the quality assurance series developed and published by the National Center for Devices and Radiological Health (NCDRH) and from material by Radiation Measurements Incorporated (RMI). These organizations have been active in promoting quality assurance and instrumental in creating a practical approach to quality assurance, allowing its concepts to be realized by *diagnostic radiology facilities** regardless of their size (Figs. 42-1 and 42-2).

*All italicized terms are defined at the end of this chapter.

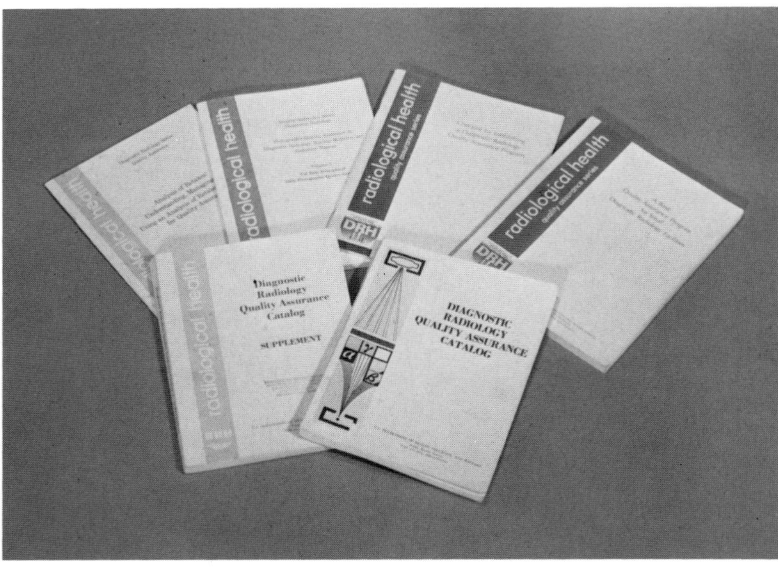

Fig. 42-1. NCDRH quality assurance publications.

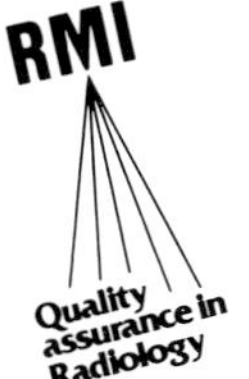

Fig. 42-2. RMI specializes in quality control test tools for radiology.

Quality Assurance Versus Quality Control

Radiographic quality assurance and radiographic quality control are terms that are often used synonymously. Both terms are concepts that define a mechanism used to enhance the quality of the services and products rendered. Their main difference is the scope of their intent.

One concept of *radiographic quality assurance* encompasses the total picture of radiographic care delivery with its primary objective being the enhancement of patient care. Patient selection parameters, management techniques, departmental polices and procedures, technical effectiveness and efficiency, and inservice education are examples of some of the elements that are included. The Joint Commission for Accreditation of Healthcare Organizations (JCAHO) uses this quality assurance concept in their hospital accreditation process.

The NCDRH's concept of radiographic quality assurance focuses primarily on the enhancement of radiographic image quality and on the reduction of unnecessary patient exposure by using quality administrative procedures and quality control techniques.

Quality control (QC) as defined by the NCDRH deals with the techniques used in the monitoring and maintenance of the technical elements of the system that affect the quality of the image. Although the idea of control is basic to this concept, the goal of optimizing the performance and assuring the accuracy of these elements must not be forgotten. This chapter uses the terms "radiographic quality assurance" and "radiographic quality control" in the context as defined by the NCDRH.

Historical Development

Quality assurance in diagnostic radiology is not new. Many radiography departments have been systematically monitoring their equipment long before "quality assurance/control" became a buzz word. The background for this interest in radiographic quality assurance can be traced to past actions taken by the federal government.

In 1968 the Radiation Control for Health and Safety Act was passed. This act required the U.S. Department of Health, Education and Welfare, now designated Health and Human Services (HHS), to conduct a radiation control program through the development and administration of standards to reduce human exposure to radiation from electronic products. The Bureau of Radiological Health (BRH), now designated The National Center for Devices and Radiological Health (NCDRH), was given the responsibility of carrying out this act.

In 1974 the BRH set forth regulatory action to control the manufacture and installation of medical/dental diagnostic x-ray equipment to reduce the production of useless radiation. This action, known as the X-ray Equipment Standard, was designed to regulate the performance of *x-ray systems,* not the use of such systems. One section of the standard requires that positive–beam-limitation (PBL) devices be included on general purpose stationary x-ray systems. This is an attempt to protect the patient from receiving unnecessary radiation by automatically adjusting the beam size to match the size of the image receptor being used. Although this ensures that the equipment is designed to accomplish this goal, in the end it is the operator who is still responsible for the proper use of the equipment.

Another approach to help realize the goal of reducing the patient's exposure to unnecessary radiation was thought to be in the development of facility-based *quality assurance programs.* Support was given this notion by results of numerous studies, which pointed out that many diagnostic radiology facilities produce subquality images and deliver unnecessary amounts of radiation while examining patients. It was believed that the best way to discourage such practices was to educate the radiologic community about the concept of radiographic quality assurance. The professional community was made aware of the BRH's intent to develop recommendations concerning quality assurance programs in 1976. The professional community was solicited for their input in the development of quality assurance recommendations, and in 1978 the proposed Recommendation for Quality Assurance Programs in Diagnostic Radiology Facilities was published. Comments on the proposal were solicited, and in 1979 the recommendation was published in its final form in the Federal Register.

The Consumer-Patient Radiation Health and Safety Act of 1981 established guidelines for further reducing unnecessary patient exposure. This act addressed issues such as unnecessary repeat examinations, quality assurance techniques, radiation exposure, referral criteria, and unnecessary mass screening programs. In addition, the act established minimum standards for accreditation of educational programs in the radiologic sciences and for the certification of radiographic equipment operators.

Benefits

The benefits of having a well-administered radiographic quality assurance program are numerous. The use of such a program in diagnostic radiology facilities is one of the methods that can minimize unnecessary radiation to patient consumers. Studies have demonstrated that the number of repeated radiographs, which result in additional radiation to the patient, can be reduced with the implementation of quality assurance procedures. Although the reduction in unnecessary patient exposure is significant, the potential to improve the overall efficiency of the radiologic service delivery can also be realized. These advantages result in satisfied patient consumers.

The radiology facility is also the beneficiary of quality assurance. Improvement of radiographic image quality is achievable, as is increased consistency of image production. Quality control procedures can increase the reliability, efficiency, and cost effectiveness of the equipment used by the facility. These are important gains, considering the current emphasis on cost containment in health care delivery. Although increased overall departmental efficiency in itself is a major advantage, the betterment of personnel morale resulting from such improvements may be the most important benefit in the long run.

Not all facilities engaged in quality assurance gain from all the benefits possible; the goal is to provide a more effective and efficient delivery of radiologic services along with a reduction in unnecessary radiation to the patient consumer. With the proper planning, design, and management of a quality assurance program, these benefits are easily achievable.

National Center for Devices and Radiological Health Quality Assurance Program Recommendation

The National Center for Devices and Radiological Health's (NCDRH) recommendation for establishing quality assurance programs in diagnostic radiology facilities was developed from research, empirical data, and feedback from the professional community. Although the recommendation is not mandatory, the NCDRH strongly believes that the establishment of quality assurance programs helps to achieve the goals of reducing unproductive patient radiation, minimizing unnecessary costs, and improving the consistency of quality images.

The NCDRH's recommendation includes 10 elements that are considered essential for a viable program. All facilities would not require an approach to quality assurance as comprehensive as that recommended; the NCDRH suggests that the size, objectives, and available resources of a facility should determine the extent to which each element should be implemented. The recommendation provides some valuable insight to the concepts of quality assurance. A brief description of each of the 10 elements follows.

RESPONSIBILITY

Although quality assurance is the responsibility of the entire staff of the diagnostic radiographic facility, an efficient and effective quality assurance program requires accountability. Distinct and documented assignments of responsibility for the program and its components are essential for success. The size of the facility, scope of the program, and available resources are some of the factors that dictate the levels to which these responsibilities are assigned (i.e., physicist, chief technologist, supervisory personnel, staff technologist, and consultant). Regardless of facility size, the primary responsibility for quality assurance is that of the owner or practitioner in charge.

EVALUATION

The element of evaluation within a quality assurance program should be addressed at different levels. First, the performance of the facility should be evaluated. This information can be used to determine the scope and design of a quality assurance program for the facility and/or provide data that can be used for comparison with data generated at future points in time. These comparison evaluations demonstrate the effectiveness of the quality assurance program. The most popular procedure used to evaluate facility performance is the analysis of rejected radiographs, commonly known as *reject analysis*. On another level, equipment monitoring results should be evaluated to assess the need for corrective action or to determine trends that may indicate that preventive maintenance is required.

PURCHASE SPECIFICATIONS

When new equipment is purchased, the facility should determine the desired performance criteria for the equipment. These performance criteria are then reflected in the purchase specifications. Before final acceptance of the equipment, it should be tested to ensure that the actual performance meets the criteria requested in the purchase specifications. The future monitoring and testing of the equipment can be compared to the equipment performance criteria to determine if the equipment is continuing to perform at the acceptable level.

STANDARDS FOR IMAGE QUALITY

Standards for image quality should be established for the performance parameters of the x-ray system that are of interest to the facility. The creation of these standards should, when possible, *objectively* indicate the amount of performance variation that can be accepted before the quality of the image is affected. A *subjective* determination of the standards is often used when objective standards cannot be defined. If the equipment monitoring results show the equipment does not meet the acceptance limits of the standard, then corrective actions are needed and should be taken.

MONITORING AND MAINTENANCE

This element is sometimes referred to as the quality control portion of the program. Equipment monitoring and maintenance is the center of a quality assurance program. The NCDRH suggests that every facility should consider monitoring the following system components:

1. Film processing
2. Performance of radiographic/fluoroscopic units
3. Cassettes and grids
4. Illuminators
5. Darkroom

The system component parameters that should be monitored vary from facility to facility, depending on such factors as program goals, available resources, and cost. The NCDRH includes a listing of parameters for all system components in their recommendation (Table 42-1). A maintenance program including both the preventative and corrective aspects of equipment maintenance is an important aspect of any quality assurance program.

TRAINING

A plan for the training of personnel with quality assurance responsibilities is recommended. A mechanism for the continuing education of these individuals should also be included. A subtle but important aspect of this element is educating the facilities staff to the importance, design, and goals of the quality assurance program. The real strength of a quality assurance program is based on the support and commitment of the entire staff.

COMMITTEE

This element might better be described as communication. Large facilities may require a quality assurance committee structure for planning, review, and evaluation purposes. Smaller facilities may not require a formal committee but instead rely on input directly from the staff. The intent of this element is to emphasize the importance of maintaining open communication among all participants in the quality assurance program.

Table 42-1. X-ray system component parameters

I. Film processing
   a. An index of speed
   b. An index of contrast
   c. Base plus fog
   d. Solution temperatures
   e. Film artifact identification

II. Fluoroscopic x-ray units
   a. Tabletop exposure rates
   b. Centering alignment
   c. Collimation
   d. kVp accuracy and reproducibility
   e. mA accuracy and reproducibility
   f. Exposure time accuracy and reproducibility
   g. Reproducibility of x-ray output
   h. Focal spot size consistency
   i. Half-value layer
   j. Representative entrance skin exposures

III. Image intensified systems
   a. Resolution
   b. Focusing
   c. Distortion
   d. Glare
   e. Low-contrast performance
   f. Physical alignment of camera and collimating lens

IV. Radiographic x-ray units
   a. Reproducibility of x-ray output
   b. Linearity and reproducibility of mA stations
   c. Reproducibility and accuracy of timer stations
   d. Reproducibility and accuracy of kVp stations
   e. Accuracy of source-to-image receptor distance indicators
   f. Light/x-ray field congruence
   g. Half-value layer
   h. Focal spot size consistency
   i. Representative entrance skin exposures

V. Automatic exposure control (AEC) devices
   a. Reproducibility
   b. kVp compensation
   c. Field sensitivity matching
   d. Minimum response time
   e. Back-up timer verification

VI. Cassettes and grids
   a. Cassettes
      1. Film/screen contact
      2. Screen condition
      3. Light leaks
      4. Artifact identification
   b. Grids
      1. Alignment and focal distance
      2. Artifact identification

VII. Illuminators
   a. Consistency of light output with time
   b. Consistency of light output from one illuminator to another
   c. Illuminator surface conditions

VIII. Darkrooms
   a. Darkroom integrity
   b. Safelight conditions

IX. Tomographic systems
   a. Accuracy of depth and cut indicator
   b. Thickness of cut plane
   c. Exposure angle
   d. Completeness of tomographic motion
   e. Flatness of tomographic field
   f. Resolution
   g. Continuity of exposure
   h. Flatness of cassette
   i. Representative entrance skin exposures

X. Computed tomography
   a. Precision (noise)
   b. Contrast scale
   c. High- and low-contrast resolution
   d. Alignment
   e. Representative entrance skin exposures

RECORDS

The documentation of equipment monitoring results, maintenance actions, and other such activities should be included in a quality assurance program. A regular and systematic method of collecting and recording data is the foundation on which the review and evaluation elements of the program are based.

MANUAL

A quality assurance program should develop and maintain a complete, comprehensive, and up-to-date manual. The manual should serve as a source document or guide for all the elements of the program. The manual should include items such as quality assurance personnel, monitoring procedures, monitoring schedules, monitoring evaluations, corrective actions, and service records.

REVIEW

Periodic review is necessary to determine the status of the quality assurance program. A look at the entire program will determine if it is operating at its maximum effectiveness or if changes have to be made. Inspection of the important program elements will reveal their currentness, appropriateness, consistency, regularity, and effectiveness in achieving the goals of the program.

Quality Assurance Program Design

Every radiographic facility is a unique entity. Although their mission may be the same, the process and environment of each are different. With this in mind, a facility must custom-fit quality assurance to its own situation. A review of the quality assurance literature provides valuable guidance for the design of a program. A systematic approach to fitting a quality assurance program to the needs of a facility makes such a seemingly large task manageable. Begin by planning an assessment of the facilities performance. This information may reveal areas that should be attended to first, along with providing documentation for supporting the program plan. One method of assessing the facilities performance is by the use of *reject analysis*. The analysis of rejected radiographs is an effective method of identifying performance problems. The establishment of a reject analysis program as a routine part of the quality assurance program can be an excellent method of evaluating the program's impact. Organizing the program plan is the next step. Training personnel, establishing image quality standards, developing and documenting monitoring procedures, and procuring the necessary monitoring equipment are some of the aspects of the organization phase. Implementation of the plan is next followed by an evaluation of the program's impact, which can be assessed by repair records, monitoring results, reject analysis results, or subjective methods. The feedback from the evaluation phase provides input to the original planning steps and should be used to make any necessary adjustments to make the program more effective and efficient.

BASIC QUALITY CONTROL TESTS

The quality control tests used to monitor x-ray system components usually require some type of device to measure the parameter being evaluated. Quality control tools range from simple homemade devices to sophisticated microprocessors (Fig. 42-3). Radiation Measurements Incorporated (RMI) manufactures a comprehensive line of quality control test tools that are relatively inexpensive and easy to use. These tools can be purchased as a complete quality control kit (Fig. 42-4) or individually. The multiple test cassette, which tests several x-ray unit parameters with a single exposure, is especially popular in smaller facilities (Fig. 42-5). The decision of what quality control tools to use depends on such factors as cost, ease of use, accuracy, and dependability. Most vendors of x-ray supplies carry a wide variety of quality control test tools. To familiarize the reader with some examples of quality control test tools, the following section briefly reviews some of the basic tests for quality control.

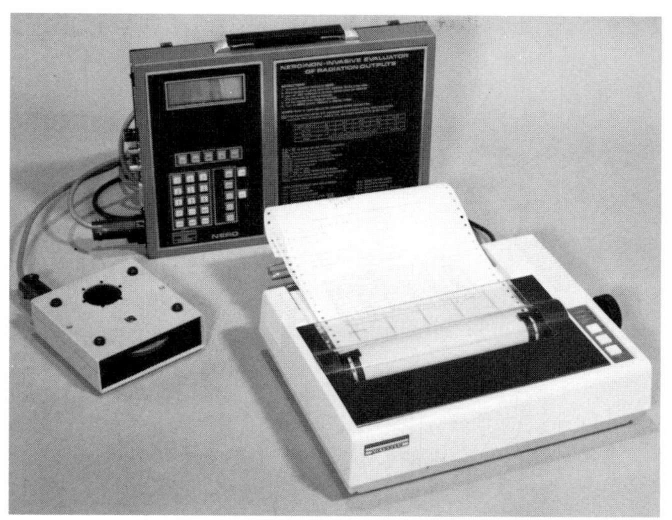

Fig. 42-3. NERO is a microprocessor that can be programmed to acquire and analyze exposure data, providing quality control test results for numerous parameters.

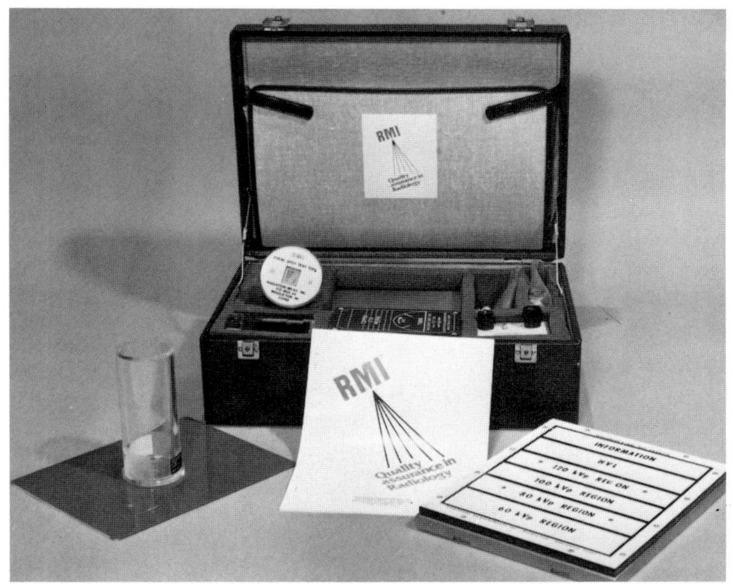

Fig. 42-4. RMI radiographic/fluoroscopic quality control kit.

A

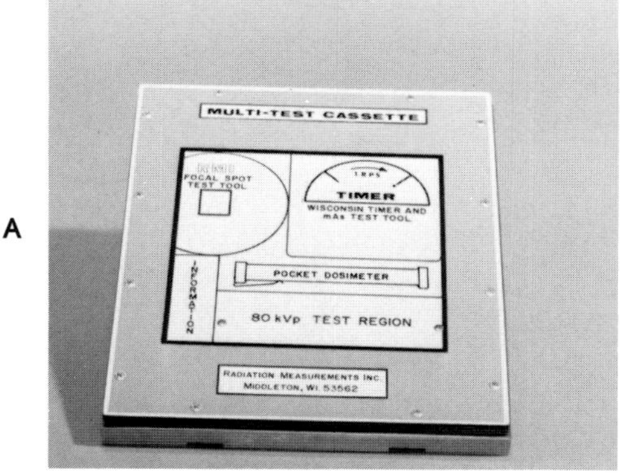

B

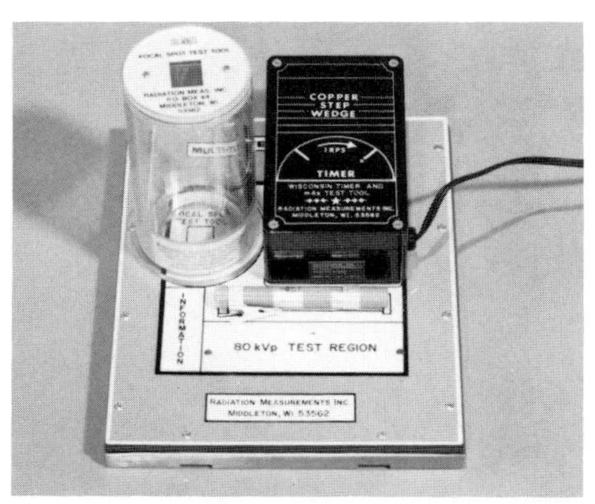

Fig. 42-5. RMI multitest cassette. **A,** Cassette only. **B,** Cassette with quality control tools in place.

Film processing

Film processors are one of the biggest contributors of variability to an x-ray system. Most authorities suggest some form of in-house sensitometric monitoring of the film processor. This approach provides a quantitative means of recording processor variability. The most accurate method of sensitometric monitoring requires the use of a *sensitometer* and a *densitometer* (Fig. 42-6). In addition, a dependable thermometer should be considered to accurately measure developer temperature, and one specific box of radiographic film should be reserved for use as control film in the testing procedure. The sensitometer is used to deliver a graduated series of controlled light intensities to a piece of radiographic control film. The exposed control film is then processed, producing a series of graduated or stepped densities known as a sensitometric *control strip* (Fig. 42-7). Control strips can also be produced by radiographing an aluminum stepwedge; however, the effects of possible x-ray generator variations may result in inaccuracies and/or inconsistencies. A densitometer is used to quantitatively measure the densities of the developed sensitometric control strip. Normally only three measurements are needed. A midrange step, which is close to having an optical density of 1, is known as the speed step. The optical density of the second step above the speed step is measured. The difference between this step and the speed step is known as the density difference, or contrast. The gross, or *base plus fog,* should also be measured. It is good practice to also measure the developer temperature at the time the sensitometric control strip is processed using an accurate thermometer. The data generated are then plotted on a processor control chart (Fig. 42-8). This procedure should be performed at least daily. By charting these processing characteristics, one can interpret the processor's operating condition on a daily basis and also detect any trends in the data that may lead to problems. The measurements should fall within the facility's film processing standard for image quality (speed, contrast, base plus fog), which are established when the processor is considered to be operating in an optimum fashion. If the measurements fall outside the standards, the situation should be analyzed and immediately corrected. The NCDRH recommends the following processing standards of quality: base plus fog ± 0.05 optical density units; contrast ± 0.10 optical density units; speed ± 0.10 optical density units. The integrity and condition of the darkroom should also be tested periodically. This is usually accomplished by visually inspecting the darkroom for light leaks and testing the safelights to determine the level of fog they contribute to the radiographic film.

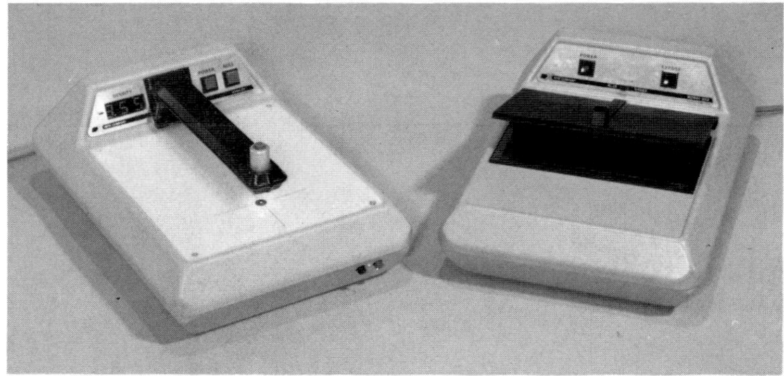

Fig. 42-6. Processor quality control program requires a sensitometer (right) and a densitometer (left).

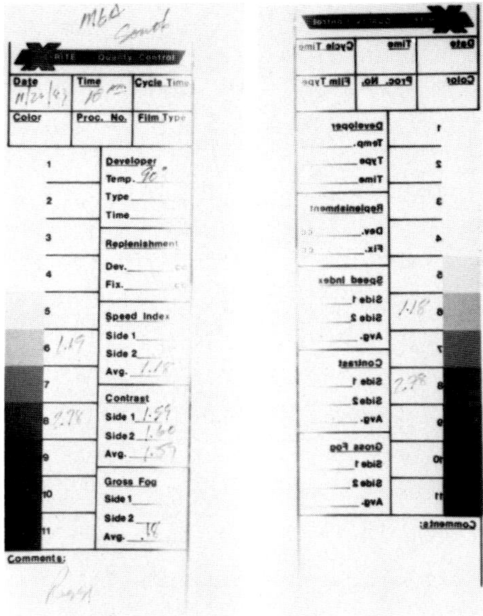

Fig. 42-7. Sensitometric control strip. Both sides of the control film emulsion are sensitometrically exposed. The densitometer measurements of both sides are averaged and recorded on the control strip.

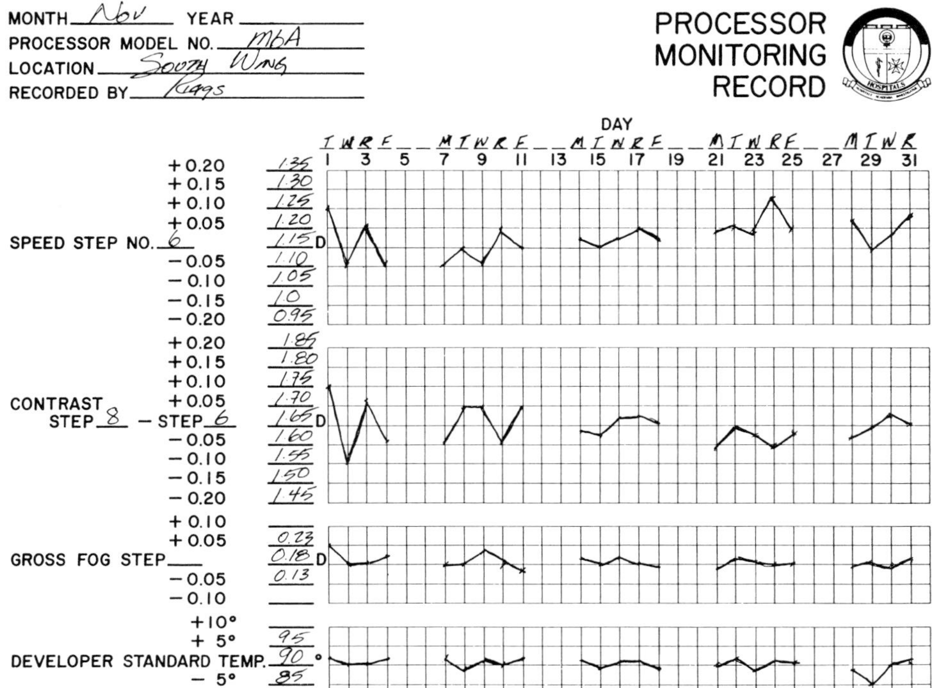

Fig. 42-8. Typical processor control chart.

Radiographic x-ray units

Numerous radiographic x-ray unit parameters can be monitored. A few of the more basic tests are described here.

Beam alignment and beam/light field congruence. This test is designed to check the centering and perpendicularity of the beam, as well as the *congruence* or the *alignment* of the collimator light field and the x-ray beam field. This is an important test since a great deal of unproductive radiation can be delivered to the patient if the system is misaligned. One tool designed to test these parameters is shown in Fig. 42-9. Light field/x-ray beam alignment is measured by exposing the collimator template. Beam alignment and perpendicularity is assessed by the plastic cylinder, which has a small metallic bead enclosed in each end. The cylinder is centered to the template and exposed. These tests are usually performed on the tabletop and can be used to test both the manual and automatic collimator modes. Beam/light field alignment should be within ± 2% of the SID. Beam perpendicularity is acceptable if both beads are protected within the center ring (Fig. 42-10).

Fig. 42-9. Beam perpendicularity and beam/light field alignment test tools.

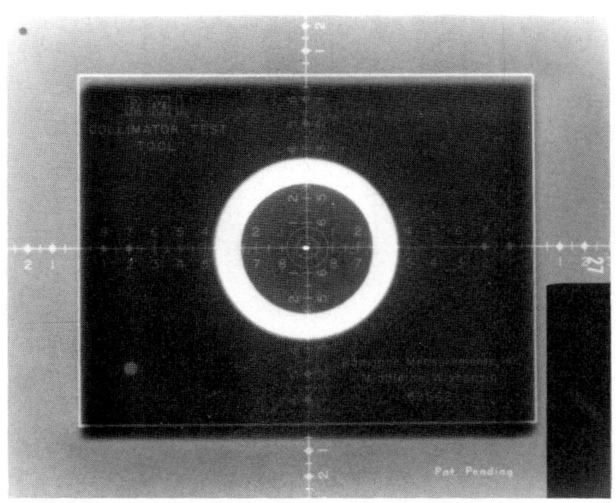

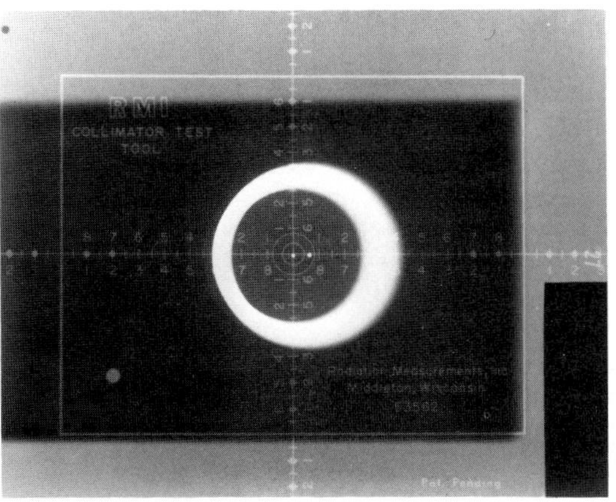

Fig. 42-10. **A,** Acceptable beam perpendicularity and beam/light field alignment. **B,** Unacceptable beam perpendicularity *(arrow)* and beam/light field alignment *(arrowheads).*

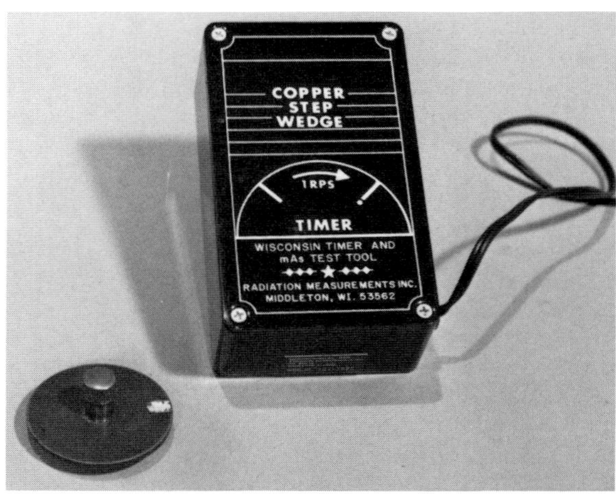

Fig. 42-11. Spinning top (left) and RMI motorized synchronous top (right).

Exposure time. This test determines if the x-ray unit is delivering the same time of exposure as indicated by the control panel's radiographic exposure time. A manually operated spinning top is appropriate for single-phase generators but three-phase generators require a motorized synchronous top (Fig. 42-11). The radiopaque face of the synchronous motor device contains a radius slit aperture. An exposure is made of the rotating top. As the slit rotates, it allows radiation to pass, producing an arc of density on the radiograph. By measuring the angle of arc, the time of exposure can be calculated and compared to the time selected on the control panel. This calculation is simplified by using a template to determine the actual exposure time as shown in Fig. 42-12.

A

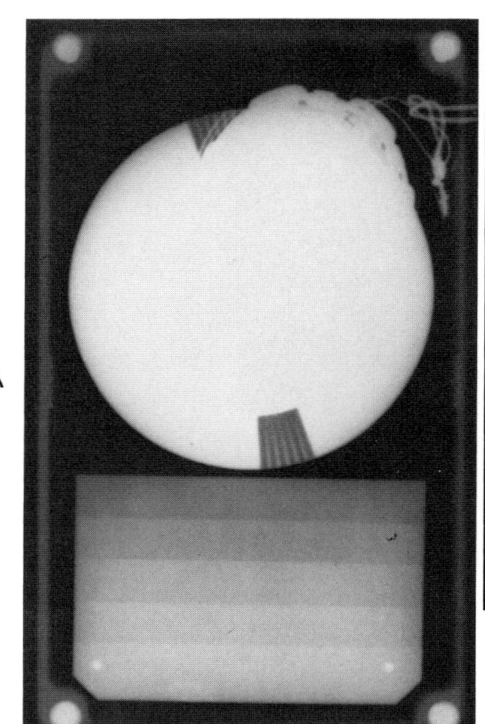

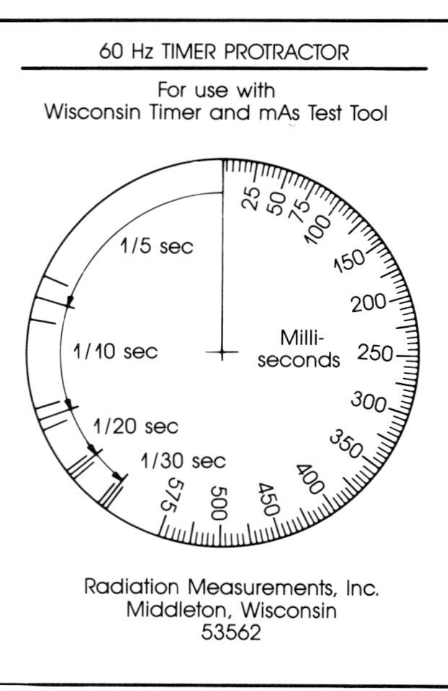

B

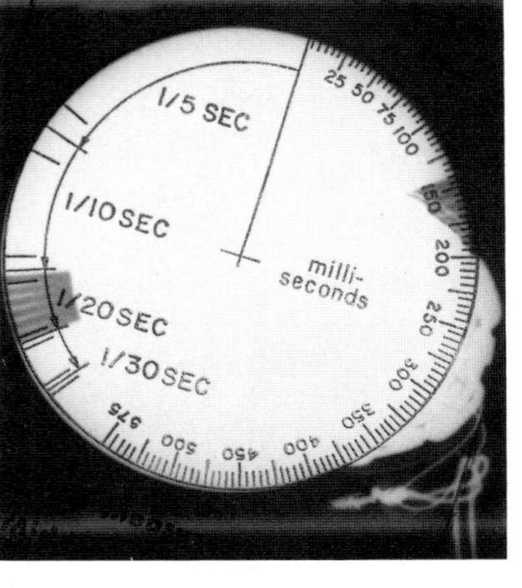

C

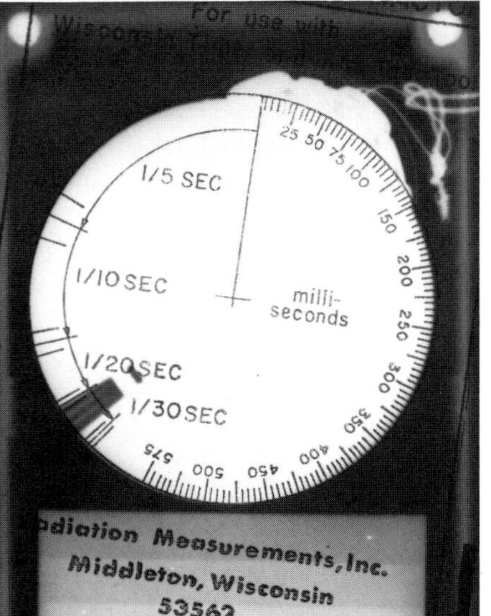

D

Fig. 42-12. A, Radiograph produced at 200 mA and 1/20-second exposure. **B,** RMI protractor template. **C,** Radiograph A with template showing acceptable results for a 1/20-second exposure. **D,** Radiograph produced at 300 mA and 1/30-second showing unacceptable results.

Beam quality. The quality of the primary x-ray beam refers to the energy of the x-ray photons that comprise it and is generally described by the *half-value layer (HVL)*. The HVL is a measurement of the x-ray beam quality or average energy. It is an indication of the total *equivalent* filtration in the path of the x-ray beam (it is not a direct measure of the total filtration). Total equivalent filtration includes the filtration properties of the x-ray glass envelope, the mirror and plastic underside of the collimator, and any added filtration at the port of the x-ray tube. Added filtration is used to increase the *beam hardness,* or average beam energy, by removing more low than high energy photons from the beam. This is an important radiation protection consideration, since low-energy x-ray photons are absorbed more readily by the patient. The *beam quality* test verifies that the beam's HVL is sufficient to reduce the patient's exposure to low-energy radiation. The HVL is determined by plotting the thickness of aluminum *attenuators* (Fig. 42-13, *A*) that are added to the beam versus the resultant exposures that are measured with a dosimeter (Fig. 42-13, *B*). The acceptable HVL for an 80 kVp beam is 2.3 mm of aluminum. An HVL less than this indicates that the total filtration of the beam must be increased (Fig. 42-13, *C*), assuming that the kVp is accurate. Inaccurate HVL values may also indicate inaccurate kVp calibration or tube problems.

A

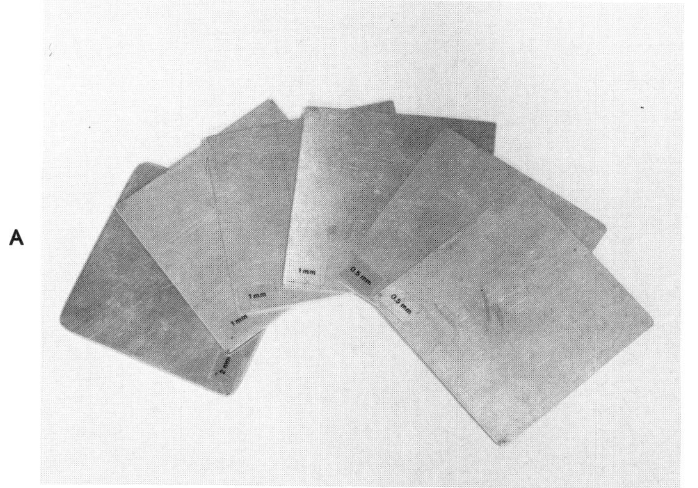

B

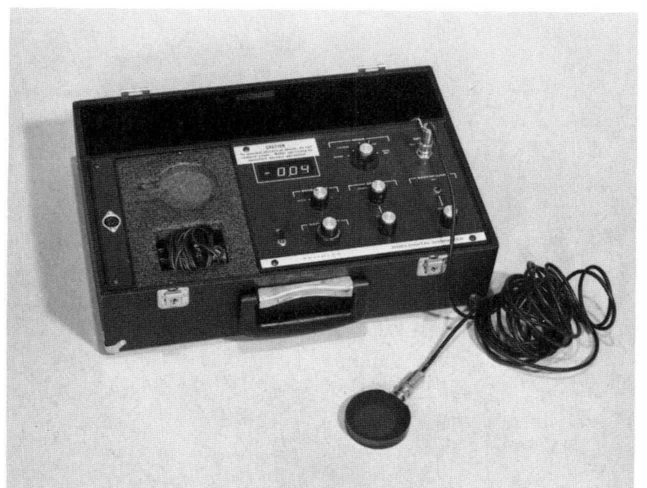

mmAl	X^1_{mR}	X^2_{mR}	X^3_{mR}	$\bar{X}_{mR}$	100 mR/mAs
0	455	454	455	454.6	4546
1	363	360	362	361.6	3.616
2	296	297	296	296.3	2.963
3	247	248	248	247.6	2.476
4	207	209	208	2080	2.08
5	178	179	178	1783	1.783

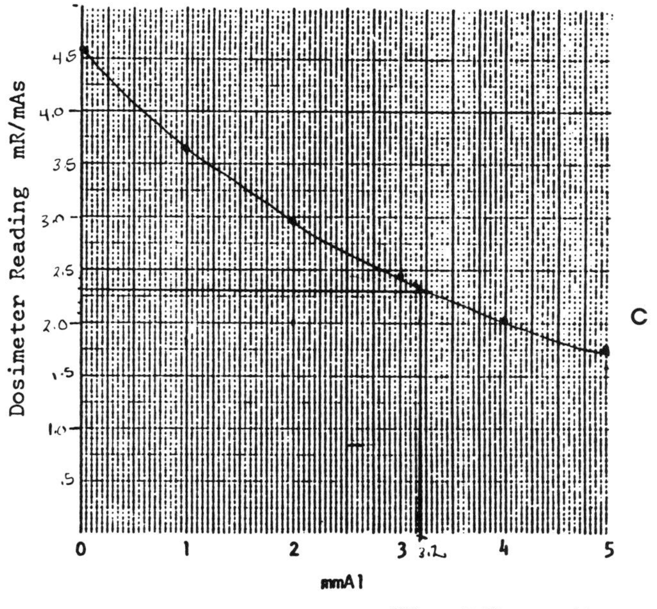

C

Fig. 42-13. A, Set of aluminum attenuators of various thicknesses. **B,** Digital dosimeter used to measure exposure output. **C,** HVL layer is calculated by plotting the average output of exposure in mR/mAs versus thickness of added A1 attenuator. Graph shows acceptable results.

kVp. The maximum or peak electrical potential (kVp) across the x-ray tube affects the radiation intensity reaching the image receptor and the subject contrast of the final image. Radiographic density and contrast can be adversely affected by inaccurate kVp calibration. One device used to test the accuracy of kVp settings is the kVp test cassette (Fig. 42-14, *A*). The cassette works on the principle that kVp can be determined by the amount of attenuation that occurs in a filtered beam. The specially designed cassette contains a copper filter, a series of *stepwedges*, and an optical attenuator built into the cassette. The cassette works on the principle that the effective kVp defines the step of the wedge that attenuates the radiation equal to the attenuation of the intensifying screen light by the optical attenuator. The attenuation effects are recorded as radiographic densities on film that has been exposed in the cassette at a given kVp setting (Fig. 42-14, *B*). By matching the step density produced by the stepwedge attenuator to the density produced by the optical attenuator the effective kVp can be determined from a calibration curve supplied with the cassette. The measured effective kVp should be within ±4 kVp of the kVp setting tested.

Exposure reproducibility and linearity. Predictable radiographic exposures are essential for consistent radiographic images. The test for *exposure reproducibility* (repeatability) determines whether the same results are attained every time the same technique factors are used. *Linearity* (reciprocity) tests are done to determine that the same exposure is obtained at a given milliampere-second selection, without regard to the combination of milliampere and exposure time selections chosen to achieve the milliampere-second setting. The reproducibility/linearity test can be accomplished qualitatively by repeatedly exposing a stepwedge with the same mA/exposure time combination to determine the exposure reproducibility. To test for exposure linearity the stepwedge should be repeatedly exposed using the same total mAs but in different mA/exposure time combinations. By matching the radiographic densities of the stepwedge images, the accuracy of the parameters can be evaluated (Fig. 42-15). A dosimeter (Fig. 42-13, *B*) can also be used to record the output of the exposures that are compared quantitatively to determine their accuracy. A x-ray unit should produce reproducible exposures to within 5% of their average. Exposure linearity should not exceed 10%.

Focal spot size. The recorded detail in a radiographic image is partially dependent on the size of the x-ray tube's focal spot. As the size of the focal spot increases, the ability to define small structures is diminished. In addition, a change in focal spot size over time may be symptomatic of the x-ray tube's deterioration. An easy test to determine the effective spot size of a tube is to evaluate its resolving capability. A *resolution* test pattern (Fig. 42-16, *A*), which is comprised of groups of different sized bar patterns (line pairs), is radiographed using a direct exposure technique (Fig. 42-16, *B*). The radiograph of the test pattern is evaluated to determine the smallest group of line pairs that can be seen clearly (Fig. 42-16, *C*, and 42-16, *D*). Tables are available that equate the effective focal spot size to the smallest pattern resolved. The star test pattern is another type of resolution test pattern that is often used. This pattern provides more accurate information but is more difficult to use.

A

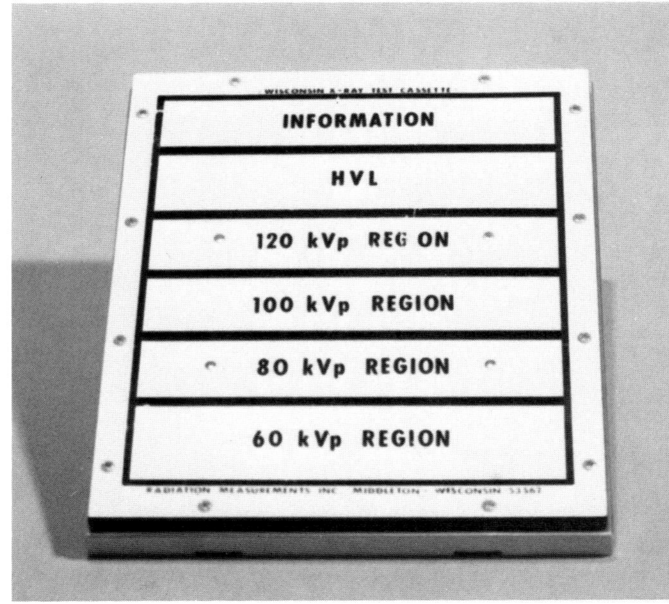

B

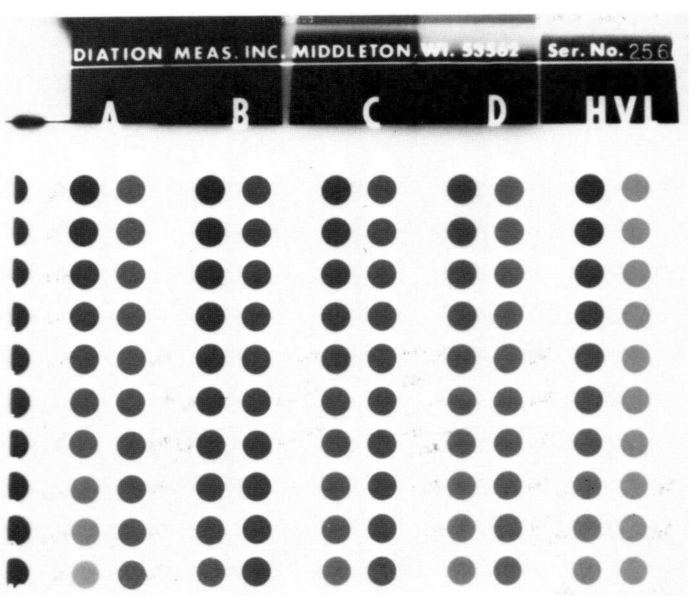

Fig. 42-14. A, RMI 8 × 10 in kVp test cassette. Can be used to measure the accuracy of 60, 80, 100, and 120 kVp settings. Cassette can also be used to measure HVL. **B,** kVp test radiograph. By measuring the densities of the adjacent dots with a densitometer, an accuracy of ±2 kVp can be achieved.

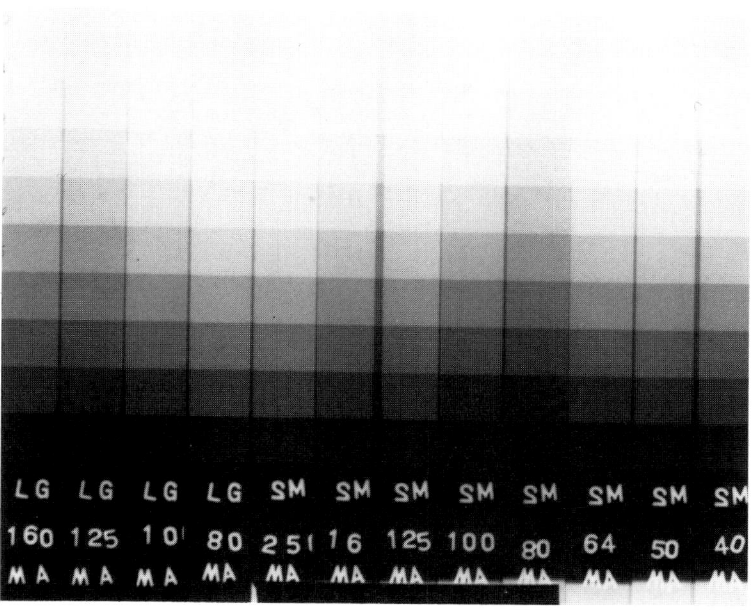

Fig. 42-15. Stepwedge exposures of various mA/time combinations, can be used to check linearity. Density should not vary more than one step between exposures.

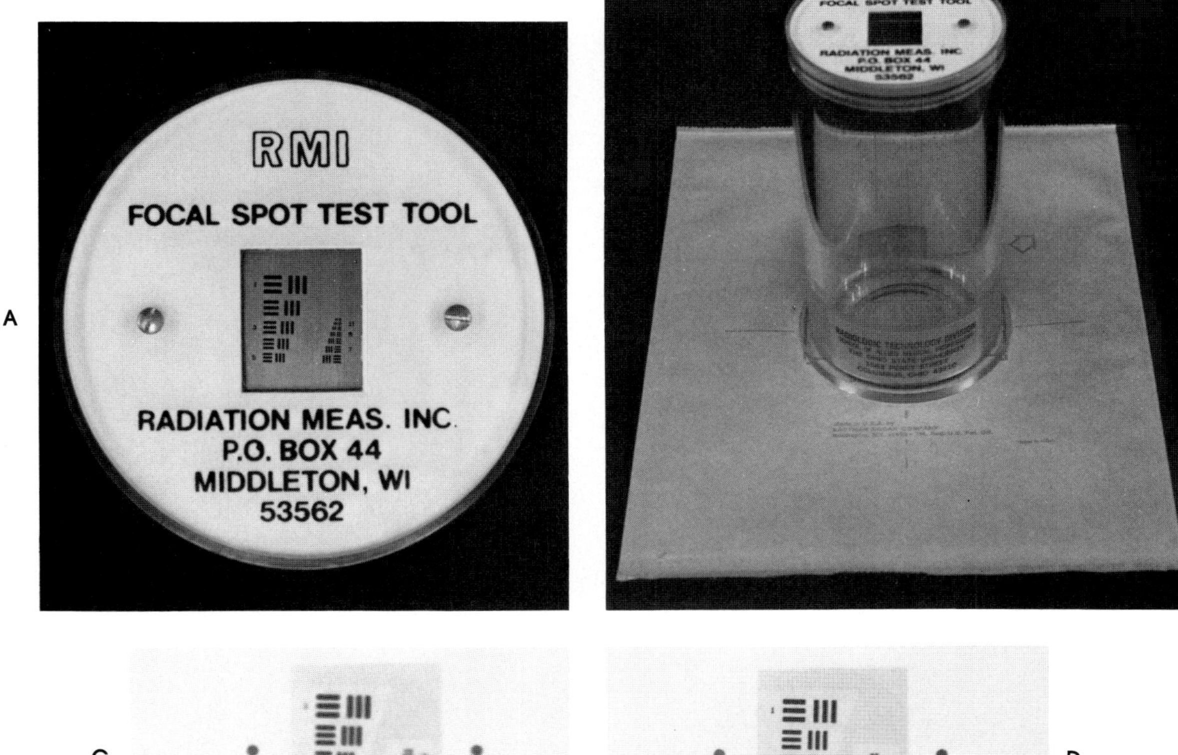

Fig. 42-16. A, RMI resolution test pattern used to measure focal spot size. **B,** Set-up of focal spot test tool. **C,** Test results on a large focal spot, showing the effective size to be 1.4 mm. **D,** Test results on a small focal spot, showing the effective size to be 0.6 mm.

Image receptors

The image receptor most commonly used in diagnostic radiology is a cassette containing intensifying screens and radiographic film. The cassette is a rigid, lightproof holder that compresses the screens and film together when closed. The care and condition of the image receptor have a direct bearing on radiographic image quality.

Cassettes: Loss of cassette integrity may produce unsharp or fogged radiographs. Cassettes should be physically inspected periodically for wearing of the latches and hinges, warping of the cassette frame, and deterioration of the foam or felt compression material. Testing for light leaks should also be a part of the inspection process. Cassettes should be repaired or replaced if they do not pass such inspections.

Intensifying screens: Dirty and worn intensifying screens can cause radiographic artifacts. It is important to visually inspect the screens for wear, abrasions, and stains and to clean them on a routine basis. Screens should be cleaned with a soft cloth and a recommended screen cleaner or a mild soap and water solution. The screens must be thoroughly dry before they are returned to service.

The speed (sensitivity) of similar intensifying screens may vary as they age or as new cassettes and screens are added to service. This lack of uniformity results in radiographic density variations. To test for screen-speed uniformity, use a reliable generator and the appropriate exposure technique to produce a radiographic density of approximately 1.5. Identify all the similar screened cassettes in service with lead markers, and expose each cassette using the same technique. Use a densitometer to measure the density of each of the radiographs and the measured density variation between the radiographs should not exceed ± 0.2.

Film-screen contact: Poor contact between the intensifying screens and the radiographic film reduces the contrast and recorded detail in the radiographic image. Radiographic cassettes should be periodically tested for poor film contact. A wire mesh test object is used for this purpose (Fig. 42-17, *A*). The wire mesh test object is placed on top of the cassette and radiographed. The radiographic image of the wire mesh should have a uniform radiographic density. Any areas that appear darker indicate poor contact (Fig. 42-17, *B* and *C*). Cassettes that exhibit areas of poor contact in the central portion of the cassette should be repaired or replaced.

A

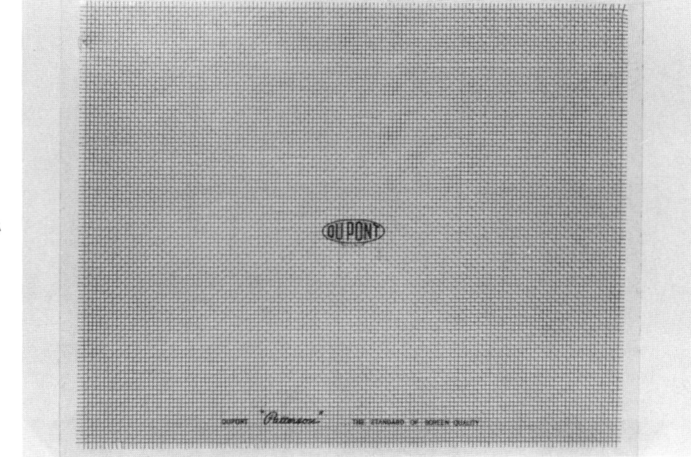

B

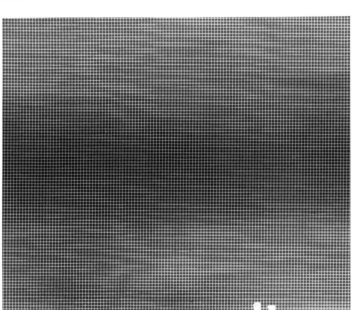

C

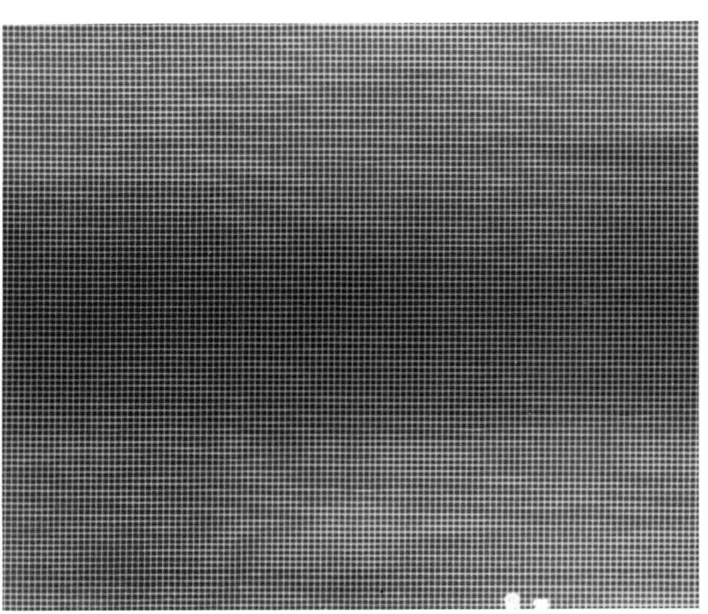

Fig. 42-17. A, Wire mesh test tool. **B,** Test radiograph exhibiting acceptable film screen contact. **C,** Test radiograph exhibiting unacceptable film screen contact.

Grids

Misaligned grids attenuate an increased portion of the primary radiation beam, resulting in increased patient radiation dose and a reduction in radiographic image quality. The loss of image quality caused by improper grid alignment can be subtle and is often attributed to other causes. A simple test to evaluate grid alignment requires radiographing a 14 × 17 inch homogeneous phantom, such as water, aluminum, or fiberboard. Expose the phantom crosswise on the radiographic table and place a 14 × 17 inch cassette crosswise in the Bucky tray. Select an exposure technique that will produce a radiographic density of approximately 1.5. A properly aligned grid will produce an even density across the radiograph. An uneven density indicates the need for corrective maintenance.

Illuminators

An important but often overlooked aspect of radiographic quality control is the evaluation of illuminator performance. Illuminator variations affect radiographic density and contrast. Illuminator output changes as the illuminator ages, and the output intensity is affected by the type of light source used. Illuminators with a reduced light intensity increase the density of the radiograph being viewed. Lack of uniformity between illuminators may cause radiographs to appear underexposed when using one illuminator and overexposed when using another, resulting in reduced contrast in both situations. A photographic or optical light meter can measure illuminator intensity and check for variation among illuminators. Gross mismatches should be corrected.

ADDITIONAL QUALITY CONTROL TESTS

The quality control tests previously described can be considered basic tests for monitoring the film processor and radiographic units. Similar quality control tests should be used to monitor fluoroscopic equipment and mobile radiographic units. Quality control tests are also designed for image intensifiers, tomographic equipment, automatic exposure control devices, computerized tomography systems, magnetic resonance imaging systems, and sonography units. Quality control should also be extended to include nuclear medicine and radiation therapy if such facilities exist.

Summary

Radiographic quality assurance programs can play a major role in the improvement of patient care, the reduction of unnecessary radiation to both personnel and patients, and the containment of costs of radiologic health care delivery. Although this chapter has dealt primarily with quality assurance in the context of the technical elements of the radiographic system, medical radiation personnel must remember that their responsibilities to the patient extend beyond the technical aspects of image production.

Definition of Terms

alignment Closeness of agreement of the centers and edges of the x-ray beam and collimator light fields.

attenuator Object that reduces the intensity of an x-ray beam.

base plus fog Density of unexposed processed radiographic film resulting from opacity of film base and density inherent to film emulsion.

beam hardening Increasing the mean energy of the x-ray beam spectrum by removal of the low-energy photons.

beam quality Energy of an x-ray beam.

congruence Closeness of agreement in position and size of x-ray beam and collimator light fields.

control strip Radiographic film that has been exposed by a sensitometer or radiation passing through a stepwedge.

densitometer A device used to measure the optical density of photographic film.

diagnostic radiology facility Any establishment using an x-ray system in procedures involving the radiation of the human body for the purpose of diagnosis or visualization.

exposure reproducibility The ability to obtain the same exposure from the same mAs over time.

half-value layer (HVL) Thickness of an absorber that will reduce the intensity of an x-ray beam by one half.

linearity The ability to obtain the same exposure for the same mAs, regardless of mA and exposure time used.

NCDRH National Center for Devices and Radiological Health, previously called the Bureau of Radiological Health (BRH).

objective Standards of image quality that relate to aspects that can be directly measured.

quality administration procedures Management procedures that provide for the organization of the quality assurance program.

quality assurance (QA) Planned and organized efforts within a diagnostic radiology facility to ensure the production of consistent optimal quality images with minimal radiation exposure and cost to the patient consumer.

quality assurance program A distinct organized structure designed to furnish quality assurance for a diagnostic radiology facility.

quality control (QC) Methods and procedures used in the testing and maintenance of the components of an x-ray system.

reject analysis The study of repeated radiographs to determine the cause for their being discarded.

resolution Ability to record separate images of small objects that are placed very close together.

sensitometer A device designed to give precise, reproducible, and graduated light exposures to photographic film.

stepwedge A device used to put a series of increasing exposures on a radiographic film when exposed by a radiographic beam.

subjective Standards of image quality that are expressed by feelings, perceptions, and thoughts of the observer rather than by direct measurement.

x-ray system The collection of components for the production, recording, and viewing of radiographic images.

SELECTED BIBLIOGRAPHY

Barber TC et al: Radiologic quality control manual, Reston, VA, 1984, Reston Publishing Co, Inc.

Basic quality control in diagnostic radiology. Report No 4, Chicago, 1978, American Association of Physicists in Medicine.

Burkhart RL: Diagnostic radiology quality assurance catalog. HEW Publication No (FDA) 77-8028. Washington, DC, 1977, US Dept of Health, Education and Welfare.

Burkhart RL: Diagnostic radiology quality assurance catalog: supplement. HEW Publication No (FDA) 78-8028. Washington, DC, 1978, US Dept of Health, Education and Welfare.

Burkhart RL: Quality assurance programs for diagnostic radiology facilities. HEW Publication No (FDA) 80-8110. Washington, DC, 1980. US Dept of Health, Education and Welfare.

Burkhart RL: Checklist for establishing a diagnostic radiology quality assurance program, HHS Publication No (FDA) 83-8219. Washington, DC, 1983, US Dept of Health and Human Services.

Burkhart RL: A basic quality assurance program for small diagnostic radiology facilities, HHS Publication No (FDA) 83-8218, Washington, DC, 1983, US Dept of Health and Human Services.

Carlton R: Establishing a total quality assurance program in diagnostic radiology, Radiol Technol 35:23-38, 1980.

Goldman LW: Analysis of retakes: understanding, managing and using an analysis of retakes program for quality assurance. HEW Publication No (FDA) 79-8097. Washington, DC, 1979, US Dept of Health, Education and Welfare.

Gray JE: Photographic quality assurance in diagnostic radiology, nuclear medicine, and radiation therapy, vol 1, The basic principles of daily photographic quality assurance. HEW Publication No (FDA) 76-8043. Washington, DC, 1976, US Dept of Health, Education and Welfare.

Gray JE: Photographic quality assurance in diagnostic radiology, nuclear medicine and radiation therapy, vol 2, Photographic processing, quality assurance and the evaluation of photographic materials. HEW Publication No (FDA) 77-8018. Washington, DC, 1977, US Dept of Health, Education and Welfare.

Gray JE et al: Quality control in diagnostic imaging, Baltimore, 1983, University Park Press.

Hendee WR et al: Quality assurance for radiographic x-ray units and associated equipment. HEW Publication No (FDA) 79-8094. Washington, DC, 1979, US Dept of Health, Education and Welfare.

Hendee WR et al: Quality assurance for fluoroscopic x-ray units and associated equipment. HEW Publication No (FDA) 80-8095, Washington, DC, 1980, US Dept of Health Education and Welfare.

Hendee WR et al: Quality assurance for conventional tomographic x-ray units. HEW Publication No (FDA) 80-8096. Washington, DC, 1980, US Dept of Health, Education and Welfare.

Lawrence DJ: A simple method of processor control, Med Radiogr Photogr 49(1):2-6, 1973.

McKinney WE: Radiographic processing and quality control, Philadelphia, 1988, JB Lippincott Co.

McLemore JM: Quality assurance in diagnostic radiology, Chicago, 1981, Year Book Medical Publishers Inc.

Nelson RE et al: Economic analysis of a comprehensive quality assurance program, Radiol Technol 49:129-134, 1977.

Noyes RS: The economics of quality assurance, RNM Mag 10(6):7-9, 24, 28, Dec. 1980.

Quality assurance programs for diagnostic radiology facilities, final recommendation, Federal Register 44:71728-71740, 1979.

Quality assurance in diagnostic radiology and nuclear medicine—the obvious decision. HHS Publication No (FDA) 81-8141. Washington, DC, 1981, US Dept of Health and Human Services.

Radiologic image quality (formerly QC News), Department of Medical Physics, Univ of Wisconsin, 1983, Madison, WI.

BIBLIOGRAPHY

AUTOTOMOGRAPHY

For bibliographic citations before 1964, please see the fifth edition of this atlas.

1977 Forman WH: Autotomography: a means of improving visualization of the upper cervical spine, Radiology 123:800-801, 1977.

1983 Doyle T and Tress B: Autotomography with metrizamide myelography: an aid to visualization of the cranio-cervical junction and cerebellar tonsils, Clin Radiol 34:401-403, 1983.

BRAIN AND SPINAL CORD

Myelography

For bibliographic citations before 1964, please see the fifth edition of this atlas.

1964 Crandall PH and Hanafee WN: Cervical spondylotic myelopathy studied by air myelography, AJR 92:1260-1269, 1964.

Di Chiro G and Fischer RL: Contrast radiography of the spinal cord, Arch Neurol 11:125-143, 1964.

1966 Epstein BS, and Epstein JA: Myelography utilizing image intensification fluoroscopy, cineradiography, and siphonage to remove the radiopaque, Med Radiogr Photogr 42:9-11, 1966.

Jacobson LH: A simple way to lower the shoulders in cervical myelography, Radiology 86:745, 1966.

Liliequist B: Gas myelography in the cervical region, Acta Radiol [Diagn] 4:79-92, 1966.

Lodin H: Two-needle oxygen myelography, Acta Radiol [Diagn] 4:62-64, 1966.

Rezende T: Double-contrast myelography, Acta Radiol [Diagn] 5:1104-1106, 1966.

Westberg G: Gas myelography and percutaneous puncture in the diagnosis of spinal cord cysts, Acta Radiol suppl:252, 1966.

Wilson G, et al: Comparison of gas and positive contrast in evaluation of cervical spondylosis, AJR 97:648-654, 1966.

1968 Ewart J: Epidural myelography, Radiography 34:93-97, 1968.

Shapiro R: Myelography, ed 2, Chicago, 1968, Year Book Medical Publishers, Inc.

Wende S and Beer K: The diagnostic value of gas myelography, AJR 104:213-218, 1968.

1969 Gilland O, et al: A cinemyelographic study of cerebrospinal fluid dynamics, AJR 106:369-375, 1969.

Jirout J: Pneumomyelography, Springfield, Ill, 1969, Charles C Thomas, Publisher.

Pribram HFW, et al: A simple biplane myelographic table, AJR 105:411-412, 1969.

Southworth LE, Jimenez JP and Goree JA: A practical approach to cervical air myelography, AJR 107:486-490, 1969.

Wendth AJ and Moriarty DJ: A simplified method for the rapid removal of myelographic contrast agent, Radiology 93:1092, 1969.

1970 Chin FK and Anderson WB: Improvements of root-sleeve filling in lumbar myelography with oil-soluble media, Radiology 96:668-669, 1970.

Kieffer SA, et al: Evaluation of dilute Pantopaque for large-volume myelography, Radiology 96:69-74, 1970.

1971 Bradac GB and Simon RS: Cervical air myelography—an improved technique, Fortschr Roentgenstr 115:73-78, 1971. (In German) Abstract: Radiology 102:489, 1972.

1972 Adams FG and Ward P: Value of lateral decubitus screening in myelography, Clin Radiol 23:427-433, 1972.

George AE and Kricheff II: A catheter technique for myelography, Radiology 104:435-436, 1972.

Haverling M: Transsacral puncture of the arachnoidal sac: an alternative procedure to lumbar puncture, Acta Radiol [Diagn] 12:1-6, 1972.

Heinz ER and Goldman RL: The role of gas myelography in neuroradiologic diagnosis, Radiology 102:629-634, 1972.

1973 Chynn KY: Painless myelography: introduction of a new aspiration cannula and review of 541 consecutive studies, Radiology 109:361-367, 1973.

Hayt DB: Remotely controlled myelography, AJR 118:677-681, 1973.

1974 Keirns M and Wiltse LL: Improved technique for injecting and removing Pantopaque in myelography, Clin Orthop 103:64-65, 1974.

Rice AC and Coyle GF: Oblique projections in cervical myelography, Radiology 113:216-218, 1974.

1975 Coin CG and Scanlan RL: Technique for internal auditory cisternography, Acta Radiol [Suppl] 347:53-57, 1975.

Novy S and Jensen KM: Filling defects and nonfilling of the internal auditory canal in posterior fossa myelography, AJR 124:265-270, 1975.

Peterson HO: The hazards of myelography, Radiology 115:237-239, 1975.

Skalpe IO and Amundsen P: Lumbar radiculography with metrizamide, a nonionic water-soluble contrast medium, Radiology 115:91-95, 1975.

1977 Boyd WR and Gardiner GA Jr: Metrizamide myelography, AJR 129:481-484, 1977.

Mosely J: The oil myelogram after operation for lumbar disc lesions, Clin Radiol 28:267-276, 1977.

Scher A and Vambeck V: An approach to the radiological evaluation of the cervicodorsal junction following injury, Clin Radiol 28:243-246, 1977.

1978 Deeb ZL, et al: Reduced morbidity in gas myelography, Neuroradiology 16:352-353, 1978.

Eldevik OP, Nakken KO and Haughton VM: The effect of dehydration on side effects of metrizamide myelography, Radiology 129:715-716, 1978.

Kieffer SA, et al: Contrast agents for myelography: clinical and radiological evaluation of Amipaque and Pantopaque, Radiology 129:695-705, 1978.

McClendon LK: Flying lateral technique for thoracic myelography, Radiol Technol 50:9-16, 1978.

McCormick CC: Radiology in low back pain and sciatica: an analysis of the relative efficacy of spinal venography, discography, and epidurography in patients with a negative or equivocal myelogram, Clin Radiol 29:393-406, 1978.

1979 Gelmers HJ: Adverse side effects of metrizamide in myelography, Neuroradiology 18:119-123, 1979.

Pilling JR: Water-soluble radiculography in the erect posture: a clinicoradiological study, Clin Radiol 30:665-670, 1979.

Rice JF and Bathia AL: Lateral C1-2 puncture for myelography: posterior approach, Radiology 132:760-762, 1979.

Schmidt RC: Cervical double contrast myelocisternography by the lateral approach, Neuroradiology 17:183-184, 1979.

1980 El Gammal T: Cervical myelography and posterior fossa examinations with Amipaque using magnification and subtraction, Radiology 136:219-222, 1980.

Taylor AJ, Haughton VM and Doust BD: CT imaging of the thoracic spinal cord without intrathecal contrast media, J Comput Assist Tomogr 4:223-224, 1980.

1981 Ahn HS, et al: Lumbar myelography with metrizamide: supplemental techniques, AJR 136:547-551, 1981.

Amundsen P: Cervical myelography with Amipaque: seven years experience, Radiologe 21:282-287, 1981.

Khan A, et al: Total myelography with metrizamide through the lumbar route, AJR 136:771-776, 1981.

Sykes RH, et al: Incidence of adverse effects following metrizamide myelography in nonambulatory and ambulatory patients, Radiology 138:625-627, 1981.

1982 Chrzanowski R: The contrast media used for myelography, Eur Neurol 21:194-197, 1982.

Drayer B, et al: Clinical trial of iopamidol for lumbar myelography, AJNR 3:59-64, 1982.

Hatten HP Jr: Routine cervical myelography with overhead oblique projections and Pantopaque, Spine 7:512-514, 1982.

Katevuo K and Kuuliala I: Lateral C1-C2 puncture: a technique to reduce adverse reactions in metrizamide sellar cisternography, Neuroradiology 24:43-44, 1982.

Lotz PR: Intracranial delivery of metrizamide from the lumbar subarachnoid space: prone versus supine positioning, J Comput Assist Tomogr 6:920-922, 1982.

Valk J: Lateral cervical, C1-C2, puncture in cervical myelography, Eur Neurol 21:175-180, 1982.

1983 Alenghat JP, Kim HS and Duda EE: Cervical and lumbar metrizamide myelography: split-dose technique, Radiology 149:852-853, 1983.

Bannon KR, et al: Comparison of radiographic quality and adverse reactions in myelography with iopamidol and metrizamide, AJNR 4:312-313, 1983.

Bockenheimer SA and Hillesheimer W: Clinical experience with iopamidol for myelography, AJNR 4:314-316, 1983.
Capek V, et al: Computed air myelography of the lumbosacral spine, AJNR 4:609-610, 1983.
Ericson K, Hindmarsh T and Hannerz J: Experience with iohexol in lumbar myelography, Acta Radiol 24:503-505, 1983.
Orrison WW, Eldevik OP and Sackett JF: Lateral C1-2 puncture for cervical myelography. Part III: Historical, anatomic, and technical considerations, Radiology 146:401-408, 1983.
Orrison WW, Sackett JF and Amundsen P: Lateral C1-2 puncture for cervical myelography. Part II: Recognition of improper injection of contrast material, Radiology 146:395-400, 1983.
Osborne D: Improved head support for prone myelographic and CT examinations, AJR 141:1025-1026, 1983.
Parks RE and Dublin AB: Residual myelographic contrast material seen on the chest radiograph, Radiology 148:617-620, 1983.
Skutta T, et al: Clinical trial of lotrol for lumbar myelography, AJNR 4:302-303, 1983.
Tan WS, et al: Computed air myelography of the lumbosacral spine, AJNR 4:609-610, 1983.
Teasdale E and Macpherson P: Incidence of side effects following direct puncture cervical myelography: bed rest versus normal mobility, Neuroradiology 25:85-86, 1983.
Virapongse C, Bhimani SM and Vliem C: Cervical metrizamide myelography via a C1-2 puncture for patients in a seated position, Radiology 149:854, 1983.
1984 Barmeir E, et al: Prone computed tomography metrizamide myelography: a technique for improved diagnosis of lumbar disc herniation, Clin Radiol 35:479-481, 1984.
Daniels DL, et al: Cervical radiculopathy: computed tomography and myelography compared, Radiology 151:109-113, 1984.
Gabrielsen TO, et al: Iohexol versus metrizamide for lumbar myelography: double-blind trial, AJR 142:1047-1049, 1984.
Shapiro R: Myelography, Chicago, 1984, Year Book Medical Publishers, Inc.
Teasdale E and Macpherson P: Guidelines for cervical myelography: lumbar versus cervical puncture, Br J Radiol 57:789-793, 1984.
1985 Laasonen EM: Iohexol and metrizamide in lumbar myelography: comparison of side effects, Acta Radiol [Diagn] (Stockh) 26:761-765, 1985.
Macpherson P and Teasdale E: Routine bed rest is unnecessary after cervical myelography, Neuroradiology 27:214-216, 1985.
Nakstad P, et al: Functional cervical myelography with iohexol, Neuroradiology 27:220-225, 1985.
Petras AF, Westmoreland LH and Sobel DF: Simplified cervical metrizamide myelography: decubitus approach, Spine 10:860-862, 1985.
1986 Burt TB, et al: Dural infolding during C1-2 myelography, Radiology 158:546-547, 1986.
Coolens D, et al: Cervical myelography and the lateral approach on a conventional examination table, J Belge Radiol 69:163-165, 1986.
Crane R and Margolis MT: Use of sitting position to relieve myelographic obstruction, AJNR 7:502-503, 1986.
Lilleas F, Bach Gansmo T and Weber H: Lumbar myelography with Omnipaque (iohexol), Neuroradiology 28:344-346, 1986.
Numaguchi Y, et al: Myelography with metrizamide: effect of contrast removal on side effects, AJNR 7:498-501, 1986.
Peeters F: Myelography using iohexol (Omnipaque), Diagn Imaging Clin Med 55:348-351, 1986.
Reicher MA, et al: The push-up view: a superior cross-table lateral projection for cervical myelography, AJNR 7:899-900, 1986.
1987 Hodges SD and Berasi CC: Complications of myelography after partial metrizamide withdrawal, Spine 12:53-55, 1987.
Raininko R and Sonninen P: Dorsal CSF space at CI-II level: technique of cervical myelography, Neuroradiology 29:73-75, 1987.
Valenti RM: Lumber myelography: contrast agents used in the past, present, and future, Radiol Technol 58(6):493-496, 1987.
Wright CJ: Epidurography, Radiography 53:131-132, 1987.
1988 Minken TJ and Ahlgren P: Cross-table cervical myelography: a technique to improve visualization, AJNR 9:874, 1988.

DISKOGRAPHY

For bibliographic citations before 1964, please see the fifth edition of this atlas.

1964 Feinberg SB: The place of diskography in radiology as based on 2,320 cases, AJR 92:1275-1281, 1964.
Schaerer JP: Cervical discography, J Int Surg 42:287-296, 1964.
1966 Butt WP: Discography: some interesting cases, J Can Assoc Radiol 17:167-175, 1966.
1967 Edholm P, Fernström I and Lindblom K: Extradural lumbar disk puncture, Acta Radiol [Diagn] 6:322-328, 1967.
Grote W and Wappenschmidt J: Ueber Technik and Indikation zur zervikalen Diskographie, Fortschr Roentgenstr 106:721-727, 1967.
1969 Jirout J: Pneumographic examination of lumbar disc lesions: a new method, Acta Radiol [Diagn] 9:727-732, 1969.
1971 Raynor RB: Discography and myelography in acute injuries of the cervical spine, J Neurosurg 35:529-535, 1971.
1975 Collins HR: An evaluation of cervical and lumbar discography, Clin Orthop 107:133-138, 1975.
Jacobs GB, Pillone PR and Mazzola R: Lumbar discography in the diagnosis of herniated disks, Int Surg 60:6-9, 1975.
1978 McCormick CC: Radiology in low back pain and sciatica: an analysis of the relative efficacy of spinal venography, discography, and epidurography in patients with a negative or equivocal myelogram, Clin Radiol 29:393-406, 1978.
1981 Mosley GT: Technical considerations of epidural venography, Radiol Technol 52:371-374, 1981.
1982 Landherr EJ and Smigiel MR, Jr: New concepts in diagnosis and treatment of back ailments in the elderly, Surg Clin North Am 62:291-295, 1982.
Raininko R and Torma T: Contrast enhancement around a prolapsed disk, Neuroradiology 24:49-51, 1982.
1983 Hartjes H, et al: Cervical disk syndromes: value of metrizamide myelography and diskography, AJNR 4:644-645, 1983.
Quinnell RC and Stockdale: Flexion and extension radiograph of the lumbar spine: a comparison with lumbar discography, Clin Radiol 34:405-411, 1983.
1987 Matsui H, et al: Significance of tangential views in lumbar discography, Clin Orthop 165-171, 1987.
1988 Buirski G and Watt I: Dynamic CT discography: an evaluation of a new technique, Australas Radiol 32:197-202, 1988.

STEREOTACTIC SURGERY

For bibliographic citations before 1964, please see the fifth edition of this atlas.

1965 Cobble SP and Brackett CE: Changes in the ventricular size during stereotaxic surgery, AJR 95:890-898, 1965.
1967 Dobben GD, Mullan S and Moseley RD: A new biplane neuroradiologic localizing instrument, Radiology 89:329-331, 1967.
1968 Fox JL and Green RC: Stereotaxic brain surgery. I. A geometric consideration of polar coordinates and polar range findings, Acta Neurochir 18:57-67, 1968.
Fox JL and Green RC: Stereotaxic brain surgery. II. Description of a method using biplane television guidance, Acta Neurochir 18:171-185, 1968.
1969 Ecker A and Perl T: Selective Gasserian injection for tic douloureaux; technical advances and results, Acta Radiol [Diagn] 9:38-48, 1969.
Fox JL and Green RC: A new method of stereotaxis, Radiology 92:259-264, 1969.
Grabow JD: Value of roentgenology in electrode placement techniques in electroencephalography, Acta Radiol [Diagn] 9:54-57, 1969.
Hodges PC and Garcia-Bengochea F: Precise alignment of x-ray beams for stereotactic surgery, AJR 105:260-269, 1969.

Rand RW, et al: Stereotaxic transsphenoidal biopsy and cryosurgery of pituitary tumors, AJR 105:273-286, 1969.
Todd EM and Crue BL: An image enlargement scale for stereotactic surgery, AJR 105:270-272, 1969.
1970 Fox JL: The central x-ray beam in stereotaxis, AJR 110:166-169, 1970.
1971 Dawson BH, Dervin E and Heywood OB: Some radiographic problems encountered in stereotactic surgery, Radiography 37:131-139, 1971.
1972 Leksell L: Stereotaxis and radiosurgery, Springfield, Ill, 1972, Charles C Thomas, Publisher.
1975 Yoshida T, et al: Stereotactic operations with the help of a skull x-ray apparatus, Confin Neurol 37:291-295, 1975.
1979 Brown RA: A computerized tomography–computer graphics approach to stereotaxic localization, J Neurosurg 50:715-720, 1979.
1980 Bergstrom M, Greitz T and Steiner L: An approach to stereotaxic radiography, Acta Neurochir 54:157-165, 1980.
Boethius J, et al: CT localization of stereotactic surgery, Appl Neurophysiol 43:164-169, 1980.
Perry JH, et al: Computed tomography/guided stereotactic surgery: conception and development of a new stereotactic methodology, Neurosurgery 7:376-381, 1980.
1981 Colombo F, et al: A new method for utilizing CT data in stereotactic surgery: measurement and transformation technique, Acta Neurochir (Wien) 57:195-203, 1981.
1982 Lunsford LD, Rosenbaum AE and Perry J: Stereotactic surgery using the "therapeutic" CT scanner, Surg Neurol 18:116-122, 1982.
Rhodes ML, et al: Stereotactic neurosurgery using 3-D image data from computed tomography, J Med Syst 6:105-119, 1982.
1983 Gildenberg PL: Stereotactic neurosurgery and computerized tomographic scanning, Appl Neurophysiol 46:170-179, 1983.
Giorgi C, et al: Neuroanatomical digital image processing in CT-guided stereotactic operations, Appl Neurophysiol 46:236-239, 1983.
Hardy TL, Koch J and Lassiter A: Computer graphics with computerized tomography for functional neurosurgery, Appl Neurophysiol 46:217-226, 1983.
Levy WJ: Simple plastic stereotactic unit for use in the computed tomographic scanner, Neurosurgery 13:182-185, 1983.
Lunsford LD, Leksell L and Jernberg B: Probe holder for stereotactic surgery in the CT scanner: a technical note, Acta Neurochir (Wien) 69:297-304, 1983.
Olivier A and Bertrand G: A new head clamp for stereotactic and intracranial procedures, Appl Neurophysiol 46:272-275, 1983.
1984 Alker G and Kelly PJ: An overview of CT based stereotactic systems for the localization of intracranial lesions, Comput Radiol 8(4):193-196, 1984.
Lunsford LD and Martinez AJ: Stereotactic exploration of the brain in the era of computed tomography, Surg Neurol 22:222-230, 1984.
1985 Fox PT, Perlmutter JS and Raichle ME: A stereotactic method of anatomical localization for positron emission tomography, J Comput Assist Tomogr 9(1):141-153, 1985.
Iseki H, et al: A new apparatus for CT-guided stereotactic surgery, Appl Neurophysiol 48(1-6):50-60, 1985.
1986 Bergstrom M, Greitz T and Ribbe T: A method of stereotaxic localization adopted for conventional and digital radiography, Neuroradiology 28(2):100-104, 1986.
Engle DJ, Lunsford LD and Panichelli T: Rigid head fixation for intraoperative computed tomography, Neurosurgery 19(2):258-262, 1986.
Lunsford LD, Martinez AJ and Latchaw RE: Stereotaxic surgery with a magnetic resonance and computerized tomography compatible system, J Neurosurg 64(6):872-878, 1986.
Patil AA and Woosley RE: Scalp marking of intracranial lesions using computed tomography (CT) images: a technical note, Acta Neurochir (Wien) 80(1-2):62-64, 1986.
1987 Watanabe E et al: Three dimensional digitizer (neuronavigator): new equipment for computed tomography–guided stereotaxic surgery, Surg Neurol 27(6):543-547, 1987.
1988 Griffin BR, et al: Stereotactic neutron radiosurgery for arteriovenous malformations of the brain, Med Dosim 13(4):179-182, 1988.
Jenny AB, et al: The computer and stereotactic surgery in neurological surgery, Comput Med Imaging Graph 12(1):75-83, 1988.
Moringlane JR, Lippitz B and Ostertag CB: Cerebral angiography under stereotactic conditions: technical note, Acta Neurochir (Wien) 91(3-4):147-150, 1988.
Redmond MJ, Saines NS and Coroneos M: The use of computed tomographic directed stereotaxis in the diagnosis of intracerebral lesions, Med J Aust 149(9):468-472, 1988.
Rossitch E Jr, et al: The use of computed tomography guided stereotactic techniques in the treatment of brainstem abscesses, Clin Neurol Neurosurg 90(4):365-368, 1988.
1989 Gower DJ: Image guided stereotaxic surgery, J Okla State Med Assoc 82(6):265-268, 1989.
Hardy TL: A method for MRI and CT mapping of diencephalic somatotopography, Stereotact Funct Neurosurg 52(2-4):242-249, 1989.
Heifetz MD, et al: Rapid method for determination of isocenter of radiation gantry and alignment of laser beams for stereotactic radiosurgery, Stereotact Funct Neurosurg 53(1):46-48, 1989.
Loeffler JS, et al: Stereotactic radiosurgery for intracranial arteriovenous malformations using a standard linear accelerator, Int J Radiat Oncol Biol Phys 17(3):673-677, 1989.
Phillips MH: Heavy charged particle stereotactic radiosurgery: cerebral angiography and CT in the treatment of intracranial vascular malformation, Int J Radiat Oncol Biol Phys 17(2):419-426, 1989.
Podgorsak EB, et al: Radiosurgery with high energy photon beams: a comparison among techniques, Int J Radiat Oncol Biol Phys 16(3):857-865, 1989.

Cerebral pneumography

For bibliographic citations before 1964, please see the fifth edition of this atlas.

1964 Alker LM: Radiography of the cerebral ventricles, Radiol Technol 35:259-266, 1964.
Diaz A and Parera CE: Radiography of the skull and brain, Wilmington, Del., 1964, EI du Pont de Nemours & Co.
Gianturco C and Miller GA: Tilt-table encephalography, Radiology 83:46-47, 1964.
Paris A: Intra-cranial investigation with the use of contrast media, Radiography 30:192-203, 1964.
Potts DG and Tavaras JM: A new somersaulting chair for cerebral pneumography, AJR 91:1144-1149, 1964.
1965 New PFJ and Webster EW: Physical and anatomical considerations in autotomography, Acta Radiol [Diagn] 3:370-384, 1965.
Potts DG: A new universal head unit, AJR 95:957-961, 1965.
1968 Fredzell G, et al: Mimer III and rotating chair, Acta Radiol [Diagn] 7:543-552, 1968.
Kieffer SA, Amplatz K and Peterson HO: Single-sweep rotation tomography in coronal and lateral planes: its value in pneumoencephalographic diagnosis, Radiology 91:372-376, 1968.
Sigueira EB, Bucy PC and Cannon AH: Positive contrast ventriculography, cisternography and myelography, AJR 104:132-138, 1968.
Stitt HL, et al: Pontocerebellar cisternography, Radiology 90:942-945, 1968.
1969 Alberti J, Andrews J and Wilson G: Posterior fossa tomography during encephalography, Acta Radiol [Diagn] 9:128-131, 1969.
Campbell CB: The value of autotomography in the demonstration of the midline ventricular system of the brain, Radiol Technol 41:65-73, 1969.
Gvozdanović V: The somersault technique in encephalography and ventriculography, Acta Radiol [Diagn] 9:160-166, 1969.

Wilkinson HA: Selective third ventricular catheterization for Pantopaque ventriculography, AJR 105:348-351, 1969.

1970 Baker HL: Pneumoencephalography: a challenge in technique, Semin Roentgenol 5:126-137, 1970.

Geilfuss CJ and Hargest TS: A modification of the Amplatz pneumographic chair for better head stabilization, Radiology 97:685-686, 1970.

Lang EK and Russell JR: Pantopaque ventriculography: demonstration and assessment of the third ventricle and posterior fossa, J Neurosurg 32:5-15, 1970.

Picaza JA, Hunter SE and Cannon BW: Axial ventriculography, J Neurosurg 33:297-303, 1970.

Pribram HFW: X-ray equipment, Semin Roentgenol 5:122-125, 1970.

1973 Morris L and Wylie IG: Tomography in cerebral pneumoencephalography, Clin Radiol 24:221-230, 1973.

White YS, Bell DS and Mellick R: Sequelae to pneumoencephalography, J Neurol Neurosurg Psychiatry 36:146-151, 1973.

1978 Swalingam S, et al: Computer assisted ventriculography, J Comput Assist Tomogr 2:162-164, 1978.

1979 Quencer RM, et al: Lateral decubitus pneumoencephalography: angiography for localizing atrial and para-atrial vascular lesions, AJR 132:617-622, 1979.

1980 Bentson JR, et al: Combined gas cisternography and edge-enhanced computed tomography of the internal auditory canal, Radiology 136:777-779, 1980.

Kricheff II, et al: Air-CT cisternography and canalography for small acoustic neuromas, AJNR 1:57-63, 1980.

Savolaine ER and Gerber AM: Need for complementary use of air ventriculography and computerized tomographic scanning in infected hydrocephalus, Neurosurgery 6:96-98, 1980.

1982 Anderson R, et al: CT air-contrast scanning of the internal auditory canal, Ann Otol Rhinol Laryngol 91:501-505, 1982.

1983 Robertson HJ, Hatten HP Jr and Keating JW: False-positive CT gas cisternogram, AJNR 4:474-477, 1983.

Ruggiero G and Manfredini M: Focused encephalography, AJNR 4:767-769, 1983.

1984 Johnson DW: Air cisternography of the cerebellopontine angle using high-resolution computed tomography, Radiology 151:401-403, 1984.

Solti-Bohman LG, et al: Gas-CT cisternography for detection of small acoustic nerve tumors, Radiology 150:403-407, 1984.

Cerebral angiography

For bibliographic citations before 1964, please see the fifth edition of this atlas.

1964 Diaz A and Parera CE: Radiography of the skull and brain, Wilmington, Del, 1964, EI du Pont de Nemours & Co.

Goree JA, et al: Percutaneous retrograde brachial angiography in the diagnosis of acoustic neurinoma, AJR 92:829-835, 1964.

Paris A: Intracranial investigation with the use of contrast media, Radiography 30:192-203, 1964.

Shenkin HA, et al: Value of routine urography during cerebral angiography, JAMA 187:207-211, 1964.

1965 Baird RM, et al: Percutaneous retrograde brachial arteriography, AJR 94:19-29, 1965.

Du Boulay GH and Jackson DC: Cranial angiotomography, Clin Radiol 16:148-153, 1965.

Hanafee W, et al: Venography of the cavernous sinus, orbital veins, and basal venous plexus, Radiology 84:751-753, 1965.

Liliequist B and Hellström L: Technique of aortocervical angiography, Acta Radiol [Diagn] 3:17-29, 1965.

Marshall TR and Ling JT: Carotid-vertebral and cerebral arteriography, J Ky Med Assoc 63:265-269, 1965.

1966 Morris L: Angiographic demonstration of the circle of Willis, Acta Radiol [Diagn] 5:424-427, 1966.

Weibel J and Fields WS: Angiography of the posterior cervicocranial circulation, AJR 98:660-671, 1966.

1967 Koch RL, Bieber WP and Hill MC: The hanging head position for detection of site of internal carotid artery occlusion, AJR 101:111-115, 1967.

Liliequist B: Capillary phase in cerebral angiography, Acta Radiol [Diagn] 6:113-125, 1967.

Rabinov K and Lavender P: The coronal tangential view for the demonstration of extracerebral hematomas, AJR 101:107-110, 1967.

1968 Leeds NE, et al: Serial magnification cerebral angiography, Radiology 90:1171-1175, 1968.

1969 Lee KF: A new head positioning device for cerebral angiography and pneumoencephalography, AJR 106:440-441, 1969.

1970 Morris L: A lateral oblique view in cerebral angiography, Radiology 96:61-65, 1970.

Sones PJ, Hoffman J and Brylski JR: Epidural subtemporal hematoma: angiographic changes involving the meningeal artery, AJR 108:756-761, 1970.

1971 Baker HL: The clinical usefulness of magnification cerebral angiography, Radiology 98:587-594, 1971.

Glickman MG, Gletne JS and Mainzer F: The basal projection in cerebral angiography, Radiology 98:611-618, 1971.

Goldman RL and Heinz ER: Technique of cerebral angiography, Semin Roentgenol 6:7-13, 1971.

Lee KF and Lin SR: An improved technique in orbital venography with the use of Innovar and compression devices, AJR 112:339-341, 1971.

Pochaczevsky R and Levine S: Skull immobilizer and positioner, AJR 112:408-410, 1971.

Smith JT, et al: Cerebral angioautotomography, AJR 112:315-323, 1971.

Wende S, Schindler K and Moritz G: The diagnostic value of the angiographic magnification technique with small focal spot tubes in two planes, Radiologe 11:471-475, 1971.

1972 Deck MDF, et al: Clinical experience with circular angiotomography, Radiology 105:591-595, 1972.

1973 Glickman MG, McNamara TO and Margolis MT: Arteriographic diagnosis of subtemporal subdural hematoma, Radiology 109:607-615, 1973.

Gold LHA, Krause D and Amplatz K: Routine biplane magnification cerebral angiography, Radiology 106:321-324, 1973.

Skelly GA and Mansour G: A simple method of stereoscopic angiography with particular reference to the posterior fossa, AJR 118:690-694, 1973.

1974 Newton TH and Potts DG, editors: Radiology of the skull and brain, vol 2, Angiography, St Louis, 1974, The CV Mosby Co.

1976 Long JM: Routine magnification cerebral angiography: a practical system designed for community hospital application, South Med J 69:911-913, 1976.

Takahashi M, et al: Serial cerebral angiography in stereoscopic magnification, AJR 126:1211-1218, 1976.

1977 Doi K, Rossmann K and Duda EE: Application of longitudinal magnification effect to magnification stereoscopic angiography: a new method for cerebral angiography, Radiology 124:395-401, 1977.

Larson EB, et al: Impact of computed tomography on utilization of cerebral angiograms, AJR 129:1-3, 1977.

1979 Quencer RM, Rosomoff HL and Green BA: Lateral decubitus pneumoencephalography-angiography for localizing atrial and para-atrial vascular lesions, AJR 132:617-622, 1979.

1980 Christenson PC, et al: Intravenous angiography using digital video subtraction: intravenous cervicocerebrovascular angiography, AJR 135:1145-1152, 1980.

Cochran RM: Determining cerebral death with radiologic diagnostic procedures, Radiol Technol 51:777-790, 1980.

Jensen HP, et al: Computerized tomography in vascular malformations of the brain, Neurosurg Rev 3:119-127, 1980.

Lantz BM, et al: Angiographic determination of cerebral blood flow, Acta Radiol [Diagn] 21:147-153, 1980.

Numaguchi Y, et al: Prolonged injection angiography for diagnosing intracranial neoplasms, Radiology 136:387-393, 1980.

Rubin JM, et al: Clinical applications of combined cerebral angiograms and brain CT scans, AJNR 1:83-87, 1980.

Savolaine ER, Gerber AM and Nowak SF: Pitfalls in the angiographic diagnosis of serious head injury, J Neurosurg 53:53-57, 1980.

Takahashi M and Ozawa Y: Routine biplane cerebral angiography with stereoscopic magnification, Radiology 136:113-117, 1980.

1981 Turnipseed WD, Sackett JF, Strother CM: Computerized arteriography of the cerebrovascular system: its use with intravenous administration of contrast material, Arch Surg 116:470-473, 1981.

1982 Ahlgren P: Iohexol compared to urografin meglumine in cerebral angiography: a randomized, double-blind cross-over study, Neuroradiology 23:195-198, 1982.

Amundsen P, et al: Cerebral angiography with iohexol: a multicentre clinical trial, Acta Radiol [Diagn] 23:529-534, 1982.

Forbes GS, et al: Digital angiography: introducing digital techniques to clinical cerebral angiography practice, Mayo Clin Proc 57:683-693, 1982.

Ingstrup HM and Hauge P: Clinical testing of iohexol, Conray meglumine and Amipaque in cerebral angiography, Neuroradiology 23:75-79, 1982.

Molyneux AJ and Sheldon PW: A randomized blind trial of iopamidol and meglumine calcium metrizoate (Triosil 280, Isopaque Cerebral) in cerebral angiography, Br J Radiol 55:117-119, 1982.

Molyneux AJ, Sheldon PW and Yates DA: A comparative trial of sodium meglumine ioxaglate (Hexabrix) and iopamidol (Niopam) for cerebral angiography, Br J Radiol 55:881-884, 1982.

Nakstad P, et al: Cerebral angiography with the non-ionic water-soluble contrast medium iohexol and meglumine-Ca-metrizoate: a randomized double-blind parallel study in man, Neuroradiology 23:199-202, 1982.

Turnipseed WD, et al: A comparison of standard cerebral arteriography with noninvasive Doppler imaging and intravenous angiography, Arch Surg 117:419-421, 1982.

Yamamoto Y, et al: Minimum dose contrast bolus in computed angiotomography of the brain, J Comput Assist Tomogr 6:575-585, 1982.

Yamamoto Y, et al: Normal anatomy of cerebral vessels by computed angiotomography in the coronal, Towne, and semisagittal planes, J Comput Assist Tomogr 6:1049-1057, 1982.

1983 Amundsen P, et al: Randomized double-blind cross-over study of iohexol and Amipaque in cerebral angiography, AJNR 4:342-343, 1983.

Brant-Zawadzki M, et al: Digital subtraction cerebral angiography by intraarterial injection: comparison with conventional angiography, AJR 140:347-353, 1983.

Bryan RN, et al: Neuroangiography with iohexol, AJNR 4:344-346, 1983.

Doi K and Duda EE: Detectability of depth information by use of magnification stereoscopic technique in cerebral angiography, Radiology 146:91-95, 1983.

Hahn FJ: "Squirt-pull" technique for left carotid catheterization, AJNR 4:1129, 1983.

Hindmarsh T, et al: Comparative double-blind investigation of meglumine metrizoate, metrizamide, and iohexol in carotid angiography, AJNR 4:347-349, 1983.

Holtas S, Cronqvist S and Renaa T: Cerebral angiography with iohexol: a comparison with metrizamide in man, Neuroradiology 24:201-204, 1983.

Ingstrup HM and Laulund S: Clinical testing of Omnipaque and Amipaque in external carotid and vertebral angiography: randomized double-blind cross-over study, AJNR 4:1097-1099, 1983.

Nakstad P, Sortland O and Aaserud O: Iohexol compared to meglumine-Cametrizoate in common carotid angiography: a randomized double-blind cross-over study in man, Neuroradiology 25:33-36, 1983.

Skalpe IO and Anke IM: Complications in cerebral angiography: a comparison between the non-ionic contrast medium iohexol and meglumine metrizoate (Isopaque Cerebral), Neuroradiology 25:157-160, 1983.

Thron A and Voigt K: Rotational cerebral angiography: procedure and value, AJNR 4:289-291, 1983.

Yamaki T, Yoshino E and Higuchi T: Extravasation of contrast medium during both computed tomography and cerebral angiography, Surg Neurol 19:247-250, 1983.

1984 Chakeres DW and Wiatrowski W: Cerebral angiography: a device to reduce exposure to the eye lens, Radiology 152:534-535, 1984.

Earnest F IV, et al: Complications of cerebral angiography: prospective assessment of risk, AJR 142:247-253, 1984.

Glover JL, et al: Duplex ultrasonography, digital subtraction angiography, and conventional angiography in assessing carotid atherosclerosis, Arch Surg 119:664-669, 1984.

Higa T, et al: A femocerebral catheter for middle-aged patients of relatively small stature, Neuroradiology 26:55-56, 1984.

Maravilla KR, et al: Digital tomosynthesis: technique modifications and clinical applications for neurovascular anatomy, Radiology 152:719-724, 1984.

O'Connor MK, et al: Digital fluoroscopy with a conventional fluoroscopic room and a nuclear medicine computer system, Br J Radiol 57:553-560, 1984.

Schonfeld SM, et al: Iopamidol and Conray 60: comparison in superselective angiography, Radiology 152:809-811, 1984.

Takahashi M, Bussaka H and Nakagawa N: Evaluation of the cerebral vasculature by intraarterial DSA—with emphasis on in vivo resolution, Neuroradiology 26:253-259, 1984.

Tsai FY, et al: Arterial digital subtraction angiography with particulate intravascular embolization and angioplasty, Surg Neurol 22:204-212, 1984.

Valk J, Crezee F and Olislagers-de Slegte RGM: Comparison of iohexol 300 mg I/ml and Hexabrix 320 mg I/ml in central angiography: a double-blind trial, Neuroradiology 26:217-221, 1984.

Zubkov YN, Nikiforov BM and Shustin VA: Balloon catheter technique for dilatation of constricted cerebral arteries after aneurysmal SAH, Acta Neurochir (Wien) 70:65-79, 1984.

1985 Karoll MP, et al: Air gap technique for digital subtraction angiography of the extracranial carotid arteries, Invest Radiol 20:742-745, 1985.

1986 Foley KT, Cahan LD and Hieshima GB: Intraoperative angiography using a portable digital subtraction unit, J Neurosurg 64:816-818, 1986.

1987 Kim KS and Weinberg PE: A simple method to form an open loop with the sidewinder catheter, Neuroradiology 29:76-77, 1987.

Kleefield J, et al: Biplane stereoscopic magnification cerebral angiography, Radiology 165:576-577, 1987.

Vandermeulen D, et al: Angiographic localizer ring for the BRW stereotactic system, Acta Neurochir Suppl (Wien) 39:15-17, 1987.

1988 Bishop S: Cerebral angiography using the femoral catheterization technique, Radiography 54:52-60, 1988.

Moringlane JR, Lippitz B and Ostertag CB: Cerebral angiography under stereotactic conditions: technical note, Acta Neurochir (Wien) 91:147-150, 1988.

1989 Mewissen MW, Zavitz WR and Lipchik EO: Brachiocephalic vessels in the elderly: technique for catheterization, Radiology 170:887, 1989.

CIRCULATORY SYSTEM
Anatomy

For bibliographic citations before 1964 please see the fifth edition of this atlas.

1979 Moncada R, et al: Normal vascular anatomy of the abdomen on computed tomography, Radiol Clin North Am 17:25-37, 1979.

VISCERAL AND PERIPHERAL ANGIOGRAPHY

For bibliographic citations before 1964, please see the fifth edition of this atlas.

1964 Ainsworth J and Gilman PW: Diagnosis of placenta previa by aortography, Proc R Soc Med 57:697-700, 1964.

Almeén T and Nylander G: False signs of thrombosis in lower leg phlebography, Acta Radiol [Diagn] 2:345-352, 1964.

Bookstein JJ and Stewart BH: The current status of renal arteriography, Radiol Clin North Am 2:461-482, 1964.

Bookstein JJ and Whitehouse WM: Splenoportography, Radiol Clin North Am 2:447-460, 1964.

Bucht H, et al: Catheterization of the left adrenal vein for contrast injection and steroid analysis in a case of Conn's syndrome, Acta Med Scand 176:233-241, 1964.

Finney LA, et al: Interosseous vertebral venography in the diagnosis of lumbar disk disease, AJR 92:1282-1292, 1964.

Glenn F, et al: Selective celiac and superior mesenteric arteriography, Surg Gynecol Obstet 118:93-100, 1964.

Guibert GE: Aortography in a small general hospital, Radiol Technol 36:172-175, 1964.

Keats TE: Trends in peripheral arteriography, Radiol Clin North Am 2:483-498, 1964.

Marshall TR and Ling JT: Percutaneous noncatheter left brachial renal arteriography, AJR 92:315-320, 1964.

Steinberg I: Method of intravenous abdominal aortography: report on present status and value in diagnosis of peripheral vascular diseases, Vasc Dis 1:233-241, 1964.

Steinberg I and Stein H: Intravenous angiocardiography, abdominal aortography, and peripheral arteriography with single arm pressure injection, AJR 92:893-906, 1964.

1965 Eiken M, et al: Intra-osseous costal venography, AJR 94:172-181, 1965.

Friedenberg MJ and Carlsson E: Bilateral aorto-ilio-femoral arteriography via unilateral common femoral artery needle, Acta Radiol [Diagn] 3:1-8, 1965.

Halpern M and Freiberger RH: Arteriography in orthopedics, AJR 94:194-206, 1965.

Hendrick CK and Schreiber MH: Intravenous placentography, AJR 93:948-954, 1965.

Riley JM: The Valsalva maneuver in renal angiography, J Urol 93:631-634, 1965.

Riley JM, et al: Left axillary approach to the abdominal aorta, Radiology 84:96-99, 1965.

Rösch J and Bret J: Arteriography of the pancreas, AJR 94:182-193, 1965.

Roy P: Percutaneous catheterization via the axillary artery, AJR 94:1-18, 1965.

Sewell WH: Coronary arteriography by the Sones technique: technical considerations, AJR 95:673-683, 1965.

Skinner GB: The use of cinefluorography in peripheral arteriography, AJR 95:745-750, 1965.

Starer F: Percutaneous suprarenal venography, Br J Radiol 38:675-681, 1965.

Steinberg I and Stein HL: Visualization of abdominal aortic aneurysms, AJR 95:684-695, 1965.

Steinberg I, et al: Thoracic aortography; intravenous and selective techniques, AJR 94:129-144, 1965.

Templeton AW: Renal aortography: advantages and technique using the Valsalva maneuver, AJR 95:383-388, 1965.

Viamonte M Jr and Stevens RC: Guided angiography, AJR 94:30-39, 1965.

Viamonte M Jr, et al: Guided catheterization of the bronchial arteries, Radiology 85:205-230, 1965.

Weidner W, et al: Percutaneous transaxillary selective coronary angiography, Radiology 85:652-657, 1965.

Wholey MH, et al: Fundamentals of angiographic techniques, Surg Gynec Obstet 121:517-527, 1965.

1966 Boijsen E and Reuter SR: Subclavian and internal mammary angiography in the evaluation of anterior mediastinal masses, AJR 98:447-450, 1966.

Hyat DB: Upright inferior vena cavography, Radiology 86:865-870, 1966.

Janover MG, et al: Azygography and lung cancer, N Engl J Med 275:803-808, 1966.

Laubenberger T and Berghaus H: The roentgenographic exploration of the prostate and the urinary bladder floor veins: periprostatic phlebography, a new method, AJR 98:208-211, 1966.

Marshall TR, et al: Hand arteriography, Radiology 86:299-304, 1966.

Nebesar RA and Pollard JJ: Portal venography by selective arterial catheterization, AJR 97:477-487, 1966.

Porstmann W, et al: Die selektive Nebennierenangiographie [selective adrenal angiography], Fortschr Roentgenstr 104:150-157, 1966. Abstract: AJR 98:262, 1966.

Puyau FA and Burko H: The tilted left anterior oblique position in the study of congenital cardiac anomalies, Radiology 87:1069-1073, 1966.

Shuford WH, et al: A comparison of carbon dioxide and radiopaque angiocardiographic methods in the diagnosis of pericardial effusion, Radiology 86:1064-1069, 1966.

Sutton D: Arterial placentography and placenta previa, Br J Radiol 39:47-51, 1966.

Turner AF, et al: Carbon dioxide cineangiocardiography in the diagnosis of pericardial disease, AJR 97:342-349, 1966.

1967 Amsler FR and Wilber MC: Intraosseous vertebral venography as a diagnostic aid in evaluating disease of the lumbar spine, J Bone Joint Surg 49-A:703-712, 1967.

Aronson KF and Nylander G: Use of direct portography in diagnosis of liver diseases, Radiology 88:40-47, 1967.

Bannister RJ: Arteriography, Radiol Technol 38:328-345, 1967.

Bayindir S and Fabbender CW: Die Bedeutung der selektive Angiographie von A. coeliaca und A. mesenterica sup. für die Diagnostik von chirurgischen Oberbaucherkrankungen, Fortschr Roentgenstr 106:13-23, 1967.

Chiandussi L, et al: Hepatic portography by direct catheterization of the portal vein through the round ligament of the liver (ligamentum teres), AJR 99:625-628, 1967.

Deutsch V: Cholecystoangiography: visualization of the gallbladder by selective celiac and mesenteric angiography, AJR 101:608-616, 1967.

Düx A, et al: Vergleichende vasographische und szintigraphische Untersuchungen bei Lebertumoren, Fortschr Roentgenstr 106:502-524, 1967.

Feldman F, et al: Arteriography of the breast, Radiology 89:1053-1061, 1967.

Hanafee W and Weiner M: Transjugular percutaneous cholangiography, Radiology 88:35-39, 1967.

Hemley SD, et al: Intravenous aortography, Med Radiogr Photogr 43:1-31, 1967.

Kahn PC and Nickrosz LV: Selective angiography of the adrenal glands, AJR 101:739-749, 1967.

Lang EK: Arteriography in gynecology, Radiol Clin North Am 5:133-149, 1967.

Nordenström B: Selective catheterization and angiography of bronchial and mediastinal arteries in man, Acta Radiol [Diagn] 6:13-24, 1967.

Wholey MH: Evaluation of arteriography in obstetrics, Radiol Clin North Am 5:121-131, 1967.

Wickbom I, Zachrisson BF and Heinmann P: Thyroid angiography, Acta Radiol [Diagn] 6:497-512, 1967.

1968 Frick PC: Translumbar aortography, Radiol Technol 39:261-266, 1968.

Herlinger H: Single film inclined angioplacentography in the diagnosis of placenta praevia, Clin Radiol 19:59-64, 1968.

Lecky JW, et al: Percutaneous intrauterine fetal transfusion; roentgenologic aspects and results, AJR 103:186-194, 1968.

McNulty JG: High dose percutaneous transsplenic portal venography, Br J Radiol 41:55-58, 1968.

Moskowitz H, et al: Prone splenoportography, Radiology 90:1132-1135, 1968.

1969 Agee OF and Kaude J: Angiography of the pelvis and lower extremities with moving table techniques, AJR 107:860-865, 1969.

Hynes DM, et al: Assessment of a technique for coronary arteriography using 70 mm films, Br J Radiol 42:736-743, 1969.

Morettin LB and Wilson M: A device for simplified femoral arteriography, AJR 107:866-868, 1969.

Ogden JA, Wade ME and Davis CD: Radiological aspects of fetal intrauterine transfusion, Radiology 93:1315-1321, 1969.

Takahashi M, Ishibashi T and Kawanami H: Angiographic diagnosis of benign and malignant tumors of the thyroid, Radiology 92:520-526, 1969.

1970 Horner RW: Angled bilateral cervical arteriography in the investigation of ischemia, Radiol Technol 42:125-132, 1970.

Kattan KR: Angled view in pulmonary angiography, Radiology 94:79-82, 1970.
1971 Eisenman JI and O'Loughlin BJ: Value of lateral abdominal aortography, AJR 112:586-592, 1971.
Di Rienzo A: Persistent portohepatography, Rev Interam Radiol 6:40-60, 1971. (In Spanish) Abstract: Radiology 100:724, 1971.
1972 Damascelli B, et al: Second thoughts on the value of selective thyroid angiography, AJR 114:822-829, 1972.
Lea TM and Andress MR: Value of oblique projections in translumbar aortography, AJR 116:187-193, 1972.
1973 Bussat P, et al: Spinal cord angiography in dorsolumbar vertebral fractures with neurological involvement, Radiology 109:617-620, 1973.
1974 Courey WR, deVillasante JM and Waltman AC: A quick, simple method of percutaneous transfemoral pulmonary arteriography, Radiology 113:475-477, 1974.
Damascelli B: A "slide rule" for angiographers, AJR 122:173-175, 1974.
Jonsson K and Lunderquist A: Angiography of the liver and spleen in Hodgkin's disease, AJR 121:789-792, 1974.
1975 Guistra PE, et al: Outpatient arteriography at a small community hospital, Radiology 116:581-583, 1975.
Sheedy FP II, Fulton RE and Atwell DT: Angiographic evaluation of patients with chronic gastrointestinal bleeding, AJR 123:338-347, 1975.
Staple TM: Vascular radiological procedures in orthopedic surgery, Clin Orthop 107:48-61, 1975.
Wendth AJ Jr: Peripheral arteriography: an overview of its origins and present status, CRC Crit Rev Radiol Nucl Med 6:369-401, 1975.
1976 Athanasoulis CA, et al: Angiography: its contribution to the emergency management of gastrointestinal hemorrhage, Radiol Clin North Am 14:265-280, 1976.
Erikson V: Technique of coronary angiography, Acta Radiol 17:781-785, 1976.
Janicki P and Alfidi RJ: Selective visceral angiography in the diagnosis and treatment of gastroduodenal hemorrhage, Surg Clin North Am 56:1365-1373, 1976.
Mojab K and Ghosh BC: Thyroid angiography, Am J Surg 132:620-622, 1976.
1977 Eisenberg RL and Mani RL: Pressure dressings and postangiographic care of the femoral puncture site, Radiology 122:677-678, 1977.
Fitzgerald DE and Carr J: Peripheral arterial disease: assessment by arteriography and alternative noninvasive measurements, AJR 128:385-388, 1977.
Leslie J, et al: A new simple power injector, AJR 128:381-384, 1977.
Tegtmeyer CJ: A simplified technique for selective and superselective abdominal angiography, J Can Assoc Radiol 28:224-226, 1977.
1978 Frasson F, et al: Angiography versus computerized tomography, Ann Radiol 21:387-392, 1978.
Holgate RC, et al: Angiography in otolaryngology: anatomy, methodology, complications, and contraindications, Otolaryngol Clin North Am 11:457-475, 1978.
Oleaga JA, et al: Renal venography: new applications in pathologic conditions, Urology 12:609-613, 1978.
Rees R, et al: Angiography in extremity trauma: a prospective study, Am J Surg 44:661-663, 1978.
1979 Boyle RN: Arteriography in the small hospital, Surg Clin North Am 59:495-500, 1979.
Cohen DB: Transcatheter therapy in angiography: indications, techniques, and illustrations, Radiol Technol 51:29-35, 1979.
Lang EK: Current and future applications of angiography in the abdomen, Radiol Clin North Am 17:55-76, 1979.
1980 Boijsen E and Gothlin J: Abdominal angiography after intra-arterial injection of vasopressin, Acta Radiol 21:523-533, 1980.
Fitzer PM: Contrast venography: a "golden oldie," Va Med 107:210-214, 1980.
Herman RJ, et al: Descending venography: a method of evaluating lower extremity venous valvular function, Radiology 137:63-69, 1980.
1981 Chuang VP: Basic rule of catheter selection for visceral angiography, AJR 136:423-433, 1981.
Elliott LP: Significance of caudal left anterior oblique view in analyzing the left main coronary artery and its major branches, Radiology 139:39-43, 1981.
Hessel SJ, et al: Complications of angiography, Radiology 138:273-281, 1981.
LeVeen RF, et al: Pressure-infusion venography of the leg with remote control fluoroscopy, Radiology 138:730-731, 1981.
Mosely GT: Technical considerations of epidural venography, Radiol Technol 52:371-374, 1981.
Nathan MH: Pressure infusion venography, Radiology 138:731-732, 1981.
Suzuki S and Mine H: Roll-film changer for whole-limb angiography: a trial production and its clinical application, Cardiovasc Intervent Radiol 4:66-70, 1981.
Turnipseed WD, et al: Computerized intravenous arteriography: a technique for visualizing the peripheral vascular system, Surgery 89:118-123, 1981.
1982 Abaskaron M: Catheter modification to improve the performance of aorto-ileo-femoral examinations, Radiology 144:420, 1982.
Gordon DH, et al: Descending varicose venography of the lower extremities: an alternative method to evaluate the deep venous system, Radiology 145:832-834, 1982.
1982 Kaseff LG: Positional variations of the common carotid artery bifurcation, Radiology 145:377-378, 1982.
Lantz BM, et al: Vasodilator response in the lower extremity induced by contrast medium, Acta Radiol [Diagn] 23:185-191, 1982.
Laskey WK, et al: A safe and rapid technique for retrograde catheterization of the left ventricle in aortic stenosis, Cathet Cardiovasc Diagn 8:429-435, 1982.
Slack JD, Slack LA and Orr C: Recurrent severe reaction to iodinated contrast media during cardiac catheterization, Heart Lung 11:348-352, 1982.
1983 Egsgaard H, Hrup A and Praestholm J: A controlled clinical trial of iohexol and diatrizoate in aortofemoral angiography, Eur J Radiol 3:14-17, 1983.
Elliott LP, Bargeron LM Jr and Green CE: Angled angiography: general approach and findings, Cardiol Clin 1:361-385, 1983.
Foley WD, et al: Digital subtraction angiography of the portal venous system, AJR 140:497-499, 1983.
Hagen B: Iohexol and iopromide—two new non-ionic water-soluble radiographic contrast media: randomized, intraindividual double-blind study versus ioxaglate in peripheral angiography, Fortschr Geb Rontgenstr Nuklearmed Erganzungsband 118:107-114, 1983.
Harrington DP, et al: Compound angulation for the angiographic evaluation of renal artery, Radiology 146:829-831, 1983.
Higgins CB and Buonocore E: Digital subtraction angiography: techniques and applications for evaluating cardiac anatomy and function, Cardiol Clin 1:413-425, 1983.
Kolbenstvedt A: Iohexol in lower extremity, renal, and visceral angiography: survey and present state, Acta Radiol 366:153-157, 1983.
Mardini MK and Rao PS: Left ventricular and aortic catheterization and angiography via a patent ductus arteriosus: a new technique, Cathet Cardiovasc Diagn 9:89-95, 1983.
Saibil EA, Maggisano R and Witchell SJ: Angiography in the diagnosis and treatment of trauma, J Can Assoc Radiol 34:218-227, 1983.
Seigel RS and Williams AG: Efficacy of prone positioning for intravenous digital angiography of the abdomen, Radiology 148:295, 1983.
Seldin DW, et al: Left ventricular volume determined from scintigraphy and digital angiography by a semiautomated geometric method, Radiology 149:809-813, 1983.
Skjennald A, Heldaas J and Hiseth A: Comparison of iohexol and meglumine-Na-Ca-metrizoate in visceral angiography, Acta Radiol 366:158-163, 1983.
Widrich WC, et al: Iopamidol and meglumine diatrizoate: comparison of effects on patient discomfort during aortofemoral arteriography, Radiology 148:61-64, 1983.

1984 Brandt PW: Axially angled angiocardiography, Cardiovasc Intervent Radiol 7:166-169, 1984.

Cragg AH, et al: Rotational kymography: technique for automated analysis of cine left ventriculograms, Radiology 150:260-262, 1984.

Hillman BJ: Digital imaging of the kidney, Radiol Clin North Am 22:341-364, 1984.

1984 Kinnunen J, et al: A double curve catheter for the left axillary artery approach to aortofemoral, selective renal, and visceral angiography, Eur J Radiol 4:229-231, 1984.

Nelson JA and Kruger RA: Digital angiography, Radiologe 24:149-154, 1984.

Schatz SL, et al: A subtraction technique in conventional angiography, Radiology 151:531, 1984.

Soto B, Coghlan CH and Bargeron LM: Present status of axially angled angiocardiography, Cardiovasc Intervent Radiol 7:156-165, 1984.

Vetrovec GW and Strash AM: Modification of cradle angiographic tables to more easily obtain axial coronary views, Cathet Cardiovasc Diagn 10:607-611, 1984.

1985 Block RW, et al: A device for positioning the breast during angiography, Radiology 155:824, 1985.

Detrano R, et al: Cardiac digital subtraction angiography: peripheral versus central intravenous dye injections, Cardiovasc Intervent Radiol 8:55-58, 1985.

Fisher M, et al: Arteriography of the carotid bifurcation: oblique projections, Neurology 35:1201-1204, 1985.

Guthaner DF, Wexler L and Bradley B: Digital subtraction angiography of coronary grafts: optimization of technique, AJR 145:1185-1190, 1985.

Karoll MP, et al: Air gap technique for digital subtraction angiography of the extracranial carotid arteries, Invest Radiol 20:742-745, 1985.

McCorkell SJ, et al: Indications for angiography in extremity trauma, AJR 145:1245-1247, 1985.

Mendelson EB, et al: Evaluation of the prone position in digital subtraction angiography, Cardiovasc Intervent Radiol 8:72-75, 1985.

Passariello R: Angio-CT techniques, Eur J Radiol 5:193-198, 1985.

Saddekni S, et al: Contrast administration and techniques of digital subtraction angiography performance, Radiol Clin North Am 23:275-291, 1985.

Smith DC and Simmons CR: The quick aortic turn: a rapid method for reformation of the sidewinder catheter, Radiology 155:247-248, 1985.

Wilson P: Equipment for digital angiography, Radiography 51:193-196, 1985.

1986 Cohen MI and Vogelzang RL: A comparison of techniques for improved visualization of the arteries of the distal lower extremity, AJR 147:1021-1024, 1986.

Favilla I, Barry WR and Turner IJ: Video and digital fluorescein angiography, Aust NZ J Ophthalmol 14:229-234, 1986.

Gerard P and Lefkovitz Z: The optical push device: an aid to the angiographer, Cardiovasc Intervent Radiol 9:111-112, 1986.

Gersten K, et al: Crossed-leg technique for digital subtraction angiography, AJR 146:843-844, 1986.

Gmelin E, Weiss HD and Buchmann F: Cardiac gating in intravenous DSA, Eur J Radiol 6:24-29, 1986.

Kimme Smith C, et al: Diagnostic effects of edge sharpening filtration and magnification, Med Phys 13:850-856, 1986.

Mills CS and Van Aman ME: Modified technique for percutaneous transfemoral pulmonary angiography, Cardiovasc Intervent Radiol 9:52-53, 1986.

Ovitt TW and Newell JD II: Digital subtraction angiography: technology, equipment, and techniques, Med Instrum 20:199-205, 1986.

Takahashi M, et al: Biplane digital subtraction angiography, Comput Radiol 10:221-225, 1986.

1987 Boesmi B, et al: Digital angiography in children, Rays 12:47-52, 1987.

Compton SC: Bit conversion of technical factors in vascular procedures, Radiol Technol 58:413-416, 1987.

Dorros G and Lewin RF: Angiography of the internal mammary artery via the contralateral brachial artery, Cathet Cardiovasc Diagn 13:138-140, 1987.

Dumoulin CL, Souza SP and Hart HR: Rapid scan magnetic resonance angiography, Magn Reson Med 5:238-245, 1987.

Interventional radiology in the thorax, J Thorac Imaging 2:1-80, 1987.

Tempkin DL and Ladika JE: New catheter design and placement technique for pulmonary arteriography, Radiology 163:275-276, 1987.

Witte G, et al: The use of the Fourier transform in cardiac digital angiography, Cardiovasc Intervent Radiol 10:59-64, 1987.

1988 Bowman LK: Peak filling rate normalized to mitral stroke volume: a new Doppler angiographic technique, J Am Coll Cardiol 12:937-943, 1988.

Delcour C, et al: Technical advances in penile arteriography, AJR 150:803-804, 1988.

Dondelinger RF and Kurdziel JC: Computed tomographic arteriography (CTA) of the liver, Bull Soc Sci Med Grand Duche Luxemb 125:27-34, 1988.

Dumay AC, et al: Three-dimensional reconstruction of myocardial contrast perfusion techniques, Int J Card Imaging 3:141-152, 1988.

Dumoulin CL, et al: Time-resolved magnetic resonance angiography, Magn Reson Med 6:275-286, 1988.

Foster CJ, Butler P and Freer CE: Digital subtraction angiography of the left ventricle, Br J Radiol 61:1009-1013, 1988.

Frahm J: Rapid line scan NMR angiography, Magn Reson Med 7:79-87, 1988.

Kozak BE and Rosch J: Curved guide wire for percutaneous pulmonary angiography, Radiology 167:864-865, 1988.

McLellan GL and Scalapino MC: Pulmonary artery catheterization: a modified technique, Radiology 169:264-265, 1988.

Nakhjavan FK: Use of angioplasty guidewire for technically difficult angiography, Cathet Cardiovasc Diagn 14:213, 1988.

Robertson HJ: Nonionic contrast media in radiology: procedural considerations, Invest Radiol 23:S374-S377, 1988.

Schnell N, et al: Requirements on resolution of digital imaging equipment in the cardiac catheterization laboratory, Int J Card Imaging 3:111-116, 1988.

Takeda T: Intraarterial digital subtraction angiography with carbon dioxide, Cardiovasc Intervent Radiol 11:101-107, 1988.

Vogel RA: Left ventricular imaging by digital subtraction angiography, Int J Card Imaging 3:29-38, 1988.

Wondrow MA, et al: Technical consideration for a new x-ray video progressive scanning, Cathet Cardiovasc Diagn 14:126-134, 1988.

1989 Anand R: Fluorescein angiography. Part I. Technique and normal study, J Ophthalmic Nurs Technol 8:48-52, 1989.

Hwang MH, et al: The potential risk of thrombosis during coronary angiography using nonionic contrast media, Cathet Cardiovasc Diagn 16:209-213, 1989.

Ireland MA, et al: Safety and convenience of a mechanical injector pump for coronary angiography, Cathet Cardiovasc Diagn 16:199-201, 1989.

Pond GD, et al: Intraoperative arteriography: comparison of conventional screen-film with photostimulable imaging plate radiographs, Radiology 170:367-370, 1989.

INTERVENTIONAL RADIOGRAPHY

1980 Abele JE: Balloon catheters and transluminal dilatation: technical considerations, AJR 135:901-906, 1980.

Athanasoulis CA: Percutaneous transluminal angioplasty: general principles, AJR 135:893-900, 1980.

Jander HP and Russinovich NA: Transcatheter gelfoam embolization in abdominal, retroperitoneal, and pelvic hemorrhage, Radiology 136:337-344, 1980.

Weber J and Novak D: Occlusion arteriography: diagnostic and therapeutic applicability of balloon catheters to arterial disease of the lower extremities, AJR 142:23-25, 1980.

1981 Ring EJ and McLean GK: Interventional radiology, Boston, 1981, Little, Brown & Co.

Vlietstra RE, et al: Percutaneous transluminal coronary angioplasty: initial Mayo clinic experience, Mayo Clin Proc 56:287-293, 1981.
1982 Miller K and Pruneau D: Transcatheter therapy in the angiographic suite, Radiol Technol 53:469-476, 1982.
Sclafani SJ, et al: Interventional radiology in trauma victims: analysis of 51 consecutive patients, J Trauma 22:353-360, 1982.
1983 Comazzi JL, et al: Percutaneous transluminal angioplasty of a large septal artery, Cathet Cardiovasc Diagn 9:181-186, 1983.
Health and Public Policy Committee, American College of Physicians: Percutaneous transluminal angioplasty, Ann Intern Med 99:864-869, 1983.
Lock JE, et al: Balloon dilatation angioplasty of hypoplastic and stenotic pulmonary arteries, Circulation 67:962-967, 1983.
Rogers PA: Percutaneous needle aspiration biopsy of pulmonary lesions, Radiol Technol 55(1):527-531, 1983.
Rose JS: Invasive radiology: risks and patient care, Chicago, 1983, Year Book Medical Publishers, Inc.
1984 Fellows KE, Jr: Therapeutic catheter procedures in congenital heart disease: current status and future prospects, Cardiovasc Intervent Radiol 7:170-177, 1984.
Katzen BT: Percutaneous transluminal angioplasty for arterial disease of the lower extremities, AJR 142:23-25, 1984.
McAuley BJ, Oesterle S and Simpson JB: Advances in guidewire technology, Am J Cardiol 53:94C-96C, 1984.
Nichols DM, et al: The safe intercostal approach? Pleural complications in abdominal interventional radiology, AJR 142:1013-1018, 1984.
O'Neill DM: Percutaneous transluminal angioplasty: development, technique, and application, Radiol Technol 55:10-16, 1984.
1986 Ingram C and Burkhalter: Percutaneous nephrostolithotomy, Radiol Technol 58(1):11-15, 1986.
1987 Interventional radiology in the thorax, J Thorac Imaging 2:1-80, 1987.
1989 Teplick SK: Diagnostic and therapeutic interventional gall bladder procedures, AJR 152:913-916, 1989.

SUBTRACTION TECHNIQUE

For bibliographic citations before 1964, please see the fifth edition of this atlas.

1964 Horenstein R, Lundh A and Sjögren SE: A subtraction method, Acta Radiol [Diagn] 2:264-272, 1964.
1965 Chynn KY: Simplified subtraction technique, AJR 95:970-975, 1965.
Oldendorf WH: A modified subtraction technique for extreme enhancement of angiographic detail, Neurology 15:366-370, 1965.
1966 Hanafee W and Shinno JM: Second-order subtraction with simultaneous bilateral carotid, internal carotid injections, Radiology 86:334-341, 1966.
Oldendorf WH: Auto-subtraction: a photographic technique for enhancement of detail in radiographic reproduction, Acta Radiol [Diagn] 4:97-104, 1966.
Wallman H and Wickbom I: Electronic subtraction, Acta Radiol [Diagn] 5:562-569, 1966.
Wise RE and Ganson J: Subtraction technic: video and color methods, Radiology 86:814-821, 1966.
1967 Dalrymple GV, et al: A rapid method for producing subtraction technic roentgenograms, Radiology 89:934-935, 1967.
Kimber PM: Routine photographic subtraction, Radiography 33:255-258, 1967.
Ruggiero G and Mazzacurati M: Subtraction technique in encephalography, Invest Radiol 2:326-331, 1967.
Tucker AK: Subtraction in radiology, Radiography 33:125-129, 1967.
1968 Winkler NT: Roentgenographic subtraction technique, Radiol Technol 39:339-346, 1968.
1969 Benness GT: Television subtraction, Australas Radiol 13:314-318, 1969.
Liliequist B and Welander U: Colour in subtraction angiography, Acta Radiol [Diagn] 8:1-4, 1969.
1970 Jenkin C, Pribram H and Eisenman JI: Light intensity variation: a novel approach to subtraction technique, Radiology 97:684-685, 1970.
Joyce JW, et al: Improved contrast in subtraction technique, Radiology 94:157-159, 1970.
Miller ER, McCurry EM and Hruska BB: Anisotrophic subtraction and edge enhancement of roentgenographic images, Radiology 97:27-32, 1970.
Thiel AJ: Photographic subtraction and color addition to enhance cut film, 35 mm slides and 16 mm cine studies of vascular systems, Radiol Technol 42:1-7, 1970.
1971 Hehman KN: Subtraction in cerebral angiography, Semin Roentgenol 6:14-16, 1971.
1972 Fiebach O and Dorr K: A simplified method for photographic subtraction using a 90 second processor, Fortschr Roentgenstr 117:476-478, 1972. (In German)
Hoffman RB and Rein B: The routine use of subtraction in aortic arch studies, Radiology 102:575-578, 1972.
1973 Athanasoulis CA, et al: Angionephrotomography and subtraction: relative value in renal mass lesions, AJR 117:108-111, 1973.
Lee I and Hunter TB: Modified subtraction technique for neuroradiology, Radiology 108:442-443, 1973.
Miller ER: Photographic anisotrophic subtraction and edge enhancement, Radiology 106:222-223, 1973.
Rothman SLG, et al: A simple technique for photographic image enhancement of subtraction films, Radiology 107:461-463, 1973.
1974 Leeds NE: Image enhancement with magnification and subtraction, Radiol Clin North Am 12:241-256, 1974.
Sucher DL and Strand RD: Composite mask subtraction: white-over-white technique, Radiology 113:470-472, 1974.
1977 Mikkelsen WJ, et al: Subtraction technique in intravenous aortography, Radiology 123:231-232, 1977.
Mojab K, Garcia L and Talge G: A new subtraction technique using duplicating film as a final print, AJR 129:528-530, 1977.
Ort MG: Subtraction radiography techniques and limitations, Radiology 124:65-72, 1977.
1980 El Gammal T: Cervical myelography and posterior fossa examinations with Amipaque using magnification and subtraction, Radiology 136:219-222, 1980.
1981 Brody WR: Hybrid subtraction for improved arteriography, Radiology 141: 828-831, 1981.
1983 Foley WD, et al: Digital subtraction angiography of the portal venous system, AJR 140:497-499, 1983.
Grondahl HG and Grondahl K: Subtraction radiography for the diagnosis of periodontal bone lesions, Oral Surg 55:208-213, 1983.
McSweeney MB, Sprawls P and Egan RL: Enhanced image mammography, AJR 140:9-14, 1983.
Thron A and Voigt K: Rotational cerebral angiography: procedure and value, AJNR 4:289-291, 1983.
1984 Fallone BG and Podgorsak EB: Image subtraction by solid state electroradiography, Phys Med Biol 29:703-709, 1984.
Fallone BG and Podgorsak EB: Radiographic image subtraction in gas ionography, Med Phys 11:47-49, 1984.
McSweeney MB, Sprawls P and Egan RL: Enhanced-image mammography, Recent Results Cancer Res 90:79-89, 1984.
Schatz SL, et al: A subtraction technique in conventional angiography, Radiology 151:531, 1984.
1986 Nelson JA: Newer subtraction and filtration techniques, Med Instrum 20:192-198, 1986.

LYMPHOGRAPHY

For bibliographic citations before 1964, please see the fifth edition of this atlas.

1964 Benninghoff DL and Herman PG: Iliopelvic abdomino-aortic lymphatic structures: a chart, Med Radiogr Photogr 40:35-37, 1964.
Brody HS, et al: Lymphangiography: an aid in urological surgery, J Urol 91:606-607, 1964.
Clouse ME, et al: Lymphangiographic criteria for diagnosis of retroperitoneal fibrosis, Radiology 83:1-5, 1964.

Herman PG, Benninghoff DL and Schwartz S: A physiologic approach to lymph flow in lymphography, AJR 91:1207-1215, 1964.

Koehler PR, et al: Lymphangiography: a survey of its current status, AJR 91:1216-1221, 1964.

Lachapèle AP, et al: De l'étude anatomoradiologique du canal thoracique d'après 60 opacifications sur l'être humain vivant, J Radiol Electr 45:1-10, 1964. Abstract: AJR 92:723, 1964.

1965 Buonocore E and Young JR: Lymphangiographic evaluation of lymphedema and lymphatic flow, AJR 95:751-765, 1965.

De Roo T: Une nouvelle technique simple pour la lymphographie, Ann Radiol 8:97-100, 1965.

De Roo T, Thomas P and Kropholler RW: The importance of tomography for the interpretation of the lymphographic picture of lymph node metastases, AJR 94:925-934, 1965.

O'Leary JA and Friedman PJ: Lymphography and pelvic carcinoma, Am J Obstet Gynecol 92:777-791, 1965.

Van Rensburg LCJ: Lymphography: its technique and value, S Afr Med J 39:271-277, 1965.

1966 Dolan PA: Lymphography: complications encountered in 522 examinations, Radiology 86:876-880, 1966.

Jackson RJA: Complications of lymphography, Br Med J 1:1203-1205, 1966.

Jing B-S: Improved technique of lymphangiography, AJR 98:952-956, 1966.

Love RW and Takaro T: Lymphangiography with direct roentgenographic magnification, Radiology 87:123-127, 1966.

1967 Ditchek T and Scanlon GT: Direct magnification lymphography, JAMA 199:654-656, 1967.

Kuisk H and Panning WP: A simple, practical technic of lymphography, Radiology 88:576-583, 1967.

Maddison FE: Lymphatic cannulation without dye, Radiology 88:362-363, 1967.

Miller WE: A simplified cannulation technique for lymphangiography, AJR 101:978-980, 1967.

1968 O'Brien PH, et al: Lymphangiography, Surg Gynecol Obstet 126:131-143, 1968.

1969 Burgener F and Fuchs WA: The importance of lymphography in the diagnosis and treatment of malignant testicular tumors, Schweiz Med Wochenschr 99:764-774, 1969. (In German) Abstract: Radiology 94:477, 1970.

1971 Lee KF, Hodes PJ and Lin SR: The value of the inlet and outlet views of the pelvis in lymphography, AJR 111:297-300, 1971.

1972 Howland WJ: A cannula method of lymphangiography, AJR 114:830-831, 1972.

1973 Bergstrom JF: A simplified and reliable cannulation technique for lymphography, AJR 117:701-703, 1973.

Bruna J: Suprailiac lymphography, Acta Radiol [Diagn] 14:157-160, 1973.

1974 Page RE: Normal lymphographic variations of lumbar, iliac, and inguinal lymph vessels, Acta Radiol 15:662-669, 1974.

1975 Göthlin J, et al: Retrograde angiography of the human thoracic duct, AJR 124:472-476, 1975.

Grant W: Lymphography: technique, indications, and principles of interpretation, S Afr Med J 49:1341-1346, 1975.

Laurin S: Cavography and lymphangiography in Hodgkin's disease, Acta Radiol 16:98-106, 1975.

1976 Beeckman P, et al: Critical evaluation of different x-ray methods in exploration of mediastinal lymphadenopathy, J Belge Radiol 59:459-465, 1976.

1977 Blank N and Castellino RA: Mediastinal lymphadenopathy, Semin Roentgenol 12:215-223, 1977.

Gandhi MG: Testicular lymphography: a clinical study, J Urol 117:174, 1977.

Kinmonth JB: Lymphography 1977: a review of some technical points, Lymphology 10:102-106, 1977.

1978 Farah RN and Cerny JC: Lymphangiography in staging patients with carcinoma of the bladder, J Urol 119:40-41, 1978.

Nuttall J, et al: Lymphography in tumours of the urogenital tract, J R Soc Med 71:41-43, 1978.

Rubin BE: Extravasation of Ethiodol into deep tissues of the foot: a complication of lymphangiography, AJR 131:342-343, 1978.

1979 Knochel JQ, Koehler PR and Miller FJ: Need for chest radiographs during and after lymphography, AJR 132:981-982, 1979.

Raghavaiah NV and Jordan WP Jr: Prostatic lymphography, J Urol 121:178-181, 1979.

1980 Carr D and Davidson JK: Magnification lymphography, Clin Radiol 31:535-539, 1980.

Castaneda-Zuniga WR, et al: Routine magnification lymphangiography with a swinging slot x-ray machine, Radiology 137:231-234, 1980.

Lee JK, et al: Limitations of the postlymphangiogram plain abdominal radiograph as an indicator of recurrent lymphoma: comparison to computed tomography, Radiology 134:155-158, 1980.

McIvor J: Changes in lymph node size induced by lymphography, Clin Radiol 31:541-544, 1980.

Ritsema GH: Ether-thinned ethiodol in lymphangiography: a prospective comparative study, Diagn Imaging 49:316-319, 1980.

Siefert HM, et al: Iotasul, a water-soluble contrast agent for direct and indirect lymphography: results of preclinical investigations, Lymphology 13:150-157, 1980.

1981 Bollinger A, et al: Fluorescence microlymphography, Circulation 64:1195-1200, 1981.

Hoekstra WJ and Schroeder FH: The role of lymphangiography in the staging of prostatic cancer, Prostate 2:433-440, 1981.

1982 Hirsch JI, et al: Use of Isosulfan Blue for identification of lymphatic vessels: experimental and clinical evaluation, AJR 139:1061-1064, 1982.

Magnusson A, et al: Computed tomography, ultrasound and lymphography in the diagnosis of malignant lymphoma, Acta Radiol [Diagn] 23:29-35, 1982.

1983 Eichner E, Danese C and Katz G: Vulvar lymphatics as demonstrated by vital dyes and lymphangiography, Int Surg 68:175-177, 1983.

Kinsman P: Lymphangiography—the last decade. Part I. Anatomy, uses, procedure, Radiography 49:203-209, 1983.

Magnusson A: Size of normal retroperitoneal lymph nodes, Acta Radiol 24:315-318, 1983.

Strijk SP, Debruyne FM and Herman CJ: Lymphography in the management of urologic tumors: radiological-pathological correlation, Radiology 146:39-45, 1983.

Zoretic SN, et al: Filling of the obturator nodes in pedal lymphangiography: fact or fiction, J Urol 129:533-535, 1983.

1984 Castellino RA, et al: Computed tomography, lymphography, and staging laparotomy: correlations in initial staging of Hodgkin disease, AJR 143:37-41, 1984.

Staton R: Lymphography, Radiol Technol 55:233-238, 1984.

1985 Groote AD, et al: Radiographic imaging of lymph nodes in lymph node dissection specimens, Lab Invest 52:326-329, 1985.

Miller DL, et al: The upright film in lymphangiographic detection of lymphangiomatosis, AJR 145:847-848, 1985.

1988 Cooper SG, Maitem AN and Richman AH: Fluorescein labeling of lymphatic vessels for lymphangiography, Radiology 167:559-560, 1988.

COMPUTED TOMOGRAPHY

1973 Ambrose J: Computerized transverse axial scanning (tomography). II. Clinical application, Br J Radiol 46:1023-1047, 1973.

Hounsfield GN: Computerized transverse axial scanning (tomography). I. Description of system, Br J Radiol 46:1016-1022, 1973.

1975 Wilson GH: Computed cerebral tomography, West J Med 122:316-317, 1975.

1976 Banna M: Basic introduction to computerized tomography, J Can Assoc Radiol 27:143-148, 1976.

Laffey P, et al: Computerized tomography in clinical medicine, Philadelphia, 1976, Medical Direction.

1977 Huckman MS, Grainer LS and Clasen RC: The normal computed tomogram, Semin Roentgenol 12:27-38, 1977.

Ledley RS, et al: Cross-sectional anatomy: an atlas for computerized tomography, Baltimore, 1977, Williams & Wilkins.

McCullough EC: Factors affecting the use of quantitative information from a CT scanner, Radiology 124:99-107, 1977.
Zata LM and Alvarez RE: An inaccuracy in computed tomography: the energy dependence of CT values, Radiology 124:91-97, 1977.
1978 Christensen EE, et al: An introduction to the physics of diagnostic radiology, ed 2, Philadelphia, 1978, Lea & Febiger.
Maravilla KR and Pastel MS: Technical aspects of CT scanning, CT 2:137-144, 1978.
Meire HB and Kreel L: Computed tomography and ultrasound: a comparison, Practitioner 220:593-597, 1978.
Thompson T: A practical approach to modern x-ray equipment, Boston, 1978, Little, Brown & Co.
Tully RJ, McFarland WD and Lodwick GS: General purpose digital display system for computed tomography images, Radiology 127:539-541, 1978.
Wackenheim A: Neuroradiology and computed tomography, J Belge Radiol 61:281-286, 1978.
1979 Cohen G: Contrast-detail-dose analysis of six different computed tomographic scanners, J Comput Assist Tomogr 3:197-203, 1979.
Cohen G: The use of contrast-detail-dose evaluation of image quality in a computed tomographic scanner, J Comput Assist Tomogr 3:189-195, 1979.
Frank E: Computed tomography of the pancreas: a new roentgenographic examination, Radiol Technol 50:403-409, 1979.
Kowalski G and Wagner W: Patient dose rate: an ultimate limit for spatial and density resolution of scanning systems, Biomed Tech 24(3):38-42, 1979.
Rice JF and Banks TE: Normal and high accuracy computed tomography of the brain: dose and imaging considerations, J Comput Assist Tomogr 3:497-502, 1979.
Rice JF, et al: Introduction to computed tomography, Milwaukee, 1979, General Electric Co.
1980 Ball WS, Wicks JD and Mettler FA Jr: Prone-supine change in organ position: CT demonstration, AJR 135:815-820, 1980.
Coin CG and Coin JT: Contact enhancement by xenon gas in computed tomography of the spinal cord and brain: preliminary observations, J Comput Assist Tomogr 4:217-221, 1980.
Computed tomography of the abdomen, Int Adv Surg Oncol 3:221-274, 1980.
Farber AL: Advantages of varient section of thickness relative to specific anatomy, Radiol Technol 51:793-796, 1980.
Fischer HW: Occurrence of seizure during cranial computed tomography, Radiology 137:563-564, 1980.
Ghoshhajra K and Rao KC: CT in spinal trauma, CT 4:309-318, 1980.
Hatfield KD, Segal SD and Tait K: Barium sulfate for abdominal computer assisted tomography, J Comput Assist Tomogr 4:570, 1980.
Hounsfield GN: Computed medical imaging: Nobel lecture, Dec 8, 1979, Comput Assist Tomogr 4:665-674, 1980.
Joseph PM, et al: Clinical and experimental investigation of a smoothed CT reconstruction algorithm, Radiology 134:507-516, 1980.
Kubota K, et al: Some devices for computed tomography radiotherapy treatment planning, J Comput Assist Tomogr 4:677-679, 1980.
Margulis AR, et al: The desirable properties of computed tomography scanners, Radiology 134:261, 1980.
Meany TF, et al: Detection of low contrast lesions in computed body tomography: an experimental study of simulated lesions, Radiology 134:149-154, 1980.
Schindler E and Reck R: Value and limits of computer-assisted tomography, Head Neck Surg 2:287-292, 1980.
Scott WR: Seizures: a reaction to contrast media for computed tomography of the brain, Radiology 137:359-361, 1980.
Termote JL, et al: Computed tomography of the normal and pathologic muscular system, Radiology 137:439-444, 1980.
van Hassel-Strijbosch M and van de Werf K: Value of reconstruction modes in CT scanning of the head, Radiography 46:209-212, 1980.
Williams AL, Haughton VM and Syvertsen A: Computed tomography in the diagnosis of herniated nucleus pulposus, Radiology 135:95-99, 1980.
Winter J: Edge enhancement of computed tomograms by digital unsharp masking, Radiology 135:234-235, 1980.
Young SW, et al: Dynamic computed tomography body scanning, J Comput Assist Tomogr 4:168-173, 1980.
1981 Cohen Z, et al: Iodinated starch particles: new contrast material for computed tomography of the liver, J Comput Assist Tomogr 5:843-846, 1981.
Egund N, et al: CT of soft tissue tumors, AJR 137:725-729, 1981.
Haaga JR, et al: The effect of mAs variation upon computed tomography image quality as evaluated by in vivo and in vitro studies, Radiology 138:449-454, 1981.
Hamlin DJ and Burgener FA: Positive and negative contrast agents in CT evaluation of the abdomen and pelvis, CT 5:82-90, 1981.
Jones ET: Use of computed axial tomography in pediatric orthopedics, J Pediatr Orthop 1:329-338, 1981.
Kuhn JP: CT in the evaluation of pediatric abdominal abnormalities, CRC Crit Rev Diagn Imaging 16:125-180, 1981.
Schoppe WD, Hessel SJ and Adams DF: Time requirements in performing body CT studies, J Comput Assist Tomogr 5:513-515, 1981.
Steele JR and Hoffman JC: Brainstem evaluation with CT cisternography, AJR 136:287-292, 1981.
Tianado J, et al: Computed tomography of the perineum, AJR 136:475-481, 1981.
Turnipseed WD, et al: Computerized arteriography of the cerebrovascular system: its use with intravenous administration of contrast material, Arch Surg 116:470-473, 1981.
1982 Beck TJ, Rosenbaum AE and Miller NR: Orbital computed tomography: technical aspects, Int Ophthalmol Clin 22:7-13, 1982.
Carmel PW and Mawad M: CT scanning of the posterior fossa, Clin Neurosurg 29:51-102, 1982.
Ekelund L, Herrlin K and Rydholm A: Comparison of computed tomography and angiography in the evaluation of soft tissue tumors of the extremities, Acta Radiol [Diagn] 23:15-27, 1982.
Friedmann G and Promper C: CT examination of the spine and the spinal canal, Eur J Radiol 2:60-65, 1982.
Hatten HP Jr, Walker ME and Covington MC: Range highlight facility within region of interest for air-CT cisternography and canalography, Radiol Technol 54:35-36, 1982.
Howard P and Sage MR: CT of the paranasal sinuses and face, Australas Radiol 26:130-136, 1982.
Hubbard LF, McDermott JH and Garrett G: Computed axial tomography in musculoskeletal trauma, J Trauma 22:388-394, 1982.
Kassel EE, Noyek AM and Cooper PW: High resolution computerized tomography in otorhinolaryngology, J Otolaryngol 11:297-306, 1982.
Kivisaari L, Makela P and Aarimaa M: Pancreatic mobility: an important factor in pancreatic computed tomography, J Comput Assist Tomogr 6:854-856, 1982.
LaMasters DL, et al: Multiplanar metrizamide-enhanced CT imaging of the foramen magnum, AJNR 3:485-494, 1982.
Larsson SG, Mancuso A and Hanafee W: Computed tomography of the tongue and floor of the mouth, Radiology 143:493-500, 1982.
Lee JK and Balfe DM: Computed tomography evaluation of lymphoma patients, CRC Crit Rev Diagn Imaging 18:1-28, 1982.
Lee JK, et al: A support device for obtaining direct coronal computed tomographic scans of the pelvis and lower abdomen, Radiology 145:209-210, 1982.
Lee KR: Computed tomography of the gastrointestinal tract, CRC Crit Rev Diagn Imaging 18:121-165, 1982.
Martinez CR, et al: Computed tomography of the neck, Ann Otol Rhinol Laryngol 99:1-31, 1982.
Olson JE, Dorwart RH and Brant WE: Use of high-resolution thin-section CT scanning of the petrous bone, Laryngoscope 92:1274-1278, 1982.

Peyster RG and Hoover ED: CT in head trauma, J Trauma 22:25-38, 1982.

Seeram E: Computed tomography technology, Philadelphia, 1982, WB Saunders Co.

Silverman PM, et al: High-resolution multiplanar CT images of the larynx, Invest Radiol 17:634-637, 1982.

van Waes PF and Zonneveld FW: Direct coronal body computed tomography, J Comput Assist Tomogr 6:58-66, 1982.

1983 Berg BC: Complementary roles of radionuclide and computed tomographic imaging in evaluating trauma, Semin Nucl Med 13:86-103, 1983.

Burgener FA and Hamlin DJ: Contrast enhancement of hepatic tumors in CT: comparison, AJR 140:291-295, 1983.

Chakeres DW and Spiegel PK: A systematic technique for comprehensive evaluation of the temporal bone, Radiology 146:97-106, 1983.

Dickson DR and Maue Dickson W: Tomographic assessment of craniofacial structures: cleft lip/palate, Cleft Palate J 20:23-34, 1983.

duBoulay GH, Teather D and Wills K: CT: to enhance or not to enhance: a computer-aided study, AJNR 4:421-424, 1983.

Dunn EL, Berry PH and Connally JD: Computed tomography of the pelvis in patients with multiple injuries, J Trauma 23:378-383, 1983.

Foley WD, et al: Contrast enhancement technique for dynamic hepatic computed tomographic scanning, Radiology 147:797-803, 1983.

Gamsu G and Webb WR: Computed tomography of the trachea and mainstem bronchi, Semin Roentgenol 18:51-60, 1983.

Glazer GM, et al: Evaluation of the pulmonary hilum: comparison of conventional radiography, 55 degrees posterior oblique tomography, and dynamic computed tomography, J Comput Assist Tomogr 7:983-989, 1983.

Goldberg HI, et al: Computed tomography in the evaluation of Crohn disease, AJR 140:277-282, 1983.

Graf von Keyserlingk D, DeBleser R and Poeck K: Stereographic reconstruction of human brain CT series, Acta Anat 115:336-344, 1983.

Hian TW: Contrast enhancement of brain tumors in computed tomography, Diagn Imaging 52:113-116, 1983.

Jazrawy H, et al: Computed tomography of the temporal bone, J Otolaryngol 12:37-44, 1983.

Kuhns L and Seeger J: Atlas of computed tomography variants, Chicago, 1983, Year Book Medical Publishers, Inc.

Lamothe A, et al: High resolution CT scan of the temporal bone, J Otolaryngol 12:119-124, 1983.

Leitman BS, et al: The use of computed tomography in evaluating chest wall pathology, CT 7:399-405, 1983.

Lipton MJ, et al: CT scanning of the heart, Cardiovasc Clin 13:385-401, 1983.

Marsh JL and Gado M: The longitudinal orbital CT projection: a versatile image for orbital assessment, Plast Reconstr Surg 71:308-317, 1983.

Marsh JL and Vannier MW: Surface imaging from computerized tomographic scans, Surgery 94:159-165, 1983.

Morgan CL: Atlas of computed body tomography, Baltimore, 1983, University Park Press.

Osborne D, et al: Assessment of craniocervical junction and atlantoaxial relation, AJNR 4:843-845, 1983.

Parvey LS, Grizzard M and Coburn TP: Use of infusion pump for intravenous enhanced computed tomography, J Comput Assist Tomogr 7:175-176, 1983.

Rajfer J, et al: The use of computerized tomography scanning to localize the impalpable testis, J Urol 129:972-974, 1983.

Naidich DP, et al: Computed tomography of the diaphragm: normal anatomy and variants, J Comput Assist Tomogr 7:633-640, 1983.

Riddlesberger MM Jr and Kuhn JP: The role of computed tomography in diseases of the musculoskeletal system, CT 7:85-99, 1983.

Silverman PM and Korobkin M: High-resolution computed tomography of the normal larynx, AJR 140:875-879, 1983.

Swindell W, et al: Computed tomography with a linear accelerator with radiotherapy applications, Med Phys 10:416-420, 1983.

Vigo M, et al: Computerized axial tomography in the evaluation of gynecologic pelvic masses, Clin Exp Obstet Gynecol 10:210-212, 1983.

Yamamoto Y, Sakurai M and Asari S: Towne (half-axial) and semisagittal computed tomography in the evaluation of blow-out fractures of the orbit, J Comput Assist Tomogr 7:306-309, 1983.

Zeitler E, et al: Experiences with Rayvist and iopromid in head and body CT, Fortschr Geb Rontgerstr Nuklearmed Erganzungsband 118:162-172, 1983.

1984 Axel L, et al: Functional imaging of the liver: new information from dynamic CT, Invest Radiol 19:23-29, 1984.

Bramwit DN: Direct sagittal (lateral) computer tomography of the temporomandibular joints, J Bergen Cty Dent Soc 50:11-13, 1984.

Burk DL Jr, et al: Pelvic and acetabular fractures: examination by angled CT scanning, Radiology 153:548, 1984.

Chakeres DW and Kapila A: Computed tomography of the temporal bone, Med Radiogr Photogr 60:1-32, 1984.

Chambers SE and Best JJ: A comparison of dilute barium and dilute water-soluble contrast in opacification of the bowel for abdominal computed tomography, Clin Radiol 35:463-464, 1984.

Curtin HD: CT of acoustic neuroma and other tumors of the ear, Radiol Clin North Am 22:77-105, 1984.

Daniels DL, Williams AL and Haughton VM: Jugular foramen: anatomic and computed tomographic study, AJR 142:153-158, 1984.

Dorwart RH: Computed tomography of the lumbar spine: techniques, normal anatomy, CRC Crit Rev Diagn Imaging 22:1-42, 1984.

Firooznia H, et al: Computed tomography in localization of foreign bodies lodged in the extremities, Comput Radiol 8:237-239, 1984.

Goldberg HI, et al: Device for performing direct coronal CT scanning of the abdomen and pelvis, AJR 143:900-902, 1984.

1984 Griffin DJ, et al: Observations on CT differentiation of pleural and peritoneal fluid, J Comput Assist Tomogr 8:24-28, 1984.

Halvorsen RA and Thompson WA: Computed tomography of the gastroesophageal junction, CRC Crit Rev Diagn Imaging 21:183-228, 1984.

Haney PJ and Whitley NO: CT of benign cystic abdominal masses in children, AJR 142:1279-1281, 1984.

Kanematsu T, et al: Transparent box enables three-dimensional viewing of CT imaging of the liver, Jpn J Surg 14:94-96, 1984.

Kearfott KJ, Rottenberg DA and Knowles RI: A new headholder for PET, CT, and NMR imaging, J Comput Assist Tomogr 8:1217-1220, 1984.

Love L, et al: Intravenous contrast bolus in computed tomography investigation of mass lesions, Diagn Imaging Clin Med 53:57-66, 1984.

Mintz MC and Seltzer SE: Oral administration of contrast medium for rectal opacification in pelvic computed tomography, CT 8:73-74, 1984.

Ohishi H, et al: Usefulness of direct coronal CT in the diagnosis of urinary bladder, Radiat Med 2:181-184, 1984.

Pastakia B and Herdt JR: Radiolucent "zones" in parietal bones seen on computed tomography: a normal anatomic variant, J Comput Assist Tomogr 8:108-109, 1984.

Patel RB, Barton P and Green L: CT of isolated elbow in evaluation of trauma: a modified technique, Comput Radiol 8:1-4, 1984.

Proto AV: Evaluation of the bronchi with CT, Semin Roentgenol 19:199-210, 1984.

Roberts D, et al: Three-dimensional imaging and display of the temporomandibular joint, Oral Surg Oral Med Oral Pathol 58:461-474, 1984.

Roberts D, et al: Radiologic techniques used to evaluate the temporomandibular joint, Anesth Prog 31:241-256, 1984.
Shetty AK, Deeb ZL and Hryshko FG: Computed tomography of spine trauma, J Comput Tomogr 8:105-112, 1984.
Symposium on CT of ear, nose, and throat, Radiol Clin North Am 22:1-284, 1984.
Tehranzadeh J and Gabriele OF: The prone position for CT of the lumbar spine, Radiology 152:817-818, 1984.
Totty WG and Vannier MW: Complex musculoskeletal anatomy: analysis using three-dimensional surface reconstruction, Radiology 150:173-177, 1984.
Whelan MA, et al: CT of the base of the skull, Radiol Clin North Am 22:177-217, 1984.
1985 Clark LR, et al: Enhanced pancreatic CT imaging utilizing a geometric magnification, Invest Radiol 20:531-538, 1985.
Conover GL: Direct sagittal CT scanning of the temporomandibular joint, CDS Rev 78:28-31, 1985.
Deutsch AL, Resnick D and Mink JH: Computed tomography of the glenohumeral and sternoclavicular joints, Orthop Clin North Am 16:497-511, 1985.
Garrett JS, Higgins CB and Lipton MJ: Computed axial tomography of the heart, Int J Card Imaging 1:113-126, 1985.
Gould R, Rosenfield AT and Friedlaender GE: Loose body within the glenohumeral joint in recurrent anterior dislocation: CT demonstration, J Comput Assist Tomogr 9:404-406, 1985.
Johnson JF, et al: Tracheoesophageal fistula: diagnosis with CT, Pediatr Radiol 15:134-135, 1985.
Knapp RH, Vannier MW and Marsh JL: Generation of three-dimensional images for CT scans: technological perspective, Radiol Technol 56:391-398, 1985.
Lau LS, Simpson L and Murphy F: High resolution CT scanning of the bronchial tree: CT bronchography—technique and clinical application, Australas Radiol 29:323-331, 1985.
Manzione JV, Rumbaugh CL and Katzberg RW: Direct sagittal computed tomography of the temporal bone, J Comput Assist Tomogr 9:417-419, 1985.
Munro CJ: Computed tomography of the adrenal glands, Radiography 51:281-285, 1985.
Noble PN: Computed tomography of the pancreas, Radiography 51:205-210, 1985.
Perkerson RB Jr, et al: CT densities in delayed iodine hepatic scanning, Radiology 155:445-446, 1985.
Sandler CM, Raval B and David CL: Computed tomography of the kidney, Urol Clin North Am 12:657-675, 1985.
Silverman PM, Dunnick NR and Ford KK: Computed tomography of the normal seminal vesicles, Comput Radiol 9:379-385, 1985.
Simon DC, et al: Direct sagittal CT of the temporomandibular joint, Radiology 157:545, 1985.
Stork J: Intraperitoneal contrast agents for computed tomography, AJR 145:300, 1985.
Zonneveld FW: The technique of direct multiplanar high resolution CT of the temporal bone, Neurosurg Rev 8:5-13, 1985.
1986 Boger DC: Traction device to improve CT imaging of lower cervical spine, AJNR 7:719-721, 1986.
Bresina SJ, et al: Three-dimensional wrist imaging: evaluation of functional and pathologic anatomy by computer, Clin Plast Surg 13:389-405, 1986.
Brody AS, et al: Artifacts seen during CT pelvimetry: implications for digital systems with scanning beams, Radiology 160:269-271, 1986.
Citrin CM: High resolution orbital computed tomography, J Comput Assist Tomogr 10:810-816, 1986.
Farmer D, et al: High-speed (cine) computed tomography of the heart, Cardiovasc Clin 17:345-356, 1986.
Helms CA, et al: Cine-CT of the temporomandibular joint, Cranio 4:246-250, 1986.
Kopelman JN, et al: Computed tomographic pelvimetry in the evaluation of breech presentation, Obstet Gynecol 68:455-458, 1986.
Kursunoglu S, et al: Three-dimensional computed tomographic analysis of the normal temporomandibular joint, J Oral Maxillofac Surg 44:257-259, 1986.
Laval Jeantet AM, et al: Influence of vertebral fat content on quantitative CT density, Radiology 159:463-466, 1986.
Leib ML: Computed tomography of the orbit, Int Ophthalmol Clin 26:103-121, 1986.
Lenke RR and Shuman WP: Computed tomographic pelvimetry, J Reprod Med 31:958-960, 1986.
Nakano Y, et al: Stomach and duodenum: radiographic magnification using computed tomography, Radiology 160:383-387, 1986.
Pozzi Mucelli RS, Muner G and Pozzi Mucelli F: Three-dimensional computed tomography of the acetabulum, Eur J Radiol 6:168-177, 1986.
Rees MR, et al: Heart evaluation by cine CT: use of two new oblique views, Radiology 159:804-806, 1986.
Schnyder P, Mansouri B and Uske A: Direct coronal computed tomography of the lumbar spine: a new technical approach in supine position, Eur J Radiol 6:248-251, 1986.
Singson RD, Feldman F and Rosenberg ZS: Elbow joint: assessment with double-contrast CT arthrography, Radiology 160:167-173, 1986.
Strickland B, Brennan J and Denison DM: Computed tomography in diffuse lung disease: improving the image, Clin Radiol 37:335-338, 1986.
Virapongse C, et al: Three-dimensional computed tomographic reformation of the spine, Neurosurgery 18:53-58, 1986.
Zeman RK, et al: Computed tomography of renal masses: pitfalls and anatomic variants, Radiographics 6:351-372, 1986.
Zonneveld FW and Koornneef L: Patient positioning for direct sagittal CT of the orbit parallel to the optic nerve, Radiology 158:547-549, 1986.
1987 Biondetti PR, et al: Wrist: coronal and transaxial CT scanning, Radiology 163:149-151, 1987.
Curnes JT, Banning BC and Robards JB: Cranial computed tomography in the morbidly obese patient, J Comput Assist Tomogr 11:920, 1987.
Gower DJ, Culp P and Ball M: Lateral lumbar spine roentgenograms: potential role in complications, Surg Neurol 27:316-318, 1987.
Heffez L, Mafee MF and Langer B: Use of a new head holder for obtaining direct sagittal CT images of the TMJ, J Oral Maxillofac Surg 45:822-824, 1987.
Honda H, et al: Optimal positioning for CT examinations of the skull base: experimental and clinical studies, Eur J Radiol 7:225-228, 1987.
Lagrange JL, et al: CT measurement of lung density: the role of patient position and value for total body irradiation, Int J Radiat Oncol Biol Phys 13:941-944, 1987.
Lipton MJ: Cine computerized tomography, Int J Card Imaging 2:209-221, 1987.
Mayo JR, et al: High-resolution CT of the lungs: an optimal approach, Radiology 163:507-510, 1987.
Moon JB and Smith WL: Application of cine computed tomography to the assessment of velopharyngeal form and function, Cleft Palate J 24:226-232, 1987.
Moore SC and Judy PF: Cardiac computed tomography using redundant-ray prospective gating, Med Phys 14:193-196, 1987.
Muranaka T, et al: CT retrograde pancreatography using an indwelling balloon catheter, Radiat Med 5:42-47, 1987.
Neufang KF, Zanella FE and Ewen K: Radiation doses to the eye lenses in computed tomography of the orbit and the petrous bone, Eur J Radiol 7:203-205, 1987.
Rhodes RA, et al: Tomographic levels for intravenous urography: CT-determined guidelines, Radiology 163:673-675, 1987.
Scott WW Jr, Fishman EK and Magid D: Acetabular fractures: optimal imaging, Radiology 165:537-539, 1987.
Stark P: Computed tomography of the sternum, CRC Crit Rev Diagn Imaging 27:321-349, 1987.

Vogelzang RL and Gore RM: Bolus-rapid infusion of contrast medium: simplified technique, J Comput Tomogr 11:1-3, 1987.

Zonneveld FW, et al: Normal direct multiplanar CT anatomy of the orbit with correlative, Radiol Clin North Am 25:381-407, 1987.

1988 Chung JW, et al: Computed tomography of cavernous sinus diseases, Neuroradiology 30:319-328, 1988.

Dondelinger RF and Kurdziel JC: Computed tomographic arteriography (CTA) of the liver, Bull Soc Sci Med Grand Duche Luxemb 125:27-34, 1988.

Fava C and Preti G: Lateral transcranial radiography of temporomandibular joints (Part I), J Prosthet Dent 59:218-227, 1988.

Heffez L, Mafee MF and Langer B: Double-contrast arthrography of the temporomandibular joint: role of direct sagittal CT imaging, Oral Surg Oral Med Oral Pathol 65:511-514, 1988.

Hishikawa Y, et al: Esophageal fistula: demonstration by CT, Radiat Med 6:115-116, 1988.

Kashiwagi T, et al: Three-dimensional demonstration of liver and spleen by a computer, Acta Radiol 29:27-31, 1988.

Levin DN, et al: Retrospective geometric correlation of MR, CT, and PET images, Radiology 169:817-823, 1988.

Mafee MF, et al: Direct sagittal CT in the evaluation of temporal bone disease, AJR 150:1403-1410, 1988.

Magid D, et al: 2D and 3D computed tomography of the pediatric hip, Radiographics 8:901-933, 1988.

Peruzzi W, et al: Portable chest roentgenography and computed tomography in critically ill patients, Chest 93:722-726, 1988.

Platt JF and Glazer GM: IV contrast material for abdominal CT: comparison of three methods, AJR 151:275-277, 1988.

Sartoris DJ and Resnick D: Computed tomography of the lower extremity (Part II), Orthop Rev 17:20-24, 1988.

Sundram SR: Direct coronal imaging of the abdomen and pelvis, Radiography 54:86-92, 1988.

Tawn DJ, Snow M and Jeans WD: Computed tomography of the internal auditory canals, Bristol Med Chir J 103:13-15, 1988.

Zinreich SJ, et al: 3-D CT for cranial, facial and laryngeal surgery, Laryngoscope 98:1212-1219, 1988.

1989 Mattrey RF: Potential role of perfluorooctylbromide in the detection and characterization of liver lesions with CT, Radiology 170:18-20, 1989.

Patel RB, Barton P and Green L: CT of isolated elbow in evaluation of trauma: a modified technique, Comput Radiol 8:1-4, 1984.

DIAGNOSTIC MEDICAL SONOGRAPHY

1964 Willocks J, et al: Foetal cephalometry by ultrasound, J Obstet Gynaecol Br Comm 71:11-20, 1964.

1966 Bernstine RL and Callagan DA: Ultrasonic Doppler inspection of fetal heart, Am J Obstet Gynecol 95:1001-1003, 1966.

Goldberg BB, Ostrum BJ and Isard HJ: Ultrasonic aortography, JAMA 198:353-358, 1966.

Gottesfeld KR, et al: Ultrasound placentography—a new method for placental localization, Am J Obstet Gynecol 96:538-547, 1966.

Grossman CC: A and B scan sonoencephalography (SEG): a new dimension in neurology. In Grossman CC, et al: editors: Diagnostic ultrasound, New York, 1966, Plenum Press, pp 130-141.

Lehman JS: Ultrasound in the diagnosis of hepatobiliary disease, Radiol Clin North Am 4:605-623, 1966.

1967 Donald I and Abdulla U: Ultrasound in obstetrics and gynaecology, Br J Radiol 40:604-611, 1967.

Ostrum BJ, Goldberg BB and Isard HJ: A-mode ultrasound differentiation of soft tissue masses, Radiology 88:745-749, 1967.

Strandness DE, Jr, et al: Ultrasonic flow detection: a useful technique in the evaluation of peripheral vascular disease, Am J Surg 113:311-320, 1967.

1968 Brown RE: Detection of intrauterine death, Am J Obstet Gynecol 102:965-968, 1968.

Brown RE: Diagnostic ultrasound associated with departments of radiology, J Can Assoc Radiol 19:83-89, 1968.

Feuerlein W and Dilling H: The echoencephalogram of the third ventricle in different age groups. In Proceedings in echoencephalography, New York, 1968, Springer-Verlag, pp 143-145.

Goldberg BB, Ostrum BJ and Isard HJ: Nephrosonography: ultrasound differentiation of renal masses, Radiology 90:1113-1118, 1968.

Goldberg BB, Sklaroff DM and Isard HJ: Echoencephalography in the management of patients receiving radiation therapy, Radiology 91:363-366, 1968.

Sigel B, et al: Comparison of clinical and Doppler ultrasound evaluation of confirmed lower extremity venous disease, Surgery 64:332-338, 1968.

Thiery M: Diagnostic uses of the fetal pulse detector, Bull Soc R Belg Gynecol Obstet 38:71-79, 1968.

1969 DeLand FH: A modified technique of ultrasonography for the detection and differential diagnosis of breast lesions, AJR 105:446-452, 1969.

Kohorn EI, et al: Ultrasonic scanning in obstetrics and gynecology, Obstet Gynecol 34:515-522, 1969.

1970 Engelhart G and Blaunstein UH: Ultrasound in the diagnosis of malignant pancreatic tumors, Gut 11:443-449, 1970.

Eycleshymer AC and Schoemaker DM: A cross-section anatomy, ed 2, New York, 1970, Appleton-Century-Crofts.

Freimanis AK: Echographic exploration of abdominal structures, CRC Crit Rev Radiol Sci 1:207, 1970.

Gottesfeld KR: Ultrasonic diagnosis of fetal death, Am J Obstet Gynecol 108:623-634, 1970.

1971 Brown RE: Doppler ultrasound in obstetrics, JAMA 218:1395-1399, 1971.

Thompson HE and Makowski EL: Estimation of birth weight and gestational age, Obstet Gynecol 37:44-47, 1971.

1972 Barnett B: Ultrasound in abdominal conditions, Radiography 38:233-241, 1972.

Falus M, Koranyi G and Sobel M: Follow-up studies on infants examined by ultrasound during fetal age, Orv Hetil 113:2119-2121, 1972 (In Hungarian).

Noah BA and Igal G: Diagnosis of placenta praevia: use of the ultrasonic method compared with the radioisotope method, J Gynecol Obstet Biol Reprod 1:361-364, 1972.

Schupbach M: Ultrasonic diagnosis of retinal detachment, Mod Probl Ophthalmol 10:443-448, 1972 (In German).

Winsberg F and Mercer EN: Echocardiography in combined valve disease, Radiology 105:405-411, 1972.

1973 Mason DT: Non-invasive methods for the assessment of cardiac function, Calif Med 119:53-55, 1973.

Reed MF: Ultrasonic placentography, Br J Radiol 46:255-258, 1973.

Watmough D: A critical assessment of ultrasonic fetal cephalometry, Br J Radiol 46:566-567, 1973.

1974 Rasmussen SN, et al: Three-dimensional imaging of abdominal organs with ultrasound, AJR 121:883-888, 1974.

1975 David H, Weaver JB and Pearson JF: Doppler ultrasound and fetal activity activity, Br Med J 2:62-64, 1975.

Fitzgerald DE and Carr J: Doppler ultrasound diagnosis and classification as an alternative to arteriography, Angiology 26:283-288, 1975.

1976 Leopold GR, et al: Gray-scale ultrasonic cholecystography: a comparison with conventional radiographic techniques, Radiology 121:445-448, 1976.

1977 Bartrum RJ, Jr, Crow HC and Foote SR: Ultrasonic and radiographic cholecystography, N Engl J Med 296:538-541, 1977.

Baum G: Ultrasound mammography, Radiology 122:199-205, 1977.

Edelstone DI: Placental localization by ultrasound, Clin Obstet Gynecol 20:285-296, 1977.

Smith RP: Basic physics of ultrasound, Clin Obstet Gynecol 20:231-241, 1977.

1978 Behan M and Kazam E: Sonography of the common bile duct: value of the right anterior oblique view, AJR 130:701-709, 1978.

Crade M, Taylor KJ and Rosenfeld AT: Water distention of the gut in the evaluation of the pancreas by ultrasound, AJR 131:348-349, 1978.

Goldberg HI, et al: Capability of CT body scanning and ultrasonography to demonstrate the status of the biliary ductal system in patients with jaundice, Radiology 129:731-737, 1978.

1979 Leopold GR and Felson B: Radiology: ultrasound, JAMA 241:1389-1390, 1979.

1980 Detwiler RP, et al: Ultrasonography and oral cholecystography: a comparison of their use in the diagnosis of gall bladder disease, Arch Surg 115:1096-1098, 1980.

Haller JO, et al: Sonographic evaluation of the chest in infants and children, AJR 134:1019-1027, 1980.

Janus C and Janus S: Ultrasound: patients' views, JCU 8:17-20, 1980.

Leslie EV, et al: Computed tomography of the abdomen, Int Adv Surg Oncol 3:221-274, 1980.

Lewis E and Ritchie WG: A simple ultrasonic method for assessing renal size, JCU 8:417-420, 1980.

Meire HB, et al: The influence of ultrasound on obstetric radiography, Br J Radiol 53:1087, 1980.

Morgan CL, et al: Ultrasound patterns of disorders affecting the gastrointestinal tract, Radiology 135:129-135, 1980.

Nudelman S and Patton DD, editors: Imaging for medicine, nuclear medicine, ultrasonics, and thermography, New York, 1980, Plenum Press.

Seltzer SE, Finberg HJ and Weissman BN: Arthrosonography—technique, sonographic anatomy, and pathology, Invest Radiol 15:19-28, 1980.

1981 Cole-Beuglet C, et al: Ultrasound mammography: a comparison with radiographic mammography, Radiology 139:693-698, 1981.

Edwards MK, et al: Cribside neurosonography: real-time sonography for intracranial investigation of the neonate, AJR 136:271-275, 1981.

Engel JM and Deitch EE: Sonography of the anterior abdominal wall, AJR 137:73-77, 1981.

Fleischer AC, et al: Sonographic assessment of the bowel wall, AJR 136:887-891, 1981.

Foley WD, et al: Reformatted coronal display of upper abdominal computed tomography: comparison with ultrasonography, J Comput Assist Tomogr 5:496-502, 1981.

Grant EG, et al: Real-time sonography of the neonatal and infant head, AJR 136:265-270, 1981.

Hessler PC, et al: High accuracy sonographic recognition of gallstones, AJR 136:517-520, 1981.

Slovis TL and Kuhns LR: Real-time sonography of the brain through the anterior fontanelle, AJR 136:277-286, 1981.

Timor-Tritsch IE, Itskovitz J and Brandes JM: Estimation of fetal weight by real-time sonography, Obstet Gynecol 57:653-656, 1981.

1982 Bernardino ME, Thomas JL and Maklad N: Hepatic sonography: technical considerations, present applications, and possible future, Radiology 142:249-251, 1982.

Burt TB, Knochel JQ and Lee TG: Gas as a contrast agent and diagnostic aid in abdominal sonography, J Ultrasound Med 1:179-184, 1982.

Cole-Beuglet C, et al: Clinical experience with a prototype real-time dedicated breast scanner, AJR 139:905-911, 1982.

McGahan JP, Phillips HE and Cox KL: Sonography of the normal pediatric gallbladder and biliary tract, Radiology 144:873-875, 1982.

Simeone JF, et al: Sonography of the bile ducts after a fatty meal: an aid in detection of obstruction, Radiology 143:211-215, 1982.

Waldman WJ: Biological interactions of ultrasound, Radiol Technol 54:106-113, 1982.

1983 Bluth EI: Ultrasound evaluation of small bowel abnormalities, Am J Gastroenterol 78:788-793, 1983.

Carroll BA and Gross DM: High-frequency scrotal sonography, AJR 140:511-515, 1983.

Dunne MG and Cunat JS: Sonographic determination of fetal gender before 25 weeks gestation, AJR 140:741-743, 1983.

Dunne MG and Weksberg AP: Portable real-time sonography—a valuable adjunct to computed tomography, CT 7:285-294, 1983.

Hagan-Ansert SL: Textbook of diagnostic ultrasonography, St. Louis, 1983, The CV Mosby Company.

Krebs CA and Carson J: Gallbladder examinations: a comparison between sonography and radiography, Radiol Technol 54:181-188, 1983.

Ralls PW: Sonography in rheumatology, Clin Rheum Dis 9:443-451, 1983.

Slasky BS, Auerbach D and Skolnick ML: Value of portable real-time ultrasound in the ICU, Crit Care Med 11:160-164, 1983.

Wicks JD and Howe KS: Fundamentals of ultrasonographic technique, Chicago, 1983, Year Book Medical Publishers, Inc.

1984 Amis ES, Jr and Hartman DS: Renal ultrasonography 1984: a practical overview, Radiol Clin North Am 22:315-332, 1984.

Barnett E and Morley P: Clinical diagnostic ultrasound, Chicago, 1984, Year Book Medical Publishers, Inc.

de Lacey G, et al: Should cholecystography or ultrasound be the primary investigation for gallbladder disease? Lancet 1:205-207, 1984.

Egan RL and Egan KL: Detection of breast carcinoma: comparison of automated water-path whole-breast sonography, mammography, and physical examination, AJR 143:493-497, 1984.

Fukuda M, et al: Endoscopic ultrasonography in the diagnosis of pancreatic carcinoma: the use of a liquid-filled stomach method, Scand J Gastroenterol 94(suppl):65-76, 1984.

Han BK, Babcock DS and Oestreich AE: Sonography of brain tumors in infants, AJR 143:31-36, 1984.

Lux G, Heyder N and Lutz H: Ultrasound tomography of the upper gastrointestinal tract: orientation and diagnostic possibilities, Scand J Gastroenterol 94:13-20, 1984.

Montalvo BM, et al: Intraoperative sonography in spinal trauma, Radiology 153:125-134, 1984.

O'Brien WF, Buck DR and Nash JD: Evaluation of sonography in the initial assessment of the gynecologic patient, Am J Obstet Gynecol 149:598-602, 1984.

Rosenberg ER, et al: Extracranial cribside sonography in infants, South Med J 77:968-971, 1984.

Shawker TH, Sonies BC and Stone M: Soft tissue anatomy of the tongue and floor of the mouth: an ultrasound demonstration, Brain Lang 21(2):335-350, 1984.

Stannard MW, Binet EF and Jimenez JF: Cranial sonography: anatomic and pathological correlation, CRC Crit Rev Diagn Imaging 22:163-268, 1984.

Strohm WD and Classen M: Anatomical aspects in ultrasonic endoscopy, Scand J Gastroenterol 94(suppl):21-33, 1984.

Valdes C, Malini S and Malinak LR: Ultrasound evaluation of female genital tract anomalies: a review of 64 cases, Am J Obstet Gynecol 149:285-292, 1984.

1985 Butch RJ, Simeone JF and Mueller PR: Thyroid and parathyroid ultrasonography, Radiol Clin North Am 23(1):57-71, 1985.

Holen J, Waag RC and Gramiak R: Representations of rapidly oscillating structures on the Doppler display, Ultrasound Med Biol 11(2):267-272, 1985.

Kimme-Smith C, et al: Ultrasound mammography: effects of focal zone placement, Radiographics 5(6):955-969, 1985.

O'Leary DH: Vascular ultrasonography, Radiol Clin North Am 23(1):39-56, 1985.

Rubin E, et al: Hand-held real-time breast sonography, AJR 144(3):623-627, 1985.

Trotnow S, et al: A new set of instruments for sonographically controlled follicular puncture, Arch Gynecol 236(4):211-217, 1985.

1986 Bartrum RJ Jr: Ultrasound instrumentation, CRC Crit Rev Diagn Imaging 25(3):279-303, 1986.

DePietro MA, Brody BA and Teele RL: Peritrigonal echogenic "blush" on cranial sonsography: pathologic correlates, AJR 146(5):1067-1072, 1986.

DiPietro MA, Faix RG and Donn SM: Procedural hazards of neonatal ultrasonography, ICU 14(5):361-366, 1986.

Kremkau FW and Taylor KJ: Artifacts in ultrasound imaging, J Ultrasound Med 5(4):227-237, 1986.

Maron BJ: Structural features of the athlete heart as defined by echocardiography, J Am Coll Cardiol 7(1):190-203, 1986.

1987 Dudley NJ, Lamb MP and Copping C: A new method for fetal weight estimation using real-time ultrasound, Br J Obstet Gynaecol 94(2):110-114, 1987.

Fornage BD: The hypoechoic normal tendon: a pitfall, J Ultrasound Med 6(1):19-22, 1987.

Pilu G, et al: Ultrasound investigation of the posterior fossa in the fetus, Am J Perinatol 4(2):155-159, 1987.

Porena M, et al: Real-time transrectal sonographic voiding cystourethrography, 30(2):171-175, 1987.

Upadhyay SS, O'Neil T, Burwell RG and Moulton A: A new method using ultrasound for measuring femoral anteversion (torsion): technique and reliability, Br J Radiol 60(714):519-523, 1987.

1988 Beynon J, Mortensen NJ and Rigby HS: Rectal endosonography, a new technique for the preoperative staging of rectal carcinoma, Eur J Surg Oncol 14(4):297-309, 1988.

Druce HM: The use of ultrasound as an imaging technique in the diagnosis of sinusitis, N Engl Reg Allergy Proc 9(2):109-112, 1988.

Fornage BD and Rifkin MD: Ultrasound examination of tendons, Radiol Clin North Am 26(1):87-107, 1988.

Fornage BD and Rifkin MD: Ultrasound examination of the hand and foot, Radiol Clin North Am 26(1):1091-1129, 1988.

Grant EB, Tessler F and Perrella R: Infant cranial sonography, Radiol Clin North Am 26(5):1089-1110, 1988.

Kimme-Smith C, et al: Ultrasound artifacts affecting the diagnosis of breast masses, Ultrasound Med Biol 1(suppl):203-210, 1988.

Quinn MK, et al: Transvaginal endosonography: a new method to study the anatomy of the lower urinary tract in urinary stress incontinence, Br J Urol 62(5):414-419, 1988.

Rouse GA, et al: Current concepts in sonographic diagnosis of fetal renal disease, Radiographics 8(1):119-132, 1988.

Wells PN: Ultrasound imaging, J Biomed Eng 10(6):548-554, 1988.

1989 Crawford ED: The role of ultrasound in prostatic imaging: introduction and overview, Urology 33(suppl 6):2-6, 1989.

Grant ES, Tessler FN and Perrella RR: Clinical Doppler imaging, AJR 152(4):707-717, 1989.

Kossoff G, et al: A sonographic technique to reduce beam distortion by curved interfaces, Ultrasound Med Biol 15(4):375-382, 1989.

Lee F, et al: Transrectal ultrasound in the diagnosis and staging of prostatic carcinoma, Radiology 170(3)(Pt 1):609-615, 1989.

Lewis BD, et al: Current applications of color Doppler imaging in the abdomen and extremities, Radiographics 9(4):599-631, 1989.

Ophir J and Parker KJ: Contrast agents in diagnostic ultrasound, Ultrasound Med Biol 15(4):319-333, 1989.

DIGITAL RADIOGRAPHY

1977 Brennecke R, et al: Computerized video-image processing with application to cardioangiographic roentgen image series. In Nagel HH, editor: Digital image processing, New York, 1977, Springer-Verlag, p 244.

1978 Kruger RA, et al: A digital video image processor for real time x-ray subtraction imaging, Opt Engl 17:652-657, 1978.

Ovitt TW, et al: Development of a digital video subtraction system for intravenous angiography. In Miller HA, Schmidt EV and Harrison DC, editors: Noninvasive cardiovascular measurements, Bellingham, Wash, 1978, Society of Photo-optical Instrumentation Engineers, pp 61-65.

1979 Amtey SR, et al: Recent and future developments in medical imaging. II. Applications of digital processing in computed radiography, Proc Soc Photo-optical Instrumentation Engineers 206:190-192, 1979.

Cohen G, et al: Applications of optical instrumentation in medicine. VII. Contrast-detail-dose evaluation of computed radiography: comparison with computed tomography (CT) and conventional radiography, Proc Soc Photo-optical Instrumentation Engineers 173:41-47, 1979.

Katragadda CS, et al: Computed radiography: a new imaging system, New York, 1979, IEEE, pp. 74-80.

Katragadda CS, et al: Digital radiography using a computed tomographic instrument, Radiology 133:83-87, 1979.

Kruger RA, et al: Computerized fluoroscopy in real time for noninvasive visualization of the cardiovascular system: preliminary studies, Radiology 130:49-57, 1979.

Kruger RA, et al: Computerized fluoroscopy techniques for intravenous study of cardiac chamber dynamics, Invest Radiol 14:279-287, 1979.

Ovitt TW, et al: Development of a digital video subtraction system for intravenous angiography, Proc Soc Photo-optical Instrumentation Engineers 206:73, 1979.

Sashin D, et al: Applications of optical instrumentation in medicine. VIII. Computer radiography for early detection of vascular disease, Proc Soc Photo-optical Instrumentation Engineers 173:88-97, 1979.

1980 Brody WR, et al: Intravenous angiography using scanned projection radiography: preliminary investigation of a new method, Invest Radiol 15:220-223, 1980.

Christenson PC, et al: Intravenous angiography using digital video subtraction: intravenous cervicocerebrovascular angiography, AJR 135:1145-1152, 1980.

Crummy AB, et al: Computerized fluoroscopy: digital subtraction for intravenous angiocardiography and arteriography, AJR 135:1131-1140, 1980.

Lawson TL, et al: Abdominal computed radiography: evaluation of low-contrast lesions, Invest Radiol 15:215-219, 1980.

Meaney TF, et al: Digital subtraction angiography of the human cardiovascular system, AJR 135:1153-1160, 1980.

Ovitt TW, et al: Intravenous angiography using digital video subtraction x-ray imaging system, Am J Neuroradiol 1:387-390, 1980.

Strother CM, et al: Clinical applications of computerized fluoroscopy: the extracranial carotid arteries, Radiology 136:781-783, 1980.

1981 Brody WR, et al: Intravenous carotid arteriography using line-scanned digital radiography, Radiology 139:297-300, 1981.

1982 Bjork L and Bjorkholm PJ: Xenon as a contrast agent for imaging of the airways and lungs using digital radiography, Radiology 144:475-478, 1982.

Brody WR, et al: Intravenous arteriography using digital subtraction techniques, JAMA 248:671-674, 1982.

Carmody RF, et al: Intracranial applications of digital intravenous subtraction angiography, Radiology 144:529-534, 1982.

Enzmann DR, et al: Intracranial intravenous digital subtraction angiography, Neuroradiology 23:241-251, 1982.

Fodor J and Malott JC: Digital video angiography, Radiol Technol 54(2):83-90, 1982.

Harrington DP, Boxt LM and Murray PD: Digital subtraction angiography: overview of technical principles, AJR 139:781-786, 1982.

Hawkins IF: Carbon dioxide digital subtraction angiography, AJR 139:19-24, 1982.

Malott JC and Fodor J: Digital video angiography, Radiol Technol 54:83-89, 1982.

Myerowitz PD: Digital subtraction angiography: present and future uses in cardiovascular diagnosis, Clin Cardiol 5:623-629, 1982.

Nelson JA, et al: Digital subtraction angiography using a temporal bypass filter: initial clinical results, Radiology 145:309-313, 1982.

Sashin D, et al: Diode array digital radiography: initial clinical experience, AJR 139:1045-1050, 1982.

Seeger JF, et al: Digital video subtraction angiography of the cervical and cerebral vasculature, J Neurosurg 56:173-179, 1982.

Tomsak RL, Modic MT and Weinstein MA: Intravenous digital subtraction angiography in neuro-ophthalmology, J Clin Neuro Ophthalmol 2:23-31, 1982.

1983 Cacayorin ED, et al: Intravenous digital subtraction angiography with iohexol, AJNR 4:329-332, 1983.

DeBrusk DP: Digital x-ray imaging: the basics, Radiol Technol 54:280-286, 1983.

Enzmann DR, et al: Low-dose, high-frame-rate versus regular-dose, low-frame-rate digital subtraction angiography, Radiology 146:669-676, 1983.

Foley WD, et al: Digital subtraction angiography of the portal venous system, AJR 140:497-499, 1983.

Grondahl HG and Grondahl K: Subtraction radiography for the diagnosis of periodontal bone lesions, Oral Surg Oral Med Oral Pathol 55:208-213, 1983.

Grondahl K, Grondahl HG and Webber RL: Digital subtraction radiography for diagnosis of periodontal bone disease, Oral Surg Oral Med Oral Pathol 55:313-318, 1983.

Harrington DP: Renal digital subtraction angiography, Cardiovasc Intervent Radiol 6:214-223, 1983.

Johnson GA and Ravin CE: A survey of digital chest radiography, Radiol Clin North Am 21:655-664, 1983.

Kaufman SL, et al: Intraarterial digital subtraction angiography: a comparative view, Cardiovasc Intervent Radiol 6:271-279, 1983.

Kollath J and Riemann H: Pulmonary digital subtraction angiography, Cardiovasc Intervent Radiol 6:233-238, 1983.

Kubal WS, Crummy AB, and Turnipseed WD: The utility of digital subtraction arteriography in peripheral vascular disease, Cardiovasc Intervent Radiol 6:241-249, 1983.

Malott JC and Fodor J: Digital vascular imaging: two years of clinical experience, Radiol Technol 55:633-638, 1983.

Mancini GB, et al: Cardiac imaging with digital subtraction angiography, Cardiovasc Intervent Radiol 6:252-262, 1983.

Maravilla KR, et al: Clinical application of digital tomosynthesis: a preliminary report, AJNR 4:277-280, 1983.

Modic MT, et al: Intravenous digital subtraction angiography: peripheral versus central injection of contrast material, Radiology 147:711-715, 1983.

Passariello R, et al: Digital subtraction angiography for examination of vessels of the leg: use of a 40-cm image intensifier, Radiology 149:669-674, 1983.

Riederer SJ, et al: The application of matched filtering to contrast material dose reduction in digital subtraction angiography, Radiology 147:853-858, 1983.

Seldin DW, et al: Left ventricular volume determined from scintigraphy and digital angiography by a semi-automated geometric method, Radiology 149:809-813, 1983.

Sider L, et al: Control of swallowing by use of topical anesthesia during digital subtraction angiography, Radiology 148:563-564, 1983.

Turski PA, et al: Limitations of intravenous digital subtraction angiography, AJNR 4:271-273, 1983.

Vizy KN: An overview of digital radiography systems, Cardiovasc Intervent Radiol 6:296-299, 1983.

1984 Anderson RE, et al: Tomographic DSA using temporal filtration: initial neurovascular application, AJNR 5:277-280, 1984.

Arnold BA and Scheibe PO: Noise analysis of a digital radiography system, AJR 142:609-613, 1984.

Hillman BJ: Digital imaging of the kidney, Radiol Clin North Am 22:341-364, 1984.

Kaufman SL, et al: Interaarterial digital subtraction angiography in diagnostic arteriography, Radiology 151:323-327, 1984.

Kinney SE and Modic MT: The role of digital subtraction angiography in diagnosis of skull-base lesions, Otolaryngol Head Neck Surg 92:151-155, 1984.

Lee BC, et al: Digital intravenous cerebral angiography in neonates, AJNR 5:281-286, 1984.

Nelson JA and Kruger RA: Digital angiography, Radiologe 24:149-154, 1984.

Partridge JB and Dickinson DF: Digital subtraction imaging in cardiac investigations, Clin Radiol 35:301-306, 1984.

Smith CB: Physical principles of digital radiography, Radiography 50:41-44, 1984.

Templeton AW, et al: Computer graphics for digitally formatted images, Radiology 151:527-528, 1984.

Tesic MM, Sones RA and Morgan DR: Single-slit digital radiography: some practical considerations, AJR 142:697-702, 1984.

1985 Adam P, et al: Pelvimetry by digital radiography, Clin Radiol 36:327-330, 1985.

Aitken AG, et al: Leg length determination by CT digital radiography, AJR 144:613-615, 1985.

Barnes GT: Detector for dual-energy digital radiography, Radiology 156:537-540, 1985.

Chakraborty DP, et al: Digital subtraction angiography apparatus, Radiology 157:547, 1985.

Claussen C, et al: Pelvimetry by digital radiography and its dosimetry, J Perinat Med 13:287-292, 1985.

Karoll MP, et al: Air gap technique for digital subtraction angiography of the extracranial carotid arteries, Invest Radiol 20:742-745, 1985.

Lavelle MI, et al: Demonstration of pancreatic parenchyma by digital subtraction techniques during endoscopic retrograde cholangiopancreatography, Clin Radiol 36:405-407, 1985.

Mendelson EB, et al: Evaluation of the prone position in digital subtraction angiography, Cardiovasc Intervent Radiol 8:72-75, 1985.

Ovitt TW and Newell JD II: Digital subtraction angiography: technology, equipment, and techniques, Radiol Clin North Am 23:177-184, 1985.

Riederer SJ: Digital radiography, Crit Rev Biomed Eng 12:163-200, 1985.

Saddekni S, et al: Contrast administration and techniques of digital subtraction, Radiol Clin North Am 23:275-291, 1985.

Schwenker RP and Eger H: Film-screen digital radiography, Radiography 51:233-235, 1985.

1986 Feldman L: Digital vascular imaging of the great vessels and heart, Cardiovasc Clin 17:357-384, 1986.

Foley KT, Cahan LD and Hieshima GB: Intraoperative angiography using a portable digital subtraction unit, J Neurosurg 64:816-818, 1986.

Gersten K, et al: Crossed-leg technique for digital subtraction angiography, AJR 146:843-844, 1986.

Kimme Smith C, et al: Diagnostic effects of edge-sharpening filtration and magnification, Med Phys 13:850-856, 1986.

Kume Y, et al: Investigation of basic imaging properties in digital radiography, Med Phys 13:843-849, 1986.

Nakstad P, et al: Intra-arterial digital subtraction angiography of the carotid artery, Neuroradiology 28:195-198, 1986.

Takahashi M, et al: Biplane digital subtraction angiography, Comput Radiol 10:221-225, 1986.

1987 Jacobs JM and Manaster BJ: Digital subtraction arthrography of the temporomandibular joint, AJR 148:344-346, 1987.

Kume Y and Doi K: Investigation of basic imaging properties in digital radiography, Med Phys 14:736-743, 1987.

Lotz H, et al: Low dose pelvimetry with biplane digital radiography, Acta Radiol 28:577-580, 1987.

Southard TE, Harris EF and Walter RG: Image enhancement of the mandibular condyle through digital subtraction, Oral Surg Oral Med Oral Pathol 64:645-647, 1987.

Trefler M and Yrizarry JM: Evaluation of dry silver hard copies in digital radiography, AJR 149:853-856, 1987.

Wilson AJ and Ramsby GR: Skeletal measurements using a flying spot digital-imaging device, AJR 149:339-343, 1987.

1988 Foster CJ, Butler P and Freer CE: Digital subtraction angiography of the left ventricle, Br J Radiol 61:1009-1013, 1988.

Harrison RM: Digital radiography, Phys Med Biol 33:751-784, 1988.

Kelly TL, et al: Quantitative digital radiography versus dual photon absorptiometry, J Clin Endocrinol Metab 67:839-844, 1988.

Perri G, et al: Digital subtraction radiography in voiding cystourethrography, Eur J Radiol 8:175-178, 1988.

Pettersson H, et al: Digital radiography of the spine, large bones and joints using stimulable phosphor: early clinical experience, Acta Radiol 29:267-271, 1988.

Rogowska J, Preston K Jr and Sashin D: Evaluation of digital unsharp masking and local contrast stretching, IEEE Trans Biomed Eng 35:817-827, 1988.

Saito H, et al: Digital radiography in an intensive care unit, Clin Radiol 39:127-130, 1988.

Sharma S, Mishra NK and Rajani M: Evaluation of the central injection technique for intravenous digital subtraction angiography—a preliminary report, Indian Heart J 40:12-16, 1988.

Shroy RE, Jr: Dependence of noise on array width and depth in digital radiography, Med Phys 15:64-66, 1988.

1989 de Monts H and Beaumont F: A new photoconductor imaging system for digital radiography, Med Phys 16:105-109, 1989.

Fraser RG, et al: Digital imaging of the chest, Radiology 171:297-307, 1989.

Gluer CC, et al: A fast low-noise line scan x-ray detector, Med Phys 16:98-104, 1989.

MAMMOGRAPHY

For bibliographic citations before 1964, please see the fifth edition of this atlas.

1964 Binzer-Pfertzel CC: Mammography and its relation to disease, Radiography 30:159-162, 1964.

Donovan RJ: A new contour cassette for mammographic roentgenography, AJR 91:917-918, 1964.

Egan RL: Mammography, Springfield, Ill., 1964, Charles C Thomas, Publisher.

Funderburk WW, Syphax B and Ruguero W: The value of contrast medium injection in locating lesions of the breast causing discharge, with particular reference to duct papillomas, J Natl Med Assoc 56:127-132, 1964.

Funderburk WW, Syphax B and Smith CW: Contrast mammography in breast discharge, Surg Gynecol Obstet 119:276-280, 1964.

Holohan F: Technical considerations in breast radiography, Radiol Technol 35:247-251, 1964.

Sherman RS: Areas of concern in mammographic techniques (editorial), AJR 91:1173-1174, 1964.

Siler WM, et al: The development and use of mammographic technique, AJR 91:910-918, 1964.

1965 Bjørn-Hansen R: Contrast mammography, Br J Radiol 38:947-951, 1965.

Gershon-Cohen J: Mammography: some remarks on techniques, Radiol Clin North Am 3:389-401, 1965.

Turner AE: A review of technique development: mammography, xeromammoradiography, and thermomammography, Radiol Technol 36:325-334, 1965.

1966 Berger SM, et al: Mammographic localization of unsuspected breast cancer, AJR 96:1046-1052, 1966.

Curcio GM: Mammography and the radiologic technologist, Radiol Technol 38: 143-151, 1966.

Egan RL: The technical aspects of mammography, Med Radiogr Photogr 42:2-5, 1966.

Lotz K, Reichel WS and Tautz M: Grundlagen der Mammographie, Fortschr Roentgenstr 105:229-239, 1966.

1967 Gershon-Cohen J, et al: Mammographic screening for breast cancer: results of a ten-year survey, Radiology 88:663-667, 1967.

Gros CM: Methodologie, J Radiol Electr 48:638-655, 1967.

Lotz K and Tautz M: Das Problem der Planparallelität bei der Mammographie, Fortschr Roentgenstr 106:276-282, 1967.

Metzenthin B, Rehm A and Fischedick O: Das Röntgenbild der männlichen Mamma, Fortschr Roentgenstr 106:567-573, 1967.

O'Mara RE, et al: Xeromammography and film mammography: completion of a comparative study, Radiology 88:1121-1126, 1967.

Scott WG: Mammography and the training program of the American College of Radiology, AJR 99:1002-1008, 1967.

1968 Ap Simon HT, Stewart HJ and Williams WJ: Recording the gross outlines of breast tumors: a pathological assessment of the accuracy of radiographs of breast cancer, Br J Cancer 22:40-46, 1968.

Egan RL: Technologist's guide to mammography, Baltimore, 1968, Williams & Wilkins.

Egan RL and Fenn JO: Phantoms for evaluating mammography techniques and roentgenographic detail, AJR 102:936-940, 1968.

Lasky HJ: A new mammographic technic, Radiology 91:381-382, 1968.

Minagi H, Tennant JC, and Youker JE: Coning and breast compression: an aid in mammographic diagnosis, Radiology 91:379-381, 1968.

O'Donnell E: Radiographic objectives of mammography, Radiol Technol 39:273-282, 1968.

Strax P and Oppenheim A: New apparatus for mass screening in mammography, AJR 102:941-945, 1968.

Wolfe JN: Xerography of the breast, Radiology 91:231-240, 1968.

1969 Gershon-Cohen J and Hermel MB: Modalities in breast cancer detection: xeroradiography, mammography, thermography and mammometry, Cancer 24:1226-1230, 1969.

Hermel MB, Gershon-Cohen J and Byrne RN: Mammographic technique: need for routine spot roentgenograms, AJR 105:880-884, 1969.

Isard HJ, Ostrum BJ and Shilo R: Thermography in breast carcinoma, Surg Gynecol Obstet 128:1289-1293, 1969.

Howland WJ, Johnson TH and Reagan TA: Laminagraphy of the breast, Radiology 92:609-612, 1969.

Stevens GM: Variations and supplementary techniques in mammography, Oncology 23:120-125, 1969.

Wallace T: Radiographic identification of calcifications in breast specimens, Radiol Technol 40:211-215, 1969.

Zippin C: The epidemiology of breast cancer, Oncology 23:93-98, 1969.

1970 Curcio B: Technique for radiographic localization of non-palpable breast tumors, Radiol Technol 42:155-160, 1970.

Gershon-Cohen J: Atlas of mammography, New York, 1970, Springer-Verlag.

Gershon-Cohen J, Hermel MB and Birsner JW: Advances in mammographic technique, AJR 108:424-427, 1970.

Gilbertson JD, Randall MG and Fingerhut AG: Evaluation of roentgen exposure in mammography. I. Six views, Radiology 95:383-394, 1970.

Gilbertson JD, Randall MG and Fingerhut AG: Evaluation of roentgen exposure in mammography. II. Four views, Radiology 97:641-648, 1970.

Jabczenski MA: Pendant mammography: a new approach to an old technique, J Can Assoc Radiol 21:43-45, 1970.

Palmer RC, Egan RL and Barrett BJ: Preliminary evaluation of absorbed dose in mammography, Radiology 95:395-397, 1970.

Price JL and Butler PD: The reduction of radiation and exposure time in mammography, Br J Radiol 43:251-255, 1970.

1971 Dowdy AH, et al: Mammography as a screening method for the examination of large populations, Cancer 28:1558-1562, 1971.

Palmer RC, et al: Absorbed dose in mammography using three tungsten and three molybdenum target tubes, Radiology 101:697-699, 1971.

Quimet-Oliva D: Air axillography, AJR 111:153-156, 1971.

Shapiro S, Strax P and Venet L: Periodic breast cancer screening in reducing mortality from breast cancer, JAMA 215:1771-1785, 1971.

Snyder RE and Rosen P: Radiography of breast specimens, Cancer 28:1608-1611, 1971.

Wolfe JN, Dooley RP and Harkins LE: Xeroradiography of the breast: a comparative study with conventional film mammography, Cancer 28:1569-1574, 1971.

1972 Gurley L and Harwood S: A practical technique for baseline mammography, Radiol Technol 44:138-145, 1972.

Nunnerley HB and Field S: Mammary duct injection in patients with nipple discharge, Br J Radiol 45:717-725, 1972.

Simon N, et al: Roentgenographic localization of small lesions of the breast by the spot method, Surg Gynecol Obstet 134:572-574, 1972.

1973 Martin JE: Xeromammography: an improved diagnostic method. AJR 117:90-96, 1973.

Ostrum BJ, Becker W and Isard HJ: Low-dose mammography, Radiology 109:323-326, 1973.

Rini JM, et al: A comparison of tungsten and molybdenum as target material for mammographic x-ray tubes, Radiology 106:657-661, 1973.

Strax P, Venet L and Shapiro S: Value of mammography in reduction of mortality from breast cancer in mass screening, AJR 117:686-689, 1973.

Threatt B and Appelman HD: Mammary duct injection, Radiology 108:71-76, 1973.

1974 Wasserman NF: Thermogram and mammogram, Minn Med 57:971-974, 1974.

Young GB: Techniques and radiation in mammography, Br J Radiol 47:811-815, 1974.

1975 Egan RL: Mammography, xeroradiography, and thermography, Clin Obstet Gynecol 18:197-209, 1975.

Lawrence W Jr and Horsley JS: The use of xeromammography in early detection of breast cancer, Va Med Mon 102:313-321, 1975.

1976 Hermel MB and Murdock MG: Microdose mammography, Cancer 38:1947-1951, 1976.

Egan RL: Mammography and radiation dose, J Med Assoc Ga 65:328-329, 1976.

Puretz DH: Mammography, history, current events, and recommendations, NY State J Med 76:1985-1991, 1976.

1977 Baum G: Ultrasound mammography, Radiology 122:199-205, 1977.

Chang CH, et al: Computed tomography of the breast: a preliminary report, Radiology 124:827-829, 1977.

Kalisher L and Schaffer D: Indications and guidelines for mammographic examinations, Am J Surg 133:326-330, 1977.

Lester RG: Risk vs. benefit in mammography, Radiology 124:1-6, 1977.

Matallana RH: Negative technique in xeroradiography of the breast, Cancer 39:112-122, 1977.

Wilson P: Some application problems and solutions in xeromammography, Radiol Technol 48:389-403, 1977.

1978 Arnold BA, Webster EW and Kalisher L: Evaluation of mammographic screen-film systems, Radiology 129:179-185, 1978.

Lundgren B: Malignant features of breast tumors at radiography, Acta Radiol 19:623-633, 1978.

Moskowitz M: Mammography in medical practice, a rational approach, JAMA 240:1898-1899, 1978.

Quimet-Oliva D, Hebert G and Ladouceur J: Radiographic characteristics of male breast cancer, Radiology 129:37-40, 1978.

1979 Askins BS, et al: Autoradiographic enhancement of mammograms: investigation of a new dose reduction technique, Radiology 130:103-107, 1979.

Bassett LW and Axelrod S: A modification of the craniocaudal view in mammography, Radiology 132:222-224, 1979.

Bigongiari L, et al: Dependent compression mammography: a new look at an old idea, J Kans Med Soc 80:336-340, 1979.

Greens RA, et al: Efficacy of the lateral view mammogram in the detection of breast malignancy, Radiology 130:793-794, 1979.

Palmer DS: Needle localization of nonpalpable breast lesions, Clin Radiol 30:291-293, 1979.

Sickles EA: Microfocal spot magnification mammography using xeroradiographic and screen recording systems, Radiology 131:599-607, 1979.

Sickles EA and Genant HK: Controlled single-blind clinical evaluation of low-dose mammographic screen-film systems, Radiology 130:347-351, 1979.

1980 Bassett LW, Pagani JJ and Gold RH: Pitfalls in mammography: demonstrating deep lesions, Radiology 136:641-645, 1980.

Chang CH, et al: Computed tomography in detection and diagnosis of breast cancer, Cancer 46:939-946, 1980.

Fatouros PP, Rao GU and Kao CC: Xeromammographic image quality, Med Phys 7:331-340, 1980.

Hassani SN, Bard RL and Flynn GS, Jr: High-resolution breast ultrasonography, Diagn Gynecol Obstet 2:303-312, 1980.

Moores BM, Ramsden JA and Asbury DL: An atmospheric pressure ionography system suitable for mammography, Phys Med Biol 25:893-902, 1980.

Pagani JJ, et al: Efficacy of combined film-screen/xeromammography: preliminary report, AJR 135:141-146, 1980.

Sickles EA: Further experience with microfocal spot magnification mammography in the assessment of clustered breast microcalcifications, Radiology 137:9-14, 1980.

Weshler Z and Sulkes A: Contrast mammography and the diagnosis of male breast cysts, Clin Radiol 31:341-343, 1980.

Wyatt CC: Xero and film mammography: two images with one exposure, Radiol Technol 51:621-625, 1980.

1981 Blomerus JM: Office mammography: report of 2,621 examinations, Appl Radiol 10:39-42, 1981.

Bragg DG: Tumor imaging in diagnostic radiology, Cancer 47:1159-1163, 1981.

Broadbent RV and Reid MH: Mammography—misunderstood and underutilized, Postgrad Med 70:93-97, 100-101, 1981.

Cole-Beuglet C, et al: Ultrasound mammography: a comparison with radiographic mammography, Radiology 139:693-698, 1981.

Dodd GD: Radiation detection and diagnosis of breast cancer, Cancer 47:1766-1769, 1981.

Doust BD, Milbrath JR and Doust VL: CT scanning of the breast using a conventional CT scanner, CT 5:296-302, 1981.

Friedrich M: The XERG-mammography system: a solution to the dose-quality problem? Eur J Radiol 1:143-151, 1981.

Goldberg IM, et al: Contact plate thermography: a new technique for diagnosis of breast masses, Arch Surg 116:271-273, 1981.

Jennings RJ, et al: Optimal x-ray spectra for screen-film mammography, Med Phys 8:629-639, 1981.

Loughry CW, et al: Breast cancer detection utilizing biostereometric analysis, Cancer Detect Prev 4:589-594, 1981.

Meyer JE and Munzenrider JE: Computed tomographic demonstration of internal mammary lymph-node metastasis in patients with locally recurrent breast carcinoma, Radiology 139:661-663, 1981.

Ouimet-Oliva D, et al: Effect of danazol on the radiographic density of breast parenchyma, J Can Assoc Radiol 32:159-161, 1981.

Schmarsow R, Wessels G and Bielke G: A new applicator for ultrasound mammography, Rev Interam Radiol 6:59-60, 1981.

Shrivastava PN: Radiation dose in mammography: an energy-balance approach, Radiology 140:483-490, 1981.

Tabar L, et al: The diagnostic and therapeutic value of breast cyst puncture and pneumocystography, Radiology 141:659-663, 1981.

1982 Alberti GP and Troiso A: Secreting breast: the role of galactography, Eur J Gynaecol Oncol 3:96-100, 1982.

Barnes GT and Chakraborty DP: Radiographic mottle and patient exposure in mammography, Radiology 145:815-821, 1982.

Beaman SA and Lillicrap SC: Optimum x-ray spectra for mammography, Phys Med Biol 27:1209-1220, 1982.

Breyer B, Cepulic E and Zunter F: Ultrasonic mammography without specialized equipment: comparison with clinical examination and x-rays, Ultrasound Med Biol 8:377-379, 1982.

Chang CH, et al: Computed tomographic mammography using a conventional body scanner, AJR 138:553-558, 1982.

Cole-Beuglet D, et al: Ultrasound mammography for male breast enlargement, J Ultrasound Med 1:301-305, 1982.
Homer MJ: Mammographic detection of breast cancer, Clin Obstet Gynecol 25:393-400, 1982.
Karila KT: Performance of automatic exposure controls in mammography, Med Phys 9:898-903, 1982.
Karila KT: Performance of x-ray generators and unnecessary dose in mammography, Radiology 144:395-401, 1982.
Lundgren B and Helleberg A: Single oblique-view mammography for periodic screening for breast cancer in women, JNCI 68:351-355, 1982.
Ross RJ, et al: Nuclear magnetic resonance imaging and evaluation of human breast tissue: preliminary clinical trials, Radiology 143:195-205, 1982.
Schuy S: Medical ultrasonic imaging, Med Prog Technol 9:161-164, 1982.
Sterns EE, et al: Thermography in breast diagnosis, Cancer 50:323-325, 1982.

1983 Symposium on mammography, Radiol Clin North Am 21:1-194, 1983.
Bassett LW and Gold RH: Breast radiography using the oblique projection, Radiology 149:585-587, 1983.
Beaman S, Lillicrap SC and Price JL: Tungsten anode tubes with K-edge filters for mammography, Br J Radiol 56:721-727, 1983.
Egan RL, McSweeney MB and Sprawls P: Grids in mammography, Radiology 146:359-362, 1983.
Fritz SL, Chang CH and Livingston WH: Scatter/primary ratios for x-ray spectra modified to enhance iodine contrast in screen-film mammography, Med Phys 10:866-870, 1983.
Jewell WR, Thomas JH and Chang CH: Computed tomographic mammography directed biopsy of the breast, Surg Gynecol Obstet 157:75-76, 1983.
Kapdi CC and Parekh NJ: The male breast, Radiol Clin North Am 21:137-148, 1983.
McSweeney MB, Sprawls P and Egan RL: Enhanced image mammography, AJR 140:9-14, 1983.
Muller JW, van Waes PF and Koehler PR: Computed tomography of breast lesions: comparison with x-ray mammography, J Comput Assist Tomogr 7:650-654, 1983.
Muntz EP, et al: On the significance of very small angle scattered radiation to radiographic imaging at low energies, Med Phys 10:819-823, 1983.
Novak D: Indications for and comparative diagnostic value of combined ultrasound and X-ray mammography, Eur J Radiol 3:299-302, 1983.
Tabar L, Dean PB and Pentek Z: Galactography: the diagnostic procedure of choice for nipple discharge, Radiology 149:31-38, 1983.

1984 Bloomberg TJ, Chivers RC and Price JL: Real-time ultrasonic characteristics of the breast, Clin Radiol 35:21-27, 1984.
Dodd GD: Mammography: state of the art, Cancer 53:652-657, 1984.
El-Yousef SJ, et al: Magnetic resonance imaging of the breast: work in progress, Radiology 150:761-766, 1984.
Feig SA: Radiation risk from mammography: is it clinically significant? AJR 143:469-475, 1984.
Hatton PD, Harford FJ Jr and Sheppard JR: Xeromammographic screening: is it helping? South Med J 77:857-859, 1984.
Kopans DB: "Early" breast cancer detection using techniques other than mammography, AJR 143:465-468, 1984.
Kopans DB, Meyer JE, and Sadowsky N: Breast imaging, N Engl J Med 310:960-967, 1984.
McLelland R: Mammography 1984: challenge to radiology, AJR 143:1-4, 1984.
McSweeney MB, Sprawls P and Egan RL: Enhanced-image mammography, Recent Results Cancer Res 90:79-89, 1984.
Muir BB, et al: Oblique-view mammography: adequacy for screening: work in progress, Radiology 151:39-41, 1984.
Rasmussen OS and Seerup A: Preoperative radiographically guided wire marking of nonpalpable breast lesions, Acta Radiol [Diagn] 25:13-16, 1984.
Schreiman JS, et al: Ultrasound transmission computed tomography of the breast, Radiology 150:523-530, 1984.
Sickles EA: Mammographic features of "early" breast cancer, AJR 143:461-464, 1984.
Stanton L, et al: Dosage evaluation in mammography, Radiology 150:577-584, 1984.

1985 Chan HP, et al: Ultra-high–strip-density radiographic grids: a new antiscatter technique for mammography, Radiology 154:807-815, 1985.
Dershaw DD, et al: Mammography using an ultrahigh-strip-density, stationary, focused grid, Radiology 156:541-544, 1985.
Kirkpatrick AE and Law J: The usefulness of a moving grid in mammography, Br J Radiol 58:257-258, 1985.
Kowalczyk N: Patients' perceptions of a mammographic examination, Radiol Technol 56(4):212-216, 1985.
Niklason LT, Barnes GT and Rubin E: Mammography phototimer technique chart, Radiology 157:539-540, 1985.

1986 Homer MJ and Pile Spellman ER: Needle localization of occult breast lesions with a curved end retractable wire: technique and pitfalls, Radiology 161:547-548, 1986.
Nielsen B and Fagerberg G: Image quality in mammography with special reference to anti-scatter, Acta Radiol [Diagn] (Stockh) 27:467-479, 1986.
Sickles EA, et al: Baseline screening mammography: one vs two views per breast, AJR 147:1149-1153, 1986.

1987 Bassett LW, et al: Breast cancer detection: one versus two views, Radiology 165:95-97, 1987.
Feig SA: Mammography equipment: principles, features, selection, Radiol Clin North Am 25:897-911, 1987.
Haus AG: Recent advances in screen-film mammography, Radiol Clin North Am 25:913-928, 1987.
Kimme Smith C, Bassett LW and Gold RH: Evaluation of radiation dose, focal spot, and automatic exposure of newer film-screen mammography units, AJR 149:913-917, 1987.
Logan WW and Janus J: Use of special mammographic views to maximize radiographic information, Radiol Clin North Am 25:953-959, 1987.
Pennes DR and Homer MJ: Disappearing breast masses caused by compression during mammography, Radiology 165:327-328, 1987.

1988 Bassett LW and Gold RH: The evolution of mammography, AJR 150:493-498, 1988.
Dhawan AP and Le Royer E: Mammographic feature enhancement by computerized image processing, Comput Methods Programs Biomed 27:23-35, 1988.
Eklund GW, et al: Improved imaging of the augmented breast, AJR 151:469-473, 1988.
Jackson VP, Lex AM and Smith DJ: Patient discomfort during screen-film mammography, Radiology 168:421-423, 1988.
LaFrance R, Gelskey DE and Barnes GT: A circuit modification that improves mammographic phototimer performance, Radiology 166:773-776, 1988.
Oestmann JW, et al: Comparison of two screen-film combinations in contact and magnification mammography: detectability of microcalcifications, Radiology 168:657-659, 1988.

1989 Chakraborty DP and Barnes GT: An energy sensitive cassette for dual-energy mammography, Med Phys 16:7-13, 1989.
Champ CS, et al: A Perspex grid for localization of non-palpable mammographic lesions, Histopathology 14:311-315, 1989.
Chen HH, et al: Needle localization of non-palpable breast lesions with a portable, Radiology 170:687-690, 1989.
Gilula LA, Destouet JM and Monsees B: Nipple simulating a breast mass on a mammogram, Radiology 170:272, 1989.
Kimme Smith C, et al: Mammographic film-processor temperature, development time, and chemistry: effect on dose, contrast, and noise, AJR 152:35-40, 1989.
Law J and Kirkpatrick AE: Films, screens and cassettes for mammography, Br J Radiol 62:163-167, 1989.
Linden SS and Sullivan DC: Breast skin calcifications: localization with a stereotactic device, Radiology 171:570-571, 1989.

Martin JE: A demonstration comparing film mammography with the new high sensitivity xeromammography, Radiographics 9:153-168, 1989.

MAGNETIC RESONANCE IMAGING

1971 Damadian R: Tumor detection by nuclear magnetic resonance, Science 171:1151-1153, 1971.

1972 Hazelwood CF, et al: Distinction between the preneoplastic and neoplastic state of murine mammary glands, Proc Natl Acad Sci USA 69:190-191, 1973.

1973 Lautebur PC: Image formation by induced local interaction: examples employing NMR, Nature 242:190-191, 1973.

1974 Hazelwood CF, et al: Relationship between hydration and proton nuclear magnetic resonance relaxation times in tissues of tumor-bearing and non tumor-bearing mice: implications for cancer detection, J Natl Cancer Inst 52(6), 1974.

1976 Lautebur PC, et al: Digest of the Fourth International Conference on Medical Physics, Phys Can 32, 1976. (Special issue.) Abstract: Phys Can 33:9, 1976.

1977 Hinshaw WS, Bottomley PA and Holland GN: Radiographic thin-section image of the human wrist by nuclear magnetic resonance, Nature 270:722-723, 1977.

1978 Damadian R, et al: Field-focusing nuclear magnetic resonance (FONAR) and the formation of chemical scans in man, Naturwissenschaften 65:250-252, 1978.

Goldsmith M, Koutcher JA and Damadian R: NMR in cancer, XIII. Application of NMR malignancy index to human mammary tumours, Br J Cancer 38:547-554, 1978.

Hinshaw WS, et al: Display of cross-sectional anatomy by nuclear magnetic resonance imaging, Br J Radiol 51:273-280, 1978.

1979 Budinger T: Thresholds for physiological effects due to RF and magnetic fields used in NMR imaging, IEEE Trans Nucl Sci NS:2821-2825, April 1979.

Mansfield P, et al: Carcinoma of the breast imaged by nuclear magnetic resonance (NMR), Br J Radiol 52:242-243, 1979.

1980 Damadian R: Field focusing NMR (FONAR) and the formation of chemical images in man, Philos Trans R Soc Lond (Biol) 289:389-500, 1980.

Goldman MR, et al: Nuclear magnetic resonance imaging: potential cardiac applications, Am J Cardiol 46:1278-1283, 1980.

Hawkes RC, et al: NMR tomography of the brain: a preliminary assessment with demonstration of pathology, J Comput Assist Tomogr 4:577-586, 1980.

Holland GN, Moore WS and Hawkes RC: Nuclear magnetic resonance tomography of the brain, J Comput Assist Tomogr 4:1-3, 1980.

Partain CL, et al: Nuclear magnetic resonance and computed tomography: comparison of normal body images, Radiology 136:767-770, 1980.

Wolff S, et al: Tests for DNA and chromosomal damage induced by nuclear magnetic resonance imaging, Radiology 136:707-710, 1980.

1981 Crooks L, et al: Nuclear magnetic resonance imaging, Prog Nucl Med 7:149-163, 1981.

Gore JC, et al: Medical nuclear magnetic resonance imaging: I. Physical principles, Invest Radiol 16:269-274, 1981.

Harwell, Dodcot and Oxon: Exposure to nuclear magnetic resonance clinical imaging, Radiography 47:258-260, 1981.

Smith FW, et al: Clinical application of nuclear magnetic resonance, Lancet 1:78-79, 1981.

Smith FW, et al: Nuclear magnetic resonance tomographic imaging in liver disease, Lancet 1:963-966, 1981.

Smith FW, et al: Oesophageal carcinoma demonstrated by whole-body nuclear magnetic resonance imaging, Br Med J 282:510-512, 1981.

1982 Brady TJ, et al: NMR imaging of forearms in healthy volunteers and patients with giant-cell tumor of the bone, Radiology 144:549-552, 1982.

Bydder GM and Steiner RE: NMR imaging of the brain, Neuroradiology 23:231-240, 1982.

Doyle FH, et al: Nuclear magnetic resonance imaging of the liver: initial experience, AJR 138:193-200, 1982.

Katims LM: Nuclear magnetic resonance imaging: methods and current status, Med Instrum 16:213-216, 1982.

Margulis AR: Nuclear magnetic resonance imaging—present status, J Can Assoc Radiol 33:131-136, 1982.

McCullough EC and Baker HL Jr: Nuclear magnetic resonance imaging, Radiol Clin North Am 20:3-7, 1982.

Rollo FD: New imaging modalities: positron emission tomography and nuclear magnetic resonance, Med Instrum 16:53-54, 1982.

Ross RJ, et al: Nuclear magnetic resonance imaging and evaluation of human breast tissue: preliminary clinical trials, Radiology 143:195-205, 1982.

1983 Brasch RC, et al: Brain nuclear magnetic resonance imaging enhanced by a paramagnetic nitroxide contrast agent: preliminary report, AJR 141:1019-1023, 1983.

Crooks LE, et al: Clinical efficiency of nuclear magnetic resonance imaging, Radiology 146:123-128, 1983.

Edelstein WA, et al: Signal, noise, and contrast in nuclear magnetic resonance (NMR) imaging, J Comput Assist Tomogr 7:391-401, 1983.

Ellis JH, Dallas CS and Russell RJ: Communications device for patients undergoing nuclear magnetic resonance imaging, Radiology 149:855, 1983.

Gamsu G, et al: Nuclear magnetic resonance imaging of the thorax, Radiology 147:473-480, 1983.

Higgins CB, et al: Clinical nuclear magnetic resonance imaging of the body, Semin Nucl Med 13:347-363, 1983.

Hricak H, et al: Anatomy and pathology of the male pelvis by magnetic resonance imaging, AJR 141:1101-1110, 1983.

Karstaedt N, et al: Nuclear magnetic resonance imaging, Surg Neurol 19:206-214, 1983.

Modic MT, et al: Nuclear magnetic resonance imaging of the spine, Radiology 148:757-762, 1983.

New PF, et al: Potential hazards and artifacts of ferromagnetic and nonferromagnetic surgical and dental materials and devices in nuclear magnetic resonance imaging, Radiology 147:139-148, 1983.

Norman D, et al: Magnetic resonance imaging of the spinal cord and canal: potentials and limitations, AJR 141:1147-1152, 1983.

Pykett IL: Instrumentation for nuclear magnetic resonance imaging, Semin Nucl Med 13:319-328, 1983.

Ratner AV, Okada RD and Brady TJ: Nuclear magnetic resonance imaging of the heart, Semin Nucl Med 13:339-346, 1983.

Rosen BR and Brady TJ: Principles of nuclear magnetic resonance for medical applications, Semin Nucl Med 13:308-318, 1983.

1984 Bradley WG, Opel W and Kassabian JP: Magnetic resonance installation: sitting and economic considerations, Radiology 151:719-721, 1984.

Brasch RC, et al: Magnetic resonance imaging of the thorax in childhood: work in progress, Radiology 150:463-467, 1984.

Crooks LE, et al: High-resolution magnetic resonance imaging: technical concepts and their implementation, Radiology 150:163-171, 1984.

Crooks LE, et al: Magnetic resonance imaging: effects of magnetic field strength, Radiology 151:127-133, 1984.

El-Yousef SJ, et al: Magnetic resonance imaging of the breast: work in progress, Radiology 150:761-766, 1984.

Fodor J and Malott JC: Magnetic resonance: a new imaging modality, Radiol Technol 56:17-21, 1984.

Han JS, et al: Magnetic resonance imaging in the evaluation of the brainstem, Radiology 150:705-712, 1984.

Hendee WR and Morgan C: Introduction to nuclear magnetic resonance imaging, Denver, 1984, Multi-Media Publications.

Higgins CB, et al: Multiplane magnetic resonance imaging of the heart and major vessels: studies in normal volunteers, AJR 142:661-667, 1984.

Hillman BJ, et al: Adoption and diffusion of a new imaging technology: a magnetic resonance imaging prospective, AJR 143:913-917, 1984.

Kearfott KJ, Rottenberg DA and Knowles RJ: A new headholder for PET, CT, and NMR imaging, J Comput Assist Tomogr 8:1217-1220, 1984.

Roberts D, et al: Radiologic techniques used to evaluate the temporomandibular joint, Anesth Prog 31:241-256, 1984.

Runge VM, et al: Intravascular contrast agents suitable for magnetic resonance imaging, Radiology 153:171-176, 1984.

Thickman D, et al: Nuclear magnetic resonance imaging in gynecology, Am J Obstet Gynecol 149:835-840, 1984.

Webb WR, et al: Nuclear magnetic resonance of pulmonary arteriovenous fistula, J Comput Assist Tomogr 8:155-157, 1984.

1985 Nelson TR, et al: Magnetic resonance imaging: the basic physical and clinical concepts (part I), Radiol Technol 56(6):410-415, 1985.

Nelson TR, et al: Magnetic resonance imaging: the basic physical and clinical concepts (part II), Radiol Technol 57(1):26-30, 1985.

Nelson TR, et al: Magnetic resonance imaging: the basic physical and clinical concepts (part III), Radiol Technol 57(2):142-150, 1985.

Stark DD, et al: Pelvimetry by magnetic resonance imaging, AJR 144:947-950, 1985.

Wedeen VJ, et al: Projective imaging of pulsatile flow with magnetic resonance, Science 230:946-948, 1985.

1986 Mezrich RS, et al: Strip scan: a method for faster MR imaging, Radiographics 6:833-845, 1986.

Mitchell MR, et al: Spin echo technique selection: basic principles for choosing MRI, Radiographics 6:245-260, 1986.

Niendorf HP, et al: Some aspects of the use of contrast agents in magnetic resonance imaging, Diagn Imaging Clin Med 55:25-36, 1986.

Revel D, et al: Gd-DTPA contrast enhancement and tissue, Radiology 158:319-323, 1986.

Rholl KS, et al: Oblique magnetic resonance imaging of the cardiovascular system, Radiographics 6:177-188, 1986.

Russell R, Dallas-Huitema C and Cohen M: Magnetic resonance imaging techniques in children, Radiol Technol 57(5):428-430, 1986.

1987 Balter S: An introduction to the physics of magnetic resonance imaging, Radiographics 7:371-383, 1987.

Brooks RA and Di Chiro G: Magnetic resonance imaging of stationary blood: a review, Med Phys 14:903-913, 1987.

Brooks WM, Brereton IM and Doddrell DM: RAPID—a new method for fast imaging using a single slice of Z-magnetization, Magn Reson Med 5:191-195, 1987.

Ceckler TL, Bryant RG and Hornak JP: Noise reduction in wide-bore magnets using a patient cage, Magn Reson Med 5:173-174, 1987.

Champetier J, et al: Magnetic resonance imaging of the liver by frontal (coronal) sections, Surg Radiol Anat 9:107-121, 1987.

Dumoulin CL, Souza SP and Hart HR: Rapid scan magnetic resonance angiography, Magn Reson Med 5:238-245, 1987.

Fraass BA, et al: Integration of magnetic resonance imaging into radiation therapy, Int J Radiat Oncol Biol Phys 13:1897-1908, 1987.

Gangarosa RE, et al: Operational safety issues in MRI, Magn Reson Imaging 5:287-292, 1987.

Hajek PC, et al: Potential contrast agents for MR arthrography: in vitro evaluation, AJR 149:97-104, 1987.

Mathur De Vre R: Safety aspects of magnetic resonance imaging and magnetic resonance: recommendations for MR exposures in clinical practice, Arch Belg 45:425-438, 1987.

Merritt CR: Magnetic resonance imaging—a clinical perspective: image quality, Radiographics 7:1001-1016, 1987.

Patton JA, et al: Techniques, pitfalls and artifacts in magnetic resonance imaging, Radiographics 7:505-519, 1987.

Pavlicek W: MR instrumentation and image formation, Radiographics 7:809-814, 1987.

Van Rossum AG, et al: Oblique views in magnetic resonance imaging of the heart by combined axial rotations, Acta Radiol 28:497-503, 1987.

Wang HZ, Riederer SJ and Lee JN: Optimizing the precision in T1 relaxation estimation using limited flip angles, Magn Reson Med 5:399-416, 1987.

Young IR and Payne JA: Slice-shape artifact changes with precession angle in rapid MR imaging, Magn Reson Med 5:177-181, 1987.

1988 Imaging strategies in MRI, Radiol Clin North Am 26:471-699, 1988.

Akber SF: Influence of anesthetics on relaxation times, Anesthesiology 69:290-291, 1988.

Atlas SW: Intracranial vascular malformations and aneurysms: current imaging, Radiol Clin North Am 26:821-837, 1988.

Atlas SW, et al: STIR MR imaging of the orbit, AJR 151:1025-1030, 1988.

Barnett GH, Ropper AH and Johnson KA: Physiological support and monitoring of critically ill patients, J Neurosurg 68:246-250, 1988.

Batra P, et al: MR imaging of the thorax: a comparison of axial, coronal, and sagittal imaging planes, J Comput Assist Tomogr 12:75-81, 1988.

Bellon EP, et al: Chemical shift imaging, J Belge Radiol 71:21-30, 1988.

Bird CR, et al: Gd-DTPA-enhanced MR imaging in pediatric patients after brain tumor, Radiology 169:123-126, 1988.

Brosnan T, et al: Noise reduction in magnetic resonance imaging, Magn Reson Med 8:394-409, 1988.

Burbank F, Parish D and Wexler L: Echocardiographic-like angled views of the heart by MR imaging, J Comput Assist Tomogr 12:181-195, 1988.

Crooks LE, et al: Echo-planar pediatric imager, Radiology 166:157-163, 1988.

Czervionke LF, et al: The MR appearance of gray and white matter in the cervical spinal cord, AJNR 9:557-562, 1988.

Dumoulin CL, et al: Time-resolved magnetic resonance angiography, Magn Reson Med 6:275-286, 1988.

Ehrhardt JC, Tian ZC and Chang W: Reduced MR acquisition time with the CROCUS technique, J Comput Assist Tomogr 12:468-473, 1988.

Enzmann DR and Rubin JB: Cervical spine: MR imaging with a partial flip angle, gradient-refocused pulse sequence. Part I. General considerations, Radiology 166:467-472, 1988.

Frahm J, et al: Rapid line scan NMR angiography, Magn Reson Med 7:79-87, 1988.

Gibby WA: MR contrast agents: an overview, Radiol Clin North Am 26:1047-1058, 1988.

Goddard P and Jackson P: The physics of magnetic resonance imaging: a simplified approach, Bristol Med Chir J 103:7, 1988.

Gyngell ML: The application of steady-state free precession in rapid 2DFT NMR, Magn Reson Imaging 6:415-419, 1988.

Hennig J and Friedburg H: Clinical applications and methodological developments of the RARE, Magn Reson Imaging 6:391-395, 1988.

Hennig J, et al: Fast and exact flow measurements with the fast Fourier flow technique, Magn Reson Imaging 6:369-372, 1988.

Higgins CB and Auffermann W: MR imaging of thyroid and parathyroid glands: a review of current, AJR 151:1095-1106, 1988.

Hinks RS and Quencer RM: Motion artifacts in brain and spine MR, Radiol Clin North Am 26:737-753, 1988.

Hyman RA and Gorey MT: Imaging strategies for MR of the brain, Radiol Clin North Am 26:471-503, 1988.

Karlik SJ, et al: Patient anesthesia and monitoring at a 1.5-T MRI installation, Magn Reson Med 7:210-221, 1986.

Krol G, Sze G and Amster J: Table-top support plate for imaging the entire spine with surface-coil MR, AJNR 9:396-397, 1988.

Levin DN, et al: Retrospective geometric correlation of MR, CT, and PET images, Radiology 169:817-823, 1988.

Lipcamon JD, et al: MRI of the upper abdomen using motion artifact suppression technique, Radiol Technol 59:415-418, 1988.

Listinsky JJ and Bryant RG: Gastrointestinal contrast agents: a diamagnetic approach, Magn Reson Med 8:285-292, 1988.

Lufkin R, et al: A technique for MR-guided needle placement, AJR 151:193-196, 1988.

Lufkin R, et al: Automated MR imaging protocols for improved patient throughout, Comput Med Imaging Graph 12:85-88, 1988.

Mitchell DG, et al: Multiple spin-echo MR imaging of the body: image contrast and motion-induced artifact, Magn Reson Imaging 6:535-546, 1988.

Muller RN, et al: The importance of nuclear magnetic relaxation dispersion (NMRD), Invest Radiol 23:6229-6231, 1988.

Norris DG, Jones RA and Hutchison JM: Projective Fourier angiography, Magn Reson Med 7:1-10, 1988.

Pusey E, et al: Aliasing artifacts in MR imaging, Comput Med Imaging Graph 12:219-224, 1988.

Redpath TW and Jones RA: FADE—a new fast-imaging sequence, Magn Reson Med 6:224-234, 1988.

Runge VM and Wood ML: Fast imaging and other motion artifact reduction schemes: a pictorial overview, Magn Reson Imaging 6:595-607, 1988.

Runge VM, et al: FLASH: clinical three-dimensional magnetic resonance imaging, Radiographics 8:947-965, 1988.

Runge VM, et al: Gd DTPA. Future applications with advanced imaging techniques, Radiographics 8:161-179, 1988.

Runge VM, et al: The straight and narrow path to good head and spine MRI, Radiographics 8:507-531, 1988.

Shetty AN: Suppression of radiofrequency interference in cardiac gated MRI, Magn Reson Med 8:84-88, 1988.

Spickler E, McKenna KM and Lufkin RB: Approaches to MR angiography, Comput Med Imaging Graph 12:211-217, 1988.

Thomson JL: A simple skin marker for magnetic resonance imaging, Br J Radiol 61:638-639, 1988.

Underwood SR, et al: Left ventricular volume measured rapidly by oblique magnetic resonance imaging, Br Heart J 60:188-195, 1988.

van der Meulen P, et al: Fast field echo imaging: an overview and contrast calculations, Magn Reson Imaging 6:355-368, 1988.

Van Hecke PE, Marchal GJ and Baert AL: Use of shielding to prevent folding in MR imaging, Radiology 167:557-558, 1988.

Wendt RE III, et al: Electrocardiographic gating and monitoring in NMR imaging, Magn Reson Imaging 6:89-95, 1988.

Williamson MR, et al: Spine: device to facilitate surface coil MR imaging, Radiology 187:273-274, 1988.

Wood ML, Runge VM and Henkelman RM: Overcoming motion in abdominal MR imaging, AJR 150:513-522, 1988.

Wright SM and Wright RM: A multi-plane scout sequence using flash imaging, Magn Reson Imaging 6:105-112, 1988.

Young IR, et al: Further technical development in magnetic resonance imaging of the brain in young children, Clin Radiol 39:651-657, 1988.

1989 Constable RT, et al: High quality zoomed MR images, J Comput Assist Tomogr 13:179-181, 1989.

Duckwiler G, Lufkin RB and Hanafee WN: MR-directed needle biopsies, Radiol Clin North Am 27:255-263, 1989.

Gift DA, Pera A and Moore JB: Introduction to magnetic resonance imaging, J Am Osteopath Assoc 89:315-321, 1989.

Hall AS, et al: Use of solvent suppression technique to enhance changes due to susceptibility variations in magnetic resonance imaging, Magn Reson Med 9:411-418, 1989.

Hatatu H, et al: Pulmonary vasculature: high-resolution MR imaging: work in progress, Radiology 171:391-395, 1989.

Johnson DW, et al: MR imaging of the pars interarticularis, AJR 152:327-332, 1989.

Makow LC: Magnetic resonance imaging: a brief review of image contrast, Radiol Clin North Am 27:195-218, 1989.

Millen SJ, Daniels DL and Meyer GA: Gadolinium-enhanced magnetic resonance imaging in the temporal bone, Laryngoscope 99:257-260, 1989.

Quirk ME, et al: Anxiety in patients undergoing MR imaging, Radiology 170:463-466, 1989.

Rusinek H, et al: Volumetric rendering of MR images, Radiology 171:269-272, 1989.

Swartz JD: Current imaging approach to the temporal bone, Radiology 171:309-317, 1989.

Vaughan B: Magnetic resonance imaging: physics and technical aspects, Australas Radiol 33:34-39, 1989.

Yoffie RL, et al: Three-dimensional magnetic resonance imaging of the heart, Radiol Technol 60:303-309, 1989.

NUCLEAR MEDICINE

1964 Price WJ: Nuclear radiation detection, ed 2, New York, 1964, McGraw-Hill Book Co.

1967 Chase G and Rabinowitz J: Principles of radioisotope methodology, ed 3, Minneapolis, 1967, Burgess Publishing Co.

Hine G, editor: Instrumentation in nuclear medicine, vol 1, New York, 1967, Academic Press, Inc.

1968 Silver S: Radioactive nuclides in medicine and biology, Medicine 3:1968.

Wagner HN, editor: Principles of nuclear medicine, Philadelphia, 1968, WB Saunders Co.

1969 Freeman L and Johnson P, editors: Clinical scintillation scanning, New York, 1969, Harper & Row, Publishers.

Maynard CD: Clinical nuclear medicine, Philadelphia, 1969, Lea & Febiger.

Sodee DB, Early PJ and Razzak MA: Textbook of nuclear medicine technology, St Louis, 1969, The CV Mosby Co.

1970 Quimby EH, Feitelberg S and Gross W: Radioactive nuclides in medicine and biology, Basic Phys Instrument 3:1970.

Simmons G: Training manual for nuclear medicine technologists, Rockville, Md., 1970, US Dept of Health, Education and Welfare, Bureau of Radiologic Health.

1971 Arena V: Ionizing radiation and life, St. Louis, 1971, The CV Mosby Co.

Beierwaltes W, Keyes J and Carey J: Manual of nuclear medicine procedures, Cleveland, 1971, Chemical Rubber Press Co.

Hoffer P, Beck R and Gottschalk A: Semiconductor detectors in the future of nuclear medicine, New York, 1971, The Society of Nuclear Medicine, Inc.

Powsner ER and Raeside DE: Diagnostic nuclear medicine, New York, 1971, Grune & Stratton, Inc.

1972 Sodee DB and Early PJ: Technology and interpretations of nuclear medicine procedures, St Louis, 1972, The CV Mosby Co.

1973 Byers BJ, Dielman RW and Mueller MI: Essentials of nuclear medicine technology, Glenview, Ill, 1973, The Society of Nuclear Medical Technologists, Inc.

Lange RC: Nuclear medicine for technologists, Chicago, 1978, Year Book Medical Publishers, Inc.

Quinn JL, III, editor: Year book of nuclear medicine, Chicago, 1973, Year Book Medical Publishers, Inc.

1976 Strauss HW: Cardiovascular nuclear medicine: a new look at an old problem, Radiology 121:257-268, 1976.

1977 Freundlich IM, O'Mara R and Pitt MJ: Thermographic, radionuclide, and radiographic detection of bone metastases, Radiology 122:665-668, 1977.

1978 Groch MW, et al: Radionuclide kymography for the assessment of regional myocardial wall motion, J Nucl Med 19:1131-1137, 1978.

1979 Maynard CD: The relationship of nuclear medicine to other diagnostic studies, Semin Nucl Med 9:4-7, 1979.

Nusynowitz ML: Nuclear medicine, JAMA 241:1388-1389, 1979.

1980 Ashare AB: Radiocolloid liver scintigraphy: a choice and an echo, Radiol Clin North Am 18:315-319, 1980.

Kaul A, Henrichs K and Roedler HD: Radionuclide biokinetics and internal dosimetry in nuclear medicine, Ric Clin Lab 10:629-660, 1980.

Nudelman S and Patton DD, editors: Imaging for medicine, nuclear medicine, ultrasonics, and thermography, New York, 1980, Plenum Press.

1981 Batillas J, et al: Bone scanning in the detection of occult fractures, J Trauma 21:564-569, 1981.

Beierwaltes WH: New horizons for therapeutic nuclear medicine in 1981, J Nucl Med 22:549-554, 1981.

Ell PJ and Khan O: Emission computerized tomography: clinical applications, Semin Nucl Med 11:50-60, 1981.

Malmud LS and Fisher RS: Scintigraphic evaluation of disorders of the esophagus, stomach, and duodenum, Med Clin North Am 65:1291-1310, 1981.

Oldendorf WH: Nuclear medicine in clinical neurology: an update, Ann Neurol 10:207-213, 1981.

Polak JF and Holman BL: Cardiac nuclear medicine, part I: the methods, Med Instrum 15:174-177, 1981.

Pollet JE, et al: Intravenous radionuclide cystography for the detection of vesicorenal reflux, J Urol 125:75-78, 1981.

Sodee DB and Early PJ: Mosby's manual of nuclear medicine, ed 3, St Louis, 1981, The CV Mosby Co.

1982 Abdel-Dayem HM, Barodawala YK and Papademetriou T: Scintographic arthrography: comparison with contrast arthrography and future applications, Clin Nucl Med 7:516-522, 1982.

Aw SE, et al: Nuclear medicine—an overview, Ann Acad Med Singapore 11:464-468, 1982.

Blahd WH and Rose JG: Nuclear medicine in diagnosis and treatment of diseases of the head and neck: II, Head Neck Surg 4:213-226, 1982.

Blaufox MD, et al: Applications of nuclear medicine in genitourinary imaging, Urol Radiol 4:155-164, 1982.

Chandra R: Introductory physics of nuclear medicine, Philadelphia, 1982, Lea & Febiger.

Doucet TW, Hurwitz JJ and Chin-Sang H: Lacrimal scintillography: advances and functional applications, Surv Ophthalmol 27:105-113, 1982.

Greer KL, Jaszczak RJ and Coleman RE: An overview of a camera-based SPECT system, Med Phys 9:455-463, 1982.

1983 Adams FG and Shirley AW: Factors influencing bone scan quality, Eur J Nucl Med 8:436-439, 1983.

Berg BC: Complementary roles of radionuclide and computed tomographic imaging in evaluating trauma, Semin Nucl Med 13:86-103, 1983.

Croll MN, Brady LW and Dadparvar S: Implications of lymphoscintigraphy in oncologic practice: principles and differences vis-a-vis other imaging modalities, Semin Nucl Med 13:4-8, 1983.

Goetz WA, Hendee WR and Gilday DL: In vivo diagnostic nuclear medicine: pediatric experience, Clin Nucl Med 8:434-439, 1983.

Lull RJ, et al: Radionuclide evaluation of lung trauma, Semin Nucl Med 13:223-237, 1983.

Rudavsky AZ and Moss CM: Radionuclide evaluation of peripheral vascular injuries, Semin Nucl Med 13:142-152, 1983.

Uthoff LB, et al: A prospective study comparing nuclear scintigraphy and computerized axial tomography in the initial evaluation of the trauma patient, Ann Surg 198:611-616, 1983.

Wilson R, McKusick K and Strauss HW: Cardiovascular nuclear medicine current applications and the outlook for 1985, Eur Radiol 3:264-267, 1983.

1984 Cowan RJ and Moody DM: Radionuclide techniques for brain imaging, Neurol Clin 2(4):835-851, 1984.

Fink-Bennett DM and Shapiro EE: The angle of Louis: a potential pitfall ("Louie's hot spot") in bone scan interpretation, Clin Nucl Med 9:352-354, 1984.

Froelich JW and Swanson D: Imaging of inflammatory processes with labeled cells, Semin Nucl Med 14(2):128-140, 1984.

Gross MD, et al: The scintigraphic imaging of endocrine organs, Endocr Rev 5:221-281, 1984.

Kramer EL and Sanger JJ: Radionuclide scanning—new applications in urology, Urology 23:468-477, 1984.

Packer S: Ocular anatomy for nuclear medicine, Semin Nucl Med 14:3-7, 1984.

Pauwels EK and Cleton FJ: Radiolabelled monoclonal antibodies: a new diagnostic tool in nuclear medicine, Radiother Oncol 1(4):333-338, 1984.

Pozen MW, et al: Cardiac nuclear imaging: adoption of an evolving technology, Med Care 22:343-348, 1984.

Sundrehagen E: A new technique for formation of 99mTc-labelled blood leucocytes and platelets, Int J Appl Radiat Isot 35(5):365-366, 1984.

1985 Clarke LP, et al: SPECT imaging of ^{131}I (364 keV): importance of collimation, Nucl Med Commun 6(1):41-47, 1985.

Dale S, et al: Ectomography—a tomographic method for gamma camera imaging, Phys Med Biol 30(11):1237-1249, 1985.

English RJ, Holman BL and Tu'meh SS: Computed tomography in nuclear medicine, Radiol Technol 56(5):291-295, 1985.

Garver PR, et al: Appearance of breast attenuation artifacts with thallium myocardial SPECT imaging, Clin Nucl Med 10(10):694-696, 1985.

Lopez-Majano V, Sansi P and Colter R: Nuclear medicine in the diagnosis of cardiac contusion, Eur J Nucl Med 11(8):290-294, 1985.

Moreno AJ, et al: The gallium-67 citrate bone scan, Clin Nucl Med 10(8):594-595, 1985.

Nimmo MKJ, Merrick MV and Millar AM: A comparison of the economics of xenon 127, xenon 133 and krypton 81m for routine ventilation imaging of the lungs, Br J Radiol 58(691):635-636, 1985.

Seagrave V: Radionuclide imaging, Radiography 51(595):55-56, 1985.

Wackers FJ, et al: Quantitative planar thallium-201 stress scintigraphy: a critical evaluation of the method, Semin Nucl Med 15(1):46-66, 1985.

1986 Brunner MC, et al: Prosthetic graft infection: limitations of indium white blood cell scanning, J Vasc Surg 3(1):42-48, 1986.

Marmor AT, et al: Improved radionuclide method for assessment of pulmonary artery pressure in COPD, Chest 89(1):64-69, 1986.

Murata K, et al: Ventilation imaging with positron emission tomography and nitrogen 13, Radiology 158(2):303-307, 1986.

Romney BM, et al: Radionuclide administration to nursing mothers: mathematically derived guidelines, Radiology 160(2):549-554, 1986.

Shore RM and Hendee WR: Radiopharmaceutical dosage selection for pediatric nuclear medicine, J Nucl Med 27(2):287-298, 1986.

Techner LM, Eiser CA and Laine W: Indium-111 imaging in osteomyelitis and neuroarthropathy: review and case report, J Am Podiatr Med Assoc 76(1):23-29, 1986.

1987 Adam WE: A general comparison of functional imaging in nuclear medicine with other modalities, Semin Nucl Med 17(1):3-17, 1987.

Franken PR, et al: Measurement of right ventricular volumes from ECG gated steady-state krypton-81m angiocardiography, Nucl Med Commun 8(5):365-373, 1987.

Murphy PH: Acceptance testing and quality control of gamma cameras, including SPECT, J Nucl Med 28(7):1221-1227, 1987.

Shulkin BL, et al: Iodine-131 MIBG scintigraphy of the extremities in metastatic pheochromocytoma and neuroblastoma, J Nucl Med 28(3):315-318, 1987.

Shulkin BL and Wahl RL: SPECT imaging of myocarditis, Clin Nucl Med 12(11):841-842, 1987.

Yano Y: Essentials of a rubidium-82 generator for nuclear medicine, Int J Rad Appl Instrum A 38(3):205-211, 1987.

1988 Bellotti C, et al: Cerebral scintigraphy with lilindium oxine-labelled leukocytes in the differential diagnosis of intracerebral cystic lesions, Acta Neurochir Suppl (Wien) 42:221-224, 1988.

Dendy PP, Barber RW and Bayliss CC: An experimental study of the relationship between image quality and spatial resolution of the gamma camera, Eur J Nucl Med 14(12):579-585, 1988.

Gainey MA and Capitanio MA: Recent advances in pediatric nuclear medicine, Radiol Clin North Am 26(2):409-418, 1988.

Halama JR, Henkin RE and Friend LE: Gamma camera radionuclide images: improved contrast with energy-weighted acquisition, Radiology 169(2):533-538, 1988.

Welch MJ: Production of positron-emitting radiopharmaceuticals, Am J Physiol Imaging 3(1):71, 1988.

1989 Deland FH: A perspective of monoclonal antibodies: past, present, and future, Semin Nucl Med 19(3):158-165, 1989.

Franken PR, et al: Clinical usefulness of ultrashort-lived iridium-191m from a carbon-based penetration system for the evaluation of the left ventricular function, J Nucl Med 30(6):1025-1031, 1989.

McAfee JG: Update on radiopharmaceuticals for medical imaging, Radiology 171(3):593-601, 1989.

Sikora K: Imaging with radiolabelled monoclonal antibodies, Clin Radiol 40(4):32-34, 1989.

Thrall JH and Swanson DP: Diagnostic interventions in nuclear medicine, Curr Probl Diagn Radiol 18(1):1-37, 1989.

Wirth V: Effective energy resolution and scatter rejection in nuclear medicine, Phys Med Biol 34(1):85-90, 1989.

Periodicals

Abbott Laboratories Radio-Pharmaceutical Bulletins, North Chicago, Ill, 1973- .

Clinical Nuclear Medicine, Philadelphia, 1976- .

International Journal of Nuclear Medicine and Biology, Elmsford, NY, 1973- .

Journal of Nuclear Medicine, New York, 1955- .

Journal of Nuclear Medicine and Allied Sciences, Turin, Italy, 1957- .

Journal of Nuclear Medicine Technology, New York, 1973- .

Progress in Nuclear Medicine, Basel, Switzerland, 1972- .

Recent Advances in Nuclear Medicine, New York, 1978- .

Seminars in Nuclear Medicine, New York, 1971- .

Vignettes in Nuclear Medicine, St Louis, 1966- .

Yearbook of Nuclear Medicine, Chicago, 1966- .

PEDIATRIC RADIOGRAPHY

For bibliographic citations before 1964, please see the fifth edition of this atlas.

1964 Franklyn PP: Paediatric radiology, Radiography 30:243-251, 1964.

Kreel L, et al: Pneumo-mediastinography by the transsternal method, Clin Radiol 15:219-223, 1964.

1965 O'Hara AE, et al: Controlled pulmonary roentgenographic exposures in newborn infants, AJR 95:99-103, 1965.

Tausend ME and Stern WZ: Thymic patterns in the newborn, AJR 95:125-130, 1965.

1968 Berdon WE, et al: The radiographic evaluation of imperforate anus: an approach correlated with current surgical concepts, Radiology 90:466-471, 1968.

1969 Kelly JH: Cine radiography in anorectal malformations, J Pediatr Surg 4:538-546, 1969.

1973 Oh KS, et al: Positive-contrast peritoneography and herniography, Radiology 108:647-654, 1973.

1975 Gooding CA, et al: Adverse reactions to intravenous pyelography in children, AJR 123:802-804, 1975.

Haller JO and Slovis TL: Importance of horizontal beam for lateral view of skull in pediatric radiography, Radiol Technol 47:150-152, 1975.

Holbert CL, et al: Radiographic technique, safety, and interpretation in the newborn nursery, J Pediatr 87:968-972, 1975.

Knake JE: A device to aid in positioning for the Andren von Rosen hip view, Radiology 117:735-736, 1975.

1976 Buckle CM: Immobilization of the patient in pediatric radiography, Radiography 42(501):195-196, 1976.

Poznanski AK: Practical approaches to pediatric radiology, Chicago, 1976, Year Book Medical Publishing, Inc.

1977 Barry JF, et al: Metrizamide in pediatric myelography, Radiology 124:409-418, 1977.

Eklof O, editor: Current concepts in pediatric radiology, New York, 1977, Springer-Verlag.

Hass EA and Solomon DJ: Telling children about diagnostic radiology procedures, Radiology 124:521, 1977.

Hirsch DJ, et al: Evaluation for hip dysplasia in infancy: the significance of x-ray in diagnosis, J Med Soc NJ 74:528-532, 1977.

1978 American Academy of Pediatrics, Committee on Radiology: Water-soluble contrast material, Pediatrics 62:114-116, 1978.

Hernandez R, Gutowski D and Poznanski AK: A simple method of using a shadow gonadal shield with closed incubators, Radiology 128:821-822, 1978.

Merten DF: Comparison radiographs in extremity injuries of childhood: current application in radiological practice, Radiology 126:209-210, 1978.

1979 Cohen MD: Intravenous urography in neonates and infants: what dose of contrast media should be used? Br J Radiol 52:942-944, 1979.

Kalender W, Reither M and Schuster W: Reduction of dose in pelvic examinations of infants using modern x-ray techniques, Pediatr Radiol 8:233-235, 1979.

1980 Anderson RE, et al: Impact of a "fast" scanner on image quality in pediatric computed tomography, Radiology 34:251-252, 1980.

Brodeur AE, et al: The many advantages of direct microfocus roentgenographic magnification in pediatric radiology, Am J Dis Child 134:245-247, 1980.

Heller RM, et al: Diagnostic imaging in pediatric emergencies, South Med J 73:844-849, 1980.

Leonidas JC: Avoiding unnecessary x-ray exposure in children, Compr Ther 6:46-54, 1980.

Lonnerholm T: Arthrography of the hip in children: technique, normal anatomy, and findings in unstable hip joints, Acta Radiol 21:279-292, 1980.

Pritchard C: Radiation protection of personnel during pediatric radiodiagnostic examination, Radiography 46:165-169, 1980.

Seibert JJ, et al: Low efficacy radiography of children, AJR 134:1219-1223, 1980.

Swischuk LE: Radiology of the newborn and young infant, Baltimore, 1980, Williams & Wilkins.

Wesenberg RL, et al: Low-dose radiography of children, Radiol Technol 51:641-648, 1980.

1981 Berger PE, Kuhn JP and Brusehaber J: Techniques for computed tomography in infants and children, Radiol Clin North Am 19:399-408, 1981.

Herbert R and McGrath A: Ultrasonic investigation of the brain in neonates, Radiography 47:187-193, 1981.

Hough S: Barium feeder for babies, Radiography 47:186, 1981.

Leonidas JC, McCauley RG and Faerber EN: Pediatric radiologists in the United States and Canada: involvement with newer imaging modalities, Radiology 138:235-237, 1981.

Milne EN and Gillan GG: Technique for improving neonatal chest roentgenograms, Appl Radiol 10:45-49, 1981.

1982 Brasch RC and Gould RG: Direct magnification radiography of the newborn infant, Radiology 143:649-655, 1982.

Cherian MJ, et al: Prone films of abdomen—a diagnostic tool in intestinal obstruction, Australas Radiol 26:255-260, 1982.

Coombs AR: Adapting a lateral cassette holder for paediatric radiography, Radiography 48:151-174, 1982.

Heller RM, Partain CL and James AE: Implications of nuclear magnetic resonance imaging for the pediatrician, Am J Dis Child 136:1045-1046, 1982.

Ferry PC: Skull roentgenograms in pediatric head trauma: a vanishing necessity? Pediatrics 69:237-238, 1982.

Kaiser MC and Martin DJ: Direct coronal images—a valuable addition to pediatric body CT-scanning, Pediatr Radiol 12:295-297, 1982.

Siegle RL, Davies P and Fullerton GD: Urography with metrizamide in children, AJR 139:927-930, 1982.

White SC: Radiation safety for children, Int Dent J 32:259-264, 1982.

1983 Diament MJ and Kangarloo H: Dosage schedule for pediatric urography based on body surface, AJR 140:815-816, 1983.

Gyll C: Preventing lordotic projection of the chest, Radiography 49:291-293, 1983.

Kaufman RA: Liver-spleen computed tomography: a method tailored for infants and children, J Comput Tomogr 7:45-57, 1983.

Kirks D: Practical techniques for pediatric computed tomography, Pediatr Radiol 13:148-155, 1983.

Leonidas JC, et al: The one-film urogram in urinary tract infection in children, AJR 141:61-64, 1983.

Ratcliffe JF: The small bowel enema in children: a description of a technique, Clin Radiol 34:287-289, 1983.

1984 Bolz KD, Skalpe IO and Gutteberg TJ: Iohexol and metrizoate in urography in children, comparison, Acta Radiol [Diagn] (Stockh) 25:155-158, 1984.
Cohen G, et al: Dose efficiency of screen-film systems used in pediatric radiography, Radiology 152:187-193, 1984.
Kuijpers D, Blickman JG and Camps JA: The five-degree rule: optimization of the paranasal sinus examination of children, Radiology 152:814, 1984.
Libson E, et al: Oblique lumbar spine radiographs: importance in young patients, Radiology 151:89-90, 1984.
McAlister WH and Siegel MJ: Fatal aspirations in infancy during gastrointestinal series, Pediatr Radiol 14:81-83, 1984.
McDaniel DL, et al: Relative dose efficiencies of antiscatter grids and air gaps in pediatric radiography, Med Phys 11:508-512, 1984.
Robey G, et al: Pediatric urography: comparison of metrizamide and methylglucamine, Radiology 150:61-63, 1984.
Smathers RL, et al: Radiation dose reduction in the neonatal intensive care unit: comparison of three gadolinium oxysulfide screen-film combinations, Invest Radiol 19:578-582, 1984.
1985 Carlsson EC, et al: Pediatric angiocardiography with iohexol, Invest Radiol 20:S75-S78, 1985.
1986 Ball WS Jr, et al: Interventional genitourinary radiology in children: a review of 61 procedures, AJR 147:791-796, 1986.
Sprigg A, et al: Compensation filtration in paediatric double-contrast barium enema, Clin Radiol 37:599-601, 1986.
Weinreb JC, et al: Imaging the pediatric liver: MRI and CT, AJR 147:785-790, 1986.
1987 Boesmi B, et al: Digital angiography in children, Rays 12:47-52, 1987.
Boothroyd AE, Carty HM and Robson WJ: 'Hunt the thimble': a study of the radiology of ingested foreign bodies, Arch Emerg Med 4:33-38, 1987.
Herman MW, Mak HK and Lachman RS: Radiation exposure reduction by use of Kevlar cassettes in the neonatal nursery, AJR 148:969-972, 1987.
Wesenberg RL, et al: Ultra-low-dose routine pediatric radiography utilizing a rare-earth filter, J Can Assoc Radiol 38:158-164, 1987.
1988 Crooks LE, et al: Echo-planar pediatric imager, Radiology 166:157-163, 1988.
Magid D, et al: 2D and 3D computed tomography of the pediatric hip, Radiographics 8:901-933, 1988.
Nahata MC: Sedation in pediatric patients undergoing diagnostic procedures, Drug Intell Clin Pharm 22:711-715, 1988.
Steiner GM: Paediatric radiology 3: genitourinary tract, Br J Hosp Med 39:518-521, 1988.
1989 Ben Ami T, Rozin M and Hertz M: Imaging of children with urinary tract infection: a tailored approach, Clin Radiol 40:64-67, 1989.
Calandrino C: Barium enema procedure for the pediatric patient, Radiol Technol 60:209-213, 1989.
Revonta M and Kuuliala I: The diagnosis and follow-up of pediatric sinusitis: Water's view, Laryngoscope 99:321-324, 1989.

POSITRON EMISSION TOMOGRAPHY

1980 Geltman EM, Roberts R and Sobel BE: Cardiac positron tomography: current status and future directions, Herz 5:107-119, 1980.
1981 Bergstrom M, et al: Head fixation device for reproducible position alignment in transmission CT and positron emission tomography, J Comput Assist Tomogr 5:136-141, 1981.
Lenzi GL, Jones T and Frackowiak RS: Positron emission tomography: state of the art in neurology, Prog Nucl Med 7:118-137, 1981.
Ter-Pogossian MM, et al: Photon time-of-flight-assisted positron emission tomography, J Comput Assist Tomogr 5:227-239, 1981.
1982 Rollo FD: New imaging modalities: positron emission tomography and nuclear magnetic resonance, Med Instrum 16:53-54, 1982.
1983 Bergstrand G, et al: Cerebrospinal fluid circulation: evaluation by single-photon and positron emission tomography, AJNR 4:557-559, 1983.
Di-Chiro G, et al: Metabolic imaging of the brain stem and spinal cord: studies with positron emission tomography using 18F-2-deoxyglucose in normal and pathological cases, J Comput Assist Tomogr 7:937-945, 1983.
Wong WH, et al: Image improvement and design optimization of the time-of-flight PET, J Nucl Med 24:52-60, 1983.
1984 Budinger TF, Derenzo SE and Huesman RH: Instrumentation for positron emission tomography, Ann Neurol 15(Suppl): 35-43, 1984.
Ginsberg MD, Howard BE and Hassel WR: Emission tomographic measurement of local cerebral blood flow in humans by an in vivo autoradiographic strategy, Ann Neurol 15(Suppl):12-8, 1984.
Hoffman EJ, et al: Prospects for both precision and accuracy in positron emission tomography, Ann Neurol 15(Suppl):25-34, 1984.
Kearfott KJ, Rottenberg DA and Knowles RJ: A new headholder for PET, CT, and NMR imaging, J Comput Assist Tomogr 8:1217-1220, 1984.
Kuhl DE: Imaging local brain function with emission computed tomography, Radiology 150:625-631, 1984.
Lockwood AH: Functional evaluation of the blood-brain barrier using positron emission tomography, Ann Neurol 15(Suppl):103-106, 1984.
1985 Correia JA and Alpert NM: Positron emission tomography in cardiology, Radiol Clin North Am 23:783-793, 1985.
1986 Muehllehner G and Karp JS: Positron emission tomography imaging—technical considerations, Semin Nucl Med 16:35-50, 1986.
1987 Chugani HT: Positron emission tomography: principles and applications in pediatrics, Mead Johnson Symp Perinat Dev Med 15-18, 1987.
Guzzardi R and Licitra G: A critical review of Compton imaging, Crit Rev Biomed Eng 15:237-268, 1987.
1988 Chen JJ, et al: Single photon emission computed tomography of the thyroid, J Clin Endocrinol Metab 66:1240-1246, 1988.
Levin DN, et al: Retrospective geometric correlation of MR, CT, and PET images, Radiology 169:817-823, 1988.
Spinks TJ, Guzzardi R and Bellina CR: Performance characteristics of a whole-body positron tomograph, J Nucl Med 29:1833-1841, 1988.
Volkow ND, Mullani NA and Bendriem B: Positron emission tomography instrumentation: an overview, Am J Physiol Imaging 3:142-153, 1988.
1989 Esser PD, Jakimcius A and Foley L: The peanut orbit: a modified elliptical orbit for single photon emission computed tomography imaging, Med Phys 16:114-118, 1989.
Mintun MA, Fox PT and Raichle ME: A highly accurate method of localizing regions of neuronal activation in the human brain with positron emission tomography, J Cereb Blood Flow Metab 9:96-103, 1989.

RADIATION THERAPY

For bibliographic citations before 1964, please see the fifth edition of this atlas.

1965 Grigg ERN: Trail of the invisible light, Springfield, Ill, 1965, Charles C Thomas, Publisher.
1966 Kaplan HS and Rosenberg SA: Treatment of Hodgkin's disease, Med Clin North Am 50:1591-1610, 1966.
Schwartz EE: The biological basis of radiation therapy, Philadelphia, 1966, JB Lippincott Co.
1967 Elkind MD and Whitmore GF: The radiobiology of cultured mammalian cells, New York, 1967, Gordon & Breach.
1968 Fenner ML: Elementary clinical radiotherapy, London, 1968, Butterworth & Co.
International Commission on Radiation Units and Measurements (ICRU); Radiation quantities and units, No 11, September 1968.
1969 Bogardus CR Jr: Clinical applications of physics of radiology and nuclear medicine, St Louis, 1969, Warren H Green, Inc.
Brecher R and Brecher E: The rays, Baltimore, 1969, Williams & Wilkins.
International Commission on Radiation Units and Measurements (ICRU): Radiation dosimetry, 0.6-50 MeV, No 14, September 1969.

Johns HE and Cunningham JR: The physics of radiology, ed 2, Springfield, Ill, 1969, Charles C Thomas, Publisher.

Stanton L: Basic medical radiation physics, New York, 1969, Appleton-Century-Crofts.

Walter J and Miller H: A short textbook of radiotherapy for technicians and students, ed 3, Boston, 1969, Little, Brown & Co.

1970 American Cancer Society, Inc: Clinical oncology for medical students and physicians, a multidisciplinary approach, ed 3, New York, 1970-1971, The Society.

Burch RJ: New approach to cancer, Nature 225:512, 1970.

Florey H: General pathology, Philadelphia, 1970, WB Saunders Co.

Goodwin P, Quimby E and Morgan R: Physical foundations of radiology, ed 4, New York, 1970, Harper & Row, Publishers.

Grant RN and Silverberg E: Cancer statistics, 1970, New York, 1970, American Cancer Society, Inc.

National Council on Radiation Protection and Measurements (NCRP): Basic radiation protection criteria, No 39, 1971.

1972 Barnes PA and Rees DJ: A concise textbook of radiotherapy, Philadelphia, 1972, JB Lippincott Co.

Pizzarello DJ and Witcofski R: Medical radiation biology, Philadelphia, 1972, Lea & Febiger.

Vaeth JM: Frontiers of radiation therapy and oncology, vol 7, The interrelationship of the immune response and cancer, Baltimore, 1972, University Park Press.

1973 Dalrymple GV, et al: Medical radiation biology, Philadelphia, 1973, WB Saunders Co.

Fletcher GH: Textbook of radiotherapy, ed 2, Philadelphia, 1973, Lea & Febiger.

1974 Abramson N: Radiation therapy: what is it? South Med J 67:1333-1336, 1974.

1975 Pizzarello DJ and Witcofski RL: Basic radiation biology, Philadelphia, 1975, Lea & Febiger.

1976 Kramer S: Definitive radiation therapy, CA 26:269-273, 1976.

Selman J: The basic physics of radiation therapy, ed 2, Springfield, Ill, 1976, Charles C Thomas, Publisher.

1977 del Regato JA and Spjut MJ: Ackerman and del Regato's cancer: diagnosis, treatment, and prognosis, ed 5, St Louis, 1977, The CV Mosby Co.

Sachs MC: Introduction to pion radiotherapy, Radiol Technol 49:11-14, 1977.

Walter J: Cancer and radiotherapy, ed 2, Edinburgh, 1977, Churchill Livingstone.

1978 Kogelnik HD and Withers HR: Radiobiological considerations in multifraction irradiation, Radiol Clin 47:362-369, 1978.

Levene MB, et al: Computer controlled radiation therapy, Radiology 129:769-775, 1978.

Rubin P, et al: Clinical oncology for medical students and physicians, ed 5, Rochester, NY, 1978, American Cancer Society, Inc.

1979 Moore JL, et al: Treatment time and sublethal repair in radiotherapy, Br J Radiol 52:978-983, 1979.

Moss WT, Brand WN and Battifora H: Radiation oncology: rationale, technique, results, ed 5, St. Louis, 1979, The CV Mosby Co.

1980 Cooper JS and Pizzarello DJ: Concepts in cancer care, Philadelphia, 1980, Lea & Febiger.

Essentials and guidelines of an accredited educational program for the radiation therapy technologist, Radiol Technol 51:651-662, 1980.

Smith LL: Cancer patients' evaluations of radiation therapy services, Radiol Technol 51:603-609, 1980.

VanDyk J, et al: A technique for the treatment of large irregular fields, Radiology 134:543-544, 1980.

Wang CC: Primer on radiation therapy technology, Boston, 1980, (pamphlet) Department of Radiation Sciences, Massachusetts General Hospital.

1981 Edwards M, et al: A computed tomography-radiation therapy treatment planning system utilizing a whole body CT scanner, Med Phys 8:242-248, 1981.

1982 Taylor HF: Intraoperative radiotherapy, Radiol Technol 54:23-25, 1982.

1983 Badcock PC: The role of computed tomography in the planning of radiotherapy fields, Radiology 147:241-244, 1983.

Bova FJ and Hill LW: Surface doses for acrylic versus lead acrylic blocking trays for Co-60, 8-MV, and 17-MV photons, Med Phys 10:254-256, 1983.

Brady LW: The changing role of radiation oncology in cancer management, Cancer 51:2506-2514, 1983.

Goitein M and Abrams M: Multi-dimensional treatment planning. I. Delineation of anatomy, Int J Radiat Oncol Biol Phys 9:777-787, 1983.

1984 Dewit L and van der Schueren E: Radiation treatment planning for the localized prostatic carcinoma: methods and rationale, Strahlentherapie 160(8):474-484, 1984.

Gerber RL: Quality assurance in radiation therapy: clinical and physical aspects: manpower requirements in training and certification of technologists and dosimetrists, Int J Radiat Oncol Biol Phys 10 (Suppl 1):127-130, 1984.

McLees E, Thompson P and Faulwell M: Radiation therapy technology: profile of a profession, Radiol Technol 55:25-33, 1984.

Pizzarello DJ, et al: The carcinogenicity of radiation therapy, Surg Gynecol Obstet 159:189-200, 1984.

Suntharalingam N: Quality assurance in radiation therapy: future plans in physics, Int J Radiat Oncol Biol Phys 10:43-44, 1984.

1985 Shuman WP, et al: The impact of CT CORRELATE ScoutView images on radiation therapy planning, AJR 145(3):633-638, 1985.

Starkschall G: Analytic evaluation of depths of dose calculation points for external beam radiation therapy treatment planning, Med Phys 12(4):477-479, 1985.

Vick NA and Wilson CB: Total care of the patient with a brain tumor with consideration of some ethical issues, Neurol Clin 3(4):705-710, 1985.

1986 Ashayer E, et al: Anesthesia in intraoperative radiotherapy patients, J Natl Med Assoc 78(3):193-199, 1986.

Brady LW, Markoe AM and Fisher S: Cancer cure with organ preservation using radiation therapy, Radiology 160(1):1-8, 1986.

Brett CM, Wara WM and Hamilton WK: Anesthesia for infants during radiotherapy: an insufflation technique, Anesthesiology 64(3):402-405, 1986.

Griffiths SE: Reproducibility in radiotherapy, Radiography 52(604):167-169, 1986.

McEwan AC and Smyth VG: The effect of scattered radiation in ^{60}Co beams on wall correction factors for ionization chambers, Med Phys 13(1):117-118, 1986.

Sause WT: Technical advances in radiation therapy, Urol Clin North Am 13(3):501-523, 1986.

1987 Bagne F and Dobelbower RR: Modified mesh panel for radiation therapy treatment table, Radiology 163(2):579-580, 1987.

Blanco S, Lopex-Bote MA and Desco M: Quality assurance in radiation therapy: systematic evaluation of errors during the treatment execution, Radiother Oncol 8(3):253-256, 1987.

Griffiths SE, Pearcey RG and Thorogood J: Quality control in radiotherapy: the reduction of field placement errors, Int J Radiat Oncol Biol Phys 13(10):1583-1588, 1987.

Jakobsen A, et al: A new system for patient fixation in radiotherapy, Radiother Oncol 8(2):145-151, 1987.

Niwa K and Fujikawa K: New equipment for a radiation therapy simulator: a device for simplifying irregular field shaping and integrating simulator and therapy machine, Radiat Med 5(1):27-29, 1987.

Rothwell BR: Prevention and treatment of the orofacial complications of radiotherapy, J Am Dent Assoc 114(3):316-322, 1987.

1988 Carabetta RJ: Island custom blocking technique, Med Dosim 13(1):13-14, 1988.

Conte S, et al: Three-field isocentric technique for breast irradiation using individualized shielding blocks, Int J Radiat Oncol Biol Phys 14(6):1299-1305, 1988.

Rozenfeld M: Treatment planning with external beams: introduction and historical overview, Radiographics 8(3):557, 1988.

Suit HD, et al: Potential for improvement in radiation therapy, Int J Radiat Oncol Biol Phys 14(4):777-786, 1988.

VanAken ML, et al: Incorporation of patient immobilization, tissue compensation and matchline junction technique for three-field breast treatment, Med Dosim 13(3):131-135, 1988.

1989 Brenner DJ: Precision and accuracy in radiotherapy, Radiother Oncol 14(2):159-167, 1989.

Chu JC, et al: Patterns of change in the physics and technical support of radiation therapy in the USA 1975-1986, Int J Radiat Oncol Biol Phys 17(2):437-442, 1989.

Ohara K, et al: Irradiation synchronized with respiration gate, Int J Radiat Oncol Biol Phys 17(4):853-857, 1989.

Harris KM, et al: The mammographic features of the postlumpectomy, postirradiation breast, Radiographics 9(2):253-268, 1989.

Periodical

Progress in Radiation Therapy, New York, 1958- .

THERMOGRAPHY

For bibliographic citations before 1964, please see the fifth edition of this atlas.

1964 Albert SM, Glickman M and Kallish M: Thermography in orthopedics, Ann NY Acad Sci 121:157-170, 1964.

Atkins E: Body temperature elevation in disease, Ann NY Acad Sci 121:26-29, 1964.

Brueschke EE, Haberman JD and Gershon-Cohen J: Relative densitometric analysis of thermograms for more precise temperature determinations, Ann NY Acad Sci 121:80-89, 1964.

Gershon-Cohen J: A short history of medical thermometry, Ann NY Acad Sci 121:4-11, 1964.

Gershon-Cohen J, et al: Thermography of the breast, AJR 91:919-926, 1964.

Minard D, Copman L and Dasler AR: Elevation of body temperature in health, Ann NY Acad Sci 121:12-25, 1964.

Stoll AM: Techniques and uses of skin temperature measurements, Ann NY Acad Sci 121:49-56, 1964.

Wolfe WL: Infrared imaging devices in infrared medical radiography, Ann NY Acad Sci 121:57-70, 1964.

1965 Birnbaum SJ and Kliot D: Thermoplacentography: placental localization by infrared sensing techniques, Obstet Gynecol 25:515-519, 1965.

Gershon-Cohen J and Barnes RG: Thermography, Gevaert X-ray Bull, No 1, pp 12-16, 1965.

Gershon-Cohen J and Haberman JD: Medical thermography, AJR 94:735-740, 1965.

Gershon-Cohen J and Haberman JD: Obstetric and gynecologic thermography, Obstet Gynecol 26:842-847, 1965.

Gershon-Cohen J, Haberman JD and Brueschke E: Medical thermography: summary of current status, Radiol Clin North Am 3:403-431, 1965.

Lawson RN and Alt LL: Skin temperature recording with phosphors: a new technique, Can Med Assoc J 92:255-260, 1965.

Smessaert A, Befeler D and Hicks RG: Use of thermography for evaluation of sympathetic blocks, Am J Surg 109:594-598, 1965.

Wood EH: Thermography in the diagnosis of cerebrovascular disease, Radiology 85:270-283, 1965.

Wright MM and Korr LM: Neural and spinal components of disease: progress in the application of thermography, J Am Osteopath Assoc 64:918-921, 1965.

1966 Crandell CE and Hill H: Thermography in dentistry, Oral Med Oral Pathol 21:316-320, 1966.

Goldberg HI, Heinz ER and Taveras JM: Thermography in neurological patients, Acta Radiol [Diagn] 5:786-795, 1966.

Johnson PM, Siarra JG and Brogg DG: Placental localization: a comparison of radiopharmaceutic and thermographic methods, AJR 96:681-689, 1966.

1967 Bjork NA: AGA Thermovision, a high speed infrared camera with instantaneous picture display, J Radiol Electr 48:30-33, 1967.

Gershon-Cohen J: Medical thermography, Sci Am 216:94-102, 1967.

Lane WZ: Infrared mapping of peripheral vascular disorders, Hosp Prac 2:36-39, 1967.

1968 Barnes BR: Diagnostic thermography, Appl Optics 7:1673-1685, 1968.

Branemark P and Johansson BW: Thermography as an aid in hibernation research, Acta Physiol Scand 73:300-304, 1968.

Edeiken J, et al: Thermography and herniated lumbar discs, AJR 102:790-796, 1968.

Freundlich I, Wallace J and Dodd G: Thermography of the venous diameter rates in the detection of non-palpable breast carcinoma, AJR 102:927-932, 1968.

Haberman JD: The present status of mammary thermography, CA 18:314-321, 1968.

Haberman JD, Ehrlich GE and Levinson C: Thermography in rheumatic diseases, Arch Phys Med Rehabil 49:187-192, 1968.

Hitchcock CR, Hitkok DF and Soucherey R: Thermography in mass screening for occult breast cancer, JAMA 204:419-422, 1968.

Mawdsley C, Samuel E and Sumerling MD: Thermography in occlusive cerebrovascular diseases, Br Med J 3:521-524, 1968.

1969 Dodd GD, et al: New developments in breast thermography, Cancer 24:1212-1221, 1969.

Isard HJ, Ostrum BJ and Shilo R: Thermography in breast carcinoma, Surg Gynecol Obstet 128:1289-1293, 1969.

Lilienfeld A, et al: An evaluation of thermography in the detection of breast cancer: a cooperative pilot study, Cancer 24:1206-1211, 1969.

Parker JE and Bradham GB: Thermographic demonstration of nicotine-induced vasoconstriction, J SC Med Assoc 65:423-425, 1969.

Thorne FL, Georgiado N and Mladick R: Use of thermography in determining viability of pedicle flaps, Arch Surg 99:97-99, 1969.

Weill F, et al: Radiology without x-rays: placenta localization by thermography and tomoechoradiography, Ann Radiol 12:797-810, 1969. (In French) Abstract: Radiology 96:235, 1970.

1970 Feasey CM, James WB and Davison M: A technique for breast thermography, Br J Radiol 43:462-465, 1970.

Gershon-Cohen J, Hermel MB and Murdock MG: Thermography in the detection of early breast cancer, Cancer 26:1153-1156, 1970.

Guibor P and Kenney AH: Ophthalmologic thermography, Trans Am Acad Ophthalmol Otolaryngol 74:1032-1043, 1970.

Ryan J: Thermography in the diagnosis of breast cancer, Australas Radiol 14:70-78, 1970.

1971 Curcio B and Haberman J: Infrared thermography: a review of current medical application, instrumentation and technique, Radiol Technol 42:233-247, 1971.

Farrell C, Wallace JD and Mansfield CM: The use of thermography in the detection of metastatic breast cancer, AJR 111:148-152, 1971.

Haberman J: Image analysis of medical infrared thermograms, CRC Crit Rev Radiol Sci 2:427-465, 1971.

1972 Haberman J, Francis J and Love TJ: Thermographic responses to local external heat sources, Radiology 102:341-348, 1972.

1974 Cooke ED, et al: Deep vein thrombosis: preclinical diagnosis by thermography, Br J Surg 61:971-978, 1974.

Wallace JD: Thermography in bone disease, JAMA 230:447-479, 1974.

Wasserman NF: Thermogram and mammogram, Minn Med 57:971-974, 1974.

1975 Egan RL: Mammography, xeroradiography, and thermography, Clin Obstet Gynecol 18:197-209, 1975.

Jones CH, et al: Thermography of the female breast: a five-year study in relation to the detection and prognosis of cancer, Br J Radiol 48:532-538, 1975.

1976 Evans AL, James WB and Forrest H: Thermography in lower limb arterial disease, Clin Radiol 27:383-388, 1976.

1977 Bergqvist D, Efsing HO and Hallböök T: Thermography: a noninvasive method for diagnosis of deep venous thrombosis, Arch Surg 112:600-604, 1977.

Freundlich IM, O'Mara R and Pitt MJ: Thermographic, radionuclide, and radiographic detection of bone metastases, Radiology 122:665-668, 1977.

1978 Buchanan JB and Weisberg BF: Breast thermography, J Ky Med Assoc 76:544-546, 1978.

1980 Barrett AH, Myers PC and Sadowsky NL: Microwave thermography in the detection of breast cancer, AJR 134:365-368, 1980.

Cooke ED, Carter LM and Pilcher MF: Identifying scoliosis in the adolescent with thermography: a preliminary study, Clin Orthop 148:172-176, 1980.

Kopecky WJ: Using liquid dielectrics to obtain spatial thermal distributions, Med Phys 7:566-570, 1980.

Liu DT and Blackwell RJ: Placental localization by liquid crystal thermography, Int J Gynaecol Obstet 17:617-619, 1980.

Nudelman S and Patton DD, editors: Imaging for medicine, nuclear medicine, ultrasonics, and thermography, New York, 1980, Plenum Press.

1981 Cacak RK, et al: Millimeter wavelength thermographic scanner, Med Phys 8:462-465, 1981.

Goldberg IM, et al: Contact plate thermography: a new technique for diagnosis of breast masses, Arch Surg 116:271-273, 1981.

Rajapakse C, et al: Thermography in the assessment of peripheral joint inflammation—a re-evaluation, Rheumatol Rehabil 20:81-87, 1981.

1982 Bosiger P and Scaroni F: A microprocessor-assisted thermography system for the online analysis of thermograms and dynamic thermogram sequences, Prog Clin Biol Res 107:329-337, 1982.

Gautherie M, et al: Long-term assessment of breast cancer risk by liquid-crystal thermal imaging, Prog Clin Biol Res 107:279-301, 1982.

Greenblatt RB, Samaras C and Vasquez J: Mastopathies: hormonology and thermography, Prog Clin Biol Res 107:303-311, 1982.

Hobbins WB: Thermography and pain, Prog Clin Biol Res 107:361-375, 1982.

Isard HJ: Breast disease and correlation of images: mammography—thermography—diaphanography, Prog Clin Biol Res 107:321-328, 1982.

Miki Y, Kawatsu T and Matsuda K: Thermographic venography in inflammatory lower leg nodules, Prog Clin Biol Res 107:439-443, 1982.

1982 Raflo GT, Chart P and Hurwitz JJ: Thermographic evaluation of the human lacrimal drainage system, Ophthalmic Surg 13:119-124, 1982.

Robillard M, et al: Microwave thermography—characteristics of waveguide applicators and signatures of thermal structures, J Microwave Power 17:97-105, 1982.

Ring EF: Thermal imaging and therapeutic drugs, Prog Clin Biol Res 107:463-474, 1982.

Rubal BJ, Traycoff RB and Ewing KL: Liquid crystal thermography: a new tool for evaluating low back pain, Phys Ther 62:1593-1596, 1982.

Wexler CE: Lumbar, thoracic, and cervical thermography, Prog Clin Biol Res 107:377-388, 1982.

Sterns EE, et al: Thermography in breast diagnosis, Cancer 50:323-325, 1982.

1983 Salisbury RS, et al: Heat distribution over normal and abnormal joints: thermal pattern and quantification, Ann Rheum Dis 42:494-499, 1983.

Soffin CB, et al: Thermography and oral inflammatory conditions, Oral Surg 56:256-262, 1983.

1984 Font-Sastre V, Jr, et al: Breast cancer screening of the high risk population with clinical examination and thermography: a combination of telethermography and plate thermography, Eur J Gynaecol Oncol 5:105-109, 1984.

Kopans DB: "Early" breast cancer detection using techniques other than mammography, AJR 143:465-468, 1984.

Kopans DB, Meyer JE and Sadowsky N: Breast imaging, N Engl J Med 310:960-967, 1984.

1985 Taylor H and Warfield CA: Thermography of pain: instrumentation and uses, Hosp Pract [Off] 20:164, 168-164, 169, 1985.

Uematsu S: Thermographic imaging of cutaneous sensory segment in patients with peripheral nerve injury: skin-temperature stability between sides of the body, J Neurosurg 62:716-720, 1985.

1986 Luk KD, Yeung PS and Leong JC: Thermography in the determination of amputation levels in ischaemic limbs, Int Orthop 10:79-81, 1986.

Theuvenet WJ, Koeyers GF and Borghouts MH: Thermographic assessment of perforating arteries: a preoperative screening method for fasciocutaneous and musculocutaneous flaps, Scand J Plast Reconstr Surg 20:25-29, 1986.

White BA, et al: The use of infrared thermography in the evaluation of oral lesions, J Am Dent Assoc 113:783-786, 1986.

1987 Fraser S, Land D and Sturrock RD: Microwave thermography—an index of inflammatory joint disease, Br J Rheumatol 26:37-39, 1987.

DIAPHANOGRAPHY

1981 Angquist KA, et al: Diaphanoscopy and diaphanography for breast cancer detection in clinical practice, Acta Chir Scand 147:231-238, 1981.

Isard HJ: A preliminary appraisal of diaphanography in diseases of the breast, Cancer Detect Prev 4:565-569, 1981.

1982 Brenner RJ: X-ray mammography and diaphanography in screening for breast cancer, J Reprod Med 27:679-684, 1982.

1983 McIntosh DM: Breast light scanning: a real-time breast-imaging modality, J Can Assoc Radiol 34:288-290, 1983.

1984 Fodor J, Malott JC and Moskowitz M: Diaphanography: transillumination of the breast, Radiol Technol 55:97-100, 1984.

Isard HJ: Other imaging techniques, Cancer 53:658-664, 1984.

Muirhead A and Seright W: Clinical experience with the diaphanograph machine, Ann R Coll Surg Engl 66:123-124, 1984.

Sickles EA: Breast cancer detection with transillumination and mammography, AJR 142:841-844, 1984.

1985 Wallberg H, Alveryd A and Carlsson K: Physical interpretation of diaphanograms using the computer-controlled image scanner OSIRIS, Acta Radiol [Diagn] (Stockh) 26:417-424, 1985.

1986 Linford J, et al: Development of a tissue-equivalent phantom for diaphanography, Med Phys 13:869-875, 1986.

1988 Navarro GA and Profio AE: Contrast in diaphanography of the breast, Med Phys 15:181-187, 1988.

TOMOGRAPHY

For bibliographic citations before 1964, please see the fifth edition of this atlas.

1965 Greenwell FP and Wright RW: Rotational tomography, Clin Radiol 16:377-389, 1965.

Landau P: La tomographie multiple simultanée unidirectionnelle: méthodes et possibilités nouvelles, J Radiol Electrol 46:299-305, 1965.

1966 Ettinger A and Fainsinger MH: Zonography in daily radiological practice, Radiology 87:82-86, 1966.

Liliequist B: Tomography with the Mimer in otosclerosis of the temporal bone, Acta Radiol [Diagn] 4:639-644, 1966.

Ring J: Elements of sectional radiography, Radiol Technol 38:17-22, 1966.

Westra D: Zonography: the narrow angle tomography, Amsterdam, 1966, Excerpta Medica Foundation.

1967 Lodin H: Tomography of the middle and lingular bronchi, Acta Radiol [Diagn] 6:26-32, 1967.

1968 Inzinna JF, Salomon H and Vazir A: The synchroplanigraphic device: a new simultaneous tomographic device, AJR 103:678-680, 1968.

Rybadova NI and Kuznetsov AA: Concerning the method of tomographic examination of the bronchial tree, Vestn Rentgenol Radiol 43:36-43, 1968, 1249, 1968.

Wright JT and Benjamin B: Cycloidal tomography of the temporal bone, Australas Radiol 12:320-327, 1968.

1969 Brünner S: Roentgen anatomy of the temporal bone using the Polytome, Semin Roentgenol 4:118-121, 1969.

Conway JJ and Cowell HR: Tarsal coalition: clinical significance and roentgenographic demonstration, Radiology 92:799-811, 1969.

du Boulay G and Bostick T: Linear tomography in congenital abnormalities of the ear, Br J Radiol 42:161-183, 1969.

Kimber PM: A thin-layer cassette for precision neuroradiology, Radiography 35:183-184, 1969.

Lame EL and Redick TJ: Autotomography applied to the pharynx and dens, AJR 105:359-360, 1969.

Mattsson O: Control of a tomographic system, Acta Radiol [Diagn] 8:433-445, 1969.

Potter GD and Trokel SL: Tomography of the optic canal, AJR 106:530-535, 1969.

1970 Brünner S and Pedersen CB: Roentgen examination of the facial canal, Acta Radiol [Diagn] 10:545-552, 1970.

Chin FK, Anderson WB and Gilbertson JD: Radiation dose to critical organs during petrous tomography, Radiology 94:623-627, 1970.

Crysler WE: Tomoscopy and related matters, AJR 109:619-623, 1970.

Frimann-Dahl J and Kühl HB: Immediate centering and tomographic cut localization by means of roentgen television, Acta Radiol [Diagn] 10:236-240, 1970.

James AE, Jr: Tarsal coalition and personal spastic flat foot, Australas Radiol 14:80-83, 1970.

1971 Lockery RM: Principles of body-section radiography, Radiol Technol 42:335-345, 1971.

Smith WVJ: A review of tomography and zonography, Radiography 37:5-15, 1971.

Ziedses des Plantes BG: Body-section radiography: history, image information, various techniques and results, Australas Radiol 15:57-64, 1971.

1972 El Gammal T and King GE: Patient positioning device for hypocycloidal tomography of the midline ventricles of the brain, Radiology 102:206-207, 1972.

Potter GD: Tomography of the orbit, Radiol Clin North Am 10:21-38, 1972.

Reichmann S: Modified theory of the development of tomographic blurring, Acta Radiol 12:457-468, 1972.

1973 Amplatz K: Autotomography AJR 117: 896-902, 1973.

Berrett A: Modern thin-section tomography, Springfield, Ill, 1973, Charles C Thomas, Publisher.

Dalinka MK, Gohel VK and Rancier L: Tomography in the evaluation of the anterior cruciate ligament, Radiology 108:31-33, 1973.

Greig JH and Musaph FW: A method of radiological demonstration of the temporomandibular joints using orthopantomography, Radiology 106:307-310, 1973.

Littleton JT, Crosby EH and Durizch ML: Adjustable- versus fixed-fulcrum tomographic systems, AJR 117:910-929, 1973.

1974 Anderson PW and Maslin P: Tomography applied to knee arthrography, Radiology 110:271-275, 1974.

Berger P, Gildersleeve S and Poznanski A: The feasibility of the PA projection for tomography of the petrous bone: significant reduction in radiation dose to the lens of the eye, AJR 122:67-69, 1974.

Bosniak MA: Nephrotomography: a relatively unappreciated but extremely valuable diagnostic tool, Radiology 113:313-321, 1974.

1975 Freedman GS, Putman CE and Potter GD: Critical review of tomography in radiology and nuclear medicine, CRC Crit Rev Clin Radiol Nucl Med 6:253-294, 1975.

Norman A: The use of tomography in the diagnosis of skeletal disorders, Clin Orthop 107:139-145, 1975.

Welander V: Layer formation in narrow beam rotation radiography, Acta Radiol 16:529-540, 1975.

1976 Harding G and Day MJ: Blurring quality in spiral tomography, Acta Radiol (Ther) 15:465-480, 1976.

Littleton JT: Tomography physical principles and clinical application, Baltimore, 1976, Williams & Wilkins.

Polga JP and Watnick M: Whole lung tomography in metastatic disease, Clin Radiol 27:53-56, 1976.

Stanson AW and Baker HL: Routine tomography of the temporomandibular joint, Radiol Clin North Am 14:105-127, 1976.

1977 Helander CG, Reichmann S and Astrand K: Xeroradiographic tomography, Acta Radiol 18:369-382, 1977.

Wayrynen RE, Holland RS and Schwenker RP: Film-screen sharpness in complex motion tomography, Invest Radiol 12:195-198, 1977.

1978 Durizch ML: Technical aspects of tomography, Baltimore, 1978, Williams & Wilkins.

1979 Palmer A and Munro L: The principles of tomographic positioning with particular reference to skull tomography, Radiography 45(531):51-60, 1979.

1980 Eckerdal O and Nelvig P: Reproducible positioning of the skull at tomography, Acta Radiol 21:557-559, 1980.

Farber AL: Advantages of variant section of thickness relative to specific anatomy, Radiol Technol 51:793-796, 1980.

Littleton JT, Durizch ML and Callahan WP: Linear vs. pluridirectional tomography of the chest: correlative radiographic anatomic study, AJR 134:241-248, 1980.

Nakamura Y, Kiyota H and Hara K: Elimination of blur in linear tomography: a simple method using the x-ray processor, Radiology 135:232-233, 1980.

1981 Bein ME and Stone DN: Full lung linear and pluridirectional tomography: a preliminary evaluation of nodule direction, AJR 136:1013-1015, 1981.

Nehen AM, et al: Computed tomography and hypocycloid tomography in lesions of the nose, paranasal sinuses, and nasopharynx, Acta Radiol 22:285-287, 1981.

Perilhou JR, et al: Intensified tomography: enhancement of soft tissue discrimination in conventional tomography of the brain, Radiology 138:689-696, 1981.

1982 Anderson LD, et al: The role of polytomography in the diagnosis and treatment of cervical spine injuries, Clin Orthop 165:64-67, 1982.

Wright JW Jr, Wright JW III and Hicks G: Polytomography and congenital anomalies of the ear, Ann Otol Rhinol Laryngol 91:480-484, 1982.

1983 Cade WJ and Haddaway MJ: Measurement of absorbed skin dose in tomography, Radiography 49:24-26, 1983.

Chasen MH and Yrizarry JM: Tomography of the pulmonary hili: anatomical reassessment of the conventional 55 degrees posterior oblique, Radiology 149:365-369, 1983.

Genereux GP: Conventional tomographic hilar anatomy emphasizing the pulmonary veins, AJR 141:1241-1257, 1983.

Glazer GM, et al: Evaluation of the pulmonary hilum: comparison of conventional radiography, 55 degrees posterior oblique tomography, and dynamic computed tomography, J Comput Assist Tomogr 7:983-989, 1983.

Gusching AC: Frontal tomography of articulating temporomandibular joint surfaces, Angle Orthod 53:234-239, 1983.

Marlowe NA: The application of blurred undersubtraction in polytomography, Radiol Technol 54:455-465, 1983.

Stigsson L and Tylen U: 55 degrees posterior oblique tomography of the pulmonary hilum in the evaluation of lung tumors, Radiologe 23:224-228, 1983.

Westesson PL: Double-contrast arthrotomography of the temporomandibular joint, J Oral Maxillofac Surg 41:163-172, 1983.

1984 Bussard DA, Yune HY and Whitehead D: Comparison of corrected-axis and straight lateral TMJ tomograms, J Clin Orthod 18:894-898, 1984.

De la Cruz A: Polytomographic evaluation of the clivus and petrous apices: a new view, Laryngoscope 94:153-164, 1984.

Moilanen A and Pitkanen M: Panoramic zonography in the radiographic diagnosis of facial and related structures: a clinical study, Rontgenblatter 37:95-99, 1984.

1985 Fileni A, et al: Tomography in the preoperative evaluation of ear malformations, J Laryngol Otol 99:432-438, 1985.

Ghosh Roy DN, et al: Selective plane removal in limited angle tomographic imaging, Med Phys 12:65-70, 1985.

Vezina JA and Beauregard CG: An update on the technique of double-contrast arthrotomography of the shoulder, J Can Assoc Radiol 36:176-182, 1985.

1986 Rosenberg HM and Graczyk RJ: Temporomandibular articulation tomography: a corrected anteroposterior and lateral cephalometric technique, Oral Surg Oral Med Oral Pathol 62:198-204, 1986.

1987 Avill R, et al: Applied potential tomography: a new noninvasive technique for measuring gastric emptying, Gastroenterology 92:1019-1026, 1987.

Fernandes RJ, et al: A cephalometric tomographic technique to visualize the buccolingual and vertical dimensions of the mandible, J Prosthet Dent 58:466-470, 1987.

Mangnall YF, et al: Applied potential tomography: a new noninvasive technique for assessing gastric function, Clin Phys Physiol Meas 8:119-129, 1987.

1988 Eyuboglu BM and Brown BH: Methods of cardiac gating applied potential tomography, Clin Phys Physiol Meas 9:43-48, 1988.

Ramthun SK and Bender CE: Tomography of the posterior cervical spine fusion: a new concept, Radiol Technol 60:27-31, 1988.

1989 Nakanishi T, et al: Sagittal tomography in the supine patient, Radiology 171:574-576, 1989.

INDEX

Index

Index

Index

Index

Index

Index

Index

P

Q

R

Index

S

Index

Index

U

V

Index

W

X

Y

Z